NUTRITION ESSENTIALS

Second Edition

A Personal Approach

WENDY J. SCHIFF, MS, RD

Mc
Graw
Hill
Education

NUTRITION ESSENTIALS: A PERSONAL APPROACH, SECOND EDITION

1 2 3 4 5 6 7 8 9 LMN 21 20 19 18 17

ISBN 978-1-259-70654-7
MHID 1-259-70654-0

Chief Product Officer, SVP Products & Markets: *G. Scott Virkler*
Vice President, General Manager, Products & Markets: *Marty Lange*
Vice President, Content Design & Delivery: *Betsy Whalen*
Managing Director: *Lynn Breithaupt*
Brand Manager: *Marija Magner*
Director, Product Development: *Rose Koos*
Product Developer: *Darlene Schueller*
Marketing Managers: *Kristine Rellihan/Jessica Cannavo*
Director of Digital Content: *Michael G. Koot, PhD*
Director, Content Design & Delivery: *Linda Avenarius*
Program Manager: *Angela R. FitzPatrick*
Content Project Managers: *Vicki Krug/Brent dela Cruz*
Buyer: *Jennifer Pickel*
Design: *Tara McDermott*
Content Licensing Specialists: *Lori Hancock/Lorraine Buczek*
Cover Image: *©McGraw-Hill Education. Mark A. Dierker, photographer*
Compositor: *MPS Limited*
Printer: *LSC Communications*

© FoodCollection/StockFood RF

All credits appearing on page or at the end of the book are considered to be an extension of the copyright page.

Library of Congress Cataloging-in-Publication Data

Schiff, Wendy.
  Nutrition essentials : a personal approach/Wendy J. Schiff, MS, RD.
  2nd edition. | New York, NY : McGraw-Hill Education, [2018] | Includes index.
  LCCN 2016058993 | ISBN 9781259706547 (alk. paper)
  LCSH: Human nutrition—Textbooks.
  LCC QP141 .S3434 2018 | DDC 612.3—dc23
  LC record available at https://lccn.loc.gov/2016058993

mheducation.com/highered

Brief Contents

© Purestock/SuperStock RF

1 Food *Is* More than Something to Eat 2

2 Nutrition Information: Fact or Fiction? 22

3 Making More Nutritious Choices 40

4 How Food Becomes You 70

5 Carbohydrates: Fuel and Fiber 100

6 Lipids: Focusing on Fats and Cholesterol 128

7 Proteins: Life's Building Blocks 160

8 Vitamins: Nutrients that Multitask 186

9 Key Minerals, Water, and the Nonnutrient Alcohol 228

10 Nutrition for a Healthy Weight and Fit Body 274

11 Nutrition for Your Life, Environment, and World 316

Appendixes

A English-Metric Conversion and Metric-to-Household Units A-3

B Canada's Food Guide A-4

C Daily Values (DVs) Table A-11

D The Basics of Energy Metabolism A-12

E Answers to *Test Yourself* Questions A-14

F References A-15

G Dietary Reference Intake (DRI) Tables A-29

H Stretching Your Food Dollars A-35

I Modifying Recipes for Healthy Living A-39

Meet the Author

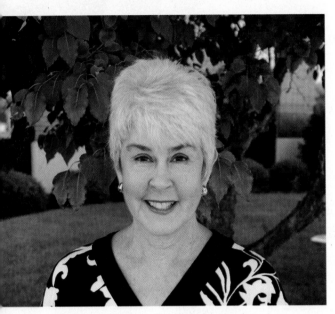

© McGraw Hill Education. Mark Dierker, photographer.

Wendy J. Schiff, MS, RD received her BS in biological health/medical dietetics and MS in human nutrition from The Pennsylvania State University. She has taught introductory food and nutrition courses at the University of Missouri–Columbia, as well as nutrition, human biology, and personal health courses at St. Louis Community College–Meramec. She has worked as a public health nutritionist at the Allegheny County Health Department (Pittsburgh, Pennsylvania) and State Food and Nutrition Specialist for Missouri Extension at Lincoln University in Jefferson City, Missouri. In addition to authoring *Nutrition Essentials: A Personal Approach,* she is author of *Nutrition for Healthy Living* and coauthor of *Human Nutrition: Science for Healthy Living*. Wendy has authored or coauthored many other nutrition- and health-related educational materials as well. She is a registered dietitian nutritionist and a member of the Academy of Nutrition and Dietetics.

To my mother (1925–2016)

© Digital Vision/Getty Images RF

A Note From the Author

A few years ago, I decided that none of the college-level personal nutrition textbooks available was "right" for most students who wanted to learn about nutrition but weren't interested in majoring in the field of nutrition and dietetics.

My goal was to create a fresh approach and prepare a personal nutrition book that was less rigorous but would still cover the essentials of nutrition science. This book would be written in a style that was engaging and easy to read and understand. To facilitate learning, the text would include relevant and interesting photos and other visuals as well as superb illustrations to help explain basic but often challenging concepts. The textbook would also include personal perspectives about diets, foods, and nutrition from real college students, and practical food and nutrition tips to help students become more informed consumers.

Nutrition Essentials: A Personal Approach

- has a consumer-oriented focus, providing practical tips for applying concepts such as ways to prepare foods to make them safer and healthier, and ways to become a savvy consumer of nutrition-related information; and

- provides non-nutrition majors with the basic scientific principles of nutrition in a highly visual, engaging context. For example, the major steps involved in complex physiological processes such as protein digestion and glucose regulation are realistically illustrated and featured as Essential Concepts.

As I prepared the second edition of **Nutrition Essentials: A Personal Approach,** new Dietary Guidelines, Daily Values, and Nutrition Facts panels for food labels were introduced. Thus, the second edition has been extensively updated to reflect these and other significant advances in the constantly changing field of nutrition.

The first edition of **Nutrition Essentials: A Personal Approach** met all of my goals for a personal nutrition textbook. Now, the instructors who teach and the students who take personal nutrition courses have a new edition to enjoy!

Best wishes, *Wendy J Schiff*

McGraw-Hill Connect®
Learn Without Limits

Connect is a teaching and learning platform that is proven to deliver better results for students and instructors.

Connect empowers students by continually adapting to deliver precisely what they need, when they need it, and how they need it, so your class time is more engaging and effective.

> 73% of instructors who use **Connect** require it; instructor satisfaction **increases** by 28% when **Connect** is required.

Analytics

Connect Insight®

Connect Insight is Connect's new one-of-a-kind visual analytics dashboard—now available for both instructors and students—that provides at-a-glance information regarding student performance, which is immediately actionable. By presenting assignment, assessment, and topical performance results together with a time metric that is easily visible for aggregate or individual results, Connect Insight gives the user the ability to take a just-in-time approach to teaching and learning, which was never before available. Connect Insight presents data that empowers students and helps instructors improve class performance in a way that is efficient and effective.

Mobile

Connect's new, intuitive mobile interface gives students and instructors flexible and convenient, anytime–anywhere access to all components of the Connect platform.

Connect's Impact on Retention Rates, Pass Rates, and Average Exam Scores

> Using **Connect** improves retention rates by **19.8%**, passing rates by **12.7%**, and exam scores by **9.1%**.

Impact on Final Course Grade Distribution

> Students can view their results for any **Connect** course.

Adaptive

THE **ADAPTIVE** READING EXPERIENCE DESIGNED TO TRANSFORM THE WAY STUDENTS READ

More students earn **A's** and **B's** when they use McGraw-Hill Education **Adaptive** products.

SmartBook®

Proven to help students improve grades and study more efficiently, SmartBook contains the same content within the print book, but actively tailors that content to the needs of the individual. SmartBook's adaptive technology provides precise, personalized instruction on what the student should do next, guiding the student to master and remember key concepts, targeting gaps in knowledge and offering customized feedback, and driving the student toward comprehension and retention of the subject matter. Available on tablets, SmartBook puts learning at the student's fingertips—anywhere, anytime.

Over **8 billion questions** have been answered, making McGraw-Hill Education products more intelligent, reliable, and precise.

www.mheducation.com

STUDENTS WANT SMARTBOOK®

95% of students reported **SmartBook** to be a more effective way of reading material.

100% of students want to use the Practice Quiz feature available within **SmartBook** to help them study.

100% of students reported having reliable access to off-campus wifi.

90% of students say they would purchase **SmartBook** over print alone.

95% of students reported that **SmartBook** would impact their study skills in a positive way.

*Findings based on 2015 focus group results administered by McGraw-Hill Education

Personalized Teaching and Learning Environment

Saves students and instructors time while improving performance.

McGraw-Hill Connect® for *Nutrition Essentials: A Personal Approach* is a digital teaching and learning environment that saves students and instructors time while improving performance over a variety of critical outcomes.

- ### First Week of Class

  LearnSmart Prep® is available to all students. No prerequsite, no problem! Assign LearnSmart Prep the first week of class to get some basic chemistry, biology, or scienctific math level-setting among your students. Or suggest it to students along the way who might benefit from the remediation.

- ### Before the Lecture

  Assign adaptive LearnSmart® questions within SmartBook® and more! Get your students into the material, learning the vocabulary and chapter basics. In an online class, consider assigning additional LearnSmart questions to ensure your students have a deeper understanding of all the content. Obtain data on the most missed learning objectives to guide your lecture or about additional learning resources you provide.

- ### Active Learning

  Instructor Resources include an instructor's manual and art, photos, tables, Power Points®, and animations to use with your students. Utilize question bank questions, assignable and assessable within Connect, or use labeling images with small groups in class.

- ### Assessment of Learning Outcomes

  All Connect questions are created by the author or nutrition instructors. They are all tagged to learning outcomes, specific section and topic, and Bloom's level of the cognitive domain. Easily create customized homework, quizzes, or tests. Customize assessments that can be automatically or manually graded.

- ### Deliver your lecture online quickly and easily

  Tegrity digital lecture capture lets students access your lecture outside of class anytime, anywhere, on just about any device.

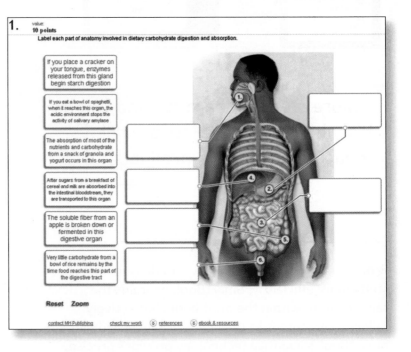

1. value: **10 points**

Label each part of anatomy involved in dietary carbohydrate digestion and absorption.

If you place a cracker on your tongue, enzymes released from this gland begin starch digestion

If you eat a bowl of spaghetti, when it reaches this organ, the acidic environment stops the activity of salivary amylase

The absorption of most of the nutrients and carbohydrate from a snack of granola and yogurt occurs in this organ

After sugars from a breakfast of cereal and milk are absorbed into the intestinal bloodstream, they are transported to this organ

The soluble fiber from an apple is broken down or fermented in this digestive organ

Very little carbohydrate from a bowl of rice remains by the time food reaches this part of the digestive tract

Reset Zoom

contact MH Publishing   check my work   references   ebook & resources

diet analysis tool
Launch NutritionCalc Plus

- ### Inspire behavior change

  NutritionCalc Plus is a suite of powerful dietary self-assessment tools that help students track their food intake and activity, and analyze their diet and health goals. Students and instructors can trust the reliability of the ESHA database while interacting with a robust selection of reports.

Campus

- ### Easily build a digitally-rich course

  Connect seamlessly integrates with every learning management system through **McGraw-Hill Education Campus**, so you can easily combine your course resources into a single platform. Instructors and students benefit from universal single sign-on, automatic registration, and gradebook synchronization.

A Visual Approach

Highly visual; designed with students in mind.

Nutrition Essentials: A Personal Approach was designed with a magazine-like influence and today's student in mind. The many photos and appealing page layouts entice students to explore and read further. The highly visual nature reduces anxiety sometimes associated with large blocks of text.

> "I definitely feel this will serve to engage the reader who is so often overwhelmed by numerous pages of text. The magazine feel is a style the students are comfortable with."
>
> **Andrea Villarreal**
> Phoenix College

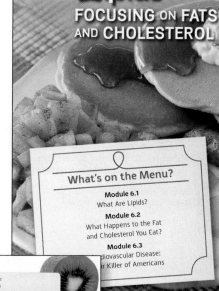

Unit **6**

Lipids
FOCUSING ON FATS AND CHOLESTEROL

What's on the Menu?

Module 6.1
What Are Lipids?

Module 6.2
What Happens to the Fat and Cholesterol You Eat?

Module 6.3
Cardiovascular Disease:
...r Killer of Americans

---

240 Unit 9   Key Minerals, Water, and the Nonnutrient Alcohol

9.2b The Fluid Balancers: Potassium and Sodium

Major minerals potassium and sodium play a vital role in maintaining normal body fluid balance. The typical American diet supplies far more sodium than potassium. This mineral imbalance may lead to high blood pressure, a serious long-term health problem. However, you can help reduce the risk that excess sodium poses to your health, by consuming more foods that supply potassium.[5]

Potassium

Potassium (K) is the major positively charged ion in the fluid that's inside cells. Fresh fruits, fruit juice, and vegetables are good dietary sources of potassium. Milk, whole grains, dried beans, and meats are also major contributors of potassium to American diets.

On average, Americans who were 2 years of age or older consumed only about 2540 mg of potassium per day in 2013–2014.[3] This amount is much lower than the Adequate Intake amount (4700 mg). According to the *Dietary Guidelines for Americans*, potassium is a nutrient of public health concern. You can raise your potassium intake by eating more fruits, vegetables, whole-grain breads and cereals, and low-fat and fat-free dairy foods. **Table 9.4** provides information about the potassium content of a few selected foods. **Figure 9.9** indicates food groups that are naturally good sources of potassium.

People who experience excessive body fluid losses through sweating, vomiting, or diarrhea are at risk for electrolyte depletion. Symptoms of low blood potassium levels generally include muscle cramps, confusion, and constipation. In severe cases, the lack of potassium causes muscular weakness and abnormal heartbeat. Therefore, it's important to seek medical treatment when potassium depletion is suspected.

TABLE 9.4 **POTASSIUM CONTENT OF SELECTED FOODS**

Food	Potassium (mg)
Beet greens, boiled, drained, 1 cup	1309
Baked potato, including skin, 6 oz	963
Spinach, cooked, drained, 1 cup	839
Coconut water, 1 cup	600
Kiwi, sliced, 1 cup	562
Banana, sliced, 1 cup	537
Sweet potato, canned, mashed, 1 cup	536
Orange juice, frozen, reconstituted, 1 cup	473
Cantaloupe, cubes, 1 cup	427
Papaya, raw, mashed, 1 cup	419
Milk, fluid, 1% fat, 1 cup	366
Salmon, sockeye, cooked, 3 oz	347
Peaches, raw, sliced, 1 cup	293
Grapes, raw, red, 1 cup	288
Yogurt, low-fat, plain, 8 oz	264
Corn, canned yellow, 1 cup	226
Tuna, canned in water, drained, 3 oz	202

AI for adults = 4700 mg/day
Source: *USDA National nutrient database for standard reference, release 2...*

Figure 9.9 MyPlate: Good food sources of potassium.

Fruits
- Pears
- Prunes
- Peaches
- Avocados
- Cantaloupes
- Bananas

Vegetables
- Spinach
- Squash
- Potatoes
- Tomatoes
- Lettuce
- Lima beans

Dairy
- Milk
- Cottage cheese
- Yogurt
- Ricotta cheese

Grains
- Whole-wheat bread
- Whole-grain products

Protein
- Meat
- Chicken
- Fish
- Shrimp
- Beans

Choose **MyPlate**.gov

Acorn squash: © Burke/Triolo Productions/Getty Images RF; Pear: © Stockbyte/Getty Images RF; Yogurt: © Ingram Publishing/SuperStock RF; Loaf of bread: © IT Stock/PunchStock RF; Shrimp: © Comstock/Jupiter Images RF; MyPlate: Source: ChooseMyPlate.gov; Kiwi, Peaches: © FoodCollection/StockFood RF

Key Nutrition Concepts

Marisa, the student quoted in this unit's opener, is concerned with the balance of n... in her diet. "I try to eat the right balance of ... vegetables, along with meats... I like beef ... chicken...." Tex-Mex dishes are usually mi... of various foods, which can make it difficult ... determine whether daily meals and snacks p... a healthful balance of nutrients. Unit 3 disc... food groups and how to plan a nutritionally ... adequate diet.

Figure 1.8 The MyPlate food guide [see Unit 3].

1.3c Food Is the Best Source of Nutrients and Phytochemicals

The most natural, reliable, and economical way to obtain nutrients and beneficial phytochemicals is to base your diet on a variety of "whole" and minimally processed foods. For most Americans, eating 100% raw foods isn't practical and, in some instances, it's unsafe. Many foods undergo some form of processing, such as peeling, refining, and heating, before they're eaten. Such treatments can make food safer and more convenient to eat.

Plant foods naturally contain a variety of nutrients and phytochemicals, but processing the foods often removes some of the most healthful parts. For example, a wheat kernel is stripped of its germ and outer hull (*bran*) during refinement into white flour (Fig. 1.9). Wheat germ is a rich source of vitamin E and beneficial ("healthy") fats. Wheat bran contains fiber and certain phytochemicals, and it's a concentrated source of several micronutrients. The endosperm is primarily starch (a form of carbohydrate) with some protein and very small amounts of micronutrients and fiber. A "whole grain" includes the bran and germ portions of the kernel along with the endosperm. By replacing refined grain products, such as white bread, with 100% whole-grain products, you can increase the likelihood of obtaining a wide variety of nutrients and phytochemicals.

TASTY Tidbits

Almonds and other nuts are nutrient and energy dense. For example, 1 ounce of almonds [about 23 whole nuts] supplies about 160 kcal, 6 g of protein, 14 g of fat, more than 7 mg of vitamin E, and small amounts of iron, calcium, B vitamins. Snack on a handful of n... them to your cereal.

Figure 1.9 **What is white flour?** During refinement, a wheat kernel is stripped of its nutrient-rich germ and bran. The endosperm [white flour] that remains is mostly starch.

▶ Why is it important to choose a variety of foods, especially those that are whole or minimally processed?

Bran
Endosperm
Germ

White Flour

MyPlate: Source: ChooseMyPlate.gov; Almonds: © FoodCollection/StockFood RF; Wheat image: © Photo/Du/PunchStock RF; White flour: © McGraw-Hill Education, Michael Scott, photographer

---

Unit 3   Making More Nutritious Choices

Vegetables

Vegetables include fresh, cooked, canned, frozen, and dried/dehydrated vegetables, and 100% vegetable juice. Vegetables can be further grouped into dark green, orange, and starchy categories. Some guides include dried beans and peas in the vegetable group. Many vegetables are good sources of micronutrients, fiber, and phytochemicals. Furthermore, most vegetables are naturally low in fat and energy.

Other Foods

Dietary guides may include an oils group and a group for sugary foods and alcoholic beverages. Oils include canola, corn, and olive oils, as well as other fats that are liquid at room temperature. Certain spreadable foods made from vegetable oils, such as mayonnaise, margarine, and salad dressing, are also classified as oils. Because nuts, olives, avocados, and some types of fish have high fat contents, a dietary guide may group these foods with oils.[6] Oils are often good sources of fat-soluble vitamins and may be sources of "healthy" fats that don't increase your risk of cardiovascular disease.

...cup equivalents: Vegetables

...er glass   6.5" diameter bowl   8.5" diameter plate

... juice   1 cup raw or cooked vegetables   2 cups raw greens   1 medium potato (3" diameter)

What *IS* That?

For centuries, the people of Central America have grown and eaten *tomatillos* ("husk-tomatoes"). After the papery husk is removed, the fruit can be roasted, chopped, and mixed with ground chili peppers to form sauces, such as *salsa verde* (green sauce).

Three medium tomatillos provide about 33 kcal, 2 g fiber, and 12 mg vitamin C.

Avocado: © Zoonar/Shellye Sorbi/AGE Fotostock; Vegetables and Tomatillos: © Wendy Schiff

What's In Your Diet?!, found at the end of most units, is a personal dietary analysis activity that offers many ways for students to apply concepts to their daily lives immediately.

Tasty Tidbits, interesting bits of information about food or nutrition, provide students with ways to be more savvy consumers and to make healthier choices.

TASTY Tidbits

Dark yellow and orange fruits and vegetables usually contain more beta-carotene and other provitamin A carotenoids than does lightly colored produce. Dark green fruits and vegetables also contain provitamin A, but their green pigment hides the yellow-orange pigments. So, don't discard the dark green leaves of cabbage, lettuce, or broccoli when preparing food. Use them in salads and soups or on sandwiches.

© FoodCollection/StockFood RF

TASTY Tidbits

Canned fruit is often packed in a sugary syrup. Consider buying canned fruit that's packed in water or its own juice. If you have canned fruit that's in syrup, rinse the fruit in plain water before serving it. Also choose frozen fruit that has no sugar added.

© Wendy Schiff

TASTY Tidbits

High temperatures used to cook meat may cause charring of the meat and the formation of a group of carcinogens called heterocyclic (*het´-eh-ro-sí-klic*) amines. Therefore, you may be able to reduce your risk of certain cancers by limiting your intake of grilled meats and avoiding charred parts of charcoal-grilled meats. Also, covering the grate with aluminum foil, poking a few holes in the foil, and placing the meat on top of it will reduce charring of the meat.

© Ingram Publishing/Alamy RF

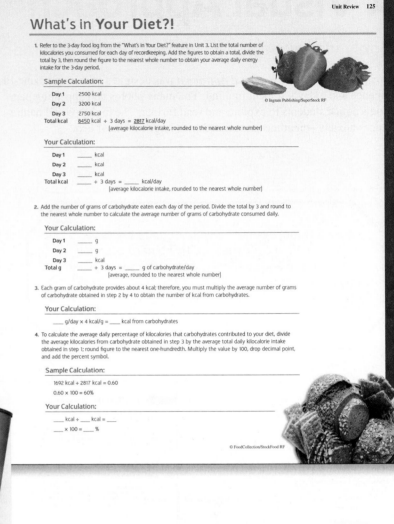

What's in **Your Diet?!**

1. Refer to the 3-day food log from the "What's in Your Diet?" feature in Unit 3. List the total number of kilocalories you consumed for each day of recordkeeping. Add the figures to obtain a total, divide the total by 3, then round the figure to the nearest whole number to obtain your average daily energy intake for the 3-day period.

Sample Calculation:

Day 1	2500 kcal
Day 2	3200 kcal
Day 3	2750 kcal
Total kcal	<u>8450</u> kcal ÷ 3 days = <u>2817</u> kcal/day

         [average kilocalorie intake, rounded to the nearest whole number]

© Ingram Publishing/SuperStock RF

Your Calculation:

Day 1	_____ kcal
Day 2	_____ kcal
Day 3	_____ kcal
Total kcal	_____ ÷ 3 days = _____ kcal/day

         [average kilocalorie intake, rounded to the nearest whole number]

2. Add the number of grams of carbohydrate eaten each day of the period. Divide the total by 3 and round to the nearest whole number to calculate the average number of grams of carbohydrate consumed daily.

Your Calculation:

Day 1	_____ g
Day 2	_____ g
Day 3	_____ kcal
Total g	_____ ÷ 3 days = _____ g of carbohydrate/day

         [average, rounded to the nearest whole number]

3. Each gram of carbohydrate provides about 4 kcal; therefore, you must multiply the average number of grams of carbohydrate obtained in step 2 by 4 to obtain the number of kcal from carbohydrates.

Your Calculation:

____ g/day × 4 kcal/g = ____ kcal from carbohydrates

4. To calculate the average daily percentage of kilocalories that carbohydrates contributed to your diet, divide the average kilocalories from carbohydrate obtained in step 3 by the average total daily kilocalorie intake obtained in step 1; round figure to the nearest one-hundredth. Multiply the value by 100, drop decimal point, and add the percent symbol.

Sample Calculation:

1692 kcal ÷ 2817 kcal = 0.60

0.60 × 100 = 60%

Your Calculation:

____ kcal ÷ ____ kcal = ____

____ × 100 = ____ %

© FoodCollection/StockFood RF

> "[Tasty Tidbits] is a great way to implement positive change. This was my favorite feature in the book. It reinforced practical nutritional changes that anyone can do."
>
> **Michelle Higgins**
> Erie Community College

What *IS* That?

Foods that contain live and active probiotics may be beneficial to your health, particularly your intestinal health. Kefir is a "cultured" milk. Cultured milks, such as kefir and cultured buttermilk, have probiotics added to them. The probiotic bacteria use the natural carbohydrate in milk for energy, and produce acid and carbon dioxide as a result. The acid curdles the milk and gives it a distinctive taste; the carbon dioxide provides some "fizz," like a carbonated soft drink. A 1 cup serving of kefir that's made from 2% milk supplies about the same energy and nutrient contents as 1 cup of 2% milk.

© Wendy Schiff

What Is That? highlights foods that are often unfamiliar to Americans and provides nutrition information about the foods. Exposing students to new food items expands their options as a consumer.

Nutrition Fact or Fiction? dispels popular food and nutrition myths such as "sugar causes hyperactivity," "the 5-second rule," and the "freshman 15."

Nutrition Fact or Fiction?

Sugar makes children hyperactive.

If you've ever attended a child's birthday party, you can understand why people often blame sugary foods for causing "hyper" behavior. The results of scientific studies, however, don't indicate that sugar is a cause of *attention deficit hyperactivity disorder*, also known as *ADHD*.[2] Children with ADHD are impulsive and have difficulty controlling their behavior and paying attention. The cause of ADHD is uncertain, but genetic and environmental factors play important roles. When children attend parties, their excitement and lack of self-control are more likely caused by the situation than by their sugar intake.

It's possible that caffeine is responsible for children's "hyper" behavior. Caffeine is a stimulant drug. Sources of caffeine in children's diets include "energy drinks"; certain sugar-sweetened soft drinks, such as colas; and chocolate.

© Digital Vision/Getty Images RF

Answer This questions give students opportunities to practice using basic skills, including math, graph reading, and critical thinking to answer questions relating to the unit's content.

Q Answer This

If your total calorie intake is 2400 kcal per day and fat provides 30% of your calories, how many grams of fat do you consume? You'll find the answer on the last page of this unit.

A Answer This (Module 3.1b)

80 g

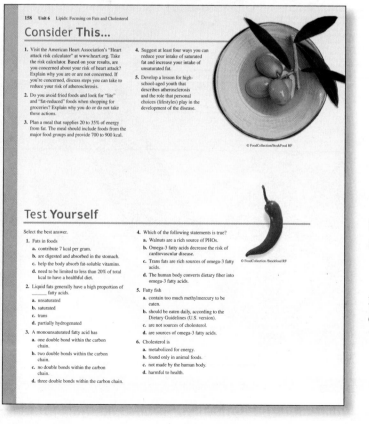

158   Unit 6   Lipids: Focusing on Fats and Cholesterol

Consider This...

1. Visit the American Heart Association's "Heart attack risk calculator" at www.heart.org. Take the risk calculator. Based on your results, are you concerned about your risk of heart attack? Explain why you are or are not concerned. If you're concerned, discuss steps you can take to reduce your risk of atherosclerosis.

2. Do you avoid fried foods and look for "lite" and "fat-reduced" foods when shopping for groceries? Explain why you do or do not take these actions.

3. Plan a meal that supplies 20 to 35% of energy from fat. The meal should include foods from the major food groups and provide 700 to 900 kcal.

4. Suggest at least four ways you can reduce your intake of saturated fat and increase your intake of unsaturated fat.

5. Develop a lesson for high-school-aged youth that describes atherosclerosis and the role that personal choices (lifestyles) play in the development of the disease.

© FoodCollection/StockFood RF

Test Yourself

Select the best answer.

1. Fats in foods
   a. contribute 7 kcal per gram.
   b. are digested and absorbed in the stomach.
   c. help the body absorb fat-soluble vitamins.
   d. need to be limited to less than 20% of total kcal to have a healthful diet.

2. Liquid fats generally have a high proportion of _____ fatty acids.
   a. unsaturated
   b. saturated
   c. trans
   d. partially hydrogenated

3. A monounsaturated fatty acid has
   a. one double bond within the carbon chain.
   b. two double bonds within the carbon chain.
   c. no double bonds within the carbon chain.
   d. three double bonds within the carbon chain.

4. Which of the following statements is true?
   a. Walnuts are a rich source of PHOs.
   b. Omega-3 fatty acids decrease the risk of cardiovascular disease.
   c. Trans fats are rich sources of omega-3 fatty acids.
   d. The human body converts dietary fiber into omega-3 fatty acids.

5. Fatty fish
   a. contain too much methylmercury to be eaten.
   b. should be eaten daily, according to the Dietary Guidelines (U.S. version).
   c. are not sources of cholesterol.
   d. are sources of omega-3 fatty acids.

6. Cholesterol is
   a. metabolized for energy.
   b. found only in animal foods.
   c. not made by the human body.
   d. harmful to health.

© FoodCollection /Stockfood RF

Consider This... presents critical thinking questions related to the unit's content that help students apply what they read.

Test Yourself at the end of each unit features multiple-choice questions designed to help students check their knowledge and prepare for exams.

Essential Concept

4.4   What Happens to Water-Soluble Nutrients?

Intestinal villus

1 Nutrients that dissolve in water, such as amino acids, glucose, and minerals, enter the capillary network of the villus.

Capillary network within villus

2 Eventually, these water-soluble nutrients are transported from the GI tract to the liver by the hepatic (liver) portal vein.

Hepatic portal vein

Essential Concept takes a complex scientific process and illustrates it in a unique, step-by-step manner to facilitate learning, especially for students who are not science majors. Topics include the scientific method, how the body digests proteins, and the role of hormones in regulating blood glucose levels. Numbered boxes contain points that relate to a particular portion of the illustration, while the large green arrow helps students visualize stepping through the process.

Essential Concept

7.1   Digesting and Absorbing Proteins

Inside the stomach

HCl   HCl   Inactive pepsin   Pepsin

Shorter polypeptide chains

Inside the small intestine

1 Protein digestion begins in the stomach. Hydrochloric acid (HCl) helps the process by changing the inactive form of pepsin to the active enzyme **pepsin**. HCl also causes proteins to unfold. This action makes it easier for pepsin to break apart the peptide bonds between amino acids. As a result, large protein chains break down into shorter polypeptide chains of several amino acids.

2 When the shortened polypeptide chains enter the small intestine, the pancreas and absorptive cells secrete protein-splitting enzymes called proteases. Proteases digest polypeptides into individual amino acids, dipeptides, and tripeptides.

Pancreas

Proteases from pancreas

Tripeptide

Dipeptide

Intestinal cell enzymes

Microvilli border

Absorptive cell

Small intestine

Tripeptides

3 Enzymes within the microvilli border of absorptive cells digest the di- and tripeptides into amino acids. Thus, amino acids are the end products of protein digestion.

To liver

Bloodstream

pepsin stomach enzyme that breaks down proteins into polypeptides

Liver

"I like the presentation of these [Essential Concept] processes and your illustrations are much better quality than most textbooks. The simplicity of the presentation aids in the students' understanding."

Johanna Donnenfield
Scottsdale Community College

Consumer Focus

Teaches students how to better evaluate nutrition information for a healthier life.

Nutrition Essentials: A Personal Approach is consumer focused, providing students with ample ways to both evaluate nutrition information as well as apply practical tips for healthier living. An entire unit (Unit 2) is devoted to understanding the scientific method and evaluating nutrition information.

Module 2.3

Becoming a More Critical Consumer of Nutrition Information

© McGraw-Hill Education. Mark A. Dierker, photographer

2.3 - Learning Outcomes

After reading Module 2.3, you should be able to

1. Define all of the key terms in this module.
2. Describe how you can become a more careful and critical consumer of nutrition information.
3. Identify common "red flags" that are signs of nutrition misinformation.
4. Describe how to identify reliable sources of nutrition information.

Source: Federal Trade Commission

The **Federal Trade Commission (FTC)** enforces U.S. consumer protection laws and investigates complaints about false or misleading health claims that are used in advertising. According to the FTC, Americans spend billions of dollars annually on fraudulently marketed and unproven health-related products and treatments that are often useless.[5] Claims for such products often promise cures for common and serious medical conditions, including obesity and cancer. When the products prove to be ineffective, the people who believed the claims and bought the products are cheated out of their money, and, in some instances, their health declines as a result of wasting time using the worthless product.

If you're like most people, you don't want to waste your money on things you don't need or that are useless or potentially harmful. Promoters of worthless nutrition products often use clever marketing methods, including sensational claims about the products' effectiveness, to attract people to make unnecessary purchases. Skeptical people don't believe the claims without checking into them.

2.3a Becoming a More Skeptical Consumer

How can you become a more careful, critical consumer of nutrition-related information, products, or services? By being more *skeptical*.

1. Don't believe everything you hear or read about nutrition, including nutrition-related products or services.
2. Ask questions about the information's source. Why should you believe and trust the source?
3. Ask questions about the source's motives for promoting the information. Radio or TV programs that promote nutrition information as facts may actually be advertisements for profitable nutrition-related products or services.
4. Be wary of

> **Federal Trade Commission (FTC)** federal agency that enforces U.S. consumer protection laws and investigates health claims

- *Salespeople.* Salespeople often have favorable biases toward the things they sell, and therefore, they may not be reliable sources of information about these products. Clerks in a dietary supplements store, for example, may wear a white lab coat to look as though they have a science or medical educational background. Keep in mind that the clerks were hired to sell dietary supplements and may have little or no scientific training. Furthermore, the clerks may receive commission for what they sell, so they might not inform you about the negative aspects of using a product or service.

32

Module 2.1

Nutrition: Science for Consumers

2.1 - Learning Outcomes

After reading Module 2.1, you should be able to

1. Define all of the key terms in this module.
2. List the basic steps of the scientific method as it relates to nutrition research in general.
3. Discuss ways that scientists conduct nutrition-related research that involves human subjects.
4. Explain why results of similar studies can provide different findings.

© Photodisc/Getty Images RF

In the past, nutrition facts and recommended dietary practices were often based on intuition, common sense, "conventional wisdom" (tradition), or **anecdotes** (reports of personal experiences). Today, registered dietitians and other nutrition experts discard conventional beliefs, explanations, and practices when the evidence obtained by current scientific research no longer supports them.

2.1a Collecting Science-Based Evidence

Scientists generally use the *scientific method* to answer questions about natural and physical observations. Scientists, for example, have answered questions such as: "How does the stomach break down food proteins?" "Why do babies need the mineral iron to develop normally?" and "Why is vitamin C necessary to maintain good health?"

An **experiment** is a way of testing a scientific question. Because of safety and ethical concerns, nutrition scientists often conduct experiments on small mammals before performing similar research on humans. Certain kinds of mice and rats are raised for experimentation purposes. The rodents are inexpensive to house in laboratories, and their food and other living conditions can be carefully controlled.

Researchers control conditions that are not being tested, such as the ways the animals are handled and the kinds of physical activity the animals receive. Otherwise, their findings are likely to be unclear or inaccurate.

Essential Concept 2.1 describes the basic steps of the scientific method as applied to a nutrition-related experiment involving laboratory mice.

Essential Concept
2.1 Applying the Scientific Method

1 Observe
Scientists observe a group of hospitalized patients who have stomach cancer. After obtaining dietary information from all the patients, the researchers determine that the patients with stomach cancer eat more charcoal-grilled meat than other people who are the same age but don't have stomach cancer.

2 Develop a question
The researchers think eating charcoal-grilled meat increases the risk of stomach cancer. They develop a question: "Chemical X is only in meat that has been charcoal grilled. If chemical X is given to a group of laboratory mice for 6 months, will they develop more cases of stomach cancer than mice that have not eaten chemical X?"

anecdotes reports of personal experiences

experiment a way of testing a scientific question

peer review expert critical analysis of a research article before it's published

24

X

Personalized Focus

The nutrition book that's all about YOU!

- The personalized, consumer focus gives plenty of practical examples to help you choose and prepare nutritious foods as well as make nutrition-related decisions that are good for your health.

- The proven successful Connect for *Nutrition Essentials: A Personal Approach* digital program, including Question Bank, Test Bank, Animations, LearnSmart Prep, LearnSmart/SmartBook adaptive reading, and NutritionCalc Plus dietary analysis, gives you access to one of the most effective and successful adaptive learning resources available on the market today.

Nutrition Essentials: A Personal Approach is uniquely designed to provide non-science majors with the basic scientific principles of nutrition in a highly visual, engaging framework focused on their personal choices and experiences. Adaptive learning resources LearnSmart and SmartBook create an individualized study plan to help you achieve success in understanding nutrition.

Each unit highlights an actual college student's nutrition concerns. These relatable accounts in a student's own words help frame the content of that unit and encourage you to think about your own dietary choices.

"My name is Abhinaya, but I usually go by "Abby" or "Abhi." I was born in Madras, India. My family moved to the United States when I was 13 years old. . . . American food is very bland. My American friends tell me that Indian food is very spicy, but I love foods seasoned with lots of chili powder and other Indian spices. Every summer, my family visits relatives in India. When we return, we bring back foods and spices that we can't find here.

Traditional Indian dishes really provide a balanced diet. They include cooked lentils, beans, greens, and lots of onion and garlic. I'm from southern India so I eat a lot of white rice topped with ghee, which has a buttery taste. . . . When I'm at home, I eat a wide variety of fruits and vegetables. My favorite fruits are mangoes, fresh pineapples, and bananas. . . . Strawberries aren't a traditional Indian fruit, but I love to eat them when they're in season here."

Abby Raghothaman

What's New in This Edition

The first edition of this textbook included visually stimulating and creative page layouts, and beautifully rendered, pedagogically based illustrations that were designed to engage students' interest in topics and facilitate learning. The second edition maintains this energetic, colorful, and appealing design. We have retained the interesting photos that help draw students' attention to the written information and enable them to relate content to the real world. It is important to note that the use of products in photos is for example representation only and does not constitute an endorsement.

The second edition of *Nutrition Essentials: A Personal Approach* has been extensively updated with new information. The following points highlight some of the significant revisions.

Many of the diagrams and illustrations throughout the textbook have been modified to increase their clarity. For example, the illustrations in Essential Concepts 7.1 (Digesting and Absorbing Proteins) and 7.2 (What Can Happen to Unneeded Amino Acids) have been revised to help students follow steps involved in the processes better.

Each unit now has an Answer This feature in which students must respond to a question using information they have just read. Most of these questions require students to use critical thinking, basic math, or graph interpretation skills. The answer is given at the end of the unit.

Three of the unit openers have been revised to feature new college students who share personal reflections about their dietary choices. These openers help draw students into the unit's content.

Unit 3 (Making More Nutritious Choices) underwent major changes.

- The *2015–2020 Dietary Guidelines for Americans*, including:
  - Five overarching guidelines that suggest basic food- and nutrition-related practices for consumers, such as "Focus on variety, nutrient density, and amount of food" and "Shift to healthier food and beverage choices."
  - Components of a healthy eating pattern, according to the new Dietary Guidelines.
  - Specific dietary recommendations, including "Choose foods that provide potassium, dietary fiber, calcium, and vitamin D, which are nutrients of public health concern … ," and, for pregnant women, "Do not consume alcohol."
  - New Table 3.2 Healthy Eating Patterns helps support the updated narrative that focuses on the *2015–2020 Dietary Guidelines for Americans.*

Chapter 3 also introduces the new Nutrition Facts panel for food labels. The panel includes information about added sugars' content and provides percentages of the new Daily Values.

TABLE 3.2 HEALTHY EATING PATTERNS

According to the Dietary Guidelines, a healthy eating pattern provides

- A variety of vegetables;
- A variety of fruit, especially whole fruit;
- Grains, especially whole grains;
- Fat-free or low-fat dairy products;
- Various protein foods; and
- Oils.

According to the Dietary Guidelines, a healthy eating pattern limits

- Unhealthy fats, added sugars, and sodium.

Unit 4 (How Food Becomes You) has expanded information about the gut microbiome, probiotics, and prebiotics.

Unit 5 (Carbohydrates: Fuel and Fiber) has a new section about FODMAPs and the low-FODMAP diet. FODMAPs are carbohydrates and sugar alcohols that can cause intestinal upsets because they're not well-digested by humans.

Unit 6 (Lipids: Focusing on Fat and Cholesterol) discusses PHOs (partially hydrogenated oils) and the ban on their use in foods.

Unit 7 (Proteins: Life's Building Blocks) has information about food allergies, including the possibility that introducing a variety of foods to babies can reduce their chances of developing food allergies.

Unit 10 (Nutrition for a Healthy Weight and Fit Body) discusses why the "3500-Calorie Rule" may not be reliable and introduces a couple of new surgical techniques for weight loss.

New Daily Values are presented in Appendix C. Appendix H (Stretching Your Food Dollars) provides tips to help students save money without sacrificing good nutrition when they purchase food. Appendix I (Modifying Recipes for Healthy Living) has basic food preparation tips and suggestions for making healthier substitutions in recipes.

Nutrition Facts

28 servings per container

Serving size	3 flatbreads (28g)

Amount Per Serving

Calories	110

	% Daily Values*
Total Fat 3g	
Saturated Fat 1g	5%
Trans Fat 0g	5%
Cholesterol 0mg	
Sodium 170mg	0%
Total Carbohydrate 19g	7%
Dietary Fiber 1g	6%
Total Sugars 1g	4%
Includes 0g Added Sugars	0%

© Wendy Schiff

Acknowledgments

My heartfelt thanks extends to everyone at McGraw-Hill Education who helped in the development and production of the second edition of *Nutrition Essentials: A Personal Approach*. I also owe a great deal of gratitude to Marisa Moreno, Damian Nguyen, Clare Chapman, Amanda Croker, McKenzie Frey, Matthew Lang, Abby Raghothaman, Olivia Coomes, Nancy Scott, Neill Warrington, and Theresa Washington. These current and former college students helped make *Nutrition Essentials* a more personal approach by contributing their quotations and photos to Unit openers.

A few members of my McGraw-Hill Education team deserve to be recognized for their hard work and commitment to the development and production of the second edition of *Nutrition Essentials: A Personal Approach*. Marija Magner, Brand Manager, took the necessary steps to move forward with the new edition. I am grateful for her guidance and willingness to continue developing the features of this unique textbook. My Content Production Manager, Vicki Krug, had one of the most difficult jobs as a member of the team. She had to make sure that production deadlines were met. Vicki also forwarded instructions for art and corrections to staff at the outside companies that prepared illustrations for and printed the textbook. Each year, she has to juggle the production of several textbooks at one time, and she did an amazing job of successfully managing the production of *Nutrition Essentials*.

Jessica Cannavo, Marketing Manager, did a great job of helping me analyze the needs of students taking personal nutrition courses so I could build on the success of the first edition. Jessica, thanks so much! Tara McDermott, Designer, developed the amazing cover and new design features for this new edition; Lorraine Buczek, Lori Slattery, and Lori Hancock, Content Licensing Specialists, handled the securing of permissions and releases. Such "behind-the-scenes" staff are critical players in the production of a high-quality textbook. My special thanks also extend to Tara, Lorraine, Lori, and Lori.

I also want to thank Marty Lange, Vice President and General Manager, and Lynn Breithaupt, Managing Director, for providing the support that was necessary for developing, publishing, and marketing the new edition of this textbook. Last, but not least, my Product Developer, Darlene Schueller, deserves my sincerest gratitude for the hard work, long hours, and extraordinary dedication she invested in the production of the second edition of *Nutrition Essentials: A Personal Approach* and the Connect and LearnSmart resources that support the textbook. Darlene's extensive experience and skills as a product developer were evident as she took over the development of the second edition of the textbook. Meeting deadlines can be very challenging for an author, but Darlene made the revision process flow smoothly. I look forward to working with her on future editions of this textbook!

Wendy J. Schiff

Contents

Preface   viii

Unit 1   Food *Is* More than Something to Eat   2

Module 1.1   Why Learn About Nutrition?   4

Module 1.2   Nutrition Basics   6

Module 1.3   Key Nutrition Concepts   13

Unit 2   Nutrition Information: Fact or Fiction?   22

Module 2.1   Nutrition: Science for Consumers   24

Module 2.2   Spreading Nutrition Misinformation   30

Module 2.3   Becoming a More Critical Consumer of Nutrition Information   32

Module 2.4   Seeking Reliable Nutrition Information   36

Unit 3   Making More Nutritious Choices   40

Module 3.1   Requirements and Recommendations   42

Module 3.2   Planning Nutritious Meals and Snacks   45

Module 3.3   Making Sense of Food Labels   57

Module 3.4   Should I Take Dietary Supplements?   60

© Lauren Burke/Getty Images RF

Unit 4   How Food Becomes You   70

Module 4.1   From Cells to Systems   72
Module 4.2   Digestive System   75
Module 4.3   Common Digestive System Disorders   87
Module 4.4   Metabolism Basics   95

Unit 5   Carbohydrates: Fuel and Fiber   100

Module 5.1   Sugars, Sweeteners, Starches, and Fiber   102
Module 5.2   What Happens to the Carbohydrates You Eat?   113
Module 5.3   Carbohydrates and Health   117

Unit 6   Lipids: Focusing on Fats and Cholesterol   128

Module 6.1   What Are Lipids?   130
Module 6.2   What Happens to the Fat and Cholesterol You Eat?   138
Module 6.3   Cardiovascular Disease: Major Killer of Americans   142

Unit 7   Proteins: Life's Building Blocks   160

Module 7.1   What Are Proteins?   162
Module 7.2   What Happens to the Protein You Eat?   164
Module 7.3   Proteins in Foods   169
Module 7.4   What's Vegetarianism?   173
Module 7.5   Proteins and Health   176

Unit 8   Vitamins: Nutrients that Multitask   186

Module 8.1   Introducing Vitamins   188
Module 8.2   Fat-Soluble Vitamins   193
Module 8.3   Water-Soluble Vitamins   205
Module 8.4   Vitamins and Cancer   220

Unit 9   Key Minerals, Water, and the Nonnutrient Alcohol   228

Module 9.1   Minerals for Life   230

Module 9.2   Key Minerals and Your Health   234

Module 9.3   Water: Liquid of Life   256

Module 9.4   Drink to Your Health?   262

Unit 10   Nutrition for a Healthy Weight and Fit Body   274

Module 10.1   Overweight or Obese?   276

Module 10.2   Factors That Influence Your Body Weight   283

Module 10.3   Managing Your Weight Safely   289

Module 10.4   Disordered Eating and Eating Disorders   297

Module 10.5   Get Moving; Get Healthy!   300

Unit 11   Nutrition for Your Life, Environment, and World   316

Module 11.1   Nutrition for a Lifetime   318

Module 11.2   How Safe Is My Food?   334

Module 11.3   Dietary Adequacy: A Global Concern   345

Appendix   A-1

A   English-Metric Conversion and Metric-to-Household Units   A-3

B   Canada's Food Guide   A-4

C   Daily Values (DVs) Table   A-11

D   The Basics of Energy Metabolism   A-12

E   Answers to *Test Yourself* Questions   A-14

F   References   A-15

G   Dietary Reference Intake (DRI) Tables   A-29

H   Stretching Your Food Dollars   A-35

I   Modifying Recipes for Healthy Living   A-39

Glossary   G-1

Index   I-1

© ballyscanlon/Getty Images RF

NUTRITION ESSENTIALS

Second Edition

A Personal Approach

Unit **1**

*F*ood *Is* More than Something to Eat

What's on the Menu?

Module 1.1
Why Learn About Nutrition?

Module 1.2
Nutrition Basics

Module 1.3
Key Nutrition Concepts

© McGraw-Hill Education. Mark A. Dierker, photographer

"My family's Hispanic, and most of my family was born in Texas, so I grew up helping my mother and grandmother cook 'Tex-Mex' food, using recipes passed down generation to generation. Now my diet isn't limited to Tex-Mex, but it's still my favorite type of food. I always associate this food with family gatherings."

Marisa Moreno

Marisa Moreno is a junior, majoring in English Literature at Loras College. Her Hispanic ethnic background greatly influences her favorite food choices, which she describes as "Tex-Mex." According to Marisa, "Tex-Mex dishes are similar to traditional Mexican dishes, such as tacos, tostadas, burritos, tamales, fajitas, and enchiladas, but Tex-Mex food preparation uses some different ingredients. Mexican tacos, for example, typically include crumbly white goat cheese, whereas Tex-Mex tacos have shredded yellow American cheese. Tex-Mex dishes are often served with *pico de gallo* on top. *Pico de gallo* is a salsalike topping that is made from fresh diced tomatoes, jalapeño and serrano peppers, chopped green onions and fresh cilantro (a leafy herb that looks like fresh parsley), lemon juice, and a little salt. Also, Tex-Mex recipes often incorporate sauces made with hot chili peppers that are popular in the southwestern United States. Cumin is the southwestern spice generally used in Tex-Mex dishes...hot chili sauce is added on nearly everything."

© Wendy Schiff

To what extent does your ethnic/cultural background influence your food choices? Have you ever thought about why you eat certain foods and not others? Overall, how would you rate the nutritional quality of the food that you eat—good, just OK, or poor?

Many factors influence what you eat **(Fig. 1.1).** Your usual food choices are likely to be foods that you enjoy, can afford, and can prepare easily or obtain quickly. Unfortunately, you weren't born with the ability to select the proper mix of substances that your body needs to function properly. To eat well, you need to learn about nutrition and the effects that your food selections can have on your health.

Income
Ethnic Background
Occupation
Nutritional and health beliefs
Moods
Food composition, convenience, and availability
Religious beliefs
Family Peers
Food flavor, texture and appearance
Childhood experiences
EDUCATION
Current health status
Rural vs. urban residence
habits
Advertising and media

Figure 1.1 Many factors influence food choices.

▪ *What influences your eating practices?*

3

Module 1.1

Why Learn About Nutrition?

© Purestock/SuperStock RF

1.1 - Learning Outcomes

After reading Module 1.1, you should be able to

1. Define all of the key terms in this module.

2. Identify the leading causes of death in the United States and lifestyle factors that contribute to the risk of these diseases.

nutrients life-sustaining chemicals in food that are necessary for proper body functioning

nutrition study of nutrients and how the body uses these substances

diet usual pattern of food choices

Food is more than just "something good to eat." Regardless of what you eat and drink, your body needs **nutrients**, the life-sustaining chemicals in food, to function properly. **Nutrition** is the scientific study of nutrients and how the body uses these chemicals.

Your **diet** is your usual pattern of food choices. Why should you care about your diet? In the United States, poor eating habits contribute to several leading causes of death, including heart disease, some types of cancer, stroke, and diabetes **(Fig. 1.2)**. Conditions such as heart disease, cancer, and diabetes are *chronic diseases*—health problems that usually take many years to develop and have complex causes.

Figure 1.2 Approximate percentages of leading causes of death (U.S.). Several lifestyle factors contribute to many of the 10 leading causes of death in the United States.

■ *Are any of these diseases in your family history?*

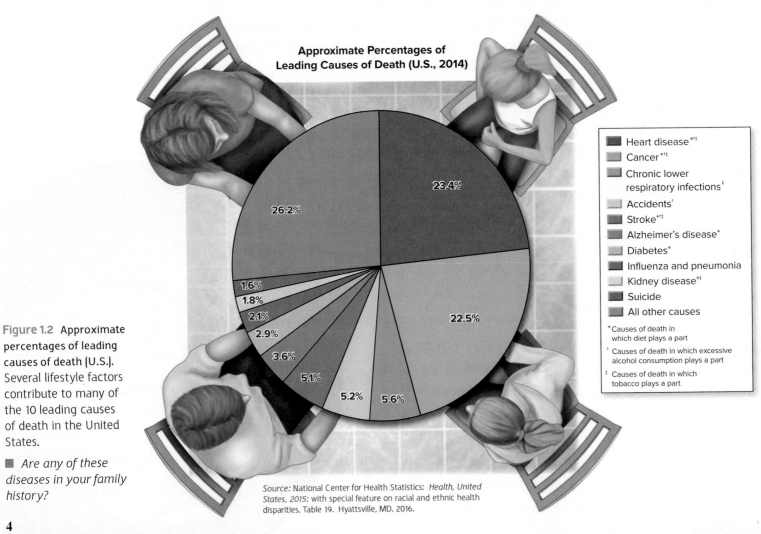

Approximate Percentages of Leading Causes of Death (U.S., 2014)

23.4%
26.2%
22.5%
1.6%
1.8%
2.1%
2.9%
3.6%
5.1%
5.2%
5.6%

- Heart disease*‡
- Cancer*†‡
- Chronic lower respiratory infections†
- Accidents†
- Stroke*†‡
- Alzheimer's disease*
- Diabetes*
- Influenza and pneumonia
- Kidney disease*‡
- Suicide
- All other causes

*Causes of death in which diet plays a part

† Causes of death in which excessive alcohol consumption plays a part

‡ Causes of death in which tobacco plays a part

Source: National Center for Health Statistics: *Health, United States, 2015:* with special feature on racial and ethnic health disparities. Table 19. Hyattsville, MD. 2016.

A **risk factor** is a personal characteristic that increases your chances of developing a chronic disease. Family history, for example, is an important risk factor for heart disease. If your father's father had a heart attack before he was 55 years old and your mother is being treated for having high blood pressure and a high blood cholesterol level (risk factors for heart disease), your family history indicates you have a higher-than-average risk of having a heart attack. For many people, however, having a family history of a chronic disease does not mean that they definitely will develop the condition. Other risk factors that contribute to health problems include age, environmental conditions, and lifestyle practices.

Lifestyle is a person's way of living that includes diet, physical activity habits, use of drugs such as tobacco and alcohol, and other typical patterns of health-related behavior. Your lifestyle may increase or reduce your chances of developing a chronic disease or delay its occurrence for years, even decades. Many people die prematurely because of their lifestyle practices. Smoking, for example, is a lifestyle. In the United States, cigarette smoking is the leading cause of preventable deaths.[1]

There are no guaranteed ways to extend your lifetime. However, you may increase your chances of living a long and healthy life by consuming more fruits, vegetables, unsalted nuts, fat-free or low-fat dairy products, seafood, dried beans and peas, and whole-grain cereals, as well as exercising regularly.[2] Reducing your intake of fatty meats, refined grain products, and sugar-sweetened foods, particularly beverages, may also improve your health.

Smoking is the leading cause of preventable death in the United States.

© Pixtal/Punchstock RF

risk factor personal characteristic that increases a person's chances of developing a disease

lifestyle way of living that includes diet, physical activity habits, use of tobacco and alcohol, and other typical patterns of behavior

Does your lifestyle include frequent meals and snacks at fast-food outlets?

© McGraw-Hill Education. Mark A. Dierker, photographer

Module 1.2

Nutrition Basics

1.2 - Learning Outcomes

After reading Module 1.2, you should be able to

1. Define all of the key terms in this module.
2. List the six classes of nutrients, and identify a major role of each class of nutrient in the body.
3. Calculate the caloric value of a serving of food based on its macronutrient (and alcohol) contents.
4. Provide examples of essential nutrients, nonnutrients, phytochemicals, and dietary supplements.
5. Explain the importance of supplying the body with antioxidants.

© FoodCollection/StockFood RF

1.2a Nutrients and Their Major Functions

There are six classes of nutrients: carbohydrates, fats and other lipids, proteins, vitamins, minerals, and water. Carbohydrates, lipids, proteins, and vitamins are **organic nutrients** because they have the element carbon in their chemical structures.

Table 1.1 presents major roles of nutrients in your body. Note that most nutrients have more than one function and some nutrients have similar roles in your body. In general, you need certain nutrients for energy, growth and development, and regulation of cellular functions, including the repair and maintenance of cells. In many instances, several nutrients work together to keep your body healthy.

Although average healthy young men and women have similar amounts of vitamins, minerals, and carbohydrates in their bodies, young women have less water and protein and more fat (**Fig. 1.3**).

organic nutrients nutrients that have carbon in their chemical structures

Male

- <1%
- 6%
- 16%
- 16%
- 62%

Female

- 5%
- 13%
- 25%
- 57%
- <1%

Legend:
- Carbohydrates
- Minerals
- Protein
- Fat and Other Lipids
- Water

Figure 1.3 **Comparing body composition.** The amount of vitamins in the human body is so small, the percentage isn't shown.

TABLE 1.1

NUTRIENTS AND THEIR MAJOR FUNCTIONS IN THE BODY

Nutrient	Major Functions
Carbohydrates	Source of energy (most forms)
Lipids	Source of energy (fats), cellular development, physical growth and development, regulation of body processes, absorption of fat-soluble vitamins
Proteins	Production of structural and functional components; cellular development, growth, and maintenance; regulation of body processes; immune function; fluid balance; source of energy
Vitamins	Regulation of body processes, maintenance of immune function, production and maintenance of tissues, protection against agents that can damage cellular components
Minerals	Regulation of body processes, including fluid balance; formation of certain chemical messengers; structural and functional components of various substances and tissues; necessary for physical growth, maintenance, and development
Water	Maintenance of fluid balance, regulation of body temperature, elimination of wastes, transportation of substances, participant in many chemical reactions

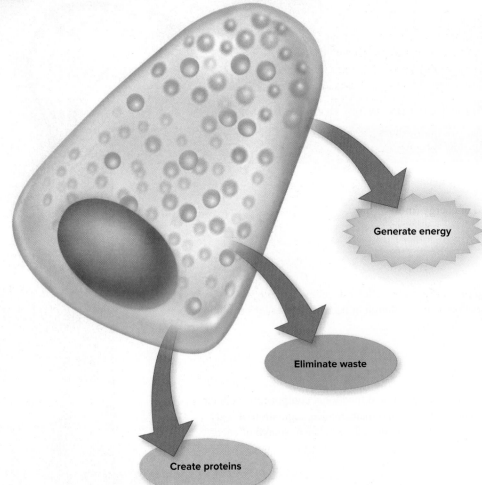

A **cell** is the smallest functional unit in a living organism, including a human being **(Fig. 1.4).** Cells do not need food to survive, but they do need the nutrients in food to carry out their metabolic activities. **Metabolism** is the total of all chemical reactions (changes) that occur in living cells, including reactions involved in generating energy, making proteins, and eliminating waste products.

1.2b Food Energy

Every cell in your body uses energy to carry out its various activities, whether you're running, sitting, or studying, and even while you're sleeping. As long as you're alive, you're constantly using energy. Foods and beverages that contain fat, carbohydrate, protein, and/or alcohol supply energy for your body. You'll learn how your cells obtain energy in Unit 4.

You're probably familiar with the term *calorie,* the unit that describes the energy content of food. The amount of energy in food is reported in 1000-calorie units called **kilocalories,** or **Calories.** If no number of kilocalories is specified, it's appropriate to use "calories." In this textbook, the term "kilocalories" (**kcal**) is interchangeable with "food energy" or simply "energy."

Figure 1.4 Some functions of a typical human cell.

cell smallest living functional unit in an organism

metabolism total of all chemical processes that take place in living cells

kilocalorie (kcal) or Calorie unit of measuring food energy

Your body uses energy even when you're sleeping.

1.2c Macronutrients and Micronutrients

Carbohydrates, fats, and proteins are sometimes called **macronutrients** because the body needs relatively large amounts of these nutrients daily. Vitamins and minerals are **micronutrients** because the body needs very small amounts of them to function properly. Macronutrients supply energy for cells, whereas micronutrients do not. Although your body requires large amounts of water, this nutrient provides no energy and isn't usually classified as a macronutrient.

Nutrition experts often use metric measurements, such as grams (g) and liters, instead of household measures, such as ounces and cups. An ounce of salt, for example, weighs about 28 g. **Table 1.2** provides the meaning of some commonly used metric prefixes, including *kilo-* and *milli-*. In general, a serving of food supplies grams of carbohydrate, fat, and protein and *milligram (mg)* or *microgram (mcg)* quantities of vitamins and minerals. Appendix A provides information about common English-to-metric and metric-to-household unit conversions.

Figure 1.5 Energy sources for the body. Alcohol isn't a nutrient.

■ *How can you estimate the amount of calories in a serving of food?*

TABLE 1.2

COMMON METRIC
PREFIXES FOR NUTRITION

kilo- (k) = one thousand (1000)

deci- (d) = one-tenth (0.1)

centi- (c) = one-hundredth (0.01)

milli- (m) = one-thousandth (0.001)

micro- (mc or μ) = one-millionth (0.000001)

A gram of carbohydrate and a gram of protein each supply about 4 kcal; a gram of fat provides about 9 kcal **(Fig. 1.5)**. Although alcohol isn't a nutrient, it does provide energy; a gram of pure alcohol furnishes 7 kcal.

If you know how many grams of carbohydrate, protein, fat, and/or alcohol are in a food, you can estimate the number of kilocalories it provides. For example, if a serving of food contains 10 g of carbohydrate and 5 g of fat, multiply 10 by 4 (the number of kcal each gram of carbohydrate supplies). Then multiply 5 by 9 (the number of kcal each gram of fat supplies). By adding the two values (40 kcal from carbohydrate and 45 kcal from fat), you'll determine that this food provides 85 kcal/serving.

A serving of food contains 30 g of carbohydrate, 10 g of fat, 5 g of protein, 60 mg of vitamin C, and 5 mg of iron. How many calories are in the serving of food? First, determine the amount of energy in each of the food's components.

30 g of carbohydrate × 4 kcal/g = 120 kcal from carbohydrate

10 g of fat × 9 kcal/g = 90 kcal from fat

5 g of protein × 4 kcal/g = 20 kcal from protein

Now, add together the calories for the three sources of energy: 120 kcal + 90 kcal + 20 kcal = 230 kcal/serving.

Q Answer This

Why don't you need to include vitamin C and iron in your calorie calculations? You'll find the answer on the last page of this unit.

macronutrients nutrients needed in gram amounts daily and that provide energy; carbohydrates, proteins, and fats

micronutrients vitamins and minerals

1.2d What's an Essential Nutrient?

Your body can make many nutrients, such as fat and cholesterol (types of lipids), but about 50 nutrients must be supplied by food because the human body does not produce the nutrient or make enough to meet its needs. Such nutrients are **essential nutrients (Table 1.3).** Water is the most essential nutrient. You can live for months without iron or vitamin C but only a few days without water.

If an essential nutrient is missing from the diet, a **deficiency disease** occurs as a result. The deficiency disease is a state of health characterized by certain abnormal *physiological* (functional) changes that result in signs and symptoms of disease. Such signs and symptoms may include skin rashes, diarrhea, and loss of night vision. Treating a deficiency disease is usually simple: when the missing essential nutrient is added to the diet, the deficiency disease is cured.

1.2e What's a Nonnutrient?

Some foods, particularly those from plants, contain nonnutrients: substances that are not nutrients, yet they may have healthful benefits. Alcohol is an energy-supplying nonnutrient that can have harmful as well as beneficial effects on your health. Plants make hundreds of **phytochemicals** *(fi'-toe-kem'-ih-kals)*. Caffeine, for example, is a phytochemical naturally made by coffee plants that has a stimulating effect on the body. Later units of this text provide more information about caffeine and alcohol.

Many phytochemicals function as **antioxidants**. An antioxidant protects cells and their components from being damaged or destroyed by chemically unstable factors that are called **free radicals**.

Not all phytochemicals have beneficial effects on the body; some are *toxic* (poisonous) or can interfere with the body's ability to absorb nutrients. **Table 1.4** lists several phytochemicals, identifies rich food sources of these substances, and indicates their effects on the body, including possible health benefits. Certain vitamins act as antioxidants. You'll learn more about them in Unit 8, which focuses on vitamins.

Water is the most essential nutrient.

© Comstock Images/PictureQuest RF

Source: USDA Natural Resources Conservation Service

essential nutrient nutrient that must be supplied by food

deficiency disease state of health that occurs when a nutrient is missing from the diet

phytochemicals substances made by plants that are not nutrients but may be healthful

antioxidant substance that protects cells and their components from being damaged or destroyed by free radicals

free radicals chemically unstable factors that can damage or destroy cells

---

TABLE 1.3   ESSENTIAL NUTRIENTS FOR HUMANS

Water

Vitamins

A				C	
B vitamins				D*	
Thiamin	Pantothenic acid	B-6		E	
Riboflavin	Biotin	B-12		K	Choline**
Niacin	Folic acid (folate)				

Glucose (from carbohydrate-containing foods)†

Minerals

Calcium	Copper	Magnesium	Phosphorus	Sodium
Chloride	Iodine	Manganese	Potassium	Sulfur
Chromium	Iron	Molybdenum	Selenium	Zinc

The following components of proteins (amino acids) are generally recognized as essential:

Histidine	Lysine	Threonine
Isoleucine	Methionine	Tryptophan
Leucine	Phenylalanine	Valine

Fats that contain linoleic and alpha-linolenic acids

*The body makes vitamin D after exposure to sunlight, but a dietary source of the nutrient is often necessary.

**The body makes choline but may not make enough to meet needs. Often classified as a *vitamin-like* substance.

†A source of glucose is needed to supply the nervous system with energy and spare protein from being used for energy.

TABLE 1.4

PHYTOCHEMICALS

Examples	Rich Food Sources	Biological Effects/ Possible Health Benefits
Alpha-carotene, beta-carotene, lutein, lycopene	Orange, red, yellow fruits and vegetables; egg yolks	May reduce risk of certain cancers and macular degeneration (cause of blindness) The body can convert alpha- and beta-carotene into vitamin A.
Quercetin	Apples, tea, red wine, onions, olives, raspberries, cocoa	Antioxidant activity, may inhibit cancer growth, may reduce risk of heart disease
Anthocyanins	Red, blue, or purple fruits and vegetables	Antioxidant activity, may inhibit cancer growth, may reduce risk of heart disease
Resveratrol	Red wine, purple grapes and grape juice, dark chocolate, cocoa	Antioxidant activity, may inhibit cancer growth, may reduce risk of heart disease
Isoflavonoids	Soybeans and other legumes	Antioxidant activity, may inhibit cancer growth, may reduce risk of heart disease
Sulfur compounds	Garlic, onions, leeks, broccoli, cauliflower, cabbage, kale, bok choy, collard and mustard greens	Antioxidant activity, may inhibit cancer growth, may reduce risk of heart disease
Caffeine	Coffee, tea, cocoa	Stimulant effects
Saponins	Chickpeas, beans, oats, grapes, olives, spinach, garlic, quinoa	May kill certain microbes, inhibit certain cancers, and reduce risk of heart disease
Capsaicin	Chili peppers	May provide some pain relief

1.2f What Are Dietary Supplements?

Many Americans take dietary supplements such as vitamin pills and herbal extracts to improve their health. A **dietary supplement** is a product (excluding tobacco) that contains a vitamin, a mineral, an herb or other plant product, an amino acid, or a dietary substance that supplements the diet by increasing total intake.[3] According to scientific evidence, some dietary supplements, such as vitamins, minerals, and certain herbs, can have beneficial effects on health. However, results of scientific testing also indicate that many popular dietary supplements are not helpful and may even be harmful. Information about specific dietary supplements is in Unit 3 and woven into other units of this textbook where appropriate.

1.2g What's Malnutrition?

Malnutrition is a state of health that occurs when the body is improperly nourished. Everyone must consume food and water to stay alive, yet despite the abundance and variety of nutritious foods, many Americans consume nutritionally poor diets and suffer from malnutrition as a result. Some people select nutritionally inadequate diets because they lack knowledge about nutritious foods or the importance of nutrition to health. Low-income people, however, are at risk for malnutrition because they have limited financial resources for making wise food purchases. Other people who are at risk of malnutrition include those who have severe eating disorders, are addicted to drugs such as alcohol, or have certain serious medical problems.

Many people associate malnutrition with *under*nutrition and starvation. *Over*nutrition, the long-term excess of energy or nutrient intake, is also a form of malnutrition. Overnutrition is often characterized by unhealthy amounts of body fat (*obesity*). You may be surprised to learn that overnutrition is more common in the United States than undernutrition. Obesity is widespread in countries where most people have the financial means to buy plenty of food, have an ample food supply, and obtain little exercise. Unit 10 provides information about obesity; Unit 11 discusses the international problem of undernutrition.

Obesity is a form of malnutrition.

dietary supplement product that contains a vitamin, a mineral, an herb or other plant product, an amino acid, or a dietary substance that supplements the diet

malnutrition state of health that occurs when the body is improperly nourished

Nutrition Fact or Fiction?

The typical college student gains 15 pounds during his or her freshman year.

Although most college students (about 61%) gain weight during their freshmen year in college, the average weight gain is 7.5 pounds.[4] Factors that are thought to contribute to the weight gain include feeling "stressed out," eating too much unhealthy food, drinking too much alcohol, and being less physically active than before they entered college.

Module 1.3
Key Nutrition Concepts

© Design Pics/Alamy RF

1.3 - Learning Outcomes

After reading Module 1.3, you should be able to

1. Define all of the key terms in this module.

2. Classify foods as nutrient-dense, energy-dense, or high in empty calories.

3. Identify key basic nutrition concepts, including (a) the importance of eating a variety of foods and (b) no naturally occurring food supplies all nutrients.

Before learning about nutrients and their roles in health, it's important to grasp some key basic nutrition concepts (**Table 1.5**). Each of the sections of this module focuses on one of these concepts. The content in the units that follow will build upon these key concepts and can help you make more informed choices concerning your dietary practices.

1.3a There Are No "Good" or "Bad" Foods

Do you refer to pizza, chips, candy, doughnuts, ice cream, and sugar-sweetened soft drinks as "bad foods" or "junk foods"? All foods have nutritional value, so no food deserves to be labeled "bad" or "junk." Although pies, doughnuts, and ice cream contain a lot of fat and sugar, these foods also supply small amounts of protein, vitamins, and minerals to diets. A chocolate doughnut, for example, provides 6 g protein, 2 mg niacin (a B vitamin), 4 mg iron, and 4 g fiber. (Most forms of fiber are classified as carbohydrates.) Even sugar-sweetened soft drinks provide two nutrients: water and the carbohydrate sugar, a source of energy. As you read this textbook, you'll learn why certain foods are healthier choices than others.

A food *is* bad for you if it contains toxic substances or is contaminated with bacteria, viruses, or microscopic animals that cause food-borne illness. You've probably suffered from a food-borne illness at least once. The abdominal cramps, nausea, vomiting, and diarrhea that usually accompany a food-borne illness occur within a few hours or days after a person eats the contaminated food. Unit 11 discusses food safety concerns, including major types of food-borne illnesses and how to prevent them.

Empty Calories

Some foods and beverages, such as candies, pastries, snack chips, sugar-sweetened drinks, and some alcoholic beverages, may be described as sources of "empty calories."[5] **Empty calories** are calories from unhealthy types of fat, added sugar, and/or alcohol. Thus, a food that contains a lot of empty calories isn't a good source of vitamins and minerals. Eating too many foods that are high in empty calories may displace more nutritious foods from your diet. In later units of this text, you'll learn more about empty calories, including alcohol.

What's a Nutrient-Dense Food?

Certain foods provide more "beneficial nutrients" than others. Such beneficial nutrients include protein, fiber, vitamins C and E, iron, calcium, and potassium. A **nutrient-dense** food or beverage contains more beneficial nutrients in relation to total calories, especially calories from unhealthy fats, added sugars, and/or alcohol. Broccoli, leafy greens, fat-free milk, orange juice, lean meats, and whole-grain cereals are examples of nutrient-dense foods.

> **empty calories** calories from unhealthy fats, added sugars, and/or alcohol
>
> **nutrient-dense** describes foods or beverages that supply more beneficial nutrients in relation to total calories

Foods that contain a lot of empty calories

© FoodCollection/StockFood RF

TABLE 1.5	KEY NUTRITION CONCEPTS

1. There are no good or bad foods.

2. Variety, moderation, and balance are features of healthy diets.

3. Food is the best source of nutrients and phytochemicals.

4. There is no "one size fits all" approach to good nutrition.

5. Foods and nutrients are not cure-alls.

83 kcal

8.26 g protein

299 mg calcium

247 mg phosphorus

0.446 mg riboflavin

91 kcal

0.17 g protein

5 mg calcium

25 mg phosphorus

0 mg riboflavin

8 fluid ounces   8 fluid ounces

Figure 1.6 Nutrient density.

■ *What distinguishes an "empty calorie" food from a nutrient-dense one?*

---

energy density energy value of a food in relation to the food's weight

variety including different foods from each food group

moderation consuming foods in reasonable amounts

balance matching calorie intake with calorie expenditure to maintain a healthy weight

---

Figure 1.6 compares amounts of energy and certain nutrients provided by 8-ounce servings of fat-free milk and a cola-type, sugar-sweetened ("regular") soft drink. Although the drinks supply similar amounts of calories, the milk provides far more protein and riboflavin, and minerals calcium and phosphorus. A healthy diet contains a variety of nutrient-dense foods and limits empty calories.

Which Foods Are Energy Dense?

Energy density describes the energy value of a food in relation to the food's weight. For example, a chocolate, yeast-type frosted doughnut that weighs about 3.5 ounces and is about 4 inches in diameter provides almost 400 kcal; eight medium strawberries also weigh about 3.5 ounces, but they provide only

32 kcal. You'd have to eat 100 of the strawberries to obtain the same amount of food energy that's in the chocolate doughnut (**Fig. 1.7**). Therefore, the doughnut is an energy-dense food in comparison to the berries. In general, high-fat foods such as doughnuts are energy dense because they're concentrated sources of energy. Most fruits aren't energy dense because they contain far more water than fat.

It's important to note that not all energy-dense foods are rich sources of empty calories. Nuts, for example, are high in fat and, therefore, energy dense. However, nuts are also nutrient dense because they contribute protein, vitamins, minerals, and fiber to diets. You can find information about the energy and nutrient contents of foods by using "What's in the Foods You Eat Search Tool" at the U.S. Department of Agriculture's website: www.ars.usda.gov/Services/docs.htm?docid=17032 .

1.3b Variety, Moderation, and Balance Are Features of Healthy Diets

Most foods are mixtures of nutrients, but no natural food is "perfect" in that it contains all nutrients in amounts that your body needs. To help ensure that your diet provides all the essential nutrients as well as beneficial phytochemicals, choose a **variety** of nutrient-dense foods from each food group (**Fig. 1.8**) and consume them in reasonable amounts (**moderation**). Furthermore, **balance** your caloric intake with enough physical activity to maintain a healthy weight. Unit 3 provides more information about food groups, including recommendations for serving sizes.

Figure 1.7 Energy density.

■ *What distinguishes an "energy-dense" food from a food that's not energy dense?*

4″ diameter

400 kcal

400 kcal

Glass of milk: © Sandy Jones/Getty Images RF; Glass of soda: © Royalty-Free/Corbis RF; Donut, Strawberries: © Wendy Schiff

Figure 1.8 The MyPlate food guide (see Unit 3).

Marisa, the student quoted in this unit's opener, is concerned with the balance of nutrients in her diet. "I try to eat the right balance of fruits, vegetables, along with meats…I like beef more than chicken…." Tex-Mex dishes are usually mixtures of various foods, which can make it difficult to determine whether daily meals and snacks provide a healthful balance of nutrients. Unit 3 discusses food groups and how to plan a nutritionally adequate diet.

1.3c Food Is the Best Source of Nutrients and Phytochemicals

The most natural, reliable, and economical way to obtain nutrients and beneficial phytochemicals is to base your diet on a variety of "whole" and minimally processed foods. For most Americans, eating 100% raw foods isn't practical and, in some instances, it's unsafe. Many foods undergo some form of processing, such as peeling, refining, and heating, before they're eaten. Such treatments can make food safer and more convenient to eat.

Plant foods naturally contain a variety of nutrients and phytochemicals, but processing the foods often removes some of the most healthful parts. For example, a wheat kernel is stripped of its germ and outer hull (*bran*) during refinement into white flour (**Fig. 1.9**). Wheat germ is a rich source of vitamin E and beneficial ("healthy") fats. Wheat bran contains fiber and certain phytochemicals, and it's a concentrated source of several micronutrients. The endosperm is primarily starch (a form of carbohydrate) with some protein and very small amounts of micronutrients and fiber. A "whole grain" includes the bran and germ portions of the kernel along with the endosperm. By replacing refined grain products, such as white bread, with 100% whole-grain products, you can increase the likelihood of obtaining a wide variety of nutrients and phytochemicals.

TASTY Tidbits

Almonds and other nuts are nutrient and energy dense. For example, 1 ounce of almonds (about 23 whole nuts) supplies about 160 kcal, 6 g of protein, 14 g of fat, more than 7 mg of vitamin E, and small amounts of iron, calcium, and B vitamins. Snack on a handful of nuts or add them to your cereal.

Bran
Endosperm
Germ

White Flour

NET WT 4 LB

Figure 1.9 **What is white flour?** During refinement, a wheat kernel is stripped of its nutrient-rich germ and bran. The endosperm (white flour) that remains is mostly starch.

■ *Why is it important to choose a variety of foods, especially those that are whole or minimally processed?*

Death

Toxic

Upper limit of safe intake

↑
Safe physiologic doses (range of safe intake for optimal body function)
↓

Marginal

Deficient

Death

For each nutrient, there is a range of safe intake.

Should You Take Nutrient Supplements?

Many people take nutrient supplements in the form of pills, powders, bars, wafers, or beverages. Your body, however, is designed to obtain nutrients from foods, not supplements. In some instances, nutrients from food are more available—that is, more easily digested and absorbed than those in supplements.

It's important to understand that nutrient supplements don't contain everything you need for optimal nutrition. For example, they don't contain the wide variety of phytochemicals found in plant foods. Although supplements that contain phytochemicals are available, they may not provide the same healthful benefits as those obtained by consuming the plants that contain these substances. Why? Nutrients and phytochemicals may need to be consumed together to provide desirable effects in the body. Food naturally contains combinations of these chemicals in very small amounts and certain proportions. There's nothing "natural" about gulping down handfuls of supplements.

For each micronutrient, there's a range of safe intake. In their natural states, most commonly eaten foods contain safe levels of micronutrients. However, you can develop health problems by taking high doses of dietary supplements that contain vitamins and/or minerals. Units 2 and 3 provide more information about nutrient supplements.

1.3d There's No "One Size Fits All" Approach to Good Nutrition

By using food guides presented in Unit 3, you can individualize your diet so that it's nutritionally adequate and suits your food likes and dislikes, budget, and lifestyle. Individualizing a diet doesn't mean only eating foods that "match" your blood type, hair color, personality, or shoe size. If someone promotes a diet based on such personal traits, steer clear of the diet and the promoter. Consider this: Human beings wouldn't have survived as a species for thousands of years if their diets had to be matched to physical characteristics or personalities.

It's important to note that nutritional needs of healthy people vary during different stages of their lives. Thus, infants, children, pregnant women, and older adults often need nutrient supplements to boost their nutrient intakes. Additionally, physicians often prescribe nutrient supplements or special diets for chronically ill people.

1.3e Foods and Nutrients Aren't Cure-Alls

Although specific nutrient deficiency diseases can be cured if you eat foods that contain the nutrient that's missing or is in short supply, nutrients don't "cure" other ailments. Diet is only one aspect of yourself that influences your health. Other lifestyle factors as well as genetics and environment also play major roles in determining your health status.

Although a pregnant woman may choose nutritious foods, she still may need to take a special nutrient supplement during this stage of her life.

What *IS* That? - - - - - - - - - - - - - →

Trees that bear lychee (*lee'-chee*) fruit are native to China, but they are also grown in Hawai'i, California, and Florida. A 100 g portion (about 3.5 ounces) of the fresh fruit supplies about 65 kcal and 24 to 60 mg vitamin C.[6] Remove the leathery peel to reveal the sweet fruit, but don't eat the seed, which is surrounded by the pulp.

Peeled and pitted lychees are used to add an interesting flavor and texture to fruit salads; the juice may also be added to other fruit drinks.

What Are Functional Foods?

Many foods are manufactured for specific health-related functions. Although there's no legal definition for *functional foods,* such products have health-related purposes.[7] Functional foods are often made to boost nutrient intakes or help manage specific health problems. For example, you can increase your calcium intake by purchasing orange juice that has the mineral added to it. Certain margarine substitutes contain phytochemicals that may lower the risk of heart disease. Many yogurt products contain specific forms of bacteria that may relieve diarrhea. These bacteria are probiotics—that is, living microorganisms that can benefit human health. Although some functional foods can help people improve their health in other ways, more research is needed to determine their benefits as well as possible harmful effects.

This "buttery spread" is an example of a functional food.

1.3f Some Closing Thoughts

By applying what you learn about nutrition and the role of diet in health, you may be able to live longer and healthier as a result. Furthermore, you may become a more careful consumer of nutrition-related information by studying the content of this textbook. You must eat to live, so you'll have plenty of opportunities to use the information and, in some instances, develop new food-related attitudes and habits. Enjoy!

Basic components of a healthy diet

In a Nutshell

© McGraw-Hill Education. Mark A. Dierker, photographer

© xefstock/Getty Images RF

Module 1.1 Why Learn About Nutrition?

- Lifestyle choices, including poor eating habits and lack of physical activity, contribute to the development of many of the leading causes of premature deaths for American adults, including heart disease, cancer, stroke, and diabetes. You may be able to live longer and be healthier by applying what you learn about nutrition and the role of diet and health.

- Chronic diseases, such as heart disease and cancer, are long-term health problems that generally have multiple risk factors. A risk factor is a personal characteristic such as family history and lifestyle practices that increases your chances of developing such diseases. There are ways you may be able to reduce your risk of developing a chronic disease, especially one that's among the leading causes of death in the United States. Such actions include modifying your diet, increasing your physical activity, and improving other aspects of your lifestyle.

Module 1.2 Nutrition Basics

- Nutrients are chemicals in foods that the body needs for proper functioning. Nutrition is the scientific study of nutrients and how the body uses them. There are six classes of nutrients: carbohydrates, lipids, proteins, vitamins, minerals, and water.

- The body needs certain nutrients for energy, growth and development, and regulation of processes, including the repair and maintenance of cells. The human body can make many nutrients, but about 50 of these chemicals are dietary essentials that must be supplied by food because the body doesn't produce them or make enough to meet its needs.

- Plant foods naturally contain a variety of phytochemicals, substances that aren't classified as nutrients yet may have healthful benefits. Many phytochemicals are antioxidants that protect cells from being damaged or destroyed by exposure to certain environmental factors. However, some phytochemicals are toxic.

© Stan Sholik/Alamy RF

- Every cell needs energy. Calories or kilocalories (kcal) are used to indicate the energy value in food. A gram of carbohydrate and a gram of protein each supply about 4 kcal; a gram of fat provides about 9 kcal. Although alcohol isn't a nutrient, a gram of pure alcohol furnishes 7 kcal.

- Carbohydrates, fats, and proteins are referred to as macronutrients because the body needs relatively large amounts of these nutrients daily. Vitamins and minerals are micronutrients because each day, the body needs very small amounts. Although the body requires large amounts of water, this nutrient provides no energy and isn't usually classified as a macronutrient.

Module 1.3 Key Nutrition Concepts

- Most naturally occurring foods are mixtures of nutrients, but no food contains all the nutrients needed for optimal health. Thus, nutritionally adequate diets include a variety of foods from all food groups that are consumed in moderation. It's also important to balance calorie intake with energy output.

- Instead of classifying foods as "good" or "bad," you can focus on eating all foods in moderation and limiting empty calories.

- For each nutrient, there's a range of safe intake.

- Healthy people should rely on eating a variety of foods to meet their nutrient needs instead of taking nutrient supplements.

- Although nutrients are vital to good health, foods and the nutrients they contain are not cure-alls. There's no "one size fits all" approach to planning a nutritionally adequate diet.

What's in Your Diet?!

1. If you purchase food regularly, keep your grocery and convenience store receipts for a week.

   a. How much money did you spend on the foods you purchased at these markets?

   b. Which foods were the most expensive?

   c. How much do you spend on food and beverages that supply a lot of empty calories, such as salty snacks, cookies, soft drinks, and candy?

   d. What percentage of your food dollars was spent on foods that were high in empty calories? _____ (Divide the amount of money you spent on such foods by the total cost of food for the week. Move the decimal point over 2 places to the right and place a percent sign after the number.)

   e. How much money did you spend on nutrient-dense foods, such as whole-grain products, peanut butter, eggs, fruits, and vegetables?

   f. What percentage of your food dollars was spent on nutrient-dense foods? _____ (Divide the amount of money you spent on nutrient-dense foods by the total cost of food for the week. Move the decimal point over 2 places to the right and place a percent sign after the number.)

© Ragnar Schmuck/Getty Images RF

2. For one week, keep a detailed log of your usual vending machine purchases, including the item(s) purchased and amount of money you spent for each purchase.

   a. What types of foods and beverages did you buy from the machines?

   b. How many soft drinks did you consume each day?

   c. How much money did you spend on vending machine foods and beverages?

   d. Based on this week's vending machine expenditures, estimate how much money you spend on such purchases in a year.

3. For one week, keep a detailed log of your usual fast-food consumption practices, including fast-food purchases at convenience stores. List the types of food and beverages you purchased and amount of money you spent.

   a. According to your weekly record, how often do you buy food from fast-food places and convenience stores?

   b. What types of foods did you usually buy?

   c. How much money did you spend on fast foods?

   d. Based on this week's expenditures, estimate how much money you spend on fast-food purchases in a year.

4. Over the past month, did you purchase dietary supplements? If your response is "Yes," which product or products did you purchase? _____

   How much did you spend on such products? _____

© Stewart Walker/fStop/Getty Images RF

5. Over the past month, did you buy coffee at commercial coffee outlets? If your response is "Yes," which kinds of coffee did you purchase and how were they prepared? _____

   How much did you spend on such products? _____

Consider **This...**

1. Identify at least six factors that influence your food and beverage selections. Which of these factors is the most important? Explain why.

2. Consider your current eating habits. Explain why you think your diet is or isn't nutritionally adequate.

3. If you were at risk of developing a chronic health condition that could be prevented by changing your diet, would you make the necessary changes? Explain why or why not.

4. "Everything in moderation." Explain what this statement means in terms of your diet.

5. Recall everything that you ate or drank in the past 24 hours. Identify the foods that were energy dense, nutrient dense, or high in empty calories. Are you interested in changing your intake of such foods? Explain why or why not.

Test **Yourself**

© FoodCollection /Stockfood RF

Select the best answer.

1. Diet is a
   a. practice of restricting energy intake.
   b. pattern of food choices.
   c. method of reducing portion sizes.
   d. technique to reduce carbohydrate intake.

2. Which of the following health conditions isn't one of the 10 leading causes of death in the United States?
   a. Cancer
   b. Diabetes
   c. Arthritis
   d. Stroke

3. Which of the following substances is a nutrient that provides energy?
   a. Glucose
   b. Water
   c. Alcohol
   d. Vitamin C

4. _____ refers to all chemical processes that occur in living cells.
   a. Physiology
   b. Catabolism
   c. Anatomy
   d. Metabolism

5. Phytochemicals
   a. are essential nutrients.
   b. generally have no effects on health.
   c. should be avoided.
   d. are in plant sources of food.

6. Which of the following foods is energy and nutrient dense?
   a. Strawberries
   b. Peanuts
   c. Fat-free milk
   d. Iceberg lettuce

7. Which of the following foods is a rich source of phytochemicals?
   a. Egg whites
   b. Blueberries
   c. Canned salmon
   d. Chicken

8. Which of the following conditions is a chronic disease?

   a. Heart disease

   b. Upset stomach

   c. Broken rib

   d. Common cold

9. In the United States, the primary cause of preventable deaths is

   a. tobacco use.

   b. auto accidents.

   c. high-fat diet.

   d. excessive alcohol intake.

10. A serving of food contains 20 g carbohydrate, 6 g protein, and 9 g fat. Based on this information, a serving of this food supplies _____ kcal.

    a. 64

    b. 124

    c. 162

    d. 185

11. Which of the following items is high in empty calories?

    a. Cottage cheese

    b. Chocolate chip cookie

    c. Green grapes

    d. Egg yolk

12. Which of the following foods is the most nutrient dense?

    a. 15 French fries

    b. 1 celery stalk

    c. 1 tablespoon butter

    d. 1/2 cup raspberries

13. Which of the following substances isn't a dietary supplement?

    a. Iron

    b. Alcohol

    c. Vitamin A

    d. Calcium

© Creatas Images/Jupiter Images/Getty Images

A Answer This (Module 1.2c)

Iron and vitamin C are micronutrients; they provide no calories.

References ➡ See Appendix F.

STUDY TIP: Quickly create a customized practice quiz for this chapter by going to your Connect SmartBook "My Reports" section.

Don't have SmartBook and want to learn more? Go to **whysmartbook.com**.

Nutrition Information
FACT OR FICTION?

What's on the Menu?

Module 2.1
Nutrition: Science for Consumers

Module 2.2
Spreading Nutrition Misinformation

Module 2.3
Becoming a More Critical Consumer
of Nutrition Information

Module 2.4
Seeking Reliable Nutrition Information

© Wendy Schiff

"One of my best friends from college is very healthy and active, and she eats very healthy foods. She's told me great things about coconut oil. It's good for your hair and skin, and it seems to have endless health benefits. She always puts it in her tea and on peanut butter sandwiches. So I started using coconut oil when I cook, and in my tea, and whatever else I can think of adding it to. I don't know if I can really tell the results of using coconut oil because I'm not sure I use it enough. But I am definitely satisfied . . . there is no question in my mind that it works."

Clare Chapman

© Goodshoot/PunchStock RF

Clare Chapman is a graduate student at Minnesota State University-Mankato. Her friend's enthusiastic claims about the benefits of coconut oil are intriguing, but they're *anecdotes*—reports of personal experiences. Anecdotes aren't scientific evidence. Would you buy coconut oil and add it to food because Clare and her friend use it? How can you find out whether the oil is safe to use and actually provides health benefits?

We consume food, and we consume nutrition information. Magazines, books, television, radio, ads, and the Internet, even family members and friends, contribute to the "flood" of nutrition information. Much of this information isn't supported by scientific evidence. The challenge is learning how to be a skeptical consumer who questions the reliability of nutrition-related information, including health claims.

This unit takes a closer look at how scientists collect information that relates to nutrition. The unit also provides practical tips for judging the honesty and reliability of popular sources of nutrition information, such as Internet sites and magazine articles.

Module 2.1

Nutrition: Science for Consumers

2.1- Learning Outcomes

After reading Module 2.1, you should be able to

1. Define all of the key terms in this module.

2. List the basic steps of the scientific method as it relates to nutrition research in general.

3. Discuss ways that scientists conduct nutrition-related research that involves human subjects.

4. Explain why results of similar studies can provide different findings.

© Photodisc/Getty Images RF

In the past, nutrition facts and recommended dietary practices were often based on intuition, common sense, "conventional wisdom" (tradition), or **anecdotes** (reports of personal experiences). Today, registered dietitians and other nutrition experts discard conventional beliefs, explanations, and practices when the evidence obtained by current scientific research no longer supports them.

2.1a Collecting Science-Based Evidence

Scientists generally use the *scientific method* to answer questions about natural and physical observations. Scientists, for example, have answered questions such as: "How does the stomach break down food proteins?" "Why do babies need the mineral iron to develop normally?" and "Why is vitamin C necessary to maintain good health?"

An **experiment** is a way of testing a scientific question. Because of safety and ethical concerns, nutrition scientists often conduct experiments on small mammals before performing similar research on humans. Certain kinds of mice and rats are raised for experimentation purposes. The rodents are inexpensive to house in laboratories, and their food and other living conditions can be carefully controlled.

Researchers control conditions that are not being tested, such as the ways the animals are handled and the kinds of physical activity the animals receive. Otherwise, their findings are likely to be unclear or inaccurate.

Essential Concept 2.1 describes the basic steps of the scientific method as applied to a nutrition-related experiment involving laboratory mice.

Essential Concept

2.1 Applying the Scientific Method

1 Observe
Scientists observe a group of hospitalized patients who have stomach cancer. After obtaining dietary information from all the patients, the researchers determine that the patients with stomach cancer eat more charcoal-grilled meat than other people who are the same age but don't have stomach cancer.

2 Develop a question
The researchers think eating charcoal-grilled meat increases the risk of stomach cancer. They develop a question: "Chemical X is only in meat that has been charcoal grilled. If chemical X is given to a group of laboratory mice for 6 months, will they develop more cases of stomach cancer than mice that have not eaten chemical X?"

anecdotes reports of personal experiences

experiment a way of testing a scientific question

peer review expert critical analysis of a research article before it's published

5 Analyze the findings

At the end of the 6-month study, the scientists review all the data and use statistical tests to analyze the findings. The researchers are particularly interested in comparing the health of the two groups of mice, especially whether any of the mice developed stomach cancer.

4 Collect information

Every month the researchers collect information (*data*) about each mouse.

3 Test

The scientists test the question by dividing a group of 100 3-week-old laboratory mice into two groups that have 50 mice in each group. One group of mice in the study (subjects) is the treatment (or experimental) group. Each of these mice is fed ½ teaspoon of charcoal-grilled meat along with their ration of regular mouse chow every day. The other group of mice is called the control group. Instead of receiving ½ teaspoon of charred meat, mice in the control group only eat the mouse chow.

FINDINGS

Mice that ate charred meat were 3x as likely to develop stomach cancer than mice that didn't eat the meat.

6 Form conclusions

After analyzing the data, the researchers form conclusions based on their findings. Now, the scientists can answer their original question. According to the results of their study, the mice that consumed the charred meat were more likely to develop stomach cancer, compared to the mice that didn't eat the charred meat.

7 Share the results

The team shares the results of their findings, usually by preparing an article that describes the study and its findings. The team submits the article to the editor of a scientific journal. The article undergoes **peer review**—that is, the editor sends copies of the article to a group of peer reviewers—scientists who are qualified to judge the findings presented in the article. The researchers don't know the identities of the peer reviewers. If the peer reviewers accept the study's findings as being scientifically reliable, the journal's editor agrees to publish the article.

8 Conduct more research

After reading the article in the journal, other researchers conduct more research to examine the original question. Scientists do not accept the results of the study until the findings are supported by evidence from more studies, especially those conducted by different researchers.

Human Intervention Studies

Researchers must be careful when applying the results of laboratory experiments involving animals to people because of the many differences between people and "lab" animals. Nutrition scientists, however, do conduct experimental (intervention) studies using humans to obtain information about health conditions (outcomes) that can result from specific dietary practices. In such instances, scientists often design a double-blind study. In a **double-blind study,** the researchers and subjects don't know which participants are assigned to the **treatment** and **control groups.** Maintaining such secrecy is important during the course of a study because researchers and subjects may try to predict their group assignments. If the investigators who interview the participants are aware of their individual group assignments during the study (a single-blind study), they may convey clues to each subject. For example, a researcher's tone of voice or body language could influence a subject's belief about being in the experimental or control group. Subjects who think they're in the control group may report no changes in their condition. Ideally, subjects shouldn't be able to figure out their group assignment during the study.

When conducting double-blind studies, researchers provide all study participants with the same instructions and a "treatment," such as a dietary supplement or experimental food. However, only members of the treatment group actually receive the treatment. Subjects in the control group are given a placebo.

Placebos are not simply "sugar pills"; they are a fake treatment, such as a sham pill, injection, or medical procedure. If the treatment is a pill, the placebo pill looks, tastes, and smells like the pill that contains the active ingredient that is given to the subjects in the treatment group. The placebo pill, however, contains substances that don't produce any measurable physical changes. Providing placebos to members of the control group enables scientists to compare the extent of the treatment's response with that of the placebo.

What Is the Placebo Effect?

People often report positive or negative reactions to a treatment even though they received the placebo. If a patient believes a medical treatment will improve his or her health, the patient is more likely to report positive results for the therapy. Such wishful thinking is called the **placebo effect.**

At the present time, there is little scientific evidence to support claims that coconut oil is a "super food" with exceptional health benefits. Clare Chapman's firm belief that the tropical oil has improved her health may be the result of the placebo effect. On the other hand, Clare's body might be experiencing positive effects of using the oil that have not been considered or measured by researchers. As more people consume coconut oil, scientists are likely to conduct studies to determine whether the oil actually has any effects on health, including negative ones.

Single purple pill, Capsules and bottle: © Wendy Schiff; Crowd walking: © Tom Mareschal/Alamy RF

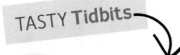

TASTY Tidbits

Placebos can produce beneficial results, particularly in subjects who have conditions that involve pain.[1] Because participants in the control group believe they are receiving a real treatment, their faith in the "treatment" can stimulate the release of chemicals in the brain that alter pain perception, reducing their discomfort. Therefore, when people report that a treatment was helpful, they may not have been imagining the positive response, even when they were taking a placebo. This is because the chemicals released in the brain actually relieved the pain.

double-blind study
experimental design in which neither the participants nor the researchers are aware of each participant's group assignment

treatment group group being studied that receives a treatment

control group group being studied that does not receive a treatment

placebo fake treatment, such as a sham pill, injection, or medical procedure

placebo effect response to a placebo

Nutrition researchers often use surveys to obtain information about a population's eating practices.

What *IS* That?- - - - - - - - - - - - - →

Pomegranate (*Punica granatum*) is a leathery-skinned fruit that is filled with pockets of edible, juicy seeds. In the United States, pomegranates are grown mostly in California, but the plant is native to northern India, the Mediterranean region, and certain Middle Eastern countries. For centuries, pomegranate has been used to treat a variety of ailments, including sore throats, wounds, and diarrhea.

When compared to other fruits, pomegranate juice has very high contents of phytochemicals with antioxidant activity. Nevertheless, results of scientific studies fail to provide good evidence that the juice is useful for reducing the risk of serious health problems such as heart disease. Pomegranate juice, however, may help prevent infections and reduce inflammation in people who have kidney disease.[2] Although pomegranate is high in phytochemicals, it's not a good source of vitamins and most minerals. A ½ cup serving of pomegranate juice supplies 70 kcal and 270 mg of potassium.

© Wendy Schiff

Population Studies

For decades, nutrition scientists have noted differences in rates of chronic diseases and causes of death among various populations. To understand why these differences exist, researchers rely on physical examinations, such as height and weight measurements, of large numbers of people to obtain health data. Additionally, they may collect information about a specific population's health and food-related practices by conducting surveys. Such surveys often question people about their personal and family medical histories, environmental exposures, and dietary practices.

The Framingham Heart Study

The Framingham Heart Study, which began in 1949 in Massachusetts, is one of the most well-known population studies that relates to nutrition. At the beginning of the study, the over 5000 healthy participants underwent physical examinations and were questioned about their family and personal medical histories as well as their lifestyle practices. Over the following years, a group of medical researchers periodically collected information concerning each participant's health and, if the person died, the cause of death. The scientists analyzed this information and found relationships among a variety of personal characteristics and health outcomes. Findings from the Framingham Heart Study identified numerous risk factors for heart disease, including high blood cholesterol levels and cigarette smoking. Today, medical researchers are still collecting information from the original Framingham Heart Study participants as well as their descendants.

2.1b Confusion and Conflict

One day, the news media highlight research about the health benefits of eating garlic, dark chocolate, brown rice, or cherries. A few weeks later, the media report the results of new scientific investigations that don't support the earlier findings. Consumers often become confused and disappointed when they learn about conflicting results generated by nutrition studies. As a result, some people think nutrition scientists don't know what they are doing. Why can't scientists agree and provide proof that eating specific foods benefits health?

Conflicting findings often result from differences in the ways that various studies are designed. Even when investigating the same question, different groups of scientists often conduct their studies and analyze the results differently. For example, the numbers, ages, and physical conditions of people who participate in each study (*subjects*), the type and length of the study, the amount of the treatment provided, and the methods used to analyze results typically vary among studies. Furthermore, situational, genetic, behavioral, and environmental differences among individuals account for much of the variation in the ways they respond to a treatment. Not only are people genetically different, they also have different lifestyles, and they typically recall or report dietary information and follow instructions concerning health care practices differently. These and other factors can influence the results of nutrition research involving human subjects. This is why dietary recommendations shouldn't be made from the results of a single study. The popular media, however, often report the findings of a study if they're sensational, that is, they grab your attention.

© Getty Images RF

What Is Research Bias?

Scientists expect other researchers to avoid relying on their personal attitudes and biases ("points of view") when collecting and analyzing data, and to evaluate and report their results objectively and honestly. However, the funding sources of scientific research may have certain expectations or biases about research outcomes. As a result, such groups are more likely to finance studies of scientists whose research efforts support their interests. The beef industry, for example, might not fund scientific investigations to find connections between high intakes of beef and the risk of certain cancers. On the other hand, the beef industry might be interested in supporting a team of scientists whose research indicates that a high-protein diet that contains plenty of beef is beneficial for people who are trying to lose weight.

Peer-reviewed journals usually require authors of articles to *disclose* (mention) their affiliations and sources of financial support. (Peer review is discussed in Essential Concept 2.1.) Such disclosures might appear on either the first page or at the end of the article. By having this information, readers can decide whether research bias may have influenced the researchers. Although peer review helps ensure that the scientists are as ethical and objective as possible, it's impossible to eliminate all research bias.

What kinds of nutrition-related research are likely to be funded by the beef industry?

© Carson Ganci/DesignPics

Cause and Effect

Population studies involving people and their eating practices generally cannot establish *cause and effect*—that is, whether a practice is responsible for an outcome. When two different natural events occur simultaneously within a population, it doesn't necessarily mean they're related to each other. For example, when a population's intake of sugar-sweetened soft drinks increases, the percentage of overweight people in the population also increases. Does this prove that drinking sugary soft drinks causes weight gain? Not necessarily. What appears to be a relationship between a dietary practice and a physical outcome could be a coincidence—that is, a chance happening.

In cases involving chronic diseases such as heart disease and cancer, it is difficult to prove that a single factor is responsible for the development of the condition. Multiple risk factors, including your *genetic susceptibility* (inherited proneness) to develop the disease, usually influence whether you'll develop a chronic disease. Other factors that play a role in the development of heart disease include high blood pressure, age, tobacco use, and intake of certain fats. Unit 6 provides more information about heart disease.

Q Answer This

Lemonade consumption increases in the summer, and drowning deaths also increase in the summer. Does this prove that drinking lemonade increases the risk of drowning? This answer is on the last page of this unit.

What *IS* That?----------→

For centuries, people in Asia have used the *rhizomes* (rye'-zhomes), fleshy underground stems, of the tropical plant ginger (*Zingiber officinale*) to treat stomach aches, nausea, diarrhea, arthritis, and muscle pain.[3] Popular forms of ginger include fresh or candied rhizomes, ginger extracts, and the dried, powdered seasoning that many Americans enjoy in pies and cakes. One teaspoon of raw, diced ginger root provides only 2 kcal.

According to results of scientific studies, eating small amounts of ginger for a short time is a safe way to relieve "morning sickness"—the nausea and vomiting that often accompany early pregnancy. However, studies also indicate that eating ginger may not be as helpful in controlling "motion sickness" and relieving arthritis and muscle pain. If you consume ginger, particularly the powdered herb, you may experience side effects, including intestinal gas, heartburn, and, ironically, nausea.

Nutrition Fact or Fiction?
Emotional stress causes stomach ulcers.

H. pylori

Not always! In 1982, Dr. Barry Marshall and Dr. Robin Warren proposed that a type of bacterium (*Helicobacter pylori*) causes gastritis, inflammation of the stomach lining.[4] Gastritis can lead to stomach ulcers. Initially, other physicians were skeptical about this notion because it challenged traditional medical beliefs. To provide support for his idea, Marshall actually swallowed some of the bacteria and developed severe stomach inflammation as a result. Physicians now know that *H. pylori* is a primary cause of gastritis and stomach ulcers. Although emotional stress may increase the risk of stomach ulcers, people who have ulcers and *H. pylori* in their stomachs are treated with antibiotics that kill the bacterium.

Module 2.2

Spreading Nutrition Misinformation

2.2 - Learning Outcomes

After reading Module 2.2, you should be able to

1. Define all of the key terms in this module.
2. Explain the difference between an anecdote and a testimonial.
3. Explain why there is so much nutrition misinformation.

If you think you already know a lot of nutrition facts, what were your sources of the information? Did you rely on magazines or the Internet? Why did you think these sources were trustworthy? In many instances, such popular sources of nutrition information are not reliable. Let's take a closer look at why you need to be careful when seeking nutrition information and advice.

2.2a Anecdotes and Testimonials

The host of a popular TV program interviews an attractive, young actress who claims to have lost a lot of weight after she started taking weight-loss pills made from a rare type of cactus. A few days later, a friend mentions that she's lost 3 pounds since she began taking this product a week ago. You'd like to lose a few pounds without restricting your food intake or exercising. Should you take this dietary supplement? It's promoted by the TV show host and helped the actress and your friend. Perhaps it will help you.

Although the TV show host is a likable person who seems to be honest and the personal experiences of the actress and your friend seem to provide evidence that the weight-loss supplement is effective, can you trust their judgment?

The actress's information is a **testimonial,** a personal endorsement of a product. People are usually paid to provide their testimonials for advertisements; therefore, their remarks might be biased in favor of the product. Your friend's experience with the weight-loss product is an anecdote, as is Clare's experience with coconut oil (see this unit's opener). When your source of nutrition information is a testimonial, advertisement, or anecdote, you cannot be sure that the information is based on scientific facts and is, therefore, reliable.

2.2b A Matter of Mistrust

Although people's lives have improved as a result of scientific advancements in medicine, many Americans mistrust the motives of scientists, dietitians, and other medical professionals. Promoters of nutrition misinformation use this mistrust to sell their products. For example, they may claim that physicians are more interested in making money than doing what's best for their patients, such as recommending dietary supplements. Are physicians driven by the desire to make money from their patients' illnesses? Do they hide information about natural cures from them?

It's true that physicians need incomes to support themselves and their families. However, people who tell you that the "medical/scientific establishment is hiding information about natural cures from you just to make money from your misery" are using *scare tactics* to build your mistrust in the medical establishment. Consider this: If your physician makes a mistake, you can sue him or her for malpractice. If you purchase a nutrition-related product or service, then your money enters the promoter's pockets. If the product or service doesn't live up to the promoter's claims or is harmful, what can you do?

As a group, physicians strive to diagnose and treat diseases using techniques that are scientifically tested for safety and effectiveness. Physicians have nothing to gain from concealing a cure from the public, but they have much to gain from treating their patients kindly and effectively. If you follow a physician's advice and have positive results, how likely are you to be that doctor's patient for a long time and recommend the practitioner to others?

---

testimonial personal endorsement of a product

TASTY Tidbits

You can often distinguish a peer-reviewed scientific journal from a popular magazine simply by looking at their covers and skimming their pages. Compared to scientific journals, popular magazines typically have

- More colorful, attractive covers and photographs;
- Articles that are shorter and easier for the average person to read; and
- Advertisements for products mentioned in articles.

If your car breaks down, you probably would want people who have the best training, tools, and equipment to determine the problem and repair it. If you think something is wrong with your body, it's wise to seek information and opinions from medical professionals who have the best scientific training and experience to diagnose and treat health disorders.

2.2c Why Is There So Much Nutrition Misinformation?

People may think they've learned facts about nutrition by reading popular magazine articles or best-selling books, by visiting Internet websites, or by watching television news, commercials, infomercials, or home shopping network programs. In many instances, however, they've been misinformed. To be a careful consumer, you shouldn't assume that all nutrition information presented in the popular media is reliable. Why?

First Amendment Freedoms

The First Amendment to the U.S. Constitution guarantees freedom of the press and freedom of speech. As a result, people can provide nutrition information that's not true. Thus, the First Amendment doesn't protect consumers with freedom from nutrition misinformation or false nutrition claims.

The **U.S. Food and Drug Administration (FDA)** can regulate nutrition- and health-related claims on product labels, but the agency cannot prevent the spread of health and nutrition misinformation published in books or pamphlets or presented in television or radio programs. People who promote nutrition misinformation often profit from these freedoms. As a consumer, you are responsible for questioning and researching the accuracy of nutrition information as well as the credentials of the people making nutrition-related claims.

U.S. Food and Drug Administration (FDA) federal agency that regulates claims on product labels

Module 2.3

Becoming a More Critical Consumer of Nutrition Information

2.3 - Learning Outcomes

After reading Module 2.3, you should be able to

1. Define all of the key terms in this module.

2. Describe how you can become a more careful and critical consumer of nutrition information.

3. Identify common "red flags" that are signs of nutrition misinformation.

4. Describe how to identify reliable sources of nutrition information.

© McGraw-Hill Education. Mark A. Dierker, photographer

Source: Federal Trade Commission

The **Federal Trade Commission (FTC)** enforces U.S. consumer protection laws and investigates complaints about false or misleading health claims that are used in advertising. According to the FTC, Americans spend billions of dollars annually on fraudulently marketed and unproven health-related products and treatments that are often useless.[5] Claims for such products often promise cures for common and serious medical conditions, including obesity and cancer. When the products prove to be ineffective, the people who believed the claims and bought the products are cheated out of their money, and, in some instances, their health declines as a result of wasting time using the worthless product.

If you're like most people, you don't want to waste your money on things you don't need or that are useless or potentially harmful. Promoters of worthless nutrition products often use clever marketing methods, including sensational claims about the products' effectiveness, to attract people to make unnecessary purchases. Skeptical people don't believe the claims without checking into them.

2.3a Becoming a More Skeptical Consumer

How can you become a more careful, critical consumer of nutrition-related information, products, or services? By being more *skeptical.*

1. Don't believe everything you hear or read about nutrition, including nutrition-related products or services.

2. Ask questions about the information's source. Why should you believe and trust the source?

3. Ask questions about the source's motives for promoting the information. Radio or TV programs that promote nutrition information as facts may actually be advertisements for profitable nutrition-related products or services.

4. Be wary of

   - ***Salespeople.*** Salespeople often have favorable biases toward the things they sell, and therefore, they may not be reliable sources of information about these products. Clerks in a dietary supplements store, for example, may wear a white lab coat to look as though they have a science or medical educational background. Keep in mind that the clerks were hired to sell dietary supplements and may have little or no scientific training. Furthermore, the clerks may receive commission for what they sell, so they might not inform you about the negative aspects of using a product or service.

Federal Trade Commission (FTC) federal agency that enforces U.S. consumer protection laws and investigates health claims

- *Nutrition "experts."* Anyone can call him- or herself a "nutritionalist" to appear to be a "nutrition expert." What is the person's educational background? Are his or her nutrition degrees from accredited institutions? What is the person's professional experience? Is it limited to the industry that's marketing nutrition-related products?

- *Claims that the product was "scientifically tested" or "clinically tested at a major university."* Where can you read the article about the study? Which university was involved in the clinical tests? Is it an accredited university? How was the testing done?

- *Citations to what appear to be scientific journal articles.* Promoters often make up journal citations or cite "journals" that were created by the products' manufacturers to provide the appearance of scientific credibility.

- *Scientific-sounding terms,* such as "enzymatic therapy," "nutritionals," or "colloidal chelated extract." Promoters typically use such vague or meaningless terms when presenting false or misleading information as factual and obtained by scientific methods. Such terms are designed to convince people without science backgrounds that the nutrition-related information is true.

- *Popular sources of nutrition information,* such as magazines and the Internet, because such sources generally don't subject articles or blogs to expert review before publishing the information. A reliable source has information about research that supports claims of a product's effectiveness as well as scientific studies that don't support its usefulness. Furthermore, reliable sources of information will alert consumers to possible health risks linked to using the products.

TASTY **Tidbits**

Practicing medicine without the proper training and licensing (**quackery**) is illegal. Quackery includes promoting useless medical treatments, such as copper bracelets to treat arthritis.

© Wendy Schiff

quackery practicing medicine without the proper training and licensing

2.3b Look for "Red Flags" of Misinformation

A *red flag* is a term or expression that draws your attention. For consumers of nutrition information, red flags are clues or signals of misinformation in media, advertising, and personal communications. Common red flags include

1. **Promises of quick and easy health remedies,** such as: "Our product helps you lose weight fast, *without* exercising or dieting."

2. **Claims that sound too good to be true,** such as: "You can eat everything you like and still lose weight," and "Garlic pills cure heart disease." These claims are rarely true. Remember, if the claim sounds too good to be true, it probably isn't true.

3. **Scare tactics,** such as: "Your liver is loaded with toxins and needs cleansing" and "There are chemicals in your food!" Your liver can't be "cleansed," and everything in your environment is chemical in nature.

World's Most Potent Energy & FAT BURNING Drink!

- A scientifically sound formula so powerful you'll see and feel its effects by taking only 1 capsule a day!
- A diet designed to burn Fat and keep it off!
- Groundbreaking tests have shown record results!

GUARANTEED RESULTS

Lose **WEIGHT** Quick

New and Improved
WEIGHT-LOSS FORMULA

You'll eat the foods you LOVE, and still lose weight!

Effective enzymatic therapy

Muscle Mania

A NEW BODY IN A BOX

- Burns FAT
- Provides
- Attacks Ce
- Increases
- Lose inches

Miracle Vitamin Formula
Reverses Aging!

Call **NOW** for immediate delivery!
1-800-555-

Everything you need to burn fat and build muscle

Muscle Mania

CD inside

This disclaimer may be a red flag that this product has little or no effectiveness.

4. **"Money back" guarantees,** such as "No risk. Just return the partially empty container and pay only shipping and handling," or "You have nothing to lose!" You *lose* money on worthless, ineffective, and potentially unsafe dietary supplements. Furthermore, you may lose valuable time trying to diagnose and treat a serious health problem on your own, rather than seeking more conventional and, usually, more effective medical care.

5. **Statements about the superiority of unconventional medical practices,** such as: "Russian scientists have discovered the countless health benefits of taking Siberian ginseng," or "Herbal tea is the only cure for intestinal cancer."

6. **Testimonials and anecdotes as evidence of effectiveness,** such as: "I lost 50 pounds in 30 days using this product," or "I rubbed this vitamin E-containing lotion on my scar and it disappeared in days." As mentioned earlier, testimonials and anecdotes are not scientific.

7. **Information that promotes a product's benefits while overlooking its risks:** "Our all-natural supplement boosts your metabolism naturally so it won't harm your body." Beware of any source of information that fails to mention the possible side effects of using a dietary supplement or nutrition-related treatment. Anything you consume, even natural substances such as water and minerals, can be toxic in high doses.

8. **Recommendations based on a single study:** "Research conducted at our private health facility proves coffee enemas can cure cancer." Results of such research are likely to be biased.

9. **Information concerning nutrients or the human body that's not supported by reliable scientific evidence:** "This book explains how to combine certain foods based on your blood type," or "Most diseases are caused by undigested food that gets stuck in your guts," or "People with alkaline bodies don't develop cancer."

10. **Disclaimers, usually in small or difficult-to-read print:** "Results may vary," "Results not typical," or "This product is not intended to diagnose, cure, or prevent any disease." Disclaimers are often clues that the product probably won't live up to your expectations or the manufacturer's claims.

Supplement label: © Wendy Schiff; Dollar bills: © Medioimages/Photodisc/Getty Images RF

bio-supplement

*Results not typical and depend on

The Internet can be a source of nutrition misinformation.

© Pixtal/AGE Fotostock RF

2.3c The Internet

You can find abundant sources of information about nutrition and the benefits of dietary supplements on the Internet. Before trusting the information, you must be careful and consider the sources. The same critical consumer tools for evaluating nutrition information from other sources can be applied to judging the reliability of information on the Internet (see Modules 2.3a and 2.3b).

A careful consumer of nutrition information

- Uses multiple sites, especially government agency sites (*.gov), such as the Centers for Disease Control and Prevention (www.cdc.gov) and the Food and Drug Administration (www.fda.gov).

- Relies primarily on sites that are sponsored by groups of qualified health professionals. In general, websites sponsored by nationally recognized health organizations (*.org) such as the Academy of Nutrition and Dietetics (www.eatright.org) and nonprofit organizations such as the American Cancer Society (www.cancer.org) and National Osteoporosis Foundation (www.nof.org) are reliable sources of nutrition information. Nationally accredited colleges and universities (*.edu) are excellent sources of credible nutrition information.

- Is skeptical of information in blogs. Blogs might be interesting to read, but they are not necessarily reliable.

- Is wary of websites that promote or sell products for profit (*.com) because such sources of information may be biased. Be wary if an *.org site sells dietary supplements online and/or includes articles that promote a products' benefits without mentioning their risks.

- Avoids sites that include disclaimers. Examples of disclaimers include "The FDA has not evaluated this website," or "The author and owner of this site are not liable for personal actions taken as a result of the site's contents."

Source: FDA

- Doesn't trust sites that include attacks on the trustworthiness of the medical or scientific establishment.

- Avoids sites that provide online diagnoses and treatments.

- Avoids giving personal information at the site because its confidentiality may not be protected.

The FTC enforces consumer protection laws and investigates complaints about false or misleading health claims that appear on the Internet. To obtain more information to help you evaluate nutrition and health-related claims, visit the agency's website. To complain about a product, you can complete and submit the FTC's complaint form at the agency's website (https://www.consumer.ftc.gov/about-us) or call the agency's toll-free line (1-877-382-4357).

TASTY Tidbits

In 2010, a federal district court ruled in favor of the FTC in a case involving companies that used unproven claims to promote "Chinese Tea Diet" and "Bio-Slim Patch." The court fined the companies nearly $2 million for claiming that the products would enable people to lose weight without exercising and cutting calories.[6]

© Wendy Schiff

Module 2.4

Seeking Reliable Nutrition Information

If you have questions about food or nutrition, where do you find factual answers? Should you ask your friends or coaches? Who can be trusted to provide the facts?

© Thinkstock/Getty Images RF

2.4a Nutrition Experts

If you pick up a fitness, food, or health magazine, you're likely to find something about nutrition. An article in a popular men's fitness magazine, for example, refers to an herbal tea recipe developed by a "physical fitness guru and nutrition expert." It seems that anyone who eats food can describe him- or herself as a nutritionist and provide nutrition- and food-related advice.

Although many states regulate and license people who call themselves nutritionists, you cannot always rely on someone who refers to him- or herself as a nutrition expert, "nutritionist," or "nutritionalist" for reliable nutrition information because there are no nationally standardized legal definitions for these descriptors.

"Doctors" may not be physicians or nutrition scientists. Most physicians aren't nutrition experts because they didn't have extensive training in human nutrition while they were in medical school. Furthermore, a so-called nutrition expert who's referred to as "Doctor" may not have a doctorate degree (PhD) in human nutrition from an accredited university. Such persons may have obtained their degrees simply by purchasing them on the Internet or through a mail-order outlet, without having taken appropriate coursework or graduated from an accredited university or college.

To obtain information about an author's or nutritionist's credentials, enter the person's name at an Internet search engine and evaluate the results. For example, is the person a scientist associated with an accredited school of higher education, such as a state or private university, or a government agency such as the U.S. Department of Agriculture? You can also visit www.quackwatch.org and submit an "Ask a Question" e-mail requesting information about a person's credentials.

If this person appeared on a television show or in a magazine advertisement, would you consider her to be a reliable source of nutrition information? Explain why you would or would not trust her nutrition-related advice.

© Purestock/SuperStock RF

Nutrition Professors and Registered Dietitian Nutritionists

If your university or college has a nutrition or dietetics department, you are likely to find nutrition experts, including nutrition professors and registered dietitians, who are faculty members. Nutrition professors generally have doctorate degrees in human nutrition from accredited universities and extensive educational backgrounds that emphasize coursework in human nutrition. Such instructors teach nutrition courses, conduct nutrition research, or do both.

A registered dietitian (RD) or a registered dietitian nutritionist (RDN) is a college-trained health care professional who has extensive knowledge of foods, nutrition, and dietetics. Dietetics is the application of nutrition and food information to treat many health-related conditions. Registered dietitian nutritionists are certified and must maintain their certification regularly by meeting nationally established standards. The titles "registered dietitian" and "registered dietitian nutritionist" are legally protected, so people cannot refer to themselves as RDs or RDNs without having the proper certification. You can also locate registered dietitians by contacting your local dietetic association or visiting the Academy of Nutrition and Dietetics website (www.eatright.org) or the dietitians of Canada's website (www.dietitians.ca).

Clare Chapman, the graduate student featured in the unit opener, believed consuming coconut oil improved her health. At the present time, however, there's little scientific evidence to support claims that the oil is a "super food" with exceptional health benefits. Clare's impressions of the tropical oil might be the result of the placebo effect. On the other hand, Clare's body may be experiencing positive effects of using the oil that researchers haven't considered or measured. As more people consume coconut oil, scientists may conduct studies to determine whether the oil actually has any effects on health, including negative ones.

In a **Nutshell**

© McGraw-Hill Education. Mark A. Dierker, photographer

Module 2.1 Nutrition: Science for Consumers

- Scientists generally use the scientific method to answer questions about natural and physical observations.

- Nutrition research relies on scientific methods that generally involve making observations, asking questions, performing tests, collecting and analyzing data, drawing conclusions from data, and reporting on the findings. Other scientists can test the findings to confirm or reject them.

- Experimental studies using humans often involve double-blind studies and placebos. In studies that don't involve experiments, nutrition scientists may collect information about a specific population's health and food-related practices by conducting surveys.

- Scientists expect other researchers to avoid relying on their personal attitudes and biases when collecting and analyzing data, and to evaluate and report their results objectively and honestly.

- Scientists share results of their findings, usually in an article that describes the study and its findings. Before publishing the article, the editor of a scientific journal sends copies of it to peer reviewers. If peer reviewers accept the study's findings as being scientifically reliable, the journal's editor agrees to publish the article.

- Conflicting research findings often result because different teams of researchers use different study designs, populations, and ways of analyzing results. Other factors, such as individual genetic and lifestyle differences, can also influence the results of nutrition research involving human subjects.

© FoodCollection/StockFood RF

- Studies involving people and their food-related practices generally cannot establish cause and effect. When two different natural events occur simultaneously within a population, it doesn't necessarily mean they're related to each other. What appears to be a relationship between a dietary practice and a physical outcome could be a coincidence.

Module 2.2 Spreading Nutrition Misinformation

- Although testimonials and anecdotes are often used to promote nutrition-related products, you cannot be sure that this information is reliable or based on scientific facts. Personal observations are not evidence of cause-and-effect relationships because many factors, such as lifestyle and environment, can influence outcomes.

- Popular magazine articles, best-selling popular books, Internet websites, television news reports, and other forms of media are often unreliable sources of nutrition information.

- The First Amendment to the U.S. Constitution guarantees freedom of the press and freedom of speech. The FDA can regulate nutrition- and health-related claims on product labels, but the agency cannot prevent the spread of health and nutrition misinformation presented in the media.

© fstop/Punchstock RF

Module 2.3 Becoming a More Critical Consumer of Nutrition Information

- To become a more critical consumer of nutrition information, consider being more skeptical about the reliability of the nutrition information that's readily available from family, friends, and the media. To determine whether a source of information is reliable, ask questions to determine the source's reasons for promoting the information. You can also look for red flags that indicate misinformation, such as claims that sound too good to be true and scare tactics.

- Much of the nutrition information that's on the Internet is unreliable and intended to promote sales. Websites sponsored by nonprofit organizations, nationally recognized health associations, government agencies, and nationally accredited colleges and universities are generally reliable sources of information.

- The FTC enforces consumer protection laws and investigates complaints about false or misleading health claims that appear on the Internet.

Module 2.4 Seeking Reliable Nutrition Information

- Many states regulate and license nutritionists, but there's no standard legal definition for "nutritionist" in the United States.

- For reliable food, nutrition, and dietary information, consult persons with degrees in human nutrition from accredited institutions of higher learning, such as nutrition instructors, RDs, and RDNs. To locate registered dietitians, contact local dietetic associations or visit the Academy of Nutrition and Dietetics website.

Consider This...

1. A news broadcaster reports the results of a study in which people who took fish oil and vitamin E supplements daily didn't reduce their risk of heart attack. Moreover, the researchers stopped the study when they determined the supplements increased the subjects' risk of stroke! Explain how you would determine whether this information is reliable.

2. Recall someone, maybe a parent or friend, who recommended that you take a dietary supplement or eat an unusual food because it provided health benefits. Describe the recommendation and explain why you did or didn't follow the advice.

3. Search the Internet for a website that promotes and sells dietary supplements. Record the URL for the site. Use the information in Module 2.3 to judge the reliability of the nutrition information provided by the site.

4. Browse through popular magazines to find an article or advertisement that relates to nutrition, and make a copy of the article or advertisement. Analyze each sentence or line of the article or advertisement for signs of unreliability. Is the article or advertisement a reliable source of information? Explain why it is or why it isn't.

© Comstock/Jupiter Images/Getty Images RF

Test **Yourself**

Select the best answer.

1. The first step of the scientific method usually involves
   a. making observations.
   b. developing a question.
   c. identifying relationships between personal characteristics.
   d. gathering data.

2. The government agency that enforces consumer protection laws by investigating false or misleading health-related claims is the
   a. Federal Bureau of Investigation (FBI).
   b. Environmental Protection Agency (EPA).
   c. Federal Trade Commission (FTC).
   d. Centers for Disease Control and Prevention (CDC).

3. A testimonial is a(an)
   a. unbiased report about a product's value.
   b. scientifically valid claim.
   c. form of scientific evidence.
   d. personal endorsement of a product.

4. Which of the following websites is most likely to provide biased and unreliable nutrition information?
   a. A site that sells dietary supplements (*.com)
   b. The site of a nationally recognized, nonprofit health association (*.org)
   c. A U.S. government agency's site (*.gov)
   d. The site of an accredited college or university (*.edu)

5. A (An) _____ is a fake treatment that may be used in nutrition-related studies that have human subjects.
   a. anecdote
   b. placebo
   c. control
   d. double blind

© FoodCollection /Stockfood RF

6. The federal agency that can regulate nutrition claims on food labels is the
   a. FSIS.
   b. FTC.
   c. EPA.
   d. FDA.

7. You read an article about vegetables grown in the United States. According to the article's author, Americans need to take dietary supplements because the vegetables lack essential nutrients. This claim is an example of a(an)
   a. scare tactic.
   b. scientific fact.
   c. anecdote.
   d. evidence-based report.

8. A nutrition scientist designs a study in which he assigns 100 people to the treatment group and 100 people to the control group. Although the scientist knows each person's group assignment, the subjects are not aware of their group placement. This is an example of a(an)
   a. double-blind study.
   b. uncontrolled study.
   c. single-blind study.
   d. biased study.

A Answer This (Module 2.1b)

There is no relationship between drinking lemonade and drowning. This observation is a coincidence and not a case of cause and effect.

References ➡ See Appendix F.

STUDY TIP: Quickly create a customized practice quiz for this chapter by going to your Connect SmartBook "My Reports" section.

Don't have SmartBook and want to learn more? Go to **whysmartbook.com**.

Making More Nutritious Choices

What's on the Menu?

Module 3.1
Requirements and Recommendations

Module 3.2
Planning Nutritious Meals and Snacks

Module 3.3
Making Sense of Food Labels

Module 3.4
Should I Take Dietary Supplements?

Bulk spices for sale at an outdoor market in India

"My name is Abhinaya, but I usually go by "Abby" or "Abhi." I was born in Madras, India. My family moved to the United States when I was 13 years old. . . . American food is very bland. My American friends tell me that Indian food is very spicy, but I love foods seasoned with lots of chili powder and other Indian spices. Every summer, my family visits relatives in India. When we return, we bring back foods and spices that we can't find here.

Traditional Indian dishes really provide a balanced diet. They include cooked lentils, beans, greens, and lots of onion and garlic. I'm from southern India so I eat a lot of white rice topped with ghee, which has a buttery taste. . . . When I'm at home, I eat a wide variety of fruits and vegetables. My favorite fruits are mangoes, fresh pineapples, and bananas. . . . Strawberries aren't a traditional Indian fruit, but I love to eat them when they're in season here."

Abby Raghothaman

Abby Raghothaman is a sophomore majoring in Aerospace Engineering at Iowa State University. Her diet is different than the typical American college student's diet, so she faces many challenges when choosing menu items in her university's dining hall. Traditional Asian diets, such as Abby's, often contain small amounts of animal foods and larger amounts of locally grown fruits, vegetables, lentils, and unrefined grains. Registered dietitians generally recommend that Americans should increase their consumption of plant foods and reduce their intake of animal products, particularly red meats and processed meats, such as sausage, bacon, hot dogs, and "deli meats." Such changes might improve the health status of many Americans.

How can you plan nutritious meals and snacks that don't rely on red meats, processed meats, fried potatoes, canned applesauce, and iceberg lettuce? Unit 3 discusses dietary standards; practical ways for you to plan a nutritionally adequate, well-balanced diet; and how you can interpret and use nutrition-related information that appears on food and dietary supplement labels.

Module 3.1

Requirements and Recommendations

3.1 - Learning Outcomes

After reading Module 3.1, you should be able to

1. Define all of the key terms in this module.
2. Differentiate among the various dietary standards of the Dietary Reference Intakes.
3. Identify and apply the Acceptable Macronutrient Distribution Ranges for carbohydrate, protein, and fat intakes for adults.

By using research methods discussed in Unit 2, scientists have been able to estimate required amounts of many essential nutrients. A **requirement** can be defined as the smallest amount of a nutrient that maintains a defined level of nutritional health.[1] This amount, when consumed daily, prevents the development of the nutrient's deficiency disease. For example, the requirement for vitamin C (generally, 10 mg/day) prevents scurvy, the vitamin's deficiency disease.[2] The requirement (need) for a particular nutrient varies to some degree from person to person. Your age, sex, general health status, physical activity level, and life cycle stage (pregnancy, for example) are among factors that influence your nutrient requirements.

Your body stores many nutrients, including vitamin D and the minerals iron and calcium. Major storage sites are your liver, body fat, and/or bones. Other nutrients, however, such as vitamin C and most B vitamins, aren't stored by your body. For optimal nutrition, you need to consume enough of these nutrients each day to maintain adequate levels of them in your body.

Your body uses its nutrient stores much like you can use a savings account to help manage your money. When you have some extra cash, it's wise to place the money in a savings account, so you can withdraw some of the reserves to meet future needs without going into debt. When your intake of certain nutrients is more than enough to meet your needs, the body stores the excess. During a serious illness or recovery from such an illness, your body's needs for many nutrients are likely to be greater than normal. However, you may not feel like eating. When this situation happens, your body can withdraw some nutrients from storage. As a result of having optimal levels of stored nutrients, you may recover more quickly.

3.1a Introducing the DRIs

Dietary Reference Intakes (DRIs) encompass a variety of energy and nutrient intake standards that can be used to help people reduce their risk of nutrient deficiencies and excesses, prevent disease, and achieve optimal health (**Fig. 3.1**).[3] Registered dietitians refer to DRIs when planning nutritious diets for groups of people and evaluating

Age, sex, life cycle stage, general health status, and physical activity are among the several factors that influence your nutritional needs.

DIETARY REFERENCE INTAKES
(DRIs)

Estimated Average Requirement (EAR)

Recommended Dietary Allowance (RDA)

Estimated Energy Requirement (EER)

Tolerable Upper Intake Level (UL)

Adequate Intake (AI)

© Ryan McVay/Getty Images RF

Figure 3.1 Dietary Reference Intakes (DRIs).

the nutritional adequacy of a population's diet. However, you can use DRIs to evaluate the nutritional quality of your diet (see Appendix G).[4]

Estimated Average Requirement (EAR)

An **Estimated Average Requirement (EAR)** is the amount of the nutrient that meets the needs of 50% of healthy people who are in a particular life stage/sex group (**Fig. 3.2**). Life stage/sex groups classify people according to age, sex, and whether females are pregnant or breastfeeding. Because the EAR for a nutrient only meets the requirements of 50% of the population, you shouldn't use the standard to judge whether your daily intake is adequate. Scientists, however, use EARs for setting nutrient recommendations.

Estimated Energy Requirement (EER)

The **Estimated Energy Requirement (EER)** is the average daily energy (calorie) intake that meets the needs of a healthy person who

is maintaining his or her weight. The EER takes into account the person's physical activity level, height, and weight, as well as sex and life stage. Because the EER is an average figure, you may have energy needs that are higher or lower.

Recommended Dietary Allowance (RDA)

Simply consuming required amounts of nutrients doesn't always result in optimal nutritional status. Some people may naturally have higher requirements. What if your requirement for a particular nutrient is higher than average? If that's the case, your body is likely to develop the nutrient's deficiency disease, unless you consume more than the typical person's required amount.

The **Recommended Dietary Allowances (RDAs)** are standards for recommending daily intakes of several nutrients. RDAs meet the nutrient needs of nearly all healthy individuals (97 to 98%) in a particular life stage/sex group (see Figure 3.2).

To establish an RDA for a nutrient, nutrition scientists add a "margin of safety" amount to the EAR that allows for individual variations in nutrient

Figure 3.2 The EAR. This graph shows the distribution of nutrient intakes within a population. Note the positions of the EAR and RDA.

■ *What is an EAR?*

requirement smallest amount of a nutrient that maintains a defined level of nutritional health

Dietary Reference Intakes (DRIs) various energy and nutrient intake standards for Americans

Estimated Average Requirement (EAR) amount of a nutrient that meets the needs of 50% of healthy people in a life stage/sex group

Estimated Energy Requirement (EER) average daily energy intake that meets the needs of a healthy person maintaining his or her weight

Recommended Dietary Allowances (RDAs) standards for recommending daily intakes of several nutrients needs and helps maintain tissue stores. For example, the adult RDA for vitamin C (nonsmokers) is 15 mg higher than the EAR—75 mg for women who aren't pregnant or breastfeeding and 90 mg for men.[3]

Adequate Intakes (AIs)

A few nutrients don't have RDAs because there's not enough information about them to determine human needs. Scientists set **Adequate Intakes (AIs)** for these particular nutrients. To establish an AI, scientists record eating patterns of a group of healthy people and estimate the group's average daily intake of the nutrient. If the group of people under observation shows no evidence of the nutrient's deficiency disorder, the average level of intake must be adequate and that amount becomes the AI (**Fig. 3.3**).

It is important to understand the difference between a person's requirement ("need") for a nutrient and his or her RDA or AI for that nutrient. For most people, the requirement for a nutrient is less than the RDA or AI for the nutrient. Thus, your diet is likely to be nutritionally adequate if your average daily intake for each nutrient meets the nutrient's RDA or AI value.

Smoking increases the body's need for vitamin C.

Tolerable Upper Intake Level (UL)

Many vitamins and minerals have a **Tolerable Upper Intake Level (Upper Level, or UL)**. The UL is the highest average amount of a nutrient that's unlikely to harm most people when the amount is consumed daily (see Figure 3.3). The risk of a *toxicity disorder* increases when a person regularly consumes amounts of a nutrient that exceed its UL. The UL for vitamin C, for example, is 2000 mg/day for adults.

3.1b Acceptable Macronutrient Distribution Ranges (AMDRs)

Acceptable Macronutrient Distribution Ranges (AMDRs) indicate ranges of carbohydrate, fat, and protein intakes that are likely to provide adequate amounts of vitamins and minerals and may reduce the risk of diet-related chronic diseases. You can use the AMDRs to determine whether your diet has a healthful balance of macronutrients. **Table 3.1** lists adult AMDRs.

Adequate Intakes (AIs) dietary recommendations that assume a population's average daily nutrient intakes are adequate because no deficiency diseases are present

Tolerable Upper Intake Level (Upper Level or UL) standard representing the highest average amount of a nutrient that's unlikely to be harmful when consumed daily

Acceptable Macronutrient Distribution Ranges (AMDRs) macronutrient intake ranges that are nutritionally adequate and may reduce the risk of diet-related chronic diseases

Intake Level of Nutrient X

Low Intake		High Intake
RDA/AI		UL
High risk of deficiency	**Low risk of deficiency or toxicity**	**High risk of toxicity**

Figure 3.3 RDAs, AIs, and ULs.

■ *What is an UL?*

How can you use the AMDRs? You'll need to translate the percentages of AMDRs into grams of carbohydrate, protein, and fat. Let's say you generally consume 1800 kcal/day to maintain your weight. You want to meet AMDR guidelines for carbohydrate and protein by making 50% (0.50) of your total kcal from "carbs" and 25% (0.25) of your kcal from protein. Let's start with carbohydrates. Multiply 0.50 X 1800 kcal, which equals 900 kcal. To figure out how many grams of carbohydrates this represents, divide 900 g by 4 kcal (each gram of carbohydrate supplies 4 kcal). Thus, you can consume 225 g of carbohydrate daily. To make 25% of your calorie intake from protein, multiply 0.25 X 1800 kcal, which equals 450 kcal. Divide 450 kcal by 4 kcal (each gram of protein provides 4 kcal). Your daily intake of protein is 112.5 g. Now, you've accounted for all but 25% of your daily calories. To figure out how many grams of fat you can eat each day, multiply 0.25 X 1800 kcal, which equals 450 kcal. Each gram of fat supplies 9 kcal, so divide 450 kcal by 9 kcal to get 50 g of fat. Now, you've accounted for 100% of your daily energy intake.

Q Answer This

If your total calorie intake is 2400 kcal per day and fat provides 30% of your calories, how many grams of fat do you consume? You'll find the answer on the last page of this unit.

TABLE 3.1

ACCEPTABLE MACRONUTRIENT DISTRIBUTION RANGES: ADULTS

Macronutrient	AMDR (% of total energy intake)
Carbohydrate	45–65
Protein	10–35
Fat*	20–35

*Fat intake should include essential fatty acids (see Unit 6).

Module 3.2

Planning Nutritious Meals and Snacks

3.2 - Learning Outcomes

After reading Module 3.2, you should be able to

1. Define all of the key terms in this module.

2. List major food groups, identify foods that are typically classified in each group, and indicate nutritional equivalents of foods in each group.

3. Discuss recommendations of the *2015–2020 Dietary Guidelines for Americans* and describe features of a healthy dietary pattern (according to these guidelines).

4. Use MyPlate and other dietary tools to develop nutritionally adequate daily menus.

3.2a Introducing the Food Groups

The DRIs aren't practical for planning menus, so nutrition experts develop more consumer-friendly food (dietary) guides. In general, food guides classify foods into major groups according to their natural origins and key nutrients. Most commonly consumed dairy foods, for example, are made from cows' milk, which is a good source of calcium. Food guides usually recommend amounts of foods from each group that should be eaten daily. You can use such guides to plan what to eat each day as well as add variety and nutritional balance and adequacy to your diet.

The serving equivalents charts on the following pages of Section 3.2a show amounts of commonly eaten foods from each group that are considered nutritionally equal to each other. These food standards have been set by the U.S. Department of Agriculture (USDA).

Grains

Grains include products made from wheat, rice, and oats. Pasta, noodles, crackers, and flour tortillas are members of this group. Cornmeal and popcorn are usually grouped with grain products. Although corn is a type of grain, it's often used as a vegetable in meals.

Carbohydrate (starch) and protein are the primary macronutrients that are naturally in grains. Dietary guides generally recommend that you choose foods made with *whole grains*. **Whole grains** are the entire, ground, cracked, or flaked seeds of cereal grains, such as wheat, buckwheat, oats, corn, rice, wild rice, rye, and barley.[5] Whole-grain foods, such as whole-grain breads and whole-grain cereals, are good sources of micronutrients and fiber.

TASTY Tidbits

Compared to refined grain products, foods made with whole grains naturally contain more fiber. Be careful of products that have the claim "Made with 18 grams of whole grains" on the label. Such claims can be misleading because whole grains aren't nutrients. You need to be concerned about amounts of fiber and other nutrients in a serving of the product. For that information, read the nutrition information on the product's label.

18g Whole Grain Per Serving

100% Oats 8

A serving of this cereal has 18 g "whole grains," but how much fiber does it provide?

whole grains the entire, ground, cracked, or flaked seeds of cereal grains, such as wheat, buckwheat, oats, corn, rice, wild rice, rye, and barley

enrichment addition of iron, thiamin, riboflavin, niacin, and folic acid to cereal grain products

fortification addition of any nutrient to food

In the United States, *enriched* grain products can also be good sources of several vitamins and minerals. **Enrichment** is the addition of iron and the B vitamins thiamin, riboflavin, niacin, and folic acid to refined cereal grain products such as flour and rice. In general, enrichment replaces some, but not all, of the nutrients that were lost during refinement. **Fortification** is the addition of any nutrient to foods. Nutrient fortification may restore nutrients in foods that were lost during processing or provide specific health benefits. Examples of fortification include the addition of vitamins and minerals to ready-to-eat cereals and granola bars, calcium to orange juice, and vitamins A and D to milk.

One-ounce equivalents: Grains

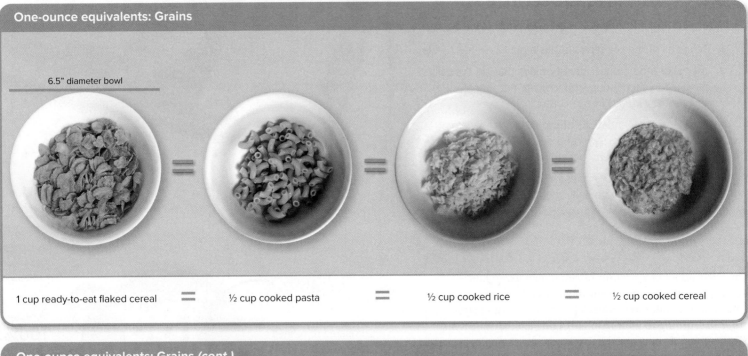

6.5" diameter bowl

| 1 cup ready-to-eat flaked cereal | = | ½ cup cooked pasta | = | ½ cup cooked rice | = | ½ cup cooked cereal |

One-ounce equivalents: Grains *(cont.)*

8.5" diameter plate

| 1 regular slice of bread | = | ½ hamburger bun | = | 5 crackers |

All images: © Wendy Schiff

One-cup equivalents: Dairy

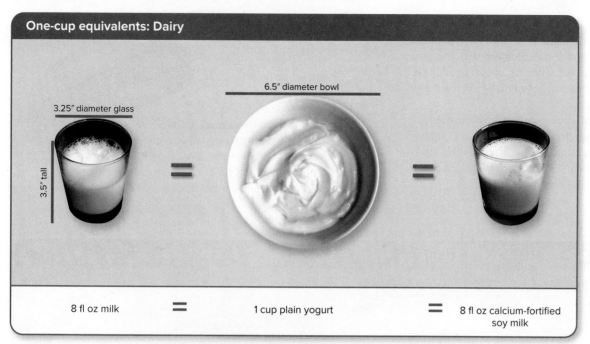

6.5″ diameter bowl

3.25″ diameter glass

3.5″ tall

| 8 fl oz milk | = | 1 cup plain yogurt | = | 8 fl oz calcium-fortified soy milk |

One-cup equivalents: Dairy (cont.)

8.5″ diameter plate

| 1.5 oz natural cheese | = | 2 oz processed cheese |

Dairy Foods

Dairy foods include milk and products made from milk that retain some or most of their calcium content after processing. In addition to calcium, many dairy foods are excellent sources of protein, phosphorus and potassium (minerals), and the vitamins A and D (if fortified), and riboflavin. Foods made from soy beans (for example, soy "milks") can substitute for cow's milk, if they are fortified with calcium and other micronutrients.

Ice cream, pudding, and frozen yogurt are often grouped with dairy foods, even though they often have high added-sugar and fat contents. Although cream cheese, cream, and butter are made from milk, they aren't included in this group because they have high amounts of fat and little or no calcium.

Dairy foods: © Wendy Schiff

TASTY Tidbits

Whole milk is about 3.25% fat by weight. Low-fat milk contains only 1% fat by weight and is often called "1% milk." Most dietary guides recommend choosing dairy products that have most of the fat removed, such as low-fat milk or *fat-free* (nonfat or skim milk), which has less than 0.5% fat.

Protein Foods

Protein-rich foods include beef, pork, lamb, fish, shellfish, liver, and poultry. Beans, eggs, nuts, tofu, and seeds are included with this group because these protein-rich foods can substitute for meats. In addition to protein, foods in this group are rich sources of many micronutrients, especially iron, zinc, and B vitamins.

In general, the body absorbs minerals, such as iron and zinc, more easily from animal foods than from plants. However, animal foods, especially red meats, often contain a lot of unhealthy kinds of fat. Diets that supply high amounts of unhealthy fat are associated with increased risk of heart and blood vessel diseases.

TASTY Tidbits

Some dietary guides use fat content to categorize meats and other protein-rich foods. According to these guides, the white meat of turkey is a *very lean* meat; ground beef that's not more than 15% fat by weight and tuna are *lean* meats. Pork sausage, bacon, and hot dogs are examples of *high-fat* meats.

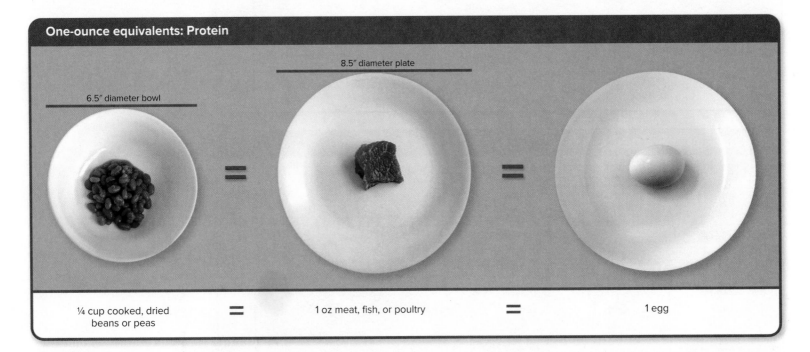

One-ounce equivalents: Protein

6.5″ diameter bowl   8.5″ diameter plate

¼ cup cooked, dried beans or peas   =   1 oz meat, fish, or poultry   =   1 egg

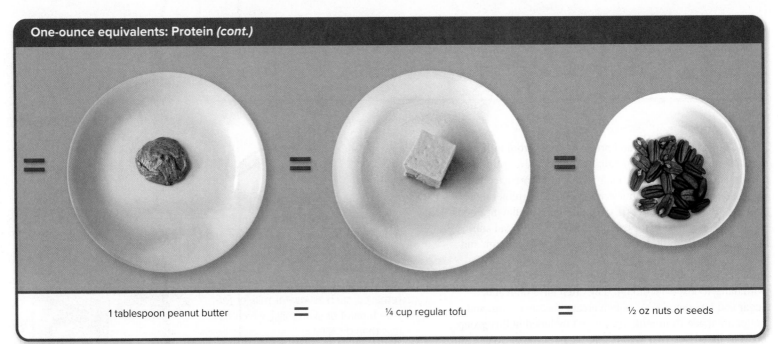

One-ounce equivalents: Protein *(cont.)*

1 tablespoon peanut butter   =   ¼ cup regular tofu   =   ½ oz nuts or seeds

Hot dog: © Comstock/Jupiter Images RF; Protein foods: © Wendy Schiff

Fruits

Fruits include fresh, dried, frozen, sauced, and canned fruit, as well as 100% fruit juice.[6] Although fruits aren't good sources of protein, most fruits are low in fat and good sources of phytochemicals and micronutrients, especially the mineral potassium and vitamins C and folate. Although 100% juice can count toward your fruit intake, the majority of your choices from this group should be whole or cut-up fruits.[7] Why? Whole or cut-up fruits are healthier options than juices because they contain more fiber.

About 4 mg vitamin C

About 46 mg vitamin C

TASTY Tidbits

The nutritional content of foods within each group often varies widely. For example, 3.5 ounces of fresh sliced apples and 3.5 ounces of fresh orange slices each supply about 50 kcal. However, the apples contribute about 4 mg of vitamin C, whereas oranges supply about 46 mg of the vitamin to diets. That's why you should eat a variety of foods from each food group.

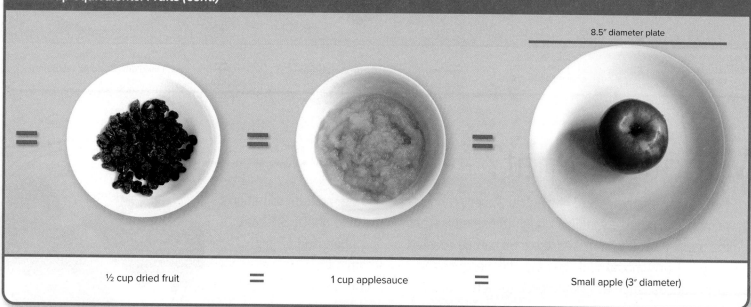

One-cup equivalents: Fruits

6.5″ diameter bowl

3.25″ diameter glass

3.5″ tall

1 cup
100% fruit juice
=
8 large strawberries

One-cup equivalents: Fruits (cont.)

8.5″ diameter plate

½ cup dried fruit
=
1 cup applesauce
=
Small apple (3″ diameter)

Vegetables

Vegetables include fresh, cooked, canned, frozen, and dried/dehydrated vegetables, and 100% vegetable juice. Vegetables can be further grouped into dark green, orange, and starchy categories. Some guides include dried beans and peas in the vegetable group as well as in the protein foods group. Many vegetables are good sources of micronutrients, fiber, and phytochemicals. Furthermore, most vegetables are naturally low in fat and energy.

Other Foods

Dietary guides may include an oils group and a group for sugary foods and alcoholic beverages. Oils include canola, corn, and olive oils, as well as other fats that are liquid at room temperature. Certain spreadable foods made from vegetable oils, such as mayonnaise, margarine, and salad dressing, are also classified as oils. Because nuts, olives, avocados, and some types of fish have high fat contents, a dietary guide may group these foods with oils.[8] Oils are often good sources of fat-soluble vitamins and may be sources of "healthy" fats that don't increase your risk of cardiovascular disease.

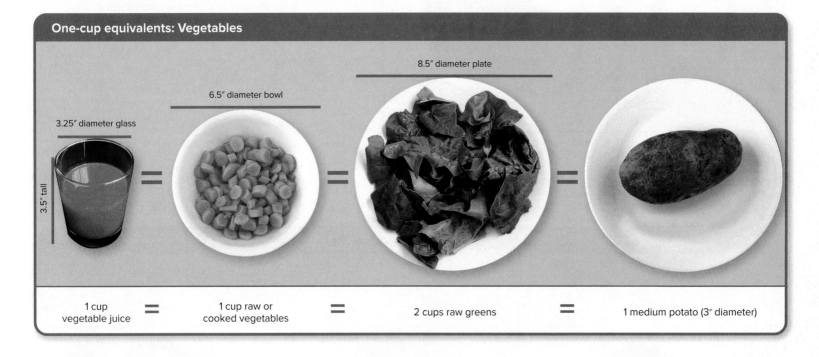

One-cup equivalents: Vegetables

8.5″ diameter plate

6.5″ diameter bowl

3.25″ diameter glass

3.5″ tall

| 1 cup vegetable juice | = | 1 cup raw or cooked vegetables | = | 2 cups raw greens | = | 1 medium potato (3″ diameter) |

What *IS* That? ------→

For centuries, the people of Central America have grown and eaten *tomatillos* ("husk-tomatoes"). After the papery husk is removed, the fruit can be roasted, chopped, and mixed with ground chili peppers to form sauces, such as *salsa verde* (green sauce).

Three medium tomatillos provide about 33 kcal, 2 g fiber, and 12 mg vitamin C.

Nutrition Fact or Fiction?

Organic foods are more nutritious than conventional foods.

The production of **organic foods** involves "environmentally friendly" (sustainable) farming methods that don't rely on the use of antibiotics, hormones, synthetic fertilizers and pesticides, genetic improvements, or ionizing radiation.[9] Results of scientific studies generally don't indicate that organic food crops are more nutritious than conventionally grown food crops.[10] However, eating organic food may reduce your exposure to pesticide residues and antibiotic-resistant bacteria.[10] To learn about organic farming methods and organic food standards, visit the USDA's website (www.usda.gov) and under "Topics," search for "Organic Agriculture."

Solid fats, such as beef fat, butter, lard (pork fat), and shortening, are fairly hard at room temperature. Solid fats contain unhealthy types of fats that may increase your risk of cardiovascular disease. Cream, cream cheese, and sour cream are liquid or soft at room temperature, but these foods are usually classified as solid fats. Unit 6 discusses how dietary fats can affect health.

Sugary foods ("sweets") include candy, regular soft drinks, jelly, and other foods that contain high amounts of sugar added during processing. Sugary foods and alcoholic beverages are sources of empty calories that supply few or no micronutrients in relation to their energy content.

3.2b How Do I Classify Combination Foods?

How do you classify menu items that combine small amounts of foods from more than one food group, such as pizza, sandwiches, and casseroles? The first step is to determine the ingredients and classify each into an appropriate food group. A slice of pizza, for example, has a crust made with wheat flour (grains), which is topped with tomato sauce (vegetable), and cheese (dairy). Estimate the number of cups or ounces of each ingredient and record the amounts contributed from a particular food group. The slice of pizza may provide ¼ cup of a vegetable, 2 ounces of grains, and ¼ cup of dairy. The familiar items in **Figure 3.4** can help you judge serving sizes without keeping handy a box of measuring cups and a scale for weighing foods.

Grain group

Vegetable group

Dairy group

© Wendy Schiff

organic foods foods produced without the use of antibiotics, hormones, synthetic fertilizers and pesticides, genetic improvements, or ionizing radiation

Figure 3.4 You can use familiar items such as these to estimate serving sizes.

Computer mouse = 1/2 to 2/3 cup (ground or chopped food)

Tennis ball = 1/2 to 2/3 cup (medium or small fruit)

4 dice = 1 oz cheese

3.2c Dietary Guidelines

About 75% of Americans have unhealthy diets. In general, Americans don't eat the recommended amounts of fruits, vegetables, dairy products, and healthy oils. On the other hand, we tend to eat a lot of foods that contain too much added sugars, saturated (unhealthy) fats, and sodium.[11] Such unhealthy food choices can lead to obesity and high blood pressure (hypertension), which are major public health problems among Americans.

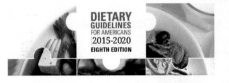

The U.S. Department of Health and Human Services (USDHHS) and the USDA publish the *Dietary Guidelines for Americans* (Dietary Guidelines), a set of general nutrition-related lifestyle recommendations that are intended for healthy people over 2 years of age.[11] The Dietary Guidelines are designed to promote adequate nutritional status and good health, and to reduce the risk of major nutrition-related, chronic health conditions, such as obesity, high blood pressure (hypertension), and cardiovascular disease. These guidelines are updated every 5 years.

The most recent version of the guidelines, the *2015–2020 Dietary Guidelines for Americans,* promotes a "healthy eating pattern" and has five overarching general guidelines:

1. Follow a healthy eating pattern across the life span;

2. Focus on variety, nutrient density, and amount;

3. Limit calories from added sugars and saturated fats, and reduce sodium intake;

4. Shift to healthier food and beverage choices; and

5. Support healthy eating patterns for all.

The features of a healthy eating pattern (diet) are listed in **Table 3.2**. The following section provides more specific advice from the Dietary Guidelines.

TABLE 3.2

HEALTHY EATING PATTERNS

According to the Dietary Guidelines, a healthy eating pattern provides

- A variety of vegetables;
- A variety of fruit, especially whole fruit;
- Grains, especially whole grains;
- Fat-free or low-fat dairy products;
- Various protein foods; and
- Oils.

According to the Dietary Guidelines, a healthy eating pattern limits

- Unhealthy fats, added sugars, and sodium.

Deli meats and dill pickles are high in sodium.

Baseball or human fist = 1 cup (large apple or orange, or 1 cup serving of ready-to-eat cereal)

Bar of soap or deck of cards = 3 oz meat

IVORY

Small yo-yo = 1 standard bagel or English muffin

Key Recommendations of the 2015–2020 Dietary Guidelines

- Increase the variety of protein foods you consume, and each week, incorporate about 8 ounces of various seafood into your meals. Avoid eating tile fish, shark, swordfish, and king mackerel because they may contain high amounts of the toxic substance methylmercury.

- Increase your intake of nutrient-dense vegetables.

- Eat more nutrient-dense fruits for snacks, desserts, or in side dishes.

- Choose enriched grain products and make at least half of your grains whole grains.

- Consume fat-free or lower-fat versions of milk, yogurt, and cheese.

- Consume less than 10% of daily calories from added sugars. Added sugars contribute calories to foods and beverages, but they lack essential nutrients. For people consuming 2000 kcal per day, the upper limit of 10% of total calories is 200 kcal, the amount of energy in about 12 teaspoons of sugar.

- Consume less than 10% of daily calories from saturated fats. Solid fats, fatty red meats, and whole-fat dairy products are generally rich sources of saturated fat.

- Consume less than 2300 mg of sodium per day. Eating too much sodium may increase your risk of high blood pressure (hypertension) and heart disease. Sodium is a mineral that's in table salt. Processed foods and fast foods (chips and French fries, for example) supply most of the salt in Americans' diets.

- Choose foods that provide potassium, dietary fiber, calcium, and vitamin D, which are "nutrients of public health concern" because Americans tend to consume them in limited amounts. Iron is an additional nutrient of public health concern for pregnant women.

- Achieve or maintain a healthy body weight. Increasing your physical activity level can help support this recommendation.

- Use vegetable oils when preparing foods. Consume as little trans fat and cholesterol as possible while following a healthy diet.

- If you consume alcohol, the beverage should be consumed in moderation and only if you are of legal drinking age. "Moderation" is up to one drink per day for women and up to two drinks per day for men. If you don't drink alcohol, you shouldn't start drinking for any reason. Furthermore, certain individuals, including pregnant women, should not consume any alcohol.

TASTY Tidbits

Many kinds of fruit make quick and easy snacks that can be carried in knapsacks, purses, and briefcases. Fresh fruit such as apples, oranges, tangerines, kiwifruit, and grapes can be kept for a few days at room temperature in a fruit bowl. You can store fresh fruits for longer periods by placing them in the refrigerator. Banana peels, however, turn dark brown when the fruit's refrigerated, but the fruit is still good to eat.

Applying the Dietary Guidelines

Table 3.3 provides some ways to incorporate the Dietary Guidelines into your diet.

TABLE 3.3

THE DIETARY GUIDELINES IN ACTION

If You Usually Eat:	Consider Replacing with:
White bread and rolls	Whole-wheat bread and rolls
Sugary ready-to-eat cereals	High-fiber cereal sweetened with fruit
Cheeseburger, French fries, and a regular soft drink	Roasted chicken or turkey sandwich, baked beans, and fat-free milk or soy milk
Potato salad or coleslaw	Leafy greens salad
Sweet rolls, doughnuts, and salty snacks	Small bran muffin or bagel topped with peanut butter and raisins
Regular soft drinks	Water, fat-free or low-fat milk, or 100% fruit juice
Fatty meats such as bacon, sausage, and hot dogs	Chicken, turkey, or fish; lean meats such as ground round
Chocolate chip or cream-filled cookies	Oatmeal cookies or fresh fruit

3.2d MyPlate

In 2011, the USDA introduced **MyPlate**. MyPlate is an interactive dietary and menu planning guide. MyPlate focuses on five different food groups: fruits, vegetables, protein foods, grains, and dairy (**Fig. 3.5**).[12] According to the USDA, "oils" isn't a food group, even though they provide some essential nutrients.[8] The government agency, however, notes the need for some fat in the diet.

To learn more about MyPlate's five food groups, visit the "ChooseMyPlate .gov" website (www.choosemyplate.gov/) and click on "MyPlate" in the menu bar to obtain a list of food groups. Then click on each food group for practical information about foods in the group, including dietary patterns (how much of the food should be eaten), scientifically supported health benefits of the food, and helpful food-related tips.

ChooseMyPlate.gov also includes a variety of food, nutrition, and physical activity resources for consumers. "SuperTracker" is handy for determining the energy and nutrient contents of your daily food choices (https://www.supertracker.usda.gov/). Within Supertracker, you can use "Food-A-Pedia" to obtain nutrition information for thousands of foods.

Using MyPlate

MyPlate has 12 different nutritionally adequate daily food patterns that supply from 1000 to 3200 kcal/day (http://www.choosemyplate.gov/MyPlate-Daily-Checklist). Each pattern can be individualized to meet your characteristics, including age, sex, physical activity level, and food likes and dislikes. The dietary patterns generally emphasize nutrient-dense foods and beverages that contain little or no empty calories.

After a person consumes recommended amounts of nutritious foods from each food group (and oils), a small number of calories remain. The 2000-kcal dietary pattern, for example, has only 260 calories remaining, which is less than the energy in two 12-ounce sugar-sweetened soft drinks. People can use up these remaining calories by choosing foods that contain a lot of solid fat and/or added sugars (empty calories) or healthy foods such as nuts and fresh fruits and vegetables.

MyPlate can be helpful for planning menus because it promotes food variety, nutritional adequacy, and moderation. You can also use MyPlate to evaluate the nutritional quality of your daily diet by recording your food and beverage choices, classifying your choices into food groups, and estimating your intake of servings from each food group. To use MyPlate as a personalized menu planning tool, visit http://www.choosemyplate.gov and click on SuperTracker and then "Create Your Profile." After you create the profile, MyPlate estimates your daily energy needs and indicates how much food you should eat from each of the food groups daily to meet your recommended energy level. **Table 3.4** shows suggested amounts of foods for average, 20-year-old adults.

Food Sources of Empty Calories

Many commonly eaten foods and beverages contain empty calories. Such foods and beverages include

- cakes, cookies, pastries, and donuts;
- sugar-sweetened soft drinks, sports drinks, and fruit drinks;
- candy
- cheese (source of solid fat);
- pizza (source of solid fat); and
- ice cream.[12]

© M. Unal Ozmen/ Shutterstock, Inc.

Figure 3.5 MyPlate is an interactive planning guide.

■ *Which MyPlate food groups are represented in a taco that contains black beans, shredded lettuce, salsa, and cheddar cheese?*

Source: ChooseMyPlate.gov

MyPlate USDA's interactive Internet dietary and menu planning guide

© Mitch Hrdlicka/Getty Images RF

Table 3.4	**MyPlate: Recommendations for Average, Healthy 20-Year-Old Young Adults**		
MyPlate Guidelines (Daily)		**Women**	**Men**
Kilocalories		1800–2400	2600–3200
Fruits		2 cups	2–2.5 cups
Vegetables		2.5–3 cups	3.5–4.0 cups
Grains		6–8 oz	9–10 oz
Protein		5.0–6.5 oz	6.5–7 oz
Dairy		3 cups	3 cups
Oils		5–7 tsp	8–11 tsp

Abby, the student featured in this unit's opener, follows a traditional Indian diet. Traditional Asian diets such as Abby's generally feature large amounts of vegetables, rice, or noodles combined with small amounts of meat, poultry, fish, or shellfish. Compare her primary food choices to the traditional Asian Diet Pyramid shown in Figure 3.7.

Other Dietary Guides and Assessment Tools

Before introducing MyPlate, the USDA promoted a food guide called the "MyPyramid Plan." The MyPyramid Plan inspired the development of other food pyramids for people who follow cultural and ethnic food traditions that differ from the mainstream American ("Western") diet. Examples of such guides include the Mediterranean Food Guide (**Fig. 3.6**) and the Asian Diet Pyramid (**Fig. 3.7**). Health Canada, the federal agency responsible for helping Canadians achieve better health, also has a dietary guide, "Eating Well with Canada's Food Guide" (see Appendix B).

In addition to www.choosemyplate.gov, the USDA sponsors other websites to help you assess your nutrient intakes. The "What's in the Food You Eat Search Tool" is one such site (www.ars.usda.gov /Services/docs.htm?docid=17032).

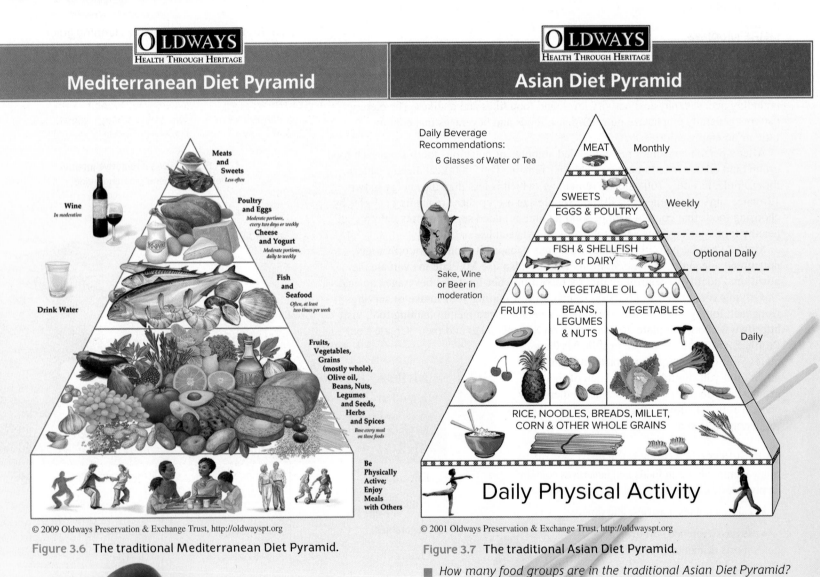

Figure 3.6 The traditional Mediterranean Diet Pyramid.

© 2009 Oldways Preservation & Exchange Trust, http://oldwayspt.org

© D. Hurst/Alamy RF

Figure 3.7 The traditional Asian Diet Pyramid.

© 2001 Oldways Preservation & Exchange Trust, http://oldwayspt.org

■ *How many food groups are in the traditional Asian Diet Pyramid?*

© Stockbyte/PunchStock RF

Module 3.3

Making Sense of Food Labels

© Fuse/Getty Images RF

3.3 - Learning Outcomes

After reading Module 3.3, you should be able to

1. Define all of the key terms in this module.
2. Use the Nutrition Facts panel to make more nutritious food choices.
3. Discuss the FDA's role in regulating food product labels.
4. Identify the types of nutrition-related claims that may be on food labels.

3.3a Nutrition Facts

Today, nearly all packaged foods and beverages must have labels that provide the product's name to identify the food. The label should also have the manufacturer's name and address, and the amount of product in the package (**Fig. 3.8a**). In addition to this information, the Food and Drug Administration (FDA) requires food manufacturers to use a special labeling format, the **Nutrition Facts panel,** to display information about the energy and nutrient contents of most packaged foods (**Fig 3.8b**).[13] You

Nutrition Facts panel information on food packaging that indicates nutrition information per serving of the food

Serving size is shown in household and metric units.

Identity of the food

Net content's weight (or volume)

Nutrition Facts

3 1/2 servings per container
Serving size 1/2 cup (126g)

Amount per serving
Calories 25

	% Daily Value*
Total Fat 0g	0%
Saturated Fat 0g	0%
Trans Fat 0g	
Cholesterol 0mg	0%
Sodium 50mg	2%
Total Carbohydrate 6g	2%
Dietary Fiber 2g	8%
Total Sugars 4g	
Includes 0g Added Sugars	0%
Protein 1g	
Vitamin D 0mcg	0%
Calcium 26mg	2%
Iron 0mg	0%
Potassium 400mg	8%

* The % Daily Value (DV) tells you how much a nutrient in a serving of food contributes to a daily diet. 2,000 calories a day is used for general nutrition advice.

NOT A SODIUM FREE FOOD
INGREDIENTS: TOMATOES, TOMATO JUICE, CALCIUM CHLORIDE, CITRIC ACID.

© WJS FOODS
DISTRIBUTED BY WJS FOODS
DUBUQUE, IA 52001 PACKED IN U.S.A.

Servings per container

Calories per serving

To reduce risk of heart disease, choose foods that are low in saturated fat, trans fat, cholesterol, and sodium.

Consider limiting your intake of foods with added sugars. Check for sugars included among the first few items in the ingredients list.

List of ingredients

Figure 3.8 Food labels are a source of nutrition and other useful information.

Consume adequate amounts of fiber and these micronutrients.

Manufacturer's name and address

Fresh and frozen fruits and vegetables; fresh poultry, fish, and shellfish; and some other food items must declare the product's *country of origin* either on the packaging or where the product is located in stores.

Daily Values (DVs) set of nutrient intake standards developed for labeling purposes

"What is my main source of nutrition information? Food labels. I use food labels to compare products. I need to eat enough food to feel full, so if a food has a low calorie count, then I feel like I can eat a little more of it."

—Amanda Croker, Kansas University

can use the information on food labels to determine ingredients and compare the energy and nutrient contents of similar packaged food products.

In 2016, the FDA introduced a new format for the Nutrition Facts panel (see Fig. 3.8b). Most food manufacturers must use the new format by August 2018. The top of the panel displays the serving size and total amount of energy, indicated as numbers of calories in a serving. The panel uses grams (g) and milligrams (mg) to indicate amounts of nutrients in a serving of food.

Products that have more than one ingredient must display a list of the ingredients in descending order according to weight. Note the list of ingredients displayed under the Nutrition Facts panel on the can of diced tomatoes shown in Figure 3.8. This particular product has tomatoes as the first ingredient. Thus, this food should contain higher amounts of tomatoes than of the remaining ingredients listed.

According to the new labeling format, the Nutrition Facts panel must provide information about the food's total fat, specific fats (saturated fat and trans fat), cholesterol, sodium, total carbohydrate, fiber, total sugars, added sugars, protein, vitamin D, potassium, calcium, and iron contents. Keep in mind, "total fat" includes amounts of saturated, monounsaturated, polyunsaturated, and trans fats. "Total carbohydrates" includes amounts of fiber and sugars. Food manufacturers can also indicate amounts of other nutrients in their products.

Be careful when using the Nutrition Facts panel; don't assume the information applies to the entire package. For example, the Nutrition Facts panel on a package of food indicates there are four servings in the container. If you eat all the container's contents, you must multiply the information concerning calories, fat, and other food components by four. Why? Because you ate four servings and the nutritional information on the Nutrition Facts panel applies to only *one* serving.

Understanding Daily Values (DV)

The RDAs and AIs are sex-, age-, and life stage-specific. Therefore, it's not practical to provide nutrient information on food labels that refers to these complex standards. To help consumers evaluate the nutritional content of food products, FDA developed the **Daily Values (DVs)** for labeling purposes. Compared to the RDAs/AIs, the DVs are a more simplified and practical set of nutrient standards. The adult DV for a nutrient is based on a diet that supplies 2000 kcal/day. Not all nutrients have DVs. For a list of DVs, see Appendix C.

Percentages of DVs are designed to help consumers compare nutrient contents of packaged foods to make more healthful choices. The general rule of thumb: A food that supplies 5%DV or less of a nutrient per serving is a *low source* of the nutrient; a food that provides 20%DV or more per serving is a *high source* of the nutrient.[13]

When evaluating or planning nutritious menus, your goal is to obtain at least 100% of the DVs for fiber, vitamins, and most minerals each day. High

Shopping for groceries can be fun at any age!

intakes of saturated fat, added sugars, and sodium may have negative effects on your health. Thus, you may need to consume *less* than 100% of the DV for these nutrients each day.

Claims on Food Labels

To make their foods more appealing to consumers, manufacturers often promote products as having certain health benefits or high amounts of nutrients. In the United States, the FDA regulates much of the information that is on food labels. The FDA permits food manufacturers to include certain *health, structure/function,* and *nutrient content claims* on labels (**Fig. 3.9**).

- A **health claim** describes the relationship between a food or food ingredient and the reduced risk of a nutrition-related condition.

- A **structure/function claim** describes the role a nutrient plays in maintaining a structure, such as bone, or promoting a normal function, such as digestion.

- A **nutrient content claim** describes levels of nutrients in packaged foods. Such claims can use terms such as "free," "high," or "low" to describe how much of a nutrient is in the product. Additionally, nutrient content claims can use terms such as "more" or

"reduced" to compare amounts of nutrients in a product to those in a similar product (*reference food*).

A *light* or lite food has

- at least one-third fewer kilocalories OR half the fat of the reference food.

A reduced-fat food contains

- less than 25% of the fat per serving than the reference food.

A low-fat food contains

- 3 g or less of fat per serving.

A low-calorie food contains

- 40 kcal or less per serving.

Lean meat or poultry provides

- less than 10 g of fat, 4.5 g of saturated fat, and 95 mg of cholesterol per serving.

The FDA regulates the use of terms such as "health" and "healthy" on food labels. In general, a serving of food that contains more than 13 g of fat, 4 g of saturated fat, 60 mg of cholesterol, or 480 mg of sodium can't have a health claim on the label.[14] As of October 2016, the FDA was reviewing its definition of a "healthy food."

In 2016, the FDA began the process of developing a standard definition for "natural food." In the past, the agency allowed manufacturers to include the term "natural" on the label if the food didn't contain food coloring agents, synthetic flavors, or other manufactured substances. For the latest information about claims that can be used for labeling purposes, visit FDA's website at www.fda.gov.

health claim statement that describes relationship between a food or food ingredient and reduced risk of a nutrition-related condition

structure/function claim statement that describes the role a nutrient plays in maintaining a structure of the body or promoting a normal body function

nutrient content claim statement that describes levels of nutrients in a packaged food

Figure 3.9 Note the claims on this food package.

■ *What kinds of claims are allowed on food labels?*

TASTY **Tidbits**

Often, the only difference between a creamy salad dressing, such as ranch or blue cheese, and the "light" version of the dressing is the amount of water they contain. Instead of paying more for calorie-reduced bottled salad dressings, make your own light salad dressing by adding about ¼ cup water to a jar of regular creamy salad dressing, then stir or shake the mixture.

Module 3.4

Should I Take Dietary Supplements?

3.4 - Learning Outcomes

After reading Module 3.4, you should be able to

1. Define all of the key terms in this module.
2. Identify popular dietary supplements and discuss the benefits and risks of taking such products.
3. Identify people who should take specific dietary supplements.

Do you think your food lacks vitamins and minerals? Do you take vitamin pills or herbal extracts because you want to improve your health? Many Americans take dietary supplements such as vitamin pills and herbal extracts because they think they are necessary or helpful. What are dietary supplements?

Recall from Unit 1 that a dietary supplement is a product (excluding tobacco) that's taken by mouth and supplements the diet by increasing total intake.

A dietary supplement can contain

- a vitamin,
- a mineral,
- an herb or other plant product, or
- an amino acid (component of proteins), enzyme, or other dietary ingredient.

The Dietary Supplement and Health Education Act (DSHEA) of 1994 allows manufacturers to classify dietary supplements as foods. As a result, manufacturers of dietary supplements don't need to test their products for safety and effectiveness. Some dietary supplements, such as vitamins and certain herbs, can have beneficial effects on health. In many instances, there's no scientific evidence that supports the usefulness as well as the safety of nonnutrient dietary supplements, including plant-based products.[15]

Supplement Facts
Serving Size 1 Tablet

Amount Per Serving		%Daily Value
Vitamin A (as Retinyl Acetate and 43% as Beta-Carotene)	3,500 IU	70%
Vitamin C (as Ascorbic Acid)	100 mg	167%
Vitamin D (as Cholecalciferol)	800 IU	200%
Vitamin E (as dl-Alpha Tocopheryl Acetate)	35 IU	117%
Vitamin K (as Phytonadione)	50 mcg	63%
Thiamin (Vitamin B-1) (as Thiamin Mononitrate)	1.1 mg	73%
Riboflavin (Vitamin B-2)	1.1 mg	65%
Niacin (as Niacinamide)	14 mg	70%
Vitamin B-6 (as Pyridoxine Hydrochloride)	5 mg	250%
Folic Acid	400 mcg	100%
Vitamin B-12 (as Cyanocobalamin)	50 mcg	833%
Biotin (as d-Biotin)	30 mcg	10%
Pantothenic Acid (as d-Calcium Pantothenate)	5 mg	50%
Calcium (as Calcium Carbonate and Dicalcium Phosphate)	500 mg	50%
Iron (as Ferrous Fumarate)	8 mg	44%

Ingredients: Cellulose (Plant Origin), Croscarmellose. Contains FD&C Blue #2 Lake, FD&C Red #40

This multivitamin-multimineral (MV/M) supplement is intended for older adults.

The FDA doesn't regulate the production of dietary supplements as strictly as it regulates the manufacturing of over-the-counter and prescription medications. As a result, you can't always be certain of the product's ingredients. Herbal products, for example, have been found to be missing the main ingredient that was listed on the label or contain ingredients that weren't listed on the label. In some instances, the extra ingredients were toxic (poisonous) or caused allergic reactions.

3.4a Popular Dietary Supplements

In the United States, the most commonly used dietary supplements are multivitamin/multimineral (MV/M) products that typically contain several vitamins and minerals.[16] Among American adults, the most popular dietary supplements that don't contain vitamins or minerals are

- fish oil or "omega 3,"
- glucosamine and/or chondroitin,
- probiotics and prebiotics, and,
- melatonin.[17]

When researchers asked a group of people why they used nonnutrient dietary supplements, the majority of the subjects (85%) reported they used the products to promote wellness; about 40% used the supplements to treat health conditions.[17]

Dietary Supplement Labels

Every dietary supplement container must be properly labeled (**Fig. 3.10**). The label must include the term "dietary supplement" or a similar term that describes the product's particular ingredient, such as "herbal supplement" or "vitamin C supplement."

Figure 3.10 Dietary supplement labels must provide information in a specific format.

Furthermore, the label must include facts about the product's contents in a special format—the "Supplement Facts" panel (see Fig. 3.10). The panel provides information about the serving size, amount per serving, and percent Daily Value (%DV) for ingredients, if one has been established. Although Daily Values (DVs) are standard desirable or maximum intakes for several nutrients, DVs have not been established for nonnutrient products, such as melatonin and cranberry fruit concentrate.

According to the FDA, dietary supplements aren't intended to treat, diagnose, cure, or alleviate the effects of diseases. Therefore, the agency doesn't permit manufacturers to market a dietary supplement product as a treatment or cure for a disease or to relieve signs or symptoms of a disease. Although such products generally cannot prevent diseases, some can improve health or reduce the risk of certain diseases or conditions. Therefore, the FDA allows supplement manufacturers to display structure/function claims on labels. Manufacturers of iron supplements, for example, may have a claim on the label that states: "Iron is necessary for healthy red blood cell formation." If the FDA has not reviewed a claim, the label must include the FDA's disclaimer indicating that the claim has not been evaluated by the agency (**Fig. 3.11**).

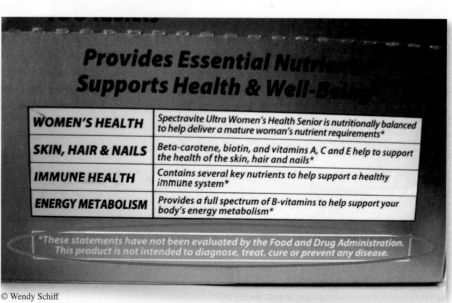

© Wendy Schiff

Figure 3.11 Disclaimers can be difficult to read on labels. This product has more than one claim.

■ *Why does the FDA require disclaimers on certain food and dietary supplement package labels?*

The FDA doesn't require dietary supplement manufacturers or sellers to provide evidence that labeling claims are accurate or truthful before they appear on product containers. However, the agency's officials may question the safety of a dietary supplement or the truthfulness of claims that appear on product labels. In such cases, the manufacturers are responsible for providing the FDA with evidence that their products are safe and the claims on labels are honest and not misleading.

Vitamin and Mineral Supplements: Safety

In their natural states, most commonly eaten foods don't contain toxic levels of nutrients. You probably don't need to worry about consuming toxic levels of micronutrients, unless you're taking *megadoses* of vitamin/mineral supplements. A **megadose** is generally defined as an amount of a vitamin or mineral that greatly exceeds the recommended amount. When taken in high amounts, many vitamins behave like drugs and can produce unpleasant and even toxic (poisonous) side effects.

Megadoses of

- B-vitamin niacin may cause painful facial flushing and liver damage;

- vitamin B6 can cause nausea, heartburn, and severe nerve damage;

- vitamin C can cause intestinal upset and diarrhea;

- vitamin A can cause birth defects and be deadly;

- vitamin D may cause intestinal upsets, weakness, confusion, disorientation, heart rhythm irregularities, and kidney damage;

megadose generally defined as an amount of a vitamin or mineral that greatly exceeds the recommended amount

Each of these vitamin C pills provides over 8 times the DV for the vitamin.

- iron may cause nausea, vomiting, constipation, diarrhea, dark-colored stools, and be deadly, especially for children;

- calcium may increase the risk of kidney stones; and

- selenium may cause gastrointestinal upsets, hair loss, fatigue, irritability, and mild nerve damage.

For most people, consuming amounts of nutrients that exceed what is necessary for good health is economically wasteful and could be harmful to the body. "More isn't always better," when it relates to optimal nutrition.

Pennyroyal

Herbal Supplements: Safety

Herbal supplements may be made from plants that have toxic parts. Comfrey, pennyroyal, sassafras, kava, lobelia, and ma huang are among the plants known to be highly toxic or cancer-causing. Products containing material from these plants should be avoided. Herbal teas may contain pollens and other parts of plants that can cause allergies, particularly in people who are sensitive to the herbs or their related species. *Echinacea* (purple cone flower) is related to ragweed, a plant that's often associated with seasonal respiratory allergies.[18] When people who are allergic to ragweed pollen take supplements that contain echinacea, they may develop allergic responses that mimic symptoms of the common cold (watery eyes, runny nose, and sneezing). In some instances, inflammatory responses, such as asthma attacks, can occur after exposure to echinacea or other plants. Asthma can be a life-threatening condition. Therefore, people who have asthma or allergies should be very careful when using plant-based supplements.

Consumers also need to be aware that medicinal herbs may contain substances that interact with prescription or over-the-counter medications as well as other herbs. Such responses can produce unwanted and even dangerous side effects (see **Table 3.5**). Ginkgo biloba, for example, can interact with aspirin, increasing the risk of bleeding. Garlic and vitamin E supplements can also increase bleeding. Kava and valerian act as sedatives (calming agents) and can amplify the effects of anesthetics used during surgery. Therefore, consult a physician or pharmacist before using any dietary supplement or giving such products to your children. Additionally, treat dietary supplements as drugs: Store them away from children and provide your physicians and other health care professionals with a list of the ones you're taking.

Echinacea flowers

3.4b Should You Take Dietary Supplements?

In 2015, sales of dietary supplements was estimated to be $37 billion in the United States.[19] In many instances, however, people don't need dietary supplements, and they are wasting their money by purchasing them—money that could be better spent on natural sources of nutrients and phytochemicals, particularly fruits, vegetables, and whole-grain cereals.

The human body is designed to obtain nutrients and phytochemicals from foods, not supplements. It's important to understand that nutrient supplements don't contain everything you need for optimal health. For example, they don't contain the wide variety of phytochemicals found in plant foods. Furthermore, supplements that contain phytochemicals may not provide the same healthful benefits as those obtained when you consume the plants that contain these substances. Why? Nutrients and phytochemicals may need to be consumed together to provide desirable effects in the body. Food naturally contains combinations of these chemicals in very small amounts and certain proportions. There's nothing "natural" about gulping down handfuls of supplements.

Some people take dietary supplements, particularly those containing nutrients, because the products are recommended by their physicians or registered dietitians. When compared to nonpregnant women, pregnant women require higher amounts of many nutrients. Thus, physicians usually recommend a special MV/M supplement for their pregnant patients. In rare cases, people are born with inherited conditions that increase their requirements for micronutrients. Older adults and people with chronic diseases may also need supplemental vitamins because their bodies don't absorb or use the nutrients normally.

Three generations of an Asian family: © Ronnie Kaufman/Blend Images LLC RF;
Ginkgo leaves: © Pixtal/AGE Fotostock RF

Most dietary supplements are available without the need for prescriptions, so people can take them without their doctors' knowledge and approval. In general, there appears to be little danger in taking a MV/M supplement that provides 100% of recommended amounts of micronutrients daily.[20] However, healthy adults should consider taking such supplements as an "insurance policy" and not a substitute for eating a variety of nutritious foods.

If you use or are thinking about using one or more dietary supplements:

- Discuss your need for the supplement with your physician or a dietitian before you purchase or use the product. This action is particularly important if you're pregnant, are breastfeeding a baby, or have a chronic medical condition such as diabetes or heart disease.

- Consult a physician as soon as you develop signs and symptoms of a serious illness. Using supplements to treat serious diseases instead of seeking conventional medical care that has proven effectiveness is a risky practice. In these instances, delaying or forgoing useful medical treatment may result in the worsening of the condition or even be life threatening.

- Be wary of claims made about a supplement's benefits and investigate the claims used to promote the product. Seek websites that provide reliable information about dietary supplements and aren't in the business of selling the products.

- Determine hazards associated with taking the supplement.

You can find information about the risks and benefits of various dietary supplements at the Office of Dietary Supplements' website: http://ods.od.nih.gov. "Herbs at a Glance," another government-sponsored website, provides information about popular plant-based dietary supplements; it can be accessed: https://nccih.nih.gov/health/herbsataglance.htm . If you experience negative side effects after using a particular dietary supplement, it's a good idea to be examined by a physician immediately. Furthermore, you, as well as your physician should report the problem to the FDA's MedWatch program by calling (800) FDA-1088 or visiting the agency's website.

Ginkgo leaves

Age influences nutrient needs.

TABLE 3.5

SOME POPULAR DIETARY SUPPLEMENTS

Dietary Supplement	Major Claims	Known Health Effects*	
		Benefits	Risks
Acidophilus (Lactobacillus)	Live bacterial culture (a probiotic) reduces risk of diarrhea and other intestinal problems	May improve health by restoring the balance of beneficial bacteria in the intestinal tract	Likely safe for most healthy people
Beta-carotene	Antioxidant Reduces risk of cancer and heart disease	Source of vitamin A Antioxidant	High doses may be unsafe. May increase risks of lung, colon, and prostate (men) cancers, especially for people who smoke and drink alcohol
Chondroitin sulfate	Relieves joint damage associated with arthritis	Some scientific evidence supports health benefit claims, but more research is needed. Often combined with glucosamine	When taken by mouth, may cause mild stomach discomfort, nausea, diarrhea, constipation, and other common physical complaints
Coenzyme Q-10	Increases exercise tolerance Prevents heart disease and cancer Reverses signs of aging and disease	Antioxidant made by the body and involved in energy metabolism; may improve immune system function Insufficient scientific evidence to support most claims	No serious side effects reported May interact with certain medications
Echinacea	Boosts immune system Prevents the common cold and reduces cold symptoms	Mixed scientific evidence to support common cold prevention claims, but research is ongoing	Generally safe but may provoke allergic response or intestinal upset
Evening primrose oil	Treats eczema (a common skin condition) Relieves arthritis and postmenopausal symptoms	Insufficient scientific evidence to support claims	May cause mild intestinal upset Safety of long-term use has not been determined.
Fish oil	Prevents heart disease and stroke Cures rheumatoid arthritis Reduces depression and risk of Alzheimer's disease	Source of omega-3 fatty acids May reduce symptoms of depression when used with antidepressant medications May provide some mild relief for symptoms of rheumatoid arthritis Lack of evidence that fish oil is beneficial for other health conditions	May interfere with blood clotting, increasing the risk of hemorrhagic stroke Cod liver oil contains vitamin A, which is toxic when taken in large doses
Flaxseed and flaxseed oil	Acts as a laxative (flaxseed) Reduces blood cholesterol levels	Nonanimal source of omega-3 fatty acids Seeds have laxative effects. May benefit people with heart disease, but more research is needed	Generally safe
Garlic	Lowers blood cholesterol levels	Doesn't lower cholesterol consistently May reduce elevated blood pressure	Can cause allergic reaction and unpleasant body odor; may increase risk of bleeding
Ginger	Treats "morning sickness" and other forms of nausea Relieves stomach upsets	Can safely treat morning sickness and may reduce other forms of nausea Lack of scientific evidence to support other health benefit claims	Mild nausea, but small amounts don't seem to cause serious side effects

Chondroitin sulfate: © McGraw-Hill Education. Jill Braaten, photographer; Echinacea in flower form: © Brand X Pictures/PunchStock RF; Primrose: © Carol Wolfe RF; Flaxseed flower: © Pixtal/SuperStock Garlic bulb: © Photodisc/Getty Images RF; Ginger: © Stockbyte/Getty Images RF

Dietary Supplement	Major Claims	Benefits	Risks
		Known Health Effects*	
Ginkgo biloba	Improves memory Reduces the risk of Alzheimer's disease and other forms of dementia	Lack of scientific evidence to support health benefit claims	May increase the risk of bleeding and cause allergic reactions, headaches, intestinal upsets, and nausea Gingko seeds are toxic.
Ginseng (Asian)	Boosts overall health Treats erectile dysfunction (male impotence) and hepatitis C	May lower elevated blood glucose levels and benefit immune system Studies are currently being conducted to determine whether the herb has other health benefits.	May cause headaches, sleep disturbances, allergic responses, and gastrointestinal upsets People with diabetes may experience low blood glucose levels, which can be dangerous.
Glucosamine hydrochloride	Relieves joint damage associated with arthritis	Some scientific evidence supports health benefit claims, but more research is needed (frequently used with chondroitin).	None identified
Green tea	Prevents or treats cancer Promotes weight loss Reduces blood cholesterol levels	Results of some laboratory studies indicate green tea protects against certain forms of cancer or reduces cancer cell growth, but results of human studies show mixed results. Lack of reliable evidence to support other health benefit claims	Green tea extracts may damage the liver. Caffeine content may cause sleep disturbances, irritability, and digestive upset.
Kava	Reduces stress	Potential harm of using kava outweighs any benefit.	Toxic—can damage the liver and cause death May cause abnormal muscle movements, yellowed skin, and sleepiness
Lavender	Reduces anxiety, treats sleep disorders	Lack of scientific evidence that supports health benefit claims	Generally considered to be safe for adults when used for aromatherapy; may be poisonous if consumed
Melatonin	Treats some sleep disorders Prevents jet lag	May be effective for treating certain sleep disorders and preventing jet lag	Questions about long-term safety
Red yeast rice	Lowers blood cholesterol, reducing risk of heart disease	May be useful, especially for people who cannot take prescription medications to lower blood cholesterol	May cause muscle pain and weakness, the breakdown of muscle tissue, and liver damage
St. John's wort	Reduces depression	Evidence to support claims is inconsistent.	May interact with other herbal products and certain medications, including prescription antidepressants and oral contraceptives
Valerian	Promotes relaxation Treats sleep disorders	Evidence to support claims is inconsistent.	Dizziness, headache, stomach upset Questions about long-term safety

**Sources:* http://ods.nih.gov; http://www.cancer.gov/about-cancer/treatment/cam/patient/coenzyme-q10-pdq ; https://www.nlm.nih.gov/medlineplus/news/fullstory_158505.html ; https://nccih.nih.gov/health/herbsataglance.htm Accessed: May 5, 2016.

In a **Nutshell**

© McGraw-Hill Education. Mark A. Dierker, photographer

Module 3.1 Requirements and Recommendations

- A requirement is the smallest amount of a nutrient that maintains a defined level of nutritional health. Numerous factors influence your nutrient requirements, including age and state of health. Scientists use information about nutrient requirements and the body's storage capabilities to establish specific dietary recommendations.

- Dietary Reference Intakes (DRIs) encompass a variety of energy and nutrient intake standards that can be used to help people reduce their risk of nutrient deficiencies and excesses, prevent disease, and achieve optimal health. An Estimated Average Requirement (EAR) is the amount of the nutrient that meets the needs of 50% of healthy people in a particular life stage/sex group. The Estimated Energy Requirement (EER) is used to evaluate a person's energy intake. The Recommended Dietary Allowances (RDAs) meet the needs of nearly all healthy individuals (97 to 98%) in a particular life stage/sex group. The RDA or AI for a nutrient is not the same as the requirement for that nutrient.

- When nutrition scientists are unable to determine an RDA for a nutrient, they establish an Adequate Intake (AI) value. The Tolerable Upper Intake Level (UL) is the highest average amount of a nutrient that's unlikely to harm most people when the amount is consumed daily.

- Acceptable Macronutrient Distribution Ranges (AMDRs) indicate ranges of carbohydrate, fat, and protein intakes that provide adequate amounts of vitamins and minerals and may reduce the risk of diet-related chronic diseases.

Module 3.2 Planning Nutritious Meals and Snacks

- Dietary guides generally classify foods into groups according to their natural origins and key nutrients. Such guides usually feature major food groups, including grains, dairy foods, and vegetables. Some dietary guides also include a group for oils.

- The Dietary Guidelines are a set of general nutrition-related lifestyle recommendations designed to promote adequate nutritional status and good health, and to reduce the risk of major chronic health conditions. These guidelines are updated every 5 years.

- The Dietary Guidelines for Americans (2015–2020 version) has five overarching concepts. These concepts are: Follow a healthy eating pattern across the life span; focus on variety, nutrient density, and amount; limit calories from added sugars and saturated fats, and reduce sodium intake; shift to healthier food and beverage choices; and support healthy eating patterns for all.

- Choosemyplate.gov is an online, interactive source of food, nutrition, and physical activity information. The MyPlate website can be helpful for planning menus because it promotes food variety, nutritional adequacy, and moderation.

Module 3.3 Making Sense of Food Labels

- Consumers can use information on food labels to determine ingredients and compare nutrient contents of packaged foods and beverages.

- Nearly all foods and beverages sold in supermarkets must be labeled with the product's name, manufacturer's name and address, amount of product in the package, ingredients listed in descending order by weight, and country of origin. Food labels must use a special format for listing specific information on the Nutrition Facts panel.

- The Daily Values (DVs) are a practical set of nutrient standards for labeling purposes. The nutrient content in a serving of food is listed on the label as a percentage of the DV (%DV). Not all nutrients have DVs. A dietary goal is to obtain at least 100% of the DVs for fiber, vitamins, and minerals (except sodium) each day.

- The FDA regulates much of the information that can be placed on food labels. The FDA permits food manufacturers to include certain health, structure/function, and nutrient content claims on food labels.

Nutrition Facts

28 servings per container

Serving size   3 flatbreads (28g)

Amount Per Serving

Calories   110

	% Daily Values*
Total Fat 3g	5%
Saturated Fat 1g	5%
Trans Fat 0g	
Cholesterol 0mg	0%
Sodium 170mg	7%
Total Carbohydrate 19g	6%
Dietary Fiber 1g	4%
Total Sugars 1g	
Includes 0g Added Sugars	0%
Protein 3g	6%
Vitamin D 0IU	0%
Calcium 0mg	0%
Iron 1.44mg	8%
Potassium 0mg	0%

* The % Daily Value (DV) tells you how much a nutrient in a serving of food contributes to a daily diet. 2,000 calories a day is used for general nutrition advice.

INGREDIENTS:
SPROUTED WHEAT FLOUR, VEGETABLE OIL

© Wendy Schiff

Module 3.4 Should I Take Dietary Supplements?

- According to the DSHEA, a dietary supplement is a product (excluding tobacco) that is taken by mouth and contains a vitamin, a mineral, an herb or other plant product, an amino acid, or a dietary ingredient that supplements the diet by increasing total intake.

- The FDA regulates the labeling of dietary supplements. According to the FDA, dietary supplements aren't intended to treat, diagnose, cure, or alleviate the effects of diseases. Therefore, the agency doesn't permit manufacturers to market a dietary supplement product as a treatment or cure for a disease, or to relieve signs or symptoms of a disease.

- According to scientific evidence, some dietary supplements can have beneficial effects on health. However, results of scientific testing also indicate that many popular dietary supplements aren't helpful and may even be harmful.

What's in **Your Diet?!**

I. Record Keeping
  A. 24-Hour Dietary Recall
  1. Recall every food and beverage that you have eaten over the past 24 hours. Recall how much you consumed and how it was prepared.
     a. How easy or difficult was it to recall your food intake?
     b. Recall your intake of nutrient supplements such as vitamin C.
  B. Three-Day Diet Record
  1. Without changing your usual diet, keep a detailed log of your food and beverage intake for 3 days; one of the days should be Friday or Saturday. Use a separate log for each day. Remember to include your daily intake of nutrient supplements in your record.

II. Analysis
  Using nutritional analysis software, analyze your daily food and nutrient supplements intakes and answer questions in Part III of this activity. Keep the record on file for future applications.

  A. Computer-Generated Dietary Analysis, such as Nutrition CalcPlus
  1. Load the software into the computer, or log on to the software website.
  2. Choose the DRIs or related nutrient standard from Appendix G, based on your life stage, sex, height, and weight.
  3. Enter the information from the 3-day food intake record. Be sure to enter each food and drink and the specific amounts. Enter your intake of nutrient supplements.
  4. The software program will give you the following results:
     a. The appropriate RDA (or related standard) for each nutrient
     b. The total amount of each nutrient and the kilocalories consumed for each day
     c. The percentage intake compared with the standard amount for each nutrient that you consumed each day
  5. Keep this assessment for activities in other units.

III. Evaluation of Nutrient Intakes
  Remember, it is not necessary to consume the maximum of your nutrient recommendations every day. A general standard is meeting at least 70% of the standards averaged over several days. It is best not to exceed the Upper Level (if set) over the long term to avoid potential toxic effects of some nutrients.

  A. For which nutrients did your average intake fall below the recommended amounts—that is, to less than 70% of the RDA/AI?
  B. For which nutrients did your average intake exceed the Upper Level (if a UL has been set)?

IV. MyPlate
  This activity determines how your diet stacks up when compared to the amounts of foods from each food group that are recommended in the USDA's www.choosemyplate.gov.

  A. Refer to your 3-day food intake record. Classify each food item in the appropriate food group of *MyPlate*. For each food group, indicate whether you ate the recommended amount daily for your sex, age, height, weight, and physical activity level. Note that some of your food choices—pizza, for example—may contribute to more than one food group. Enter a minus sign (−) if your total falls below the MyPlate recommendation or a plus sign (+) if it equals or exceeds the daily recommendation for each food group.

Consider This...

1. Your friend takes several dietary supplements daily and, as a result, his vitamin B-6 intake is 50 times higher than the RDA for the vitamin. You would like to convince him to stop taking the supplements. To support your advice, which nutrient standards would you show him? Explain why.

2. Why should you use MyPlate to plan menus instead of the DRIs?

3. How do your sodium, saturated fat, and added sugar intakes compare to the recommendations of the latest Dietary Guidelines?

4. How can you determine whether the wheat crackers that are made by a company in England have animal or vegetable fat in them?

© Royalty-Free/Corbis RF

5. Visit the USDA's website to access "What's in the Foods You Eat *Search Tool,*" a database for searching the nutritional content of foods. To practice using this search tool, find the number of kilocalories and the amounts of fiber, potassium, iron, sodium, and calcium in 1 cup of raw jicama, 1 cup of 2% milk with added vitamin A, and ¼ cup of dry roasted, salt-added sunflower seed kernels (no hulls).

Test Yourself

Select the best answer.

1. The amount of a nutrient that should meet the needs of half of the healthy people in a particular group is the

   a. Estimated Average Requirement (EAR).

   b. Recommended Dietary Allowance (RDA).

   c. Adequate Intake (AI).

   d. Tolerable Upper Intake Level (UL).

2. Which of the following statements is false?

   a. RDAs are standards for daily intakes of certain nutrients.

   b. RDAs meet the nutrient needs of nearly all healthy people.

   c. RDAs contain a margin of safety.

   d. RDAs are requirements for nutrients.

3. The Estimated Energy Requirement (EER)

   a. has a margin of safety.

   b. doesn't account for a person's height, weight, or physical activity level.

   c. is based on the average daily energy needs of a healthy person.

   d. reflects a person's actual daily energy needs.

4. A diet is likely to be unsafe if

   a. average daily intakes for nutrients meet RDA or AI values.

   b. intakes of various nutrients are slightly less than EAR amounts.

   c. nutrient intakes are consistently above ULs.

   d. MV/M supplements aren't included.

5. According to MyPlate, which of the following foods is grouped with dairy products?

   a. Eggs

   b. Yogurt

   c. Butter

   d. Sour cream

© FoodCollection/Stockfood RF

6. Protein-rich food sources that also contain saturated fat and cholesterol include

   a. peanut butter.

   b. dry beans.

   c. nuts.

   d. beef.

7. In general, whole fruits are a good source of all of the following substances, except

   a. fiber.

   b. vitamin C.

   c. phytochemicals.

   d. protein.

8. The new Nutrition Facts panel on a package of food must display amounts of vitamin ___ in a serving of the food.

   a. D

   b. C

   c. A

   d. E

© D. Hurst/Alamy RF

9. Which of the following statements is true?

   a. According to MyPlate, vegetable oils are grouped into the "Fats and Oils" food group.

   b. The MyPlate menu planning guide cannot be individualized to meet a person's food preferences.

   c. A person can use www.choosemyplate.gov to evaluate his or her diet's nutritional adequacy.

   d. MyPlate was the first food guide developed for Americans.

10. Which of the following information isn't provided by the Nutrition Facts panel?

    a. Percentage of calories from fat

    b. Amount of carbohydrate per serving

    c. Serving size

    d. Amount of protein per serving

11. Daily Values are

    a. for people who consume 1200 to 1500 kilocalorie diets.

    b. based on the lowest RDA or AI for each nutrient.

    c. dietary standards developed for food-labeling purposes.

    d. used to evaluate the nutritional adequacy of a population's diet.

12. When consumed, which of the following dietary supplements isn't likely to cause serious side effects?

    a. Pennyroyal

    b. Flaxseed oil

    c. Lobelia

    d. Ma huang

© A. Huber/U. Starke/Corbis RF

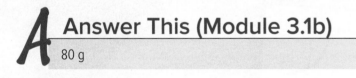

A Answer This (Module 3.1b)

80 g

References ➡ See Appendix F.

Connect

STUDY TIP: Quickly create a customized practice quiz for this chapter by going to your Connect SmartBook "My Reports" section.

Don't have SmartBook and want to learn more? Go to **whysmartbook.com**.

© Royalty-Free/Corbis RF

How Food Becomes You

What's on the Menu?

Module 4.1
From Cells to Systems

Module 4.2
Digestive System

Module 4.3
Common Digestive System Disorders

Module 4.4
Metabolism Basics

© Wendy Schiff

"I considered myself a pretty healthy person throughout high school and the first year of college. But during my sophomore year, I experienced lower abdominal pain and some intestinal bleeding. . . . I went to the university's hospital to have the problem checked out. It turned out that I had ulcerative colitis. I had no idea what this meant, but the doctor explained that my large intestine was inflamed and swollen—the disease is long-term, with little likelihood of a cure.

My doctor thinks diet has nothing to do with ulcerative colitis, but I have noticed that if I eat red meat, citrus fruits, and dairy foods, especially ice cream, some slight abdominal discomfort returns. Carbonated drinks seem to bother me a lot. I used to drink one or two cans of regular soft drinks a day. Now I've all but eliminated them from my diet, because I get abdominal cramps about 30 minutes after drinking them. Beer bothers me, too. But I have not eliminated beer from my diet."

Matthew Lang

Matthew Lang is a graduate student majoring in Accounting at the University of Missouri-Columbia. His chronic health problem, ulcerative colitis, usually develops in young people between the ages of 15 and 30.[1] If your intestinal tract ("gut") functions normally, you probably eat whatever you want. How would you react if you developed ulcerative colitis or another chronic intestinal disease? Would you follow your doctor's recommendations and, if necessary, avoid troublesome foods? Or would you continue your usual lifestyle, including diet?

Unit 4 focuses primarily on the digestive system, including how your body obtains and delivers nutrients to where it needs them. Module 4.3 provides general information about ulcerative colitis and some common intestinal problems, including constipation and heartburn.

Module 4.1

From Cells to Systems

4.1a The Organization of Your Body

By learning about your body, you may appreciate its complexity and be amazed at the variety of metabolic activities that keep you alive, physically active, mentally alert, and healthy. As mentioned in Unit 1, a cell is the smallest living functional unit in your body. Your body has about 100 *trillion* cells that can be classified into numerous cell types. Each type of cell has a specific function. For example, muscle cells are necessary for movement; nerve cells send messages; red blood cells transport oxygen; and certain white blood cells protect your body from disease-causing bacteria and viruses. Each human cell has a membrane that surrounds it and controls the passage of nutrients and other substances into and out of the cell.

Blood cells

Nerve cells

Smooth muscle cells

Essential Concept

4.1 Your Body's Organization

tissues masses of cells that have similar characteristics and functions

organ collection of tissues that function in a related fashion

organ system group of organs that work together for a similar purpose

1 Cell
For example, muscle cells are necessary for movement and nerves send messages.

2 Tissue
Cells that have similar characteristics and functions are usually joined together into larger masses called **tissues.**

3 Organ
An **organ** is composed of various tissues that function in a related fashion. The stomach, for example, is an organ because it contains different kinds of tissue that work together to churn food and break down the food's components.

4 Organ system
An **organ system** is a group of organs that work together for a similar purpose. The digestive system, for example, includes several organs, including the stomach and intestines.

5 Organism
A healthy person is composed of organ systems that function together properly.

4.1b Your Body's Organ Systems

The organ systems are dependent on each other. If your liver, for example, isn't functioning properly, the rest of your body won't be able to function properly. By following a nutritionally adequate diet, you may be able to achieve better health. **Table 4.1** lists each system's major organs or tissues and summarizes their primary functions.

TABLE 4.1

THE ORGAN SYSTEMS OF YOUR BODY

System	Major Organs or Tissues	Primary Functions
Digestive	Mouth, salivary glands, esophagus, stomach, intestines, pancreas, liver, gallbladder	Digestion and absorption of nutrients
Cardiovascular	Heart, blood vessels, blood	Circulation of blood throughout the body
Respiratory	Nose, pharynx, larynx, trachea, bronchi, lungs	Exchange of oxygen and carbon dioxide
Lymphatic and Immune	Lymphatic fluid, white blood cells, lymph vessels and nodes, spleen, thymus	Defense and immunity against infectious agents, fluid balance, white blood cell production, and absorption of fat-soluble nutrients from intestinal tract
Urinary	Kidneys, bladder	Elimination of salts, water, and wastes; and maintenance of fluid balance
Muscular	Muscles	Movement and stability of the body
Skeletal	Bones, tendons, ligaments	Support, movement, protection, and production of blood cells
Nervous	Brain, spinal cord, nerves, sensory receptors	Thought processes, regulation and coordination of many body activities, and detection of changes in external and internal environments
Endocrine	Glands or organs that secrete hormones (chemical messengers)	Regulation and coordination of many body activities, including growth, nutrient balance, and reproduction
Integumentary	Skin, hair, nails	Protection and immunity, regulation of body temperature, and vitamin D synthesis
Reproductive	Gonads and genitals	Procreation (creating children)

Adapted from: Widmaier EP, and others: *Vander's human physiology*, 12th ed. Boston: McGraw-Hill Publishing Company, 2011.

Module 4.2
Digestive System

4.2 - Learning Outcomes

After reading Module 4.2, you should be able to

1. Define all of the key terms in this module.

2. Explain the difference between mechanical and chemical digestion and provide an example of each.

3. Identify organs and structures of the digestive system and describe their primary functions.

4. Discuss the overall process of digestion and absorption.

4.2a Overview of Digestion

Grizzly bears are omnivores. In addition to salmon, they eat other animals, but fruit, nuts, leaves, and roots form the foundation of their diet. You're an **omnivore,** an organism that can digest and absorb nutrients from plants; animals; fungi, which include mushrooms; and even bacteria. The human digestive system is designed to receive food from all of these sources, process it into nutrients, transport the nutrients into the bloodstream, and eliminate the waste products. Your body doesn't need food—your cells need the nutrients that are in food to carry out their work.

Digestion is the process of breaking down large food components into smaller substances (**molecules**), including individual nutrients. This process involves mechanical and chemical digestion.

- **Mechanical digestion** involves the physical breakdown of foods, including the biting action of teeth and mixing movements of the stomach.

- **Chemical digestion** refers to the chemical breakdown of foods by substances secreted into the **digestive tract,** which is sometimes called the "GI" (gastrointestinal) tract.

Absorption is the process by which nutrients and other substances are taken up by the digestive tract and enter the bloodstream or lymphatic system (see Table 4.1). This module focuses on the functions of your digestive system.

omnivore organism that can digest and absorb nutrients from plants, animals, fungi, and bacteria

digestion process by which large food components are mechanically and chemically broken down

molecules basic chemical units that make up substances

mechanical digestion physical breakdown of foods

chemical digestion chemical breakdown of foods by substances secreted into the digestive tract

digestive tract muscular tube that extends from the mouth to the anus

absorption process by which substances are taken up from the digestive tract and enter the bloodstream or the lymph

An omnivore's food includes plants, animals, fungi, and bacteria , such as certain live bacteria in the yogurt.

accessory organs organs of the digestive system that assist digestive tract function

4.2b Your Digestive Tract

The mouth, esophagus, stomach, and small and large intestines are the major organs of the digestive tract and components of the digestive system **(Fig. 4.1a).** The digestive tract forms a continuous muscular tube that begins at the mouth and ends with the anus.

The teeth, tongue, salivary glands, liver, gallbladder, and pancreas are **accessory organs** of the digestive system that assist the functioning of the digestive tract **(Fig. 4.1b)**. The liver, gallbladder, and pancreas play major roles in digestion, even though food doesn't move through them.

Figure 4.1 Your digestive tract. [a] The major organs of the digestive system. [b] Accessory organs of the digestive system.

Mouth

Digestion actually starts in the mouth:

- Teeth begin the mechanical digestion of food by biting, tearing, and grinding chunks of food into smaller pieces that are easier to swallow.

- Salivary glands secrete **saliva**, a watery fluid that mixes with food and makes it easier to swallow. Saliva contains an enzyme that enables a minor amount of starch to undergo chemical digestion. **Enzymes** are proteins that help certain chemical changes occur, such as the breakdown of large substances.

- The tongue senses the taste and texture of foods and directs food to the back of the mouth where it can be swallowed.

A Matter of Taste

Taste buds that are located primarily on the tongue have specialized cells that help you distinguish sweet, sour, salty, bitter, and umami (*ew-mom'-ē*) tastes. Umami is often described as a meaty taste. Taste buds may also be able to sense fat in foods.[2]

The entire tongue can detect the five known tastes, but certain areas are particularly sensitive to specific tastes.[3]

- The tip of the tongue is most likely to detect sweet-tasting foods.

- The sides of the tongue are more sensitive to salty and sour items.

- The rear portion of the tongue is more likely to detect bitter substances than are other regions of the organ.

The sense of smell also contributes to your ability to taste. As you chew food, it releases chemicals that become airborne and stimulate nerves inside your nose. Your brain receives this information and combines it with information about taste sensations from your mouth to identify foods' flavors. Thus, favorite foods may seem tasteless and unappealing when you have an upper respiratory tract infection and the inside of your nose is congested.

saliva watery fluid secreted by the salivary glands that mixes with food in the mouth

enzymes proteins that help chemical reactions occur

TASTY **Tidbits**

Children have more taste buds than do adults, which may explain why they often reject strong-flavored foods such as liver, cooked broccoli, and raw onion. As you age, the number of taste buds in your mouth declines, and as an older adult, you might find yourself adding more seasoning to food to improve its taste.

Essential Concept

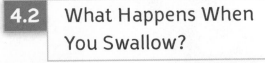

4.2 What Happens When You Swallow?

Esophagus

The **esophagus** (*eh-sof´-ah-gus*) is a muscular tube that extends about 10 inches from the back of the mouth to the top of the stomach. **Essential Concept 4.2** illustrates what happens to the material that's in your mouth when you swallow.

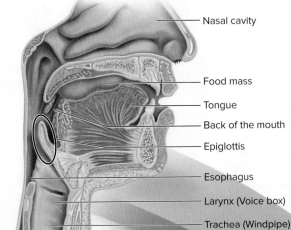

— Nasal cavity

— Food mass

— Tongue

— Back of the mouth

— Epiglottis

— Esophagus

— Larynx (Voice box)

— Trachea (Windpipe)

1 The esophagus transfers a mass of swallowed food into the stomach. The entrance to the esophagus is near the larynx and the opening of the trachea.

esophagus tubular organ of the digestive tract that connects the back of the mouth with the stomach

epiglottis flap of tissue that folds down over the trachea (windpipe) to keep food from entering the lungs during swallowing

— Epiglottis

2 When you swallow, the **epiglottis** *(ep-eh-glot´-tis)* closes over the trachea. This prevents the food from "going down the wrong pipe" (entering the larynx and trachea), which can cause choking.

Swallowing safely requires the steps that are shown in Essential Concept 4.2.

— Epiglottis

3 After swallowing the mass of food, the epiglottis returns to its usual position. Now, you can talk and breathe again, because the larynx and trachea are able to obtain air.

Swallowing food stimulates **peristalsis** (*per-uh-stall´-sis*), waves of muscular activity along the digestive tract that help propel food material through the tract. **Figure 4.2** shows how peristalsis moves a mass of food through the esophagus and to the stomach. Peristalsis also occurs in the stomach and intestines.

Peristalsis is an involuntary response, which means the muscular movements happen without the need to think about them.

Lifesaving Lesson

Accidental choking is a major cause of preventable deaths. A common distress sign of choking is grabbing the throat with one or both hands. Choking danger signs include bluish skin color, difficulty breathing, inability to speak, and weak, ineffective coughing.[4] The **Heimlich maneuver** (also called "abdominal thrusts") is a first aid technique that can help clear the blocked airway of a choking person. By learning the simple Heimlich maneuver, you can save a life, perhaps even your own.

Essential Concept

4.3 First Aid for Choking: The Heimlich Maneuver

Figure 4. 2. **What's peristalsis?** Peristalsis moves food material through the esophagus.

■ *What could happen if peristalsis didn't occur?*

Contraction

Food mass

Esophagus

Stomach

peristalsis type of muscular contraction of the digestive tract

Heimlich maneuver life-saving technique for people who are choking

1 Hands wrapped around the throat is a common sign of choking.

2a Performing the Heimlich maneuver on someone else. The abdominal thrusts may may need to be repeated at least five times.

2b Performing the Heimlich maneuver on yourself. This procedure may need to be repeated at least five times.

© Nick Koudis/Getty Images RF

Stomach

The stomach is a muscular sac that can expand and hold about 4 to 6 cups of food after a typical meal.[3] The **gastroesophageal sphincter** (*gas´-tro-eh-sof-ah-jee´-al sfink´-ter*) is the ring of muscular tissue at the lower end of the esophagus that controls the opening to the stomach (**Fig. 4.3**). After food enters the stomach, this sphincter constricts, so the food remains in the organ.

Certain cells within the stomach secrete gastric juice, a watery solution that contains hydrochloric acid (HCl) and enzymes. The enzymes break down some protein and fat. HCl helps make proteins easier to digest. The acid also kills many dangerous, disease-causing microorganisms that may be in food.

As you can see in Figure 4.3, the stomach's walls consist of layers of muscle. Muscle contains protein—so how does the stomach avoid digesting itself? Special cells that line the inside of the stomach produce a thick layer of **mucus.** Mucus is a slippery substance that protects the stomach wall from its acid and enzymes.

Stimulated by the presence of food, the stomach's churning movements mix food with gastric juice. At this point, the food is a semisolid liquid called **chyme** (*kime*). Although the stomach absorbs very few nutrients from chyme, a few drugs, including some alcohol, can pass through the organ's walls and enter the bloodstream.

The **pyloric** (*pie-lor´-ic*) **sphincter** is the ring of muscular tissue at the base of the stomach. This sphincter allows small amounts of chyme to leave the stomach and enter the small intestine (see Figure 4.3).

Following a meal, the stomach empties in about 3 to 4 hours, depending on the contents and size of the meal. Watery meals such as soups spend less time in the stomach; fatty meals spend more time there. As you'd expect, larger meals take longer to empty from the stomach than smaller meals.

© McGraw-Hill Education. Matt Meadows, photographer

gastroesophageal sphincter ring of muscle in the lower part of the esophagus; controls the opening between the esophagus and stomach

mucus slippery fluid that protects certain cells

chyme mixture of gastric juice and partially digested food

pyloric sphincter ring of muscle at the base of the stomach that controls the rate at which chyme leaves the stomach

Figure 4.3 **The stomach.**

■ *What structure controls the entrance to the stomach?*

■ *What is the function of the pyloric sphincter?*

Small Intestine

The small intestine is a highly coiled tube that extends from the stomach to the large intestine. Most nutrient digestion and absorption occurs in the small intestine. The small intestine has three sections (**Fig. 4.4**):

- **duodenum** (*do-wah-dee´-num*)
- **jejunum** (*jeh-ju´-num*)
- **ileum** (*il´-lee-um*)

What Are Villi?

The lining of the small intestine is covered by tiny, fingerlike projections called **villi** (singular, **villus**) (**Fig. 4.5a**). A villus has an outer layer of special cells called **absorptive cells** (**Fig. 4.5b**). Absorptive cells have tiny structures called microvilli that are exposed to chyme. Villi and microvilli increase the surface area of the small intestine, which increases your body's ability to digest and absorb nutrients.

Absorptive cells secrete enzymes that complete digestion. As a result of this enzyme action, macronutrients are broken down into their basic components. Proteins break down into amino acids, fats into fatty acids and glycerol, and most dietary carbohydrates into glucose. You will learn more about the digestion of these nutrients in Units 5, 6, and 7.

Absorptive cells remove (*absorb*) the breakdown products of digestion from chyme. Within each villus are tiny blood vessels that form a capillary network; and a **lacteal**, a lymphatic system vessel that carries fluid called **lymph.**

Figure 4.4 The three sections of the small intestine. This illustration shows the positions of the duodenum, jejunum, and ileum. The appendix makes immune system cells, but you can live without it.

Figure 4.5 Villi. (a) Villi cover the lining of the small intestine. (b) An intestinal absorptive cell has microvilli that help digest and absorb nutrients.

■ *What would happen if your small intestine didn't have villi?*

duodenum first segment of the small intestine

jejunum middle segment of the small intestine

ileum last segment of the small intestine

villi (singular, **villus**) tiny, fingerlike projections of the small intestinal lining that participate in digesting and absorbing food

absorptive cells digestive tract cells that absorb nutrients

lacteal lymphatic system vessel in villus that absorbs most lipids

lymph fluid in the lymphatic system

4.4 What Happens to Water-Soluble Nutrients?

1 Nutrients that dissolve in water, such as amino acids, glucose, and minerals, enter the capillary network of the villus.

Intestinal villus

Capillary network within villus

2 Eventually, these water-soluble nutrients are transported from the GI tract to the liver by the hepatic (liver) portal vein.

Liver

Hepatic portal vein

3 The liver has many functions, including monitoring the blood's nutrient contents, detoxifying many harmful substances, making glucose, and storing various nutrients.

Nutrients that don't dissolve in water (water-insoluble nutrients), such as cholesterol and fatty acids, need special treatment before they can enter the bloodstream. Absorptive cells use the water-insoluble nutrients to form chylomicrons (*ky'-lo-my'-crons*). A **chylomicron** is a lipid-rich particle that's coated with protein and phospholipids, which makes the fatty acids and cholesterol easier to transport in blood.

Chylomicrons are too large to enter the capillary network, but they can move into a lacteal (**Fig. 4.6**). The lymphatic system transports chylomicrons away from the small intestine. Eventually, the chylomicron-rich lymph enters the circulatory system by way of a major vein (subclavian vein) that's located near the heart (see Fig. 4.6). The circulatory system conveys chylomicrons to the liver where they undergo processing.

What if you had a peanut butter sandwich and a glass of milk for lunch? Within a few hours, your intestinal tract has digested this food and absorbed its nutrients. Now, these nutrients are available for your cells to use. The calcium that was in the milk can be added to your bones. The amino acids that were in the peanut butter, milk, and bread can be used for making proteins that you need. The fat and carbohydrates that were in these foods can be burned for energy. Thus, you are what you eat!

It takes about 3 to 5 hours for chyme to move through the small intestine. When chyme reaches the large intestine, most of its nutrient contents have been digested and absorbed. The water and undigested material that remains now enter the large intestine.

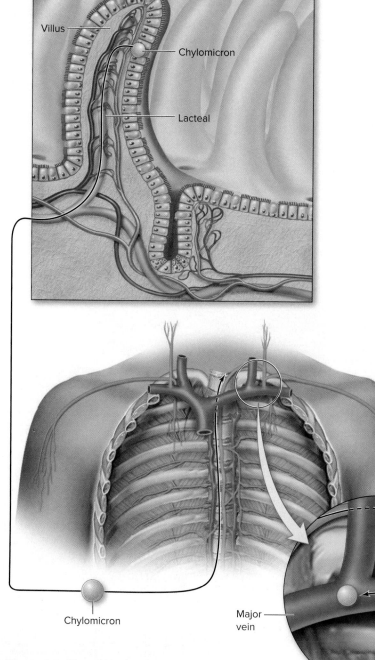

© Hera Food/Alamy RF

Figure 4.6 **Absorbing lipids.**

■ *What is the function of a chylomicron?*

chylomicron particle formed by small intestinal absorptive cells that transports lipids in the bloodstream

Accessory Organs

In addition to the stomach and small intestine, the following accessory organs are involved in the process of digesting food.

Essential Concept

4.5 The Liver, Gallbladder, and Pancreas

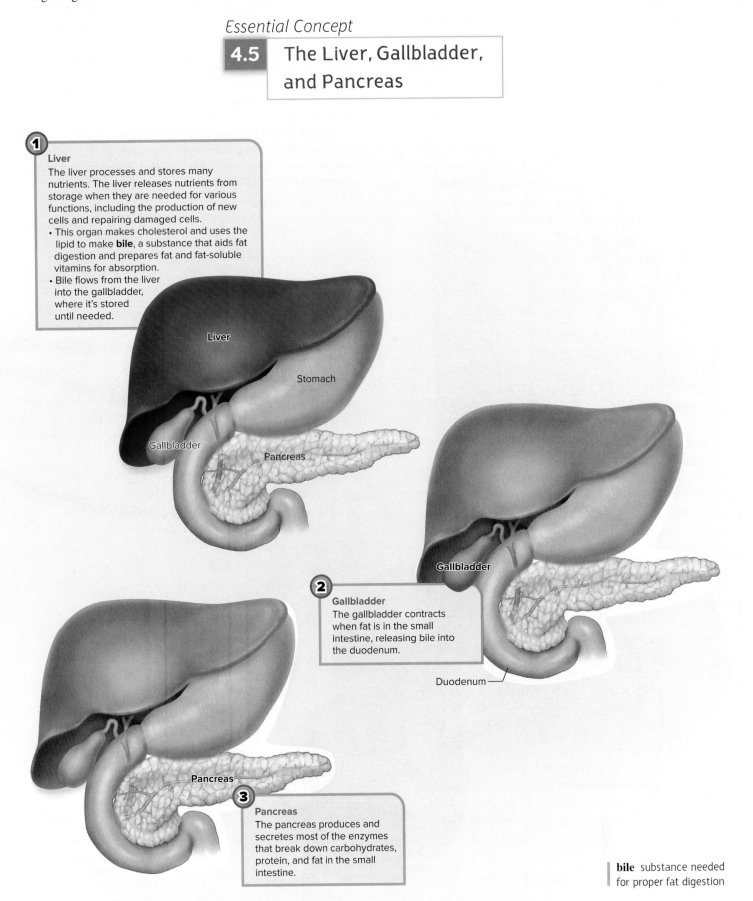

1

Liver
The liver processes and stores many nutrients. The liver releases nutrients from storage when they are needed for various functions, including the production of new cells and repairing damaged cells.
- This organ makes cholesterol and uses the lipid to make **bile**, a substance that aids fat digestion and prepares fat and fat-soluble vitamins for absorption.
- Bile flows from the liver into the gallbladder, where it's stored until needed.

Liver

Stomach

Gallbladder

Pancreas

Gallbladder

2

Gallbladder
The gallbladder contracts when fat is in the small intestine, releasing bile into the duodenum.

Duodenum

Pancreas

3

Pancreas
The pancreas produces and secretes most of the enzymes that break down carbohydrates, protein, and fat in the small intestine.

bile substance needed for proper fat digestion

Large Intestine

The two major sections of the large intestine are the **colon** and the **rectum (Fig. 4.7).** The colon is the primary section of the large intestine. The colon is connected to the rectum, a lower section of the large intestine.

Under normal circumstances, very little carbohydrate (other than dietary fiber), protein, and fat enter the large intestine. The large intestine has no villi, so little additional absorption, other than that of some water and minerals, takes place in this structure.

As chyme passes through the large intestine, most of its water content is absorbed. As a result, the residue becomes semisolid and is called *feces* or stools. Feces consist primarily of bacteria that normally live in the large intestine. Feces also contain undigested fiber from plant foods; some protein, water, and mucus; a small amount of fat; and cells that have been shed from the walls of the intestinal tract. Feces remain in the rectum until muscular contractions move the material into the anal canal and then out of the body through the anus.

Intestinal Bacteria

A healthy person's large intestine is home to vast numbers and many types of bacteria, the "gut microbiome." These bacteria use *fermentation*, a chemical process that converts undigested food material to substances the bacteria can use for their nutrient needs. Intestinal bacteria can make vitamins B-12, K, and biotin, which you may be able to absorb. These bacteria also produce substances that your colon cells and possibly, the rest of your body can use for energy. As a result of their metabolic activity, the bacteria also contribute to *flatulence*—the release of intestinal gases that are expelled through your anus.

The gut microbiome plays a role in your immunity to infectious diseases. Furthermore, your risk of developing obesity, cancer, heart disease, and certain intestinal diseases may be linked to the diversity of your gut bacteria.[5, 6] Because your diet influences the kinds of bacteria that make up your gut microbiome, scientists are studying which foods support the growth of the beneficial bacteria. **Prebiotics** are forms of dietary fiber that promote a diverse population of healthful bacteria in the large intestine.

Under normal conditions, the different bacterial populations that live in your gut maintain a balance that benefits your body. When you take an antibiotic for a bacterial infection, you kill the harmful bacteria that are making you sick as well as the beneficial bacteria in your large intestine. As a result, the harmful bacteria may flourish in the colon and limit the growth of the "good" bacteria. **Probiotics** are live, active cultures of beneficial microbes that may help maintain or re-establish the normal balance of bacterial populations in your colon. Certain brands of yogurt contain probiotics. Check the label to learn whether the product contains "live and active" cultures. You can take dietary supplements that contain probiotics, but information about their long-term safety is unknown.[7] It's a good idea to check with your physician before taking such supplements.

Starvation, antibiotic use, and excessive emotional stress can upset the normal balance of intestinal bacteria and result in intestinal infections. Some kinds of intestinal bacteria can be quite harmful if they enter other parts of your body or contaminate food. People should wash their hands after having bowel movements to reduce the likelihood of spreading dangerous microbes from their intestinal tract. Unit 11 discusses microorganisms that cause common food-borne infections and ways to limit your exposure to them.

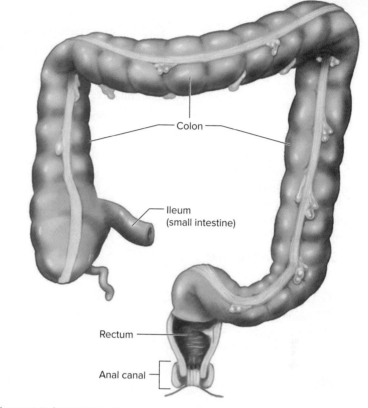

Colon

Ileum (small intestine)

Rectum

Anal canal

Figure 4.7 Large intestine.

MADE WITH 2% MILK

Fortified with Vitamins A, C, D & E

Excellent source of protein

Live and active cultures

100% of profits go to our FARMERS Supporting our Communities Supporting US

NT. 2 LBS (907g)

© Wendy Schiff

colon major structure of the large intestine

rectum lower section of the large intestine

prebiotics forms of dietary fiber that promote the growth of healthful intestinal bacteria

probiotics live and active cultures of beneficial bacteria

4.2c Digestive System Summary

Your digestive system breaks down food into nutrients that can be absorbed and used by your body. **Figure 4.8** summarizes major functions of the organs and structures of the digestive system, including the accessory organs. The following module discusses some disorders of the digestive system, including constipation and diarrhea. Celiac disease (gluten intolerance) also affects the GI tract. You'll learn more about this condition in Unit 7.

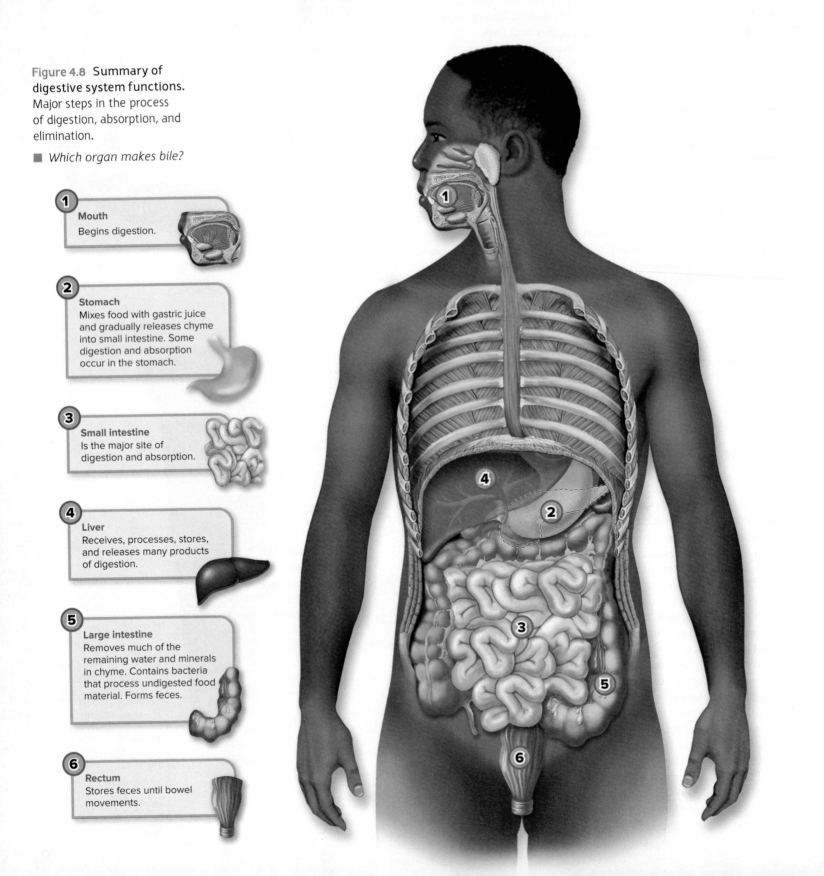

Figure 4.8 Summary of digestive system functions. Major steps in the process of digestion, absorption, and elimination.

■ *Which organ makes bile?*

1 Mouth
Begins digestion.

2 Stomach
Mixes food with gastric juice and gradually releases chyme into small intestine. Some digestion and absorption occur in the stomach.

3 Small intestine
Is the major site of digestion and absorption.

4 Liver
Receives, processes, stores, and releases many products of digestion.

5 Large intestine
Removes much of the remaining water and minerals in chyme. Contains bacteria that process undigested food material. Forms feces.

6 Rectum
Stores feces until bowel movements.

Module 4.3

Common Digestive System Disorders

4.3 - Learning Outcomes

After reading Module 4.3, you should be able to

1. Define all of the key terms in this module.

2. Identify some common as well as serious digestive system problems; and discuss risk factors, preventive measures, and typical treatments for these conditions.

4.3a Constipation

Although the normal frequency of bowel movements varies individually, a healthy person should have a bowel movement at least every three days.[8] When bowel movements occur less frequently and/or feces are difficult to eliminate, a condition called **constipation** develops.

Many factors influence your frequency of bowel movements, including

- lack of dietary fiber,
- low water intake,
- lack of exercise, and
- changes in your typical routine, such as taking a long trip or having major surgery.

Furthermore, constipation can result if you regularly ignore your normal bowel urges and avoid making a trip to the bathroom when it's not convenient.

Chronic constipation can cause discomfort and may contribute to the development of hemorrhoids and diverticula. **Hemorrhoids** are swollen veins in the anal canal that can cause itching and bleeding (**Fig. 4.9**). **Diverticula** are small pouches that can form in the lining of the large intestine (**Fig. 4.10**). Diverticula can trap bacteria and feces, causing painful inflammation or infection. If diverticula become inflamed or infected, antibiotics are used, but sometimes, surgery may be necessary to treat the condition (diverticulitis).

Figure 4.9 Hemorrhoids.

■ *What are hemorrhoids?*

Scientists don't know what causes diverticula to form, but constipation, lack of physical activity, and low intake of water may be risk factors.[9]

If you're often constipated, discuss the matter with your physician. In many instances, exercising regularly, and adding more water and fiber-rich foods to your diet is the first step to bowel "regularity." Unit 5 provides information about fiber, including rich food sources.

constipation condition that occurs when bowel movements occur less frequently than normal and/or are difficult to eliminate

hemorrhoids swollen veins in the anal canal that can cause itching and bleeding

diverticula small pouches that can form in the lining of the large intestine

Figure 4.10 In this color-enhanced x-ray, diverticula appear to be blue.

■ *What are diverticula?*

What *IS* That? - - - - - - - - - - - →

Foods that contain live and active probiotics may be beneficial to your health, particularly your intestinal health. Kefir is a "cultured" milk. Cultured milks, such as kefir and cultured buttermilk, have probiotics added to them. The probiotic bacteria use the natural carbohydrate in milk for energy, and produce acid and carbon dioxide as a result. The acid curdles the milk and gives it a distinctive taste; the carbon dioxide provides some "fizz," like a carbonated soft drink. A 1 cup serving of kefir that's made from 2% milk supplies about the same energy and nutrient contents as 1 cup of 2% milk.

© Wendy Schiff

4.3b Diarrhea

Diarrhea is a condition characterized by frequent, loose stools. Diarrhea occurs when more water than normal is secreted into the GI tract or the tract absorbs less water than normal. Most cases of diarrhea result from bacterial or viral infections of the intestinal tract. The infectious bacteria or viruses produce irritating or toxic substances that increase the movements (motility) of the GI tract. As a result, the GI tract propels chyme more rapidly through it, absorbing less water than normal in the process. Increased GI motility also enables the large intestine to eliminate the watery feces and the toxic material it contains rapidly.

Loperamide, an over-the-counter medication, can be helpful for relieving an occasional bout of mild diarrhea. Cases of severe diarrhea, however, require more immediate medical attention. Frequent watery stools can deplete the body's fluid volume (dehydration) and cause excessive losses of the minerals sodium and potassium. Therefore, treatment of severe diarrhea generally includes drinking watery replacement fluids that contain sodium, potassium, and simple sugars such as glucose.

Prompt treatment of severe diarrhea—within 24 to 48 hours—is especially crucial for infants and the elderly because they can become dehydrated quickly. In adults, diarrhea that's accompanied by bloody stools or lasts more than 7 days may be a sign of a serious intestinal disease, and a physician should be consulted.

Foods that contain probiotics, such as certain brands of cultured milk and yogurt, may help restore the normal bacterial population of your large intestine. More research, however, is needed to determine the most effective forms and doses of probiotics.

4.3c Vomiting

Not long after eating something toxic or drinking too much alcohol, you begin to feel queasy, or "sick to your stomach." Soon you become well aware that your body has an effective way of removing the harmful food or beverage—vomiting. Although vomiting is an unpleasant experience, it prevents toxic substances from entering your small intestine, where they can do more harm or be absorbed. Vomiting can also be a response to a food allergy, intense pain, "motion sickness," seasickness, migraine headaches, and hormonal changes in pregnancy (morning sickness).[10]

Treatment includes avoiding solid food until the vomiting resolves. Sipping small amounts of water or clear liquids, including noncarbonated soft drinks such as sports drinks, can help maintain body water. If you're able to drink small amounts of fluid without vomiting, you can try to drink increasing amounts of fluid until the vomiting subsides completely.

Vomiting generally doesn't last more than 24 hours. Repeated vomiting, however, can result in dehydration, especially if it's accompanied by diarrhea. Contact a physician when vomiting lasts longer than a day (adults) or is accompanied by

- signs of dehydration,
- headache or stiff neck,
- severe abdominal pain, and/or
- failure to urinate for 8 hours.

Call 911 or have someone take you to an emergency room if you think you've been poisoned, there's blood in your vomit, or the vomit looks like coffee grounds (a sign of blood that has been partially digested).

TASTY Tidbits

As mentioned in Module 4.2b, taking antibiotics can destroy healthful bacteria that normally reside in your colon. This situation can cause an imbalance in the colon's bacterial populations, resulting in diarrhea. You may be able to reduce the risk of diarrhea by consuming dairy foods or dietary supplements that contain probiotics.[7]

Source: CDC/Janice Hadey Carr

***E. coli* bacteria normally live in your colon.**

4.3d Acid Reflux

If the gastroesophageal sphincter doesn't function properly and opens when it should be closed, the stomach's contents can flow back into the esophagus. This condition, gastroesophageal reflux (GER), irritates the lining of the esophagus, causing symptoms that are often referred to as "acid indigestion" or heartburn. **Heartburn** is a gnawing pain or burning sensation generally felt in the upper chest, under the breastbone. Despite the name, heartburn isn't a heart problem—it's the result of acid reflux.

Many factors can contribute to acid reflux or worsen the condition:

- pregnancy;
- having excess body fat, especially in the middle of the body;
- drinking alcohol;
- smoking cigarettes;
- lying down soon after eating a large meal; and
- consuming certain foods.

Commonly consumed foods and beverages that can contribute to acid reflux are

- fatty or greasy foods,
- tomatoes and tomato-based sauces,
- peppermint,
- coffee,
- alcohol, and
- chocolate[11]

This combination is an invitation to acid reflux.

Gastroesophageal Reflux Disease

Many people think heartburn is a minor health problem that can be ignored. Frequent acid reflux, however, can be a symptom of a chronic condition—**gastroesophageal reflux disease (GERD).** Symptoms of GERD include

- acid reflux that occurs more than twice a week,
- nausea and vomiting,
- painful swallowing,
- chronic dry cough, and
- hoarse voice.[11]

heartburn backflow of irritating stomach contents into the esophagus

gastroesophageal reflux disease (GERD) chronic condition characterized by frequent heartburn

Onion rings: © FoodCollections/StockFood RF;
Peppermint: © Pixtal/AGE Fotostock RF;
Pasta with tomato sauce: © Jonelle Weaver/Getty Images RF;
Chocolate: © FoodCollection/StockFood RF

Foods that are made with tomato-based sauces, peppermint, or chocolate can contribute to acid reflux.

TASTY **Tidbits**

If you have mild heartburn, you can take an antacid to relieve the discomfort. Popular antacids usually include magnesium, calcium, and aluminum in forms that neutralize stomach acid. Antacids, however, can have side effects. Products that contain magnesium can cause diarrhea; aluminum- or calcium-containing antacids may cause constipation. In addition to neutralizing stomach acid, antacids that contain calcium can be a source of calcium, a mineral nutrient. Even though you can buy many kinds of antacids without prescriptions, it's a good idea to check with your physician before using them.

© Wendy Schiff

To reduce your risk of heartburn and manage GERD:

- Take over-the-counter antacids to neutralize excess stomach acid and relieve heartburn after eating.

- Lose the excess weight, if you have too much belly fat.

- Do not lie down within 2 to 3 hours after eating.

- Do not overeat at mealtimes.

- Avoid smoking cigarettes.

- Elevate the head of your bed 6 to 8 inches higher than the foot of the bed.

- Do not wear tight belts, undergarments that flatten the abdomen, or clothes with tight waistbands.

- Avoid foods that often cause acid reflux.[11]

If you suffer from frequent heartburn and have other GERD symptoms, let your physician know about it. GERD can damage the lining of the esophagus and contribute to the development of sores called *ulcers*.

People who suffer from GERD have a higher risk of esophageal cancer than people who do not have a history of this condition. You can manage GERD by making lifestyle changes and taking medications that inhibit stomach acid production, thus preventing heartburn.

4.3e Peptic Ulcers

A **peptic ulcer** is a sore that occurs in the lining of the upper digestive tract, especially in the duodenum, stomach, and sometimes the esophagus. If the layer of mucus that protects the stomach and small intestine breaks down, HCl and protein-digesting enzymes can reach the stomach and intestinal walls, destroying the tissue. Such destruction can cause one or more ulcers to form in the damaged tissues. If an ulcer injures the wall of a blood vessel, the sore can cause

serious, even life-threatening, bleeding. Therefore, it's important to recognize peptic ulcer signs and symptoms and obtain professional medical treatment.

The typical sign of peptic ulcers is "dull" or burning pain that is felt in the stomach area. Pain typically begins when the stomach is empty, and the discomfort eases for awhile after food is eaten or antacids are taken.[12] Uncommon but more serious signs are

- vomiting fresh blood or vomit that looks like "coffee grounds," and

- black tarry stools (sign of digested blood).

As mentioned in Unit 2's "Nutrition Fact or Fiction?" feature, stress isn't a major cause of peptic ulcers. Factors that increase the risk of peptic ulcers include

- *H. pylori* infection (a bacterial infection),

- tumors of the pancreas or duodenum that cause excessive stomach acid production,

- smoking cigarettes,

- heavy consumption of alcohol, and

(Continued)

peptic ulcer a sore that occurs in the lining of the upper GI tract

The arrow points to a peptic ulcer.

Image courtesy of Robert D. Fusco, MD, Three Rivers Endoscopy Center, Moon Township, PA www.gihealth.com

- frequent use of nonsteroidal anti-inflammatory drugs (NSAIDs) such as aspirin, ibuprofen, and naproxen.

Treatment for peptic ulcers may include antibiotics that kill *H. pylori* and medications that control stomach acid production.

4.3f Gallstones

If you experience severe pain in the upper right area of your midsection within an hour or two after eating a fatty meal, you may have gallstones.

Recall that the gallbladder stores bile, which is needed to digest fats properly. Gallstones form in the gallbladder. The stones usually consist of cholesterol and can be small and grainy, like particles of sand, or as large as a coin **(Fig. 4.11)**. If a person has gallstones, they cause pain when the gallbladder contracts to release bile into the small intestine.

Sometimes a gallstone blocks the small passageway that carries bile to the duodenum. When this occurs, bile can back up into the liver or pancreas, injuring these organs. Surgery to remove the diseased gallbladder is necessary to relieve the pain and prevent damage to the liver or pancreas. After surgery, bile drips from the liver directly into the small intestine.

Having excess body fat increases the risk of gallstones. To reduce your risk of gallstones, keep your weight at a healthy level.

Figure 4.11 Gallbladder and gallstones. This gallbladder has been cut to expose the gallstones that formed inside of it. Most gallstones contain cholesterol.

■ *Where do gallstones form?*

Q Answer This

Which of the following organs is not essential for good health: the liver, gallbladder, pancreas, or small intestine? You can find the answer on the last page of this unit.

Eating a fatty meal might cause a gallbladder "attack" if you have gallstones.

irritable bowel syndrome (IBS) chronic condition characterized by frequent bouts of intestinal cramps with diarrhea or constipation

ulcerative colitis form of inflammatory bowel disease

4.3g Irritable Bowel Syndrome (IBS)

Many adult Americans suffer from **irritable bowel syndrome (IBS).** People with IBS experience frequent bouts of abdominal pain and bloating with diarrhea and/or constipation. The cause of IBS is unknown, but certain foods and beverages as well as emotional stress, anxiety, and depression may trigger the disorder.

Treatment for IBS is individualized and may include

- eliminating foods that seem to trigger IBS symptoms;

- taking medications to relieve constipation, diarrhea, and abdominal pain;

- learning stress management strategies;

- obtaining psychological counseling and taking antidepressants; and

- using certain probiotics.[13]

Although irritable bowel syndrome can be uncomfortable and upsetting, the condition doesn't appear to permanently harm the large intestine or increase the risk of colorectal cancer.[14]

4.3h Ulcerative Colitis

Matthew Lang, the student featured in this unit's opener, was diagnosed with **ulcerative colitis (UC)** when he was a sophomore in college. UC is a chronic inflammatory bowel disease that causes ulcers in the inner lining of the large intestine. As a result of the inflammation, the colon's lining erodes away, leading to abdominal cramping, rectal bleeding, and diarrhea. Other signs and symptoms include

- anemia,

- fatigue,

- fever,

- nausea, and

- appetite loss and weight loss.

Medical experts don't know what causes UC. People with the disease may have immune systems that react abnormally to bacteria in their digestive tract. UC tends to "run in families," so genetic factors are suspected to play a role in its development.

"I feel a lot healthier now than when I was first diagnosed . . . the medication seems to have stabilized the disease . . . as long as I take my medicine and take care of myself, I'm fine."

Matthew Lang

© Randy Allbritton/Getty Images RF

© Wendy Schiff

Nutrition Fact or Fiction?

Regular colon cleansing is necessary for good health.

A healthy large intestine doesn't store toxins or large amounts of feces. Using "high colonics" and other types of enemas to "cleanse" your colon isn't necessary because the large intestine doesn't need to be cleansed. Furthermore, frequent enemas may deplete the body of water and minerals, including sodium and potassium.

Although emotional stress doesn't cause UC, people with the disease report that stressful situations seem to worsen their symptoms. Furthermore, food allergies aren't the cause of UC. However, some people with the disease, including Matthew Lang, learn to avoid certain foods and beverages because consuming them seems to trigger bouts of the illness. Dietary recommendations generally include eating smaller meals more often, drinking more liquids but avoiding carbonated drinks, and avoiding high-fiber foods, especially when symptoms occur. Currently, scientists are studying probiotics to see if they can be helpful in treating UC.

As Matthew noted in the unit opener, there's no cure for UC. Treatment generally includes medications to reduce inflammation. People with UC generally must take the medication for the rest of their lives, unless their large intestine is so severely diseased that surgical removal of the organ is necessary.

Patients with UC have an increased risk of colon cancer, especially when their entire colon is affected and they've had the disease for 8 or more years.[15] Patients can reduce their risk of colon cancer by managing the inflammation with medication and having regular screening (testing) to detect colon cancer.

4.3i Colorectal Cancer

Normally, cells grow and divide to form new cells as the body needs them. When cells grow old, they die. Sometimes, new cells divide and grow more rapidly than normal cells. Furthermore, these cells don't function normally, and they invade nearby tissues, often forming a mass of tissue called a *tumor*. Such abnormal cells are cancer cells.

Cancerous (*malignant*) cells spread (*metastasize*) to other parts of the body, may grow back after being removed surgically, and can be life-threatening. Cancer that starts in either the colon or the rectum is often called **colorectal cancer (Fig. 4.12).**

Figure 4.12 This illustration shows a large cancerous tumor in the colon.

■ *What steps can you take to reduce your risk of colorectal cancer?*

In the United States, colorectal cancer is the second-leading cause of cancer deaths among adults.[16] Lung cancer is the leading cause of cancer deaths among Americans. Unit 8 provides more information about cancer and the role of diet in cancer development.

What Are the Signs and Symptoms of Colorectal Cancer?

Signs and symptoms of colorectal cancer include

- having diarrhea or constipation that persists,
- feeling that your bowel doesn't empty completely after bowel movements,
- finding blood (either bright red or very dark) in your stools,
- noticing that your stools are narrower than usual,

(Continued)

colorectal cancer cancer that starts in either the colon or the rectum

Group of cancer cells

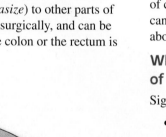

© Science Photo Library RF/Getty Images RF

Microscopic view of cancer cells

© Adam Gault/Getty Images RF

© FoodCollection/StockFood RF

Eating lots of fatty meat may increase your risk of colorectal cancer.

- losing weight without trying,
- feeling very tired all the time, and
- having abdominal cramps or pain.

Who Is at Risk?

The following characteristics increase a person's risk of developing colorectal cancer:

- being over 50 years of age;
- having colorectal *polyps*. Polyps (*paw´-lips*) are small clumps of tissue that grow on the inner wall of the colon or rectum. Most polyps are not cancerous, but some can become cancer;
- having a family history of colorectal cancer. If your close relatives have had colorectal cancer, your risk of the disease is high;
- having a personal history of cancer. If you've already had colorectal cancer, you're at risk of developing colorectal cancer again;
- having ulcerative colitis or Crohn's disease, another type of inflammatory bowel disease (IBD);
- eating a lot of red and processed meats;[16]
- being obese and/or physically inactive;
- smoking cigarettes; and
- drinking alcohol.

If you have a high risk of colorectal cancer, check with your physician. The doctor may have you undergo colorectal screenings and more frequent checkups. If tests show a polyp or an abnormal area in your colon or rectum, you may need to have some of the

affected tissue removed (a *biopsy*). With the aid of a microscope, a physician can look for cancer cells in the tissue.

Treatment Options

Treatment for colorectal cancer usually involves surgery, chemotherapy, biological therapy, or radiation therapy. Surgery removes the diseased areas of the large intestine. Chemotherapy uses drugs to kill cancer cells. Biological therapy involves using antibodies, which are special proteins that detect and bind to colorectal cancer cells. This treatment interferes with the cancer cells' ability to grow and spread. Radiation therapy uses high-energy rays to kill cancer cells. Although surgery is the most common treatment for colorectal cancer, people often undergo a combination of treatments.

Figure 4.13 shows the digestive system organs that are affected by the health problems discussed in this module. Some other disorders that affect the digestive system, such as food allergies and celiac disease, are discussed in Unit 7.

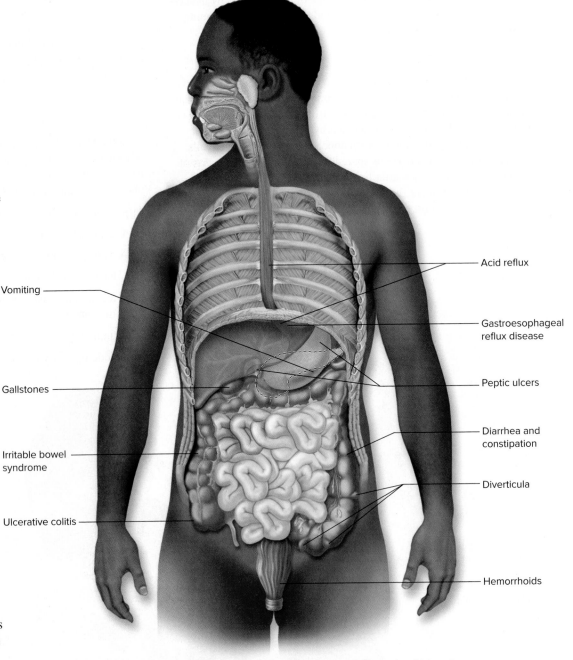

Vomiting

Gallstones

Irritable bowel syndrome

Ulcerative colitis

Acid reflux

Gastroesophageal reflux disease

Peptic ulcers

Diarrhea and constipation

Diverticula

Hemorrhoids

Figure 4.13 Sites of common health problems that affect the GI tract.

Module 4.4

Metabolism Basics

4.4 - Learning Outcomes

After reading Module 4.4, you should be able to

1. Define all of the key terms in this module.
2. Identify anabolic and catabolic processes.
3. Identify factors that influence the amount of ATP production.

© Diane Collins and Jordan Hollender/Getty Images RF

4.4a A Remarkable Machine

In essence, your body is very much like a car engine—both are complex systems that need to generate energy, remove wastes, store excess energy until needed, and maintain a proper running temperature. Your body, the "human machine," is even more amazing than a car because it can repair, maintain, and even build itself. Furthermore, the human machine can run on a variety of "biological" fuels derived from the foods and beverages it consumes: glucose (a carbohydrate), fat, and protein. Although you don't have a section of your body that is a fuel reservoir (like a gas tank), you can store large amounts of energy in your liver, muscles, and body fat. When you use your muscles for a long period of time without consuming food, you may feel as though you've "run out of gas." You can, of course, replenish your fuel supply by resting and consuming food. Like a car, your body's performance can be improved dramatically when it has access to an adequate and high-quality fuel supply.

energy capacity to perform work

Energy Metabolism

Energy is the capacity to perform work. There are several forms of energy, including chemical, mechanical, electrical, heat, solar, and nuclear. Human cells use chemical energy to perform work. Although energy can neither be created nor destroyed, it can undergo transformations. Chemical energy, for example, can change into heat energy, which explains why a car's engine heats up as it burns gasoline and your muscles warm up during exercise.

The cells in your body release, transfer, and use energy constantly. Energy enables you to move, breathe, and perform other familiar activities. Your cells obtain energy by breaking down certain nutrients to release the chemical energy that's stored in them. It's important to remember that only carbohydrates, lipids, proteins, and alcohol can be *metabolized* ("burned") for energy; cells cannot release energy from vitamins, minerals, or water.

Metabolism is the sum of all chemical reactions that occur in living cells, including the reactions that release energy from macronutrients, make proteins, and eliminate waste products. Energy

© Jack Star/PhotoLInk/Getty Images RF

catabolism metabolic processes that break down larger substances into smaller ones

anabolism metabolic processes that build larger substances from smaller ones

hormones chemical messengers

adenosine triphosphate (ATP) "energy currency" of cells

aerobic metabolism metabolic pathways that require oxygen

anaerobic metabolism metabolic pathway that functions without oxygen

metabolism involves metabolic pathways that enable your body to obtain and use energy from macronutrients. A metabolic pathway is a step-by-step process that converts compounds to new compounds. During the process, energy can be released from or gained by the compounds. Metabolic reactions may be catabolic or anabolic.

- **Catabolism** (*kuh-tab'-oh-lizm*) refers to metabolic processes that break down larger substances into smaller ones. Examples of catabolic reactions include the breakdown of a fatty acid to release energy. As a result, cells form waste products, carbon dioxide and water. When you exhale, your lungs remove excess carbon dioxide. Your body can use the water that was formed during catabolic reactions in other chemical reactions. Otherwise, the excess water is removed when you exhale, sweat, or urinate. Heat comprises some of the energy that's released—"heat of metabolism" helps the body maintain its normal temperature.

- **Anabolism** (*an-ab'-oh-lizm*) refers to metabolic processes that build larger substances from smaller ones. Such processes generally store energy for future use. Anabolic reactions include those involved in making proteins, bones, and hormones. **Hormones** are chemicals that your body uses to transmit messages.

What Is ATP?

Much of the energy released by catabolic reactions is captured in a chemical form in the energy molecule **adenosine triphosphate** (*ah-den'-oh-seen try-fos'-fate*) (**ATP**). ATP is often referred to as "energy currency" because it functions like money. Just as you save money until it's needed to make a purchase, your cells save energy in ATP until it's needed to power cellular work. Your cells "earn" ATP in energy-releasing catabolic reactions and "spend" ATP in energy-requiring anabolic reactions.

Aerobic and Anaerobic Energy Metabolism

Cells require oxygen to produce the maximum number of ATP molecules from the catabolism of macronutrients. When adequate oxygen is present in a cell, the cell can make lots of ATP (**aerobic metabolism**). When the ATP supply is inadequate, cells can still obtain the molecule using a metabolic pathway that doesn't require oxygen (**anaerobic metabolism**). Compared to aerobic metabolism, however, much less ATP is made under low-oxygen conditions. When you exercise vigorously for an extended period, your lungs and circulatory system cannot deliver enough oxygen to your muscle cells to maintain adequate ATP production. As a result, you can't sustain the vigorous physical activity. You "run out of gas" and must slow down your pace. In Unit 10, Module 10.5 provides more information about energy metabolism, including how exercise can influence the proportions of macronutrients used for energy.

"Seeing your breath" occurs when the warm water vapor that's in your exhaled breath condenses when it reaches cold air.

© McGraw-Hill Education. Christopher Kerrigan, photographer

© Comstock Images/Alamy RF

Biological Fuels

Your cells rely heavily on fat and glucose for energy. Under normal conditions, your cells don't metabolize much protein for energy. Cells in the central nervous system (CNS) depend primarily on glucose, rather than fats or proteins, to meet their energy needs. If glucose is unavailable, however, most cells (including those of the CNS) are resourceful in that they can burn more than one fuel, especially fat, for energy. **Figure 4.14** provides a basic summary of some metabolic pathways that dietary protein, carbohydrate, and fat follow during energy metabolism. For more detailed information about major metabolic pathways that cells use to obtain ATP, see Appendix D.

Figure 4.14 Summary of energy metabolism.

■ *Which of these macronutrients is not a major source of ATP energy?*

In a **Nutshell**

© McGraw-Hill Education. Mark A.
Dierker, photographer

Module 4.1: From Cells to Systems

- Cells are the basic living units of the body. Masses of cells that have similar characteristics and functions form tissues. An organ is a collection of tissues that function in a related way. An organ system is a collection of organs that work together for a similar purpose.

Module 4.2: Digestive System

- Your digestive system processes food into nutrients, absorbs the nutrients into the bloodstream, and eliminates the waste products. During digestion, large food components are broken down into smaller substances, including individual nutrients. This process involves mechanical and chemical digestion.

- The mouth, esophagus, stomach, and small and large intestines are the major organs of the digestive system. The teeth, tongue, salivary glands, liver, gallbladder, and pancreas are accessory organs of the digestive system that assist the functioning of the digestive tract.

- Digestion begins in the mouth. Teeth begin the mechanical digestion of food by biting, tearing, and grinding chunks of food into smaller pieces.

- Some mechanical and chemical digestion occurs in the stomach. The enzymes in gastric juice break down some protein and fat; hydrochloric acid in the juice helps make proteins easier to digest. The acid also kills many dangerous disease-causing microorganisms that may be in food.

- Most nutrient digestion and absorption occurs in the small intestine. The lining of the small intestine is covered by villi. Villi secrete enzymes that complete digestion. Proteins break down into amino acids, fats into fatty acids and glycerol, and most dietary carbohydrates into glucose.

- Absorptive cells remove the breakdown products of digestion from chyme. Nutrients that dissolve in water enter the capillary network and are transported to the liver by a large vein. Water-insoluble nutrients are formed into chylomicrons that move into lacteals. The lymphatic system transports chylomicrons away from the small intestine.

- The liver processes and stores many nutrients and makes cholesterol and bile. The gallbladder stores bile until it is needed. The pancreas produces and secretes most of the enzymes that break down carbohydrates, protein, and fat in the small intestine.

- Little additional absorption other than water and some minerals takes place in the large intestine. Feces consist primarily of bacteria that normally live in the large intestine. Feces also contain undigested fiber from plant foods; a small amount of fat, protein, and water; and mucus and cells shed from the walls of the intestinal tract.

Module 4.3: Common Digestive System Disorders

- Chronic constipation may contribute to the development of hemorrhoids and diverticula.

- Frequent acid reflux can be a symptom of GERD. People with GERD are at risk of esophageal cancer. Peptic ulcers can cause life-threatening bleeding.

- Although irritable bowel syndrome is common, the condition doesn't cause cancer of the large intestine. Ulcerative colitis is an inflammatory disease of the large intestine. In the United States, colorectal cancer is the second-leading cancer killer of adults.

Module 4.4: Metabolism Basics

- Metabolism is the sum of all chemical reactions that occur in living cells. Your cells obtain energy by breaking down macronutrients to release the chemical energy that's stored in them. Metabolic reactions can be catabolic or anabolic.

- Much of the energy released by catabolic reactions is captured in ATP. Cells use "ATP-energy" to power chemical reactions. Your cells "earn" ATP in energy-releasing catabolic reactions, and "spend" ATP in energy-requiring anabolic reactions. Glucose and fat are major sources of ATP-energy for your cells.

© I. Rozenbaum/PhotoAlto RF

Consider This...

1. When you were 5 years old, why did you use the tip of your tongue to taste a new food?

2. Your sister hasn't been feeling well lately. This morning, she vomited what appears to be coffee grounds, but she doesn't drink coffee. Based on this information, your sister should see a physician because she might have which common digestive tract disorder?

3. Taylor had a serious condition that required removal of the upper third of his small intestine. Based on this information, is Taylor at risk for developing multiple nutrient deficiencies? Explain why or why not.

4. Your mother complains of having persistent heartburn, but she doesn't think her discomfort is serious enough to be investigated by her physician. Do you agree or disagree with her attitude about heartburn? Explain your position.

5. Twenty-year-old Barry is worried about his risk of colorectal cancer because one of his grandfathers died of the disease. What steps can he take to reduce his risk of the disease?

Test Yourself

Select the best answer.

1. A _____ is a group of similar cells that perform similar functions.
   a. ribosome   c. cytoplasm
   b. tissue   d. system

2. Which of the following organs isn't an accessory organ of the digestive system?
   a. Stomach   c. Liver
   b. Pancreas   d. Gallbladder

3. Hydrochloric acid production occurs in the
   a. mouth.   c. small intestine.
   b. stomach.   d. liver.

4. Chemicals that help break down or make substances are called
   a. enzymes.   c. capillaries.
   b. cells.   d. hormones.

5. Tiny, fingerlike projections of the small intestine that absorb nutrients are called
   a. capillaries. c. duodenum.
   b. villi.   d. chyme.

6. A lacteal is a
   a. special structure in the small intestine that digests milk proteins.

   b. form of carbohydrate in milk.
   c. muscular structure that regulates the movement of chyme in the large intestine.
   d. lymph vessel in a villus.

7. Glands in the mouth secrete
   a. saliva.   c. bile.
   b. hydrochloric acid. d. hormones.

© FoodCollection /Stockfood RF

8. Peristalsis
   a. is a common intestinal infection.
   b. interferes with lipid absorption in the small intestine.
   c. stimulates cancer formation in the colon.
   d. helps move food/chyme through the digestive tract.

9. Your cells use _____ as a source of direct energy.
   a. ATP   c. amino acids
   b. bile   d. GERD

10. Which of the following practices increases the risk of peptic ulcers?
    a. Chewing gum   c. Drinking milk
    b. Smoking cigarettes d. Eating prebiotics

© Darren Greenwood/
DesignPics RF

A Answer This (Module 4.3f)

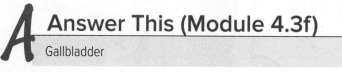
Gallbladder

References ➡ See Appendix F.

STUDY TIP: Quickly create a customized practice quiz for this chapter by going to your Connect SmartBook "My Reports" section.

Don't have SmartBook and want to learn more? Go to **whysmartbook.com**.

Unit 5

Carbohydrates
FUEL AND FIBER

What's on the Menu?

Module 5.1
Sugars, Sweeteners, Starches, and Fiber

Module 5.2
What Happens to the Carbohydrates You Eat?

Module 5.3
Carbohydrates and Health

© Pixtal/AGE Fotostock RF

© Heidi Ann Waarington

"I'd like to think my diet is pretty healthy. I like fruit, especially strawberries and bananas, and I love sandwiches made with whole-grain bread, turkey, and chicken. I try to avoid soft drinks because they have a lot of high-fructose corn syrup. From what I understand, high-fructose corn syrup is one of the leading causes of obesity. I avoid foods that contain the syrup, and I use honey to sweeten foods instead of sugar. I love honey! I think it's a healthier substitute for sugar, and I like the taste. I try not to eat sweets, but I'm not some kind of health guru. . . . I love cake! My favorite food is chocolate cake with white frosting and colored sprinkles."

Neill Warrington

If you're like **Neill Warrington,** a junior who's majoring in Math and Physics at Syracuse University, you enjoy eating cake, but you're concerned about your intake of other "sweets," especially soft drinks that are sweetened with high-fructose corn syrup. On average, an American consumed about 77 pounds of added caloric sweeteners in 2014.[1] Such sweeteners include high-fructose corn syrup as well as honey and table sugar that are added to foods to sweeten them. Added caloric sweeteners are "empty calories" that offer little nutritional value other than carbohydrates to your diet. Eating too much food that contains such sweeteners may reduce your desire to eat more nutritious foods.

Are all carbohydrates unhealthy? How many "carbs" does the body need? Is honey a more nutritious sweetener than sugar? Does eating too much high-fructose corn syrup cause excess weight gain or any other health problems? In Unit 5, you'll learn about carbohydrates, including which carbohydrates are better sources of nutrients than others.

Module 5.1

Sugars, Sweeteners, Starches, and Fiber

5.1 - Learning Outcomes

After reading Module 5.1, you should be able to

1. Define all of the key terms in this module.

2. Identify the major carbohydrates in your diet as well as their primary food sources and functions in your body.

3. Recognize chemical and common names of nutritive sweeteners and identify common alternative sweeteners.

Why do people, even newborn infants, prefer foods that taste sweet? The pleasant and sometimes irresistible taste of sugar is a clue that the food contains **carbohydrates,** a major source of energy for cells. Without a steady supply of energy, cells cannot function and they die.

Sugars, starches, and most kinds of fiber are carbohydrates. Plants make carbohydrates by using the sun's energy to combine the carbon, oxygen, and hydrogen atoms from carbon dioxide (*carbo-*) and water (*-hydrate*). Thus, plants are rich sources of carbohydrates. A carbohydrate is an organic nutrient because it contains carbon.

Your cells can metabolize ("burn") the basic chemical units of most carbohydrates. This vital process releases energy that powers various forms of cellular work, including muscle contraction, enzyme production, and bone growth. Although you need some carbohydrates for energy, consuming too much carbohydrates, as well as the other macronutrients, can lead to extra body fat. This section of Unit 5 introduces the major types of carbohydrates and their primary food sources.

Sunlight

Carbohydrates:
• Fiber
• Sugars
• Starch

CO_2

O_2

H_2O

Cupcakes: © McGraw-Hill Education; Corn plant: © Pixtal/AGE Fotostock RF

carbohydrates class of nutrients that is a major source of energy for the body

5.1a Simple Carbohydrates: Sugars

You probably think of *sugar* as the sweet, white, granulated crystals that you sprinkle on cereal or into iced tea. However, this sweetener, which is commonly called "table sugar," is only one type of sugar. Sugars are a group of carbohydrates—simple carbohydrates.

You can often identify simple carbohydrates by their chemical names. If you read the ingredients on a food label and you see a substance that has "ose" at the end of its name, it's probably a carbohydrate. For example, the chemical name for table sugar is sucrose.

Monosaccharides

The simplest type of sugar, the **monosaccharide**, a "single sugar," is the basic chemical unit of carbohydrates. The three most important dietary monosaccharides are

- **Glucose,** which is commonly called "blood sugar," is a primary fuel for muscle and other cells. Red blood cells and nervous system cells, including your brain, must use glucose for energy under normal conditions. Thus, a healthy body maintains its blood glucose levels carefully. Fruits and vegetables, especially grapes, berries, corn, and carrots, are good food sources of glucose.

Glucose

- **Galactose** isn't commonly found as a single sugar in foods. The monosaccharide, however, is a component of lactose, the form of carbohydrate in milk.

Galactose

- **Fructose** ("fruit sugar" or levulose) is found naturally in fruit, honey, and a few vegetables, particularly cabbage, green beans, and asparagus. Your body has little use for fructose but can convert the simple sugar into glucose. Note that the chemical structure of fructose is different than that of glucose and galactose. This difference explains why fructose tastes sweeter than other natural sugars.

Fructose

Sugar bowl: © FoodCollection/SuperStockRF; Honey and dish of yogurt: © Wendy Schiff; Carrots: © I. Rozenbaum & F. Cirou/PhotoAlto RF; Strawberries in bowl: © Ingram Publishing/SuperStock RF; Mixed fruit: © Davod Cook/blueshiftstudios/Alamy RF

monosaccharide simple sugar that's the basic molecule of carbohydrates

glucose monosaccharide that is a primary fuel for muscles and other cells; "blood sugar"

galactose monosaccharide that is a component of lactose

fructose monosaccharide in fruits, honey, and certain vegetables; "levulose" or "fruit sugar"

disaccharide simple sugar comprised of two monosaccharides

lactose disaccharide comprised of a glucose and a galactose molecule; "milk sugar"

maltose disaccharide comprised of two glucose molecules; "malt sugar"

sucrose disaccharide comprised of a glucose and a fructose molecule; "table sugar"

Disaccharides

A **disaccharide** is a simple sugar comprised of two monosaccharides. Disaccharides include maltose, lactose, and sucrose.

- **Lactose,** which can be referred to as "milk sugar," is comprised of a galactose molecule and a glucose molecule.

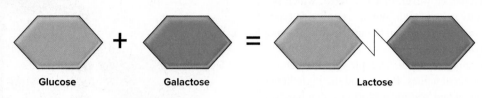

Glucose + Galactose = Lactose

Although most animal foods aren't sources of carbohydrate, milk and some products made from milk, such as ice cream, contain lactose.

- **Maltose** ("malt sugar") has two glucose molecules bonded together. Few foods contain maltose naturally, but the monosaccharide can be made from the breakdown of certain, more complex, carbohydrates. Food manufacturers use high-maltose syrup as a flavoring ingredient in sweets. High-maltose syrup is also used to brew beer.

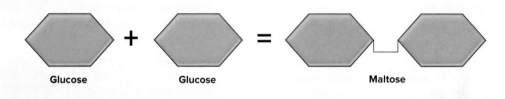

Glucose + Glucose = Maltose

- **Sucrose** ("table sugar"), the familiar sweetener, consists of one molecule of glucose and one of fructose.

Glucose + Fructose = Sucrose

Although sucrose occurs naturally in foods such as honey, maple syrup, carrots, and pineapples, much of the sucrose in the American diet is refined from sugar cane and sugar beets. The refining process strips away the small amounts of vitamins and minerals in sugar cane and sugar beets. This explains why refined sugars such as table sugar are called empty calories.

The GI tract digests sucrose into glucose and fructose molecules. Therefore, your body can't distinguish whether the glucose or fructose came from table sugar or honey.

Sugar cane field in Hawai'i

Nutrition Fact or Fiction?

Sugar makes children hyperactive.

If you've ever attended a child's birthday party, you can understand why people often blame sugary foods for causing "hyper" behavior. The results of scientific studies, however, don't indicate that sugar is a cause of *attention deficit hyperactivity disorder*, also known as *ADHD*.[2] Children with ADHD are impulsive and have difficulty controlling their behavior and paying attention. The cause of ADHD is uncertain, but genetic and environmental factors play important roles. When children attend parties, their excitement and lack of self-control are more likely caused by the situation than by their sugar intake.

It's possible that caffeine is responsible for children's "hyper" behavior. Caffeine is a stimulant drug. Sources of caffeine in children's diets include "energy drinks"; certain sugar-sweetened soft drinks, such as colas; and chocolate.

Natural sugars, such as the lactose in milk, fructose in orange juice, and glucose in grapes, make up a small percentage of all sugars in our diet. Most of the sugars that Americans eat are added to foods to sweeten them. Such refined sugars (**added sugars**) include sucrose and high-fructose corn syrup (HFCS), which Neill mentioned in the unit opener.

Table 5.1 provides a comparison of the energy and selected nutrient contents of various sweeteners, including table sugar and honey. A tablespoon of white table sugar is almost 100% sucrose; a tablespoon of honey has glucose, fructose, water, and a small amount of sucrose. A tablespoon of honey contains more protein and micronutrients than a tablespoon of white sugar, but the amounts are insignificant. For example, you would have to eat about a cup of honey to obtain 1 g protein, 1.6 mg vitamin C, and 1.4 mg iron. That amount of honey supplies over 1000 kcal! Although honey contains beneficial phytochemicals, the amounts are too small to make the sweetener a valuable source of these substances. All of the sweeteners listed in Table 5.1 are sources of empty calories.

added sugars sugars added to foods during processing or preparation

TABLE 5.1

NUTRITIONAL COMPARISON OF SELECTED SWEETENERS

Sugar/Syrup 1 Tablespoon	Water %	Kcal	Protein g	Carb g	Vit. C mg	Calcium mg	Niacin mg	Potassium mg	Iron mg	Zinc mg
Honey	17	64	0.06	17.3	0.1	1	0.025	11	0.09	0.05
White granulated sugar	0	49	0	12.6	0	0	0	0	0.01	0
Maple syrup (100% maple)	32	52	0.01	13.4	0	20	0.016	42	0.02	0.29
High-fructose corn syrup (HFCS)	24	53	0	14.4	0	0	0	0	0.01	0
Brown sugar	1	52	0.02	13.5	0	11	0.015	18	0.10	0
Molasses	22	58	0	15.0	0	41	0.186	293	0.94	0.06

Source: Data from *USDA National nutrient database for standard reference, release 28.*

Children at party: © Digital Vision/Getty Images RF; Karo and molasses, Maple syrup: © Wendy Schiff

What *IS* That?------→

When dried, the leaves of the South American shrub *Stevia rebaudiana* Bertoni are very sweet. *Rebiana* is the common name for the highly purified form of the chemical (rebaudioside A) in stevia leaves that's responsible for their intense sweetness. The Food and Drug Administration (FDA) considers rebiana safe for use as an all-purpose sweetener.

You may be able to buy stevia plants at nurseries. By placing the plants in a sunny location and watering them when necessary, you can encourage the plants to grow in your garden or home. To enjoy this natural sweetener, pick the leaves and allow them to dry. Then crush some dried leaves and use a small amount to sweeten drinks and foods.

TASTY **Tidbits**

Agave nectar is a nutritive sweetener made from the blue agave, a plant that is native to southwestern United States and Mexico. The nectar is produced from mature agaves and refined into a mild-flavored syrup that can be used like honey to sweeten foods and beverages. Nutritionally, agave nectar is similar to honey, and as an added sugar, it provides no remarkable health benefits.[3] Because the body can convert excess carbohydrates, including fructose, to fat, you should use small amounts of the sweetener.

© Wendy Schiff

Young blue agave

Answer This

According to Table 5.1, which nutritive sweetener provides the most potassium per tablespoon? You can find the answer on the last page of this unit.

5.1b Nutritive Sweeteners

Sugars and syrups are nutritive sweeteners because they contribute energy to foods. Each gram of a mono- or disaccharide supplies 4 kcal. If one of the nutritive sweeteners listed in **Figure 5.1** is the first or second ingredient listed on a product's label, the food probably contains a high amount of sugar.

Fructose tastes much sweeter than glucose and is easily made from corn. Therefore, food manufacturers often add large amounts of HFCS when they make sugar-sweetened "regular" soft drinks, candies, and baked goods. **Table 5.2** indicates the amounts of added sugars, such as table sugar and HFCS, that are in typical servings of commonly consumed foods and beverages.

*The % DV (DV) tells you how much a nutrient in a serving of food contributes to a daily diet. 2000 calories a day is used for general nutrition advice.

INGREDIENTS: Raw sugar, brown sugar, table sugar, turbinado sugar, confectioner's or powdered sugar, coconut sugar, date sugar, corn sweeteners, corn syrup, high-fructose corn syrup (HFCS), cultured corn syrup, high-maltose corn syrup, agave nectar, maple syrup, molasses, honey, fruit juice concentrate, fruit juice sweetener, glucose, dextrose, polydextrose, fructose (levulose), invert sugar, lactose, maltose, maltodextrin, sorbitol, mannitol, xylitol, erythritol

Figure 5.1 Sugars and other nutritive sweeteners. You can determine the sources of added sugars in a product by reading the ingredients list on the label.

TABLE 5.2

HOW MUCH ADDED SUGAR IS IN THAT FOOD?

Food	Serving Size	Kcal	Approximate Teaspoons Added Sugars
Doughnut, cake	3¼″ diameter	226	🥄🥄
Chocolate chip cookies, commercial brand	2 medium (50 g)	239	🥄🥄🥄🥄
Sugar-frosted cornflakes	¾ cup	114	🥄🥄🥄
Chocolate-flavored 2% milk	1 cup	158	🥄🥄🥄
Ice cream, vanilla, light, soft-serve	½ cup	111	🥄🥄
Chocolate candy bar with almonds	1.76 oz	235	🥄🥄🥄🥄🥄
Apple pie, double crust	⅙ 8″ diameter pie	277	🥄🥄🥄🥄
Snack sponge cake with cream filling	1 cake (43 g)	157	🥄🥄🥄🥄
Yogurt, vanilla low-fat	8 oz	193	🥄🥄🥄🥄
Cola, canned	12 fl oz	136	🥄🥄🥄🥄 🥄🥄🥄🥄
Fruit punch drink	12 fl oz	175	🥄🥄🥄🥄 🥄🥄🥄🥄
Chocolate milkshake, fast food	16 fl oz	580	🥄🥄🥄🥄🥄 🥄🥄🥄🥄🥄

Adapted from: Krebs-Smith SM: Choose beverages and foods to moderate your intake of sugars:
Measurement requires quantification. *Journal of Nutrition* 131: 527S, 2006.

alternative sweeteners
substances that are added to
sweeten foods while providing
few or no kilocalories

**nonnutritive ("artificial")
sweeteners** group of
manufactured alternative
sweeteners that are intensely
sweet-tasting compared to sugar

Alternative Sweeteners

Alternative sweeteners are substances added to food that sweeten the item while providing fewer calories per serving than sucrose or no calories. Alternative sweeteners that provide calories include sugar alcohols: *sorbitol, xylitol, erythritol* (Nectresse™), and *mannitol*. Unlike sugars, sugar alcohols don't promote dental decay. Thus, these compounds are used to replace sucrose in products such as sugar-free chewing gums, breath mints, and "diabetic" candies. Sugar alcohols aren't fully absorbed by the intestinal tract, and as a result, they supply an average of 2 kcal/g. Except for erythritol, sugar alcohols can cause diarrhea when consumed in large amounts.

Nonnutritive ("artificial") sweeteners are a group of manufactured alternative sweeteners that include

- saccharin,
- aspartame,
- acesulfame-K,
- sucralose,
- neotame,
- Monk fruit extract, and
- stevia leaf extracts.

Nonnutritive sweeteners taste very sweet when compared to the taste of the same amount of sugar (**Table 5.3**). Thus, a very small amount of a nonnutritive sweetener is needed to sweeten a food. These sweeteners supply no energy per serving as a result.

Nonnutritive sweeteners may help people control their energy intake and manage their body weight without increasing their appetite.[4] However, most "sugar-free" or "diabetic" foods aren't calorie free. Furthermore, results of some studies suggest that artificially sweetened foods and beverages can promote excess calorie consumption. Why? More research is needed, but the taste of products that contain artificial sweeteners may interfere with a person's ability to learn how to regulate his or her intake of sugary foods and beverages.[5]

TABLE 5.3

COMPARING ALTERNATIVE SWEETENERS

Sweetener	Comparison to Sugar/Serving*	Brand Name	Kilocalories/serving
Aspartame	160–220 times sweeter	NutraSweet®, Equal®	Nearly 0
Saccharin	300 times sweeter	Sweet'N Low®, Sugar Twin®, Necta Sweet®	0
Acesulfame-K	200 times sweeter	Sunett®, Sweet One®	0
Neotame	7,000–13,000 times sweeter	Neotame	0
Sucralose	600 times sweeter	Splenda®	0
Stevia leaf extracts such as rebaudioside A	250 times sweeter	Truvia®, SweetLeaf®, Rebiana	0
Erythritol	60 to 80% as sweet	Nectresse™	<5

*Source: Position of the Academy of Nutrition and Dietetics: Use of nutritive and nonnutritive sweeteners. *Journal of the Academy of Nutrition and Dietetics*, 112(5): 739, 2012.

TASTY Tidbits

Honey can contain spores of the deadly bacterium *Clostridium botulinum* that resist being destroyed by food preservation methods.[6] These spores can become active within an infant's intestinal tract and produce a poison that's extremely toxic to nerves. Therefore, honey shouldn't be fed to children younger than 12 months of age or used to sweeten infant foods because it may cause botulism poisoning.[6] Older children and adults can eat honey safely because the mature stomach produces enough acid to destroy the bacterial spores.

Are Artificial Sweeteners Safe?

According to the Academy of Nutrition and Dietetics, all nonnutritive sweeteners that have been approved by the U.S. Food and Drug Administration are safe.[4] A group of international health and safety organizations, including the FDA, have established *Acceptable Daily Intakes* (*ADIs*) for certain nonnutritive sweeteners (**Table 5.4**). An ADI is the amount of an artificial sweetener that you can consume safely on a daily basis, throughout your life.[4]

What About Aspartame?

Aspartame consists of two amino acids (the building blocks of proteins): phenylalanine and aspartic acid. Some people must avoid aspartame and certain protein-rich foods because they have *phenylketonuria* (*PKU*) (*fen´-il-kee´-toe-nur´-e-ah*). PKU is a rare, inherited disorder that results in the body's inability to use phenylalanine properly. To diagnose PKU, physicians generally rely on a simple blood test that's conducted on infants within 48 hours after their birth. If an infant with PKU isn't treated with a special diet, phenylalanine accumulates in the child's bloodstream and causes severe brain damage. The FDA requires the following warning statement on the label of any food that contains aspartame:

PHENYLKETONURICS: CONTAINS PHENYLALANINE.[7]

Baby: © Stacy Schmitt; Dr. Pepper & warning statement: © Wendy Schiff; Placemat: © McGraw-Hill Education. Mark A. Dierker, photographer

Source: Mattes RD, Popkin BM: Non-nutritive sweetener consumption in humans: Effects on appetite and food intake and their putative mechanisms. *American Journal of Clinical Nutrition* 89(1): 1, 2009.

TABLE 5.4

ACCEPTABLE DAILY INTAKES FOR SOME NONNUTRITIVE SWEETENERS

Food/Beverage	Nonnutritive Sweetener	Amount
Diet cola	Aspartame	18 to 19 12-oz cans
Packets	Saccharin	9 to 12 packets
Lemon-lime soft drink	Acesulfame-K	30 to 32 12-oz cans
Diet cola	Sucralose	6 12-oz cans

polysaccharides compounds comprised of more than 10 monosaccharides bonded together

starch storage form of glucose in plants

glycogen storage form of glucose in humans and other animals

dietary fiber (fiber) indigestible plant material; most types are polysaccharides

soluble fiber forms of dietary fiber that dissolve or swell in water

insoluble fiber forms of dietary fiber that generally don't dissolve in water

5.1c Starches

Plant and animal cells can combine glucose molecules into long chains called **polysaccharides.** Cells use polysaccharides to store energy; plant cells also use polysaccharides to make structural components such as stems and leaves. The most common dietary polysaccharides consist of hundreds of glucose molecules and include digestible and indigestible forms.

Starch and Glycogen

Plants store glucose as polysaccharides called **starch.** Your intestinal tract can digest starch into individual glucose molecules that can be absorbed.

Glycogen

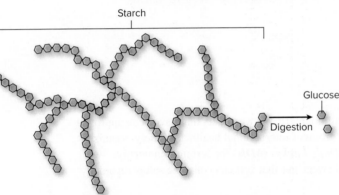

Starch digestion results in glucose molecules.

Seeds, roots, and fleshy underground stems called *tubers* often contain starch. Thus, starchy foods include:

- bread and cereal products made from wheat, rice, barley, and oats;

- vegetables such as corn, squash, beans, and peas;

- *tubers* such as potatoes, yams, taro, cassava, and jicama.

Animals store glucose as the polysaccharide **glycogen** ("animal starch"). The human body stores limited amounts of glycogen. Muscles and the liver are the major sites for glycogen formation and storage. Although muscles contain glycogen, most animal foods (for example, meat or the flesh of fish and poultry) aren't sources of carbohydrate because muscle glycogen breaks down soon after an animal dies.

5.1d Fiber

Most forms of **dietary fiber** ("fiber") are comprised of monosaccharides, such as glucose, but they're in a form that people can't digest. Cellulose, hemicellulose, pectin, gums, and mucilages are carbohydrate forms of fiber. Lignin, which is in woody parts and seeds of plants, is the only type of fiber that isn't carbohydrate.

When the undigested fiber is in the large intestine, it serves as an energy source for the bacteria that normally live there. Any fiber that the bacteria don't use is eliminated in feces. Keep in mind that only plant foods provide fiber; animal flesh contains *muscle* fibers, which are digestible proteins.

There are two types of fiber: **soluble fiber** and **insoluble fiber**:

- Soluble fiber dissolves or swells in water.

- Insoluble fiber generally doesn't dissolve in water.

TABLE 5.5

CLASSIFYING FIBER

Type	Component(s)	Physiological Effects	Food Sources
Insoluble	Cellulose, hemicelluloses	Increases fecal bulk and speeds fecal passage through large intestine	All plants Wheat, rye, brown rice, vegetables
	Lignin	Increases fecal bulk, may ease bowel movements	Whole grains, wheat bran
Soluble	Pectins, gums, mucilages, some hemicelluloses	Delays stomach emptying; slows glucose absorption; can lower blood cholesterol	Apples, bananas, citrus fruits, carrots, oats, barley, psyllium seeds, beans, and thickeners added to foods

Although fiber isn't digested by humans, soluble and insoluble fiber provide important health benefits. Soluble fiber binds cholesterol and slows glucose absorption. As a result, soluble fiber can help reduce blood cholesterol and glucose levels. Insoluble fiber increases fecal "bulk," which contributes to good health by easing bowel movements. **Table 5.5** provides information about the solubility of various types of fiber, effects of fiber in the body, and major food sources of soluble and insoluble fiber. It's important to note that plant foods usually contain both forms. **Table 5.6** lists some foods and their fiber contents.

TABLE 5.6

DIETARY FIBER CONTENT OF COMMON FOODS

Food	Fiber (g)	Food	Fiber (g)
Split peas, cooked (1 cup)	16.3	Beans, green snap, cooked (1 cup)	4.0
Black beans, cooked (1 cup)	15.0	Banana, sliced (1 cup)	3.9
Oat bran, raw (1 cup)	14.5	Prunes, dried uncooked (5 prunes)	3.5
Kidney beans, canned (1 cup)	11.0	Orange, raw (1 orange)	3.4
Chickpeas, canned (1 cup)	10.6	Strawberries, raw, sliced (1 cup)	3.3
Baked beans, canned (1 cup)	10.4	Carrots, raw, grated (1/2 cup)	3.1
Kellogg's All-Bran cereal (1/2 cup)	9.1	Barley, cooked (½ cup)	3.0
Raspberries, raw (1 cup)	8.0	Almonds (1 ounce)	2.8
Blackberries (1 cup)	7.6	Broccoli, chopped, cooked (1/2 cup)	2.6
Green peas, frozen, cooked (1/2 cup)	7.2	Whole-grain bread, toasted (1 slice)	1.9
Kellogg's Raisin Bran (1 cup)	6.7	Romaine lettuce, shredded (1 cup)	1.0
Apple, raw, with skin (3" diameter)	4.4	Iceberg lettuce, shredded (1 cup)	0.9
Baked potato, with skin (approx. 6.5 oz)	4.0	White bread (1 slice)	0.8

Source: Data from U.S. Department of Agriculture, Agricultural Research Service, USDA National Nutrient Data Laboratory: *USDA Nutrient database for standard reference, release 28,* 2015.

Fruit, nut, and vegetable display: Source: Keith Weller/USDA/ARS; Pea pod, Almonds, Romaine lettuce: © Food Collection/StockFood RF

5.1e How Much Carbohydrate Should You Eat?

Nutritionally adequate diets should provide 45 to 65% of total energy from carbohydrates.[8] The average diet of adult Americans supplies about 48% of calories from carbohydrates (**Fig. 5.2**).[9] This amount includes calories from complex carbohydrates as well as sugars.

Added Sugars

In 2014, Americans, on average, consumed almost 23 teaspoons of added sugars per person per day, which is a little more than 18% of the energy in a diet that supplies 2000 kcal/day.[1] According to the U.S. Dietary Guidelines, people should limit their added sugars intake to less than 10% of total calories. If you follow a 2000 kcal/day diet, you should limit your added sugars intake to 12 teaspoons per day.[10]

The main source of added sugars in Americans' diets is sugar-sweetened beverages, which include carbonated regular soft drinks, fruit "ades," sweetened coffees and teas, and energy drinks.[10] A 12-ounce can of a cola-flavored, sugar-sweetened soft drink contains about 33 g of HFCS, which is about 8 teaspoons of table sugar.[11] A 12-ounce serving of 100% orange juice supplies 31 g of natural sugars. They both contain similar amounts of sugars, so should you drink sugar-sweetened soft drinks instead of fruit juices? Unlike colas and other soft drinks, 100% fruit juices, such as orange, grapefruit, and cranberry juice, contribute water-soluble vitamins and antioxidant phytochemicals to your diet. According to MyPlate, adults should consume 1½ to 2 cups of fruit or fruit equivalents each day, some of which can be 100% fruit juice.

TASTY Tidbits

Canned fruit is often packed in a sugary syrup. Consider buying canned fruit that's packed in water or its own juice. If you have canned fruit that's in syrup, rinse the fruit in plain water before serving it. Also choose frozen fruit that has no sugar added.

© Wendy Schiff

The following tips can help you reduce your intake of sugar-sweetened drinks:

- Replace soft drinks with a naturally calorie-free thirst-quencher—plain water. Make plain water more interesting to drink by adding to it a slice of lemon or lime, or a few fresh or frozen berries.

- Add 1 part club soda to 1 part orange or other 100% fruit juice to make a refreshing carbonated drink.

- Avoid fruit "drinks," "punches," "blends," "cocktails," or "ades" because they often contain high amounts of added sugars and very little fruit juice.

- Limit your intake of pre-sweetened flavored coffees and teas. To save money, make your own coffee and tea, so you can control the amount of table sugar added. An even better idea: Learn to drink tea and coffee without sugar!

Appendix I has tips for reducing the amount of sugar in your favorite recipes.

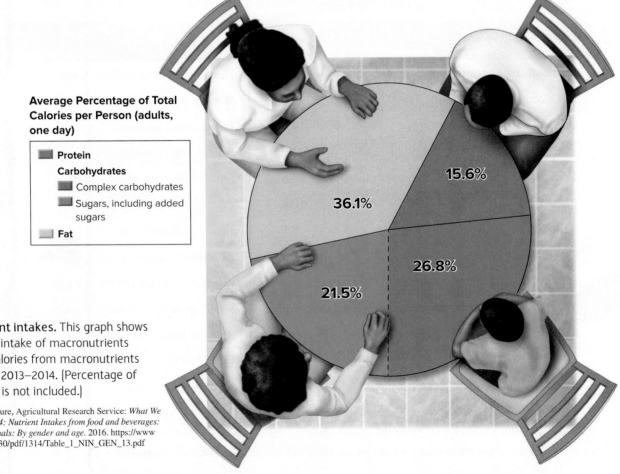

Average Percentage of Total Calories per Person (adults, one day)

- Protein
- Carbohydrates
  - Complex carbohydrates
  - Sugars, including added sugars
- Fat

15.6%
36.1%
26.8%
21.5%

Figure 5.2 Macronutrient intakes. This graph shows adult Americans' average intake of macronutrients as percentages of total calories from macronutrients (2064 kcal) on one day in 2013–2014. (Percentage of total energy from alcohol is not included.)

Source: U.S. Department of Agriculture, Agricultural Research Service: *What We Eat in America, NHANES 2013–2014: Nutrient Intakes from food and beverages: Mean amounts consumed by individuals: By gender and age.* 2016. https://www.ars.usda.gov/ARSUserFiles/80400530/pdf/1314/Table_1_NIN_GEN_13.pdf Accessed: November 14, 2016

Module 5.2

What Happens to the Carbohydrates You Eat?

© John A. Rizzo/Getty Images RF

5.2 - Learning Outcomes

After reading Module 5.2, you should be able to

1. Define all of the key terms in this module.

2. Describe how the body digests carbohydrates and uses the macronutrient for energy.

3. Explain how the body regulates its blood glucose level.

If you eat cooked oatmeal made with milk and sweetened with a little brown sugar for breakfast, what happens to the carbohydrates in these foods? The carbohydrates in oats are primarily starch and fiber; mixing milk and brown sugar with the cereal adds lactose and sucrose. **Figure 5.3** indicates the main steps of digesting carbohydrates, including the kinds that are in this meal. Note the enzymes, such as **salivary amylase**, that are involved in this process.

Figure 5.3, step 5, shows that bacteria in your large intestine metabolize (ferment) some fiber for their nutrient needs. The metabolic by-products that result can be used for energy by the cells that line your large intestine. However, a gram of fiber adds less than 3 kcal to human diets.[8] Americans, on average, consume only about 17 g of fiber daily; therefore, fiber contributes relatively little to a typical person's total energy intake.[9]

salivary amylase enzyme secreted by the salivary glands that begins starch digestion in the mouth

maltase enzyme that breaks down maltose into two glucose molecules

sucrase enzyme that breaks down sucrose into a glucose and a fructose molecule

lactase intestinal enzyme that breaks down lactose into glucose and galactose

1 **Mouth**
Some starch is broken down to maltose by salivary amylase.

2 **Stomach**
The activity of salivary amylase soon stops in the acidic environment of the stomach.

3 **Small intestine**
The small intestine is the primary site of carbohydrate digestion and absorption. The pancreas releases pancreatic amylase into the small intestine that continues the breakdown of starches into maltose molecules. The microvilli (see Unit 4) release enzymes that digest maltose and other dissacharides. **Maltase** digests maltose into glucose. **Sucrase** digests sucrose into glucose and fructose. **Lactase** breaks down lactose into glucose and galactose. Small intestinal cells absorb glucose, fructose, and galactose.

4 **Liver**
Glucose, fructose, and galactose are transported to the liver. The liver converts fructose and galactose to glucose.

5 **Large intestine**
Some soluble fiber is fermented by bacteria in the large intestine. This process results in intestinal gas production.

6 **Rectum**
Very little dietary carbohydrate is excreted in feces. Intestinal gas is expelled via the anus.

Figure 5.3 Carbohydrate digestion, absorption, and elimination.

■ *What are the end products of carbohydrate digestion?*

5.2a Maintaining Normal Blood Glucose Levels

Glucose is a major fuel for your cells. Therefore, hormones carefully maintain your blood glucose level. Your pancreas contains various types of cells, including beta and alpha cells. Beta cells produce **insulin**, and alpha cells make **glucagon**. These two hormones play key roles in regulating blood glucose levels. If you're healthy, insulin and glucagon help maintain your blood glucose level between 70 and 110 milligrams per deciliter of blood (mg/dl).[12] **Essential Concept 5.1** illustrates how insulin and glucagon help regulate your body's blood glucose level.

insulin hormone that helps regulate blood glucose levels

glucagon hormone that helps raise blood glucose levels

Essential Concept

5.1 How Your Body Regulates Your Blood Glucose

Blood vessel

Glucose

2 You may grab a piece of fruit, some crackers, or a sandwich to eat, and as the carbohydrates in these foods are digested, glucose is absorbed into your bloodstream. Now, your blood glucose level begins to rise.

1 If you haven't eaten for a while, your blood glucose level begins to fall, you start to feel hungry, and your stomach growls.

Range of healthy blood glucose level

3 Your pancreas responds by releasing insulin into the bloodstream.

4 Insulin helps lower blood glucose levels because the hormone enables glucose to enter most cells. One result of insulin's action—you feel satisfied with your snack or meal and are no longer hungry.

2a If you ignore the hunger signals and don't eat, your blood glucose level drops. Your pancreas responds by releasing glucagon into the bloodstream.

3a Glucagon opposes insulin's effects by promoting the breakdown of glycogen in the liver. This process adds glucose to the bloodstream, boosting your blood glucose level.

Pancreas

Insulin

Cell

Pancreas

Glucagon

Liver

Glycogen

5.2b The Fate of Glucose

What happens to glucose after it enters a cell? If your muscles and other cells that use glucose need energy, they'll metabolize the simple sugar for energy. When you're well fed and resting, your body stores the extra glucose as glycogen. When glycogen storage reaches maximum capacity, your liver can convert the excess glucose into fat and release it into the bloodstream. Fat cells remove and store the fat. Thus, eating too many foods that are sources of glucose may contribute to excess energy intakes and weight gain.

Glucose for Energy

Cells metabolize glucose to release the energy that's stored in the molecule. Glucose is a primary fuel for the body's cells. Furthermore, red blood cells as well as brain and other nervous system cells burn mostly glucose for energy. Regardless of its source, each gram of glucose supplies 4 kcal. Glucose is a "clean-burning" fuel—cells can burn it completely, releasing carbon dioxide gas and water as waste products. Units 4 and 10 provide more information about energy metabolism. Appendix D summarizes the primary chemical pathways that cells use to metabolize glucose for energy.

Cells need a small amount of glucose to metabolize fat for energy properly. When a person is fasting, starving, or following a very low-carbohydrate/high-protein diet (the Atkins diet, for example), his or her cells must use greater-than-normal amounts of fat for

© Alan Marsh/DesignPics RF

"Fat burns in a flame of carbohydrate."

energy. When this situation occurs, there isn't enough glucose available for cells to metabolize the fat efficiently. As a result, excessive amounts of *ketone bodies* ("ketones") form.

Ketone bodies are chemicals that result from the incomplete metabolism of fat for energy. Muscle and brain cells can use ketone bodies for energy. People who have poorly controlled diabetes form too many ketone bodies. The excess ketone bodies disrupt the body's ability to maintain normal blood chemistry, resulting in loss of consciousness and even death. This serious condition is called ketoacidosis. The Recommended Dietary Allowance (RDA) for carbohydrate is 130 g/day.[8] This amount of carbohydrate is enough to prevent excess ketone body formation.

Amino acids are the "building blocks" of proteins. Under normal conditions, your cells obtain a small proportion of their energy needs by converting certain amino acids into glucose. Starvation diets lack sources of energy such as glucose and amino acids. To meet the body's energy needs, the starving person's skeletal muscles and other tissues sacrifice amino acids from their proteins for glucose production. Using muscle proteins for energy extends the person's survival time, but results in muscle wasting, weakness, and eventually, death. Thus, you need some carbohydrate in your diet to "spare" your body's tissue proteins from being used for energy.

ketone bodies chemicals that result from the incomplete breakdown of fat for energy

© Don Hammond/DesignPics RF

Module 5.3

Carbohydrates and Health

5.3 - Learning Outcomes

After reading Module 5.3, you should be able to

1. Define all of the key terms in this module.

2. Discuss the effects of excess carbohydrate consumption on health.

3. Discuss differences between type 1 and type 2 diabetes and list common signs and symptoms of each disorder.

4. Identify risk factors for type 2 diabetes and measures that may prevent this disease.

5. Explain how carbohydrates can contribute to dental decay.

6. Explain the health benefits of soluble and insoluble fiber.

7. Explain why lactose intolerance occurs, and discuss dietary measures that will reduce signs and symptoms of the disorder.

© McGraw-Hill Education. Ken Carp, photographer

5.3a Are Carbohydrates Fattening?

Americans are fatter now than they were 20 years ago. Do carbohydrates cause obesity? Excess calorie intakes from carbohydrates, as well as fat, protein, and alcohol, contribute to excess body fat. When a person consumes excess carbohydrate, his or her body converts some of the glucose into fat, but much of the excess is "burned" as a biological fuel. As a result, dietary fat is spared from being used as a fuel, and it's stored in fat cells. Thus, eating too much digestible carbohydrate contributes to unwanted weight gain.

Foods that contain large amounts of refined carbohydrates, especially added sugars, may not satisfy hunger as well as those that contain more protein, fat, and/or fiber. As a result, you may become hungrier sooner after eating a meal or snack that contains a lot of added sugars and refined starches than if you ate a high-protein, high-fat, or high-fiber meal or snack.

Some nutrition scientists think Americans' love of soft drinks that are sweetened with HFCS is largely responsible for the population's rising rate of obesity.[13, 14] People who drink sugar-sweetened soft drinks ("liquid candy") may not reduce their energy intake from solid food accordingly, so they consume too many calories and gain body fat.

Thus, drinking sugar-sweetened soft drinks may increase the risk of type 2 diabetes.[13] More research is needed to understand how sugary soft drinks might contribute to obesity.

Recall that each gram of fat supplies more than twice the calories as a gram of carbohydrate. People, however, often blame carbohydrates for their unwanted weight gain. Why? Starches and sugars are often combined with "hidden fats" such as butter, oil, or shortening in processed foods. Fats make foods taste rich and creamy, and are difficult to resist. By adding sugar to the food, the sweet taste masks the bland taste of fat. How easy is it for you to limit your intakes of eating energy-dense foods that combine "carbs" with fat, such as snack chips, candy bars, cakes, cookies, and pies?

Can you eat just one?

© Darren Greenwood/DesignPics RF

5.3b What Is Diabetes?

Diabetes mellitus (diabetes) is a serious chronic disease in which the body is unable to regulate its blood glucose level properly. The disease is characterized by blood glucose levels that remain abnormally high, even in the fasting state. There are two major types of diabetes mellitus—type 1 and type 2. Among adults with diabetes, 5% have

Should you be like Neill Warrington, who was quoted in the opener of this unit, and use honey to sweeten foods? Is honey a more nutritious sweetener than table sugar? Would you recommend that Neill use agave syrup as a sweetener instead of honey? Explain why you would or wouldn't make this recommendation.

type 1.[15] The majority of adults with diabetes have type 2. Both types of diabetes can affect any person, regardless of age.

Fasting blood glucose levels that are

- 70 to 99 mg/dl are normal;
- 100 to 125 mg/dl indicate pre-diabetes;
- 126 mg/dl or more indicate diabetes.

One out of three adult Americans has pre-diabetes.[16] People with pre-diabetes are very likely to develop diabetes within 5 years, unless they take steps to lower their risk.[16] Some people with diabetes have high blood glucose levels because their bodies don't produce any insulin or don't produce enough to meet their needs. In other cases, the people with the disease produce insulin, but their cells don't respond properly to the hormone (insulin resistance).

In addition to high fasting blood glucose levels, people with diabetes usually experience

- excessive thirst,
- frequent urination,
- blurry vision,
- vaginal yeast infections (adult women),
- foot pain, abdominal pain,
- impotence (male), and
- sores that don't heal.

People with poorly controlled type 1 diabetes also tend to have

- increased appetite with weight loss,
- breath that smells like fruit,
- fatigue, and
- confusion.

© Mark Schiff

Device that's used for testing blood glucose level

Over time, untreated or poorly controlled diabetes damages nerves, organs, and blood vessels. For adult Americans, diabetes is a major cause of heart disease, kidney failure, blindness, and lower limb amputations. The disease is the seventh-leading cause of death in the United States.[15]

The number of people with diabetes is increasing at an alarming rate. In 2014, an estimated 29.1 million Americans had diabetes; 21 million of these persons were diagnosed with diabetes, and the remainder didn't know they had the disease.[15]

Type 1 Diabetes

Type 1 diabetes is an *autoimmune* disease. Such diseases occur when certain immune system cells don't recognize the body's own insulin-producing cells of the pancreas (beta cells). As a result, the immune system cells attack and destroy the pancreatic cells. It isn't clear why the immune cells malfunction, but genetic susceptibility and environmental factors, particularly exposure to certain viral intestinal infections, are associated with the development of type 1 diabetes.[17]

A person with type 1 diabetes must obtain insulin by injections or via a device that's commonly called an "insulin pump." The device, which is usually worn on a waistband or belt, has a container for insulin. The insulin pump is programmed to deliver the hormone through a small tube that's inserted under the patient's skin.

© Realistic Reflections RF

An insulin pump in use

Type 2 Diabetes

The most common form of diabetes is type 2 diabetes. Beta cells of people with type 2 diabetes usually produce insulin, but the body's cells are *insulin-resistant*, which means they don't respond properly to the hormone. As a result, the blood glucose level rises to abnormal levels, and the signs of diabetes occur.

People at high risk for type 2 diabetes are

- physically inactive,
- overweight or obese,
- genetically related to a close family member with type 2 diabetes, or
- Americans with Hispanic, Native American, certain Asian, African, or Pacific Islander ancestry.[15]

Some people with type 2 diabetes can control their disease by exercising regularly and losing weight. Other persons with the condition rely on a special diet as well as medications that stimulate the pancreas to secrete insulin. The American Diabetes Association has more in-depth information about both types of diabetes. The association also has an online questionnaire that you can take to determine your risk of type 2 diabetes. You can access this questionnaire by visiting the association's website (www.diabetes.org).

Diabetes During Pregnancy

A woman who has poorly controlled diabetes can experience serious health problems, such as high blood pressure, during pregnancy. Her developing offspring (*embryo* or *fetus*) can also be harmed by its mother's lack of good blood glucose control. The first 8 weeks of pregnancy are a critical period in a human embryo's development because its organs are forming. If a pregnant woman with diabetes has poor control of her blood glucose level, her embryo/fetus can develop birth defects, grow too fat, and have abnormal blood glucose levels as a result.[18]

Women may develop diabetes during pregnancy (*gestational diabetes*). This type of diabetes usually begins around the middle of pregnancy and ends with the birth of the baby. However, women who've had gestational diabetes often experience the condition again with future pregnancies. They also have a higher risk of developing type 2 diabetes later in life, when compared to women who had healthy pregnancies.

A pregnant woman with poorly controlled diabetes or gestational diabetes is more likely to have miscarriages (death of an embryo/fetus before the 20th week of pregnancy), stillbirth (delivery of a dead baby), and premature delivery (fetus born before the 37th week of pregnancy) than a pregnant woman with diabetes who manages her blood glucose properly. Thus, pregnant women who have diabetes should monitor their blood glucose levels carefully to increase their chances of having trouble-free pregnancies and healthy newborns.

Monitoring Diabetes

To avoid or delay serious health complications, people who have diabetes need to achieve and maintain normal or near-normal blood glucose levels. This can be accomplished by carefully planning and spacing out meals and snacks as well as following treatment that is individualized to meet the patient's needs.

Many people with diabetes rely on daily blood testing to monitor their blood glucose levels (**Fig. 5.4**). Such blood tests provide a "snapshot" of a single blood glucose value at a moment in time. Physicians should also measure hemoglobin A1c ("A1c") to determine their patients' average blood glucose levels over the past 3 months.

Hemoglobin is the compound in red blood cells that carries oxygen. A very small percentage of a healthy person's hemoglobin is a form called A1c. **Table 5.7** indicates how diabetes is classified according to A1c values. In general, people with diabetes should strive to maintain their HbA1c level below 7%.[19]

People with diabetes can use another method of understanding their blood glucose control. The estimated glucose average (eGA) is a way of relating A1c to the value provided by a blood glucose meter. For more information about the eGA, visit the American Diabetes Association website: www.diabetes.org.

Can Diabetes Be Prevented?

There is no way to prevent type 1 diabetes. However, you may reduce your risk of type 2 diabetes by

- losing excess weight (if necessary),
- exercising regularly, and
- following a diet that contains less red meat and processed meats and more poultry, fish, fiber-rich whole grains, beans, fruits, and vegetables.[20]

What's the Glycemic Index?

The body digests carbohydrate-rich foods at different rates, and its blood glucose response to each food varies. This response can be rated by the glycemic index. The **glycemic index (GI)** is a value that reflects the body's blood glucose response after eating a food that supplies 50 g of digestible carbohydrates as compared to a standard amount of glucose or white bread. Foods with high GIs have values above 70. A carbohydrate-rich food such as cornflakes (GI = 80) contains large amounts of refined carbohydrates, so the cereal is digested rapidly. As a result, glucose enters the bloodstream quickly, raising blood glucose and insulin

© Wendy Schiff

Figure 5.4 **Carson Smith has type 1 diabetes.** He tests his blood glucose level at least four times a day.

■ *Why do many people with diabetes monitor their blood glucose levels?*

diabetes mellitus (diabetes) group of serious chronic diseases characterized by abnormal glucose, fat, and protein metabolism

glycemic index (GI) measure of the body's blood glucose response after eating a food that supplies 50 g of digestible carbohydrates as compared to a standard amount of glucose or white bread

TABLE 5.7	CLASSIFYING DIABETES ACCORDING TO A1C VALUES[19]	
	Diagnosis*	**A1c Level**
	Normal	Below 5.7%
	Pre-diabetes	5.7 to 6.4%
	Diabetes	6.5% or above

*Any test for diagnosing diabetes requires a second test to confirm the diagnosis, unless the patient has signs and symptoms of diabetes.

glycemic load (GL) value determined by multiplying the glycemic index of a carbohydrate-containing food by the amount of carbohydrate in a typical serving of the food

hypoglycemia condition that occurs when the blood glucose level is abnormally low

metabolic syndrome condition that increases risk of CVD

levels rapidly.[21] Carbohydrate-rich foods that have high fiber content, such as raw carrots, are digested slowly. By slowing down the rate of carbohydrate digestion, low-GI foods don't cause a dramatic increase in blood glucose and insulin levels. As a result, a person's blood glucose level is more likely to remain in the healthy range.

A related value, the **glycemic load (GL)**, is determined by multiplying a food's glycemic index by the amount of carbohydrate that's in a typical serving of the food. **Essential Concept 5.2** lists average GIs and GLs of several commonly eaten foods. High GL foods have values of more than 20.

GI and GL values can vary greatly, depending on where the food was grown, its degree of ripeness,

or the extent of its processing. Furthermore, GI and GL values reflect a *single* food's effect on blood glucose levels. The increase in blood glucose levels is often less dramatic when the food is eaten as part of a meal that contains a mixture of macronutrients. Nevertheless, you may be able to reduce your risk of type 2 diabetes by following a low GI/GL diet.[21]

5.3c What Is Hypoglycemia?

If you're healthy and haven't eaten for a while, your blood glucose level falls, and you become hungry. Eating a meal or snack raises your blood glucose. (See Essential Concept 5.1 in Module 5.2a.) **Hypoglycemia** occurs when the blood glucose level is less than 70 mg/dl.[22] In response to rapidly

Essential Concept

5.2   Glycemic Index and Glycemic Load: Average Values of Selected Foods

Glycemic Index*
(High is >70)

Glycemic Load
(High is >20)

90 | 16 (8 fl oz) — Coca-Cola

46 | 4 (8 fl oz) — Fat-free milk

89 | 16 (5 oz) — Banana

56 | 6 (4 oz) — Apple, raw

66 | 7 (1 2/3 oz) — Ice cream, vanilla reduced fat

50 | 2 (3 oz) — Carrots, raw

43 | 3 (4 oz) — Peach, canned in natural juice

79 | 6 (2/3 oz) — Popcorn

*Compared to white bread (GI = 100)

declining blood glucose levels, the body secretes the hormone epinephrine, which is also called *adrenaline*. Like glucagon, epinephrine increases the supply of glucose and fatty acids in the bloodstream, but the hormone can also make a person feel irritable, restless, shaky, and sweaty. If the blood glucose level drops too low, cells cannot obtain enough glucose for energy. The affected person becomes confused, and he or she may lose consciousness and die.

Hypoglycemia rarely affects healthy persons. Some people develop *reactive hypoglycemia* after they eat a lot of highly refined carbohydrates because the pancreas responds by releasing too much insulin. People with reactive hypoglycemia may feel better if they avoid eating large amounts of sugary foods and instead eat smaller, more frequent meals that contain a mixture of macronutrients.

5.3d Metabolic Syndrome

Do you or does someone you know have a "spare tire," a "beer belly," "love handles," or an "apple shape"?

People who are too fat often have excess abdominal fat, which can be dangerous, especially when it's accompanied by high blood pressure (*hypertension*) and high blood fat and cholesterol levels.

You have **metabolic syndrome** if you have three or more of the following signs:

- large waist circumference—equal or greater than 40 inches (men); equal to or greater than 35 inches (women),
- chronically high blood pressure,
- chronically high fasting blood fats (*triglycerides*) level,
- high fasting blood glucose level,
- high LDL cholesterol ("bad cholesterol") level.

If you have a parent, brother, or sister with type 2 diabetes, you are at risk of developing metabolic syndrome.[23]

High blood pressure may be a sign of metabolic syndrome.

Orange juice — 66 — 12 (8 fl oz)

French fries — 90 — 21 (2 oz)

Spaghetti (cooked) — 68 — 23 (6 oz)

Bagel, white plain — 99 — 24 (2 oz)

Cornflakes cereal — 80 — 21 (1 oz)

Peanuts — 10 — 0 (2 oz)

Potato, baked — 158 — 33 (5 oz)

Jelly beans — 114 — 22 (1 oz)

Source: Data from Atkinson FS and others: International tables of glycemic index and glycemic load values: 2008. *Diabetes Care* 31(12): 2281, 2008.

Compared to people who don't have metabolic syndrome, individuals with this condition have a greater risk of heart and blood vessel diseases. To lower your likelihood of developing metabolic syndrome, maintain a healthy weight; exercise regularly; increase your intake of seafood and fiber-rich foods such as fruits and vegetables; and choose fat-free or low-fat dairy foods.[23]

5.3e Sugar and Health

The body can convert excess fructose into fat, which can be stored or circulate in the bloodstream. Eating too much sugar, especially fructose, may be a risk factor for heart disease, obesity, and type 2 diabetes. Furthermore, consuming high amounts of fructose may harm the liver. Under normal conditions, the liver doesn't store fat, but the organ can accumulate the lipid in response to excess alcohol consumption. This condition is called "fatty liver." The buildup of fat can damage and kill liver cells.

Fatty liver also occurs in people who drink little or no alcohol but are obese or have diabetes. The medical term for this condition is *nonalcoholic fatty liver disease* (*NAFLD*). Although there's no specific treatment for NAFLD, losing excess body fat, avoiding alcohol, and eating a healthy diet pattern may allow the liver to heal. According to experts at the National Institutes of Health, an estimated 10 to 20% of Americans have NAFLD.[24]

5.3f Lactose Intolerance

Millions of Americans suffer from **lactose intolerance**. Lactose-intolerant people don't produce enough lactase, the enzyme that breaks down lactose into glucose and galactose. When a lactase-deficient person consumes lactose, the disaccharide isn't completely digested and absorbed by the time it enters the large intestine. Bacteria that reside in the large intestine break down lactose and produce irritating gases and acids as metabolic by-products. As a result, a lactose-intolerant person usually experiences intestinal cramps, bloating, gas, and diarrhea within a couple of hours after consuming milk or other lactose-containing products.

Normally, infants produce lactase, but by the time children are 2 years old, their small intestine begins to produce less of the enzyme. Many older children and adults, particularly those with African, Asian, and Eastern European ancestry, are lactose intolerant and experience some degree of abdominal discomfort after drinking milk. Lactose intolerance isn't the same as milk allergy. Milk allergy is an immune system response to proteins in cow's milk.

Milk and milk products are excellent sources of protein, many vitamins, and the minerals calcium and phosphorus. Some lactose-intolerant people can eat hard cheeses and yogurt without experiencing any digestive tract problems.[25] Why? Milk loses most of its lactose content when it's processed to make aged cheeses, such as cheddar and Swiss. The

lactose intolerance inability to digest lactose properly

TASTY Tidbits

Carbohydrates, especially simple sugars that stick to your teeth, contribute to tooth decay. Bacteria that live on your teeth and gums use the carbohydrate in foods for their energy needs. The bacteria produce acid that damages tooth enamel and results in decay.

Infants and young children who drink bedtime bottles of milk, juice, or other beverages that contain sugars are likely to have "nursing bottle syndrome." When a sleepy child sucks slowly on the bottle, the carbohydrate-rich solution stays in contact with teeth, increasing the likelihood of dental decay. To reduce the risk of nursing bottle syndrome, offer a young child a bottle of plain water to drink at bedtime.

bacteria used to make yogurt convert much of the lactose in milk to lactic acid.

If you suspect you cannot digest lactose, try consuming a smaller-than-usual size serving of milk and note if you have intestinal discomfort within a few hours. If you cannot tolerate even small amounts of fresh fluid milk, you can substitute soy milk for cows' milk, because soy milk doesn't contain lactose. Another choice is to drink milk that's been pretreated with lactase. Most supermarkets sell fresh lactase-treated milk in the dairy food section.

What Are FODMAPs?

Can you recall having a bellyache and/or diarrhea after eating too much candy on Halloween? FODMAPs in candy may have been the source of your discomfort. FODMAPs are carbohydrates and sugar alcohols that your GI tract may not fully digest or absorb, especially when you eat too much of them. These substances attract water while passing through the intestines, and the bacteria that reside in the large intestine can ferment FODMAPs for their energy needs. Side effects of the bacteria's activity often include abdominal cramps, intestinal bloating and gas, and diarrhea.

FODMAPs include fructose, lactose, and sugar alcohols such as xylitol and sorbitol. Wheat products, various kinds of fruit, high-lactose dairy foods, and onions are often excluded in low-FODMAP diets, because they are rich sources of FODMAPs. Although a low-FODMAP diet can be difficult to follow for a long period, people with irritable bowel syndrome and, possibly, inflammatory bowel disease may benefit from such diets.[26]

5.3g Fiber and Health

Fiber isn't an essential nutrient because you can live without it. You can live *better*, however,

© Wendy Schiff

by adding fiber-rich foods to your diet. Eating high-fiber foods may reduce your risk of certain intestinal tract disorders, obesity, diabetes, and cardiovascular disease, which includes heart disease and stroke.

Fiber and the Digestive Tract

A high-fiber diet can help prevent constipation and the development of diverticula and hemorrhoids (see Unit 4). When the insoluble fiber in undigested food is in the large intestine, it promotes the formation of a large, soft fecal mass. This fecal mass applies pressure to the inner muscular walls of the large intestine. The pressure stimulates the muscles to push the residue quickly through the colon, easing elimination. Thus, you probably don't need to rely on over-the-counter laxatives to treat constipation. Try consuming more fiber-rich foods along with adequate amounts of water—it's the natural way to become "regular."

Fiber and Colorectal Cancer

Eating a diet that contains plenty of dietary fiber may reduce your risk of colorectal cancer.[27] According to some studies, the fiber in cereal grains and fruit is more protective than the fiber in vegetables. As is often the case, more research is needed to determine which forms of fiber protect against colorectal cancer and how much should be eaten.

Fiber and Heart Health

High blood levels of cholesterol are associated with increased risks of cardiovascular disease. Diets rich in fiber, particularly soluble types of fiber, can reduce the risk of cardiovascular disease by reducing blood cholesterol levels.[27] In Unit 4, we mentioned that the intestinal tract breaks bile down and absorbs its components, which eventually enter the liver. The liver recycles bile components to make new bile. When you eat sources of soluble fiber, however, the fiber binds to the bile components and prevents them from being absorbed. Thus, the bile components are eliminated in bowel movements. As a result, blood cholesterol levels drop as the liver removes cholesterol from the blood to make new bile.

Fiber and Weight Control

Populations that consume high amounts of dietary fiber tend to have healthier body weights than populations with low fiber intakes.[27] Furthermore, people who want to lose excess weight may experience some greater weight loss by increasing their intake of dietary fiber. The reasons for this healthful effect are unclear, so more research is needed to understand the relationship between dietary fiber intake and body weight.

Increasing Your Fiber Intake

The recommended Adequate Intakes (AIs) for fiber are 38 and 25 g/day for young men and women, which is much higher than what the typical American eats.[9] According to the Dietary Guidelines, fiber is a nutrient of "public health concern" because Americans generally don't eat enough of it.[10] The following tips can help you increase your fiber intake:

- Read the ingredient label to find out if a bread or cereal product is whole grain; *whole grain* or *bran* should be the first ingredient.

- When comparing bread or cereal products, don't rely on the product's name or appearance. Check the ingredients. Terms such as "100% wheat," "multigrain," or "stone-ground wheat" are misleading because the product may contain little or no whole grain.

- Brown rice has more fiber and flavor than white rice. Instant-cooking brown rice takes less time to cook than regular brown rice.

- Substitute whole-wheat pasta for regular pasta or use half whole-wheat and half regular pasta in pasta dishes.

- Snack on pieces of fresh, frozen, or dried fruit.

- Instead of removing them, eat the edible peels, pulp, and seeds of fruits and vegetables. Eat vegetables as snacks.

- Include more nuts, beans, and seeds in your diet.

- Spread peanut or soy butter on whole-grain crackers for a fiber-filled snack.

- Sprinkle unsalted nuts or hulled sunflower seeds on pancakes, waffles, or salads.

- Add frozen, dried, or fresh fruit such as berries, raisins, or bananas instead of sugar or honey to sweeten cereal or plain yogurt.

- Add a small amount of uncooked oatmeal and wheat germ to raw ground meats when making hamburgers or meatloaf.

- Add bran, wheat germ, and uncooked oatmeal to pancake or waffle batter.

- Choose packaged foods that contain at least 2.5 g of fiber per serving. You can determine the food's fiber content by reading the Nutrition Facts panel on the product label.

Eating excessive amounts of fiber may interfere with the intestinal absorption of certain minerals. You can estimate your daily carbohydrate intake, which includes fiber, by completing the Personal Dietary Analysis assignment in Connect®.

Bacteria that live in the colon produce gases when they metabolize fiber, so high-fiber diets can increase intestinal gas. To reduce the likelihood of experiencing *flatulence* (uncomfortable and embarrassing intestinal gas), you can add products such as Beano® to dishes that contain beans before eating them. Beano® contains natural enzymes that break down undigested complex carbohydrates before they can be metabolized by intestinal bacteria. Practices that result in swallowing air, such as eating quickly, drinking carbonated beverages (especially with a straw), and chewing gum, also contribute to intestinal gas.

In a Nutshell

© McGraw-Hill Education. Mark A. Dierker, photographer

Module 5.1 Sugars, Sweeteners, Starches, and Fiber

- Sugars, starches, and most kinds of fiber are carbohydrates. Carbohydrates are an important source of energy for the body. Plants make carbohydrates by using the sun's energy to combine the carbon, oxygen, and hydrogen atoms from carbon dioxide and water.

- The three most important dietary monosaccharides are glucose, fructose, and galactose. Glucose is a primary fuel for muscles and other cells; nervous system and red blood cells rely on glucose for energy under normal conditions. Fruits and vegetables, especially grapes, berries, corn, and carrots, are good food sources of glucose.

- Lactose and sucrose are major dietary disaccharides. Most animal foods aren't sources of carbohydrate, but milk and some products made from milk contain lactose. Much of the sucrose in the American diet is refined from sugar cane and sugar beets.

- Nutritionally adequate diets should provide 45 to 65% of total energy from carbohydrates. The main sources of added sugars in Americans' diets are beverages sweetened with sucrose or high-fructose corn syrup.

- Alternative sweeteners sweeten food while providing fewer calories per serving than sucrose. Alternative nutritive sweeteners include sugar alcohols: sorbitol, xylitol, and mannitol. Nonnutritive sweeteners may help people control their energy intake and manage their body weight without increasing their appetite. People with PKU must avoid consuming the nonnutritive sweetener aspartame.

- Starch, glycogen, and most forms of dietary fiber are polysaccharides. Your intestinal tract can digest starch into individual glucose molecules that can be absorbed. Muscles and the liver are the major sites for glycogen formation and storage. Fiber isn't digested by humans, but soluble and insoluble fiber provide important health benefits. Soluble fiber can help reduce blood cholesterol levels, insoluble fiber may ease bowel movements, and fiber promotes a healthy balance of gut bacteria.

Module 5.2 What Happens to the Carbohydrates You Eat?

- Glucose is the primary end product of carbohydrate digestion and an important cellular fuel. Insulin and glucagon maintain normal blood glucose levels. Cells need a small amount of glucose to metabolize fat for energy properly. When glucose is unavailable, ketone bodies result from the incomplete metabolism of fat.

Module 5.3 Carbohydrates and Health

- Excess calorie intakes from carbohydrates, as well as fat, protein, and alcohol, contribute to excess body fat. The body converts some excess dietary glucose into fat, but much of it is burned as a biological fuel. As a result, dietary fat is spared from being used as a fuel, and it's stored in fat cells. Thus, eating too many carbohydrates indirectly contributes to unwanted weight gain.

- Foods that contain large amounts of refined carbohydrates may contribute to unwanted weight gain because they are often combined with hidden fats in processed foods. Fats combined with added sugars make foods taste rich and creamy, and are difficult to resist.

- Diabetes is characterized by high blood glucose levels. Poorly controlled diabetes can result in cardiovascular disease, kidney failure, blindness, and lower limb amputations. People who are physically inactive, are overweight, and have a close relative with type 2 diabetes are at risk of developing this form of the disease.

- The glycemic index (GI) and glycemic load (GL) are ways of classifying certain foods by their effect on blood glucose levels. By following a low GI/GL diet, you may be able to reduce your risk of type 2 diabetes.

- To lower your likelihood of developing metabolic syndrome, maintain a healthy weight, be more physically active, increase your intake of fiber-rich foods and seafood, and consume more fat-free or low-fat dairy foods.

- Eating fiber-rich foods may reduce your risk of obesity, type 2 diabetes, cardiovascular disease, and certain intestinal tract disorders. Eating more foods that contain insoluble fiber may lower your risk of constipation and hemorrhoids. Eating foods that contain soluble fiber may improve your cardiovascular health by reducing cholesterol absorption in the small intestine.

© FoodCollection/StockFood RF

What's in Your Diet?!

1. Refer to the 3-day food log from the "What's in Your Diet?" feature in Unit 3. List the total number of kilocalories you consumed for each day of recordkeeping. Add the figures to obtain a total, divide the total by 3, then round the figure to the nearest whole number to obtain your average daily energy intake for the 3-day period.

Sample Calculation:

Day 1	2500 kcal
Day 2	3200 kcal
Day 3	2750 kcal
Total kcal	<u>8450</u> kcal ÷ 3 days = <u>2817</u> kcal/day

(average kilocalorie intake, rounded to the nearest whole number)

Your Calculation:

Day 1	_____ kcal
Day 2	_____ kcal
Day 3	_____ kcal
Total kcal	_____ ÷ 3 days = _____ kcal/day

(average kilocalorie intake, rounded to the nearest whole number)

2. Add the number of grams of carbohydrate eaten each day of the period. Divide the total by 3 and round to the nearest whole number to calculate the average number of grams of carbohydrate consumed daily.

Your Calculation:

Day 1	_____ g
Day 2	_____ g
Day 3	_____ kcal
Total g	_____ ÷ 3 days = _____ g of carbohydrate/day

(average, rounded to the nearest whole number)

3. Each gram of carbohydrate provides about 4 kcal; therefore, you must multiply the average number of grams of carbohydrate obtained in step 2 by 4 to obtain the number of kcal from carbohydrates.

Your Calculation:

____ g/day × 4 kcal/g = ____ kcal from carbohydrates

4. To calculate the average daily percentage of kilocalories that carbohydrates contributed to your diet, divide the average kilocalories from carbohydrate obtained in step 3 by the average total daily kilocalorie intake obtained in step 1; round figure to the nearest one-hundredth. Multiply the value by 100, drop decimal point, and add the percent symbol.

Sample Calculation:

1692 kcal ÷ 2817 kcal = 0.60

0.60 × 100 = 60%

Your Calculation:

____ kcal ÷ ____ kcal = ____

____ × 100 = ____ %

5. On average, did you consume *at least* the RDA of 130 g of carbohydrate? Yes ____ No ____

6. Did your average carbohydrate intake meet the recommended 45 to 65% of total energy? Yes ____ No ____

    a. If your average carbohydrate intake was less than 130 g or below 45% of total calories, list five nutrient-dense, carbohydrate-rich foods you could eat that would boost your intake of carbohydrates.

    Foods: _____

7. Review the log of your 3-day food intake. Calculate your average daily intake of fiber by adding the grams of fiber consumed over the 3-day period and dividing the total by three.

Your Calculation:

Day 1	____ g
Day 2	____ g
Day 3	____ g
Total =	____ g
Total g	____ ÷ 3 days = ____ g of fiber daily

    a. What was your average daily fiber intake? ____ g

    b. Did your average daily fiber intake meet the recommended Adequate Intakes of 38 and 25 g/day for young men and women, respectively? Yes ____ No ____

    c. If your response is yes, list foods that contributed to your fiber intake.

    d. If you did not meet the recommended level of fiber intake, list at least five foods that you would eat to increase your fiber intake to the recommended level.

8. Review the log of your 3-day food intake. Calculate your average daily intake of added sugars by adding the grams of added sugars consumed over the 3-day period and dividing the total number by three.

    a. What was your average daily intake of added sugars? ____ g

    b. Calculate the average number of kcal that you consumed from added sugars. ____ kcal

    c. Calculate your average percentage of daily kcal from added sugars by dividing the average number of kcal that you consumed from added sugars by your average daily total kcal intake. ____ %

    Is your average number of kcal consumed from added sugars less than 10% of your average total kcal intake? ____ Yes ____ No

Consider This...

1. One of your friends thinks honey is more nutritious and safer to eat than table sugar. He wants you to avoid table sugar and use only honey as a sweetener. What would you tell this person about the nutritive value and safety of honey compared to sugar?

2. Prepare a pamphlet that describes the health benefits of dietary fiber. In addition to English, you may prepare the pamphlet in Spanish, Vietnamese, or another modern language.

3. How did you feel about drinking sugar-sweetened soft drinks before reading Unit 5? Has your opinion changed? If so, explain how.

4. If you were 25 pounds overweight, explain why you would or wouldn't follow a weight-loss diet that supplied less than 15% of calories from carbohydrate.

5. Consider the fiber content of your diet. Do you consume enough fiber each day? If your fiber intake is adequate, what foods do you eat regularly that contribute fiber to your diet? If your dietary fiber intake is low, list foods you would consume to increase your intake.

Test Yourself

Select the best answer.

1. Which of the following substances is a disaccharide?
   a. Fructose
   b. Glucose
   c. Galactose
   d. Lactose

2. Which of the following substances is a primary fuel for muscles and other cells?
   a. Glucose
   b. Glycerol
   c. Fructose
   d. Mannitol

3. Which of the following substances is a polysaccharide?
   a. Glucagon
   b. Starch
   c. Lactose
   d. Aspartame

4. Dietary fiber
   a. is a source of energy for bacteria in the large intestine.
   b. is digested by enzymes produced by the human intestinal tract.
   c. promotes tooth decay.
   d. is only in animal sources of food.

5. Dietary fiber is
   a. in beef and pork.
   b. the primary carbohydrate in dairy foods.
   c. needed for good bowel health.
   d. an essential nutrient.

6. Which of the following substances is the hormone that enables glucose to enter cells?
   a. Glucagon
   b. Adrenaline
   c. Glycerol
   d. Insulin

© FoodCollection /Stockfood RF

7. The primary sources of added sugars in the typical American diet are
   a. candies.
   b. sugar-sweetened soft drinks.
   c. refined cereals.
   d. baked beans.

8. Type 1 diabetes is
   a. a disease that primarily affects elderly people.
   b. characterized by severe hypoglycemia.
   c. often associated with excess body weight.
   d. an autoimmune disease.

9. Which of the following signs is associated with metabolic syndrome?
   a. High blood pressure
   b. Hypoglycemia
   c. Low hemoglobin
   d. High fasting HDL cholesterol

10. Which of the following substances is an enzyme that breaks down lactose?
    a. Galactose
    b. Hydrochloric acid
    c. Lactase
    d. Lactic acid

© Wendy Schiff

A Answer This (Module 5.1b)

Molasses

References ➡ See Appendix F.

STUDY TIP: Quickly create a customized practice quiz for this chapter by going to your Connect SmartBook "My Reports" section.

Don't have SmartBook and want to learn more? Go to **whysmartbook.com**.

Lipids
FOCUSING ON FATS AND CHOLESTEROL

What's on the Menu?

Module 6.1
What Are Lipids?

Module 6.2
What Happens to the Fat and Cholesterol You Eat?

Module 6.3
Cardiovascular Disease: Major Killer of Americans

© Wendy Schiff

"I eat all the wrong foods. I like butter on everything! For breakfast, my mom usually makes sausage, fried eggs, and pancakes. For lunch, I try to eat salads, but sometimes, I just grab some potato chips or "hot fries." We eat dinner late—around 10 at night—when my mother brings fast food home. I eat cereal daily; I'm trying to get more fiber in my system. I like the high-fiber, high-antioxidant cereals. My mother takes medication to control her high cholesterol and blood pressure. . . . I'm healthy, but I don't like my pudgy belly. I would like to lose 20, maybe 30 pounds. I just don't have the motivation to eat better and exercise more."

Nancy Scott

Nancy Scott is majoring in nursing at Florissant Valley Community College. As a nontraditional college student and the mother of two preschool-age children, Nancy is extremely busy with her job, family, and school responsibilities. It's difficult for her to plan nutritious meals for herself and her children. Should she be more concerned about her diet, especially her fat intake?

What do you think when you hear the word *fat* or *cholesterol*? Does "bad" or "overweight" or "heart disease" enter your mind? If your answer is yes, are you concerned about the amounts and types of fat in your diet? Why?

You may be surprised to learn that having some fat ("healthy fats") in your diet is essential to good health. However, consuming high amounts of certain fats ("unhealthy fats") may increase your risk of serious health conditions, especially heart disease.[1] By reading Unit 6, you'll learn about fats and other lipids in your food and body as well as their major food sources. Additionally, you'll learn how these nutrients may influence your health.

Module 6.1

What Are Lipids?

© Ingram Publishing RF

lipids class of organic nutrients that generally don't dissolve in water (water-insoluble)

triglyceride lipid that has three fatty acids attached to a three-carbon compound called glycerol; fats and oils

Lipids, such as vegetable oils, generally don't dissolve in water.

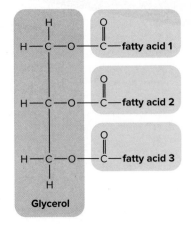

© Photodisc/Getty Images RF

Fats, oils, and cholesterol are **lipids,** a class of organic nutrients that generally don't dissolve in water (*water-insoluble*). Despite all the "bad press," fat and cholesterol are very important nutrients. Fat is a major source of energy for the body; recall from Unit 1 that each gram of fat supplies 9 kcal. Fats and other lipids play many other important roles in your body, including

- maintaining cell membranes,
- producing certain hormones,
- insulating against cold temperatures,
- regulating blood pressure and inflammation, and
- cushioning against bumps, blows, and falls.

Dietary fat helps your body absorb fat-soluble vitamins and phytochemicals. Dietary lipids also contribute to the rich flavor, smooth texture, and appetizing aroma of foods. That's why foods that contain some fat often taste more enjoyable than foods that lack the nutrient. What do you like to add to a baked potato—butter, margarine, sour cream, or some other fatty food?

6.1a Triglycerides

Triglycerides comprise about 95% of lipids in your body and food. Triglycerides are often referred to as *fats* and *oils*. In this textbook, triglycerides, fats, and oils may be referred to simply as "fats."

A **triglyceride** is composed of three fatty acid molecules attached to a glycerol (*glis'-er-ol*) "backbone" molecule (**Fig. 6.1**).

Triglyceride

Figure 6.1 Basic parts of a triglyceride. Chemists often use straight lines to show bonds between carbon, hydrogen, and oxygen atoms.

Each fatty acid (FA) has a chain of carbon atoms bonded to each other and to hydrogen atoms (**Fig. 6.2**). At one end of the chain, the first carbon has three hydrogen atoms attached to it. This part of the chain is called the *omega end*. At the other end of the fatty acid chain, the last carbon has two oxygen atoms and one hydrogen atom in a special arrangement that's called an "acid group."

What's Saturated Fat and Unsaturated Fat?

Fatty acids can be saturated or unsaturated. Furthermore, unsaturated fatty acids can be either mono-unsaturated or polyunsaturated. In foods, the three different types of fatty acids usually occur in different proportions.

Figure 6.2 Fatty acid.

The fatty acid shown in Figure 6.2 has single bonds holding each carbon in the carbon chain together. Note that each of these carbons has two hydrogen atoms attached to it. This is a **saturated fatty acid (saturated FA)** because each carbon within the chain is completely filled (*saturated*) with hydrogen atoms. Animal fats tend to contain more saturated FAs than plant oils. Important exceptions are the highly saturated "tropical" plant oils—coconut, palm, and palm kernel oils.

A **monounsaturated fatty acid (monounsaturated FA)** has two neighboring carbons within the carbon chain that each lack a hydrogen atom. When this occurs, a double bond holds those particular carbons together (**Fig 6.3**). Avocados, and olive, peanut, and canola oils are rich sources of monounsaturated FAs.

A **polyunsaturated fatty acid (polyunsaturated FA)** has more than one double bond in the carbon chain (**Fig. 6.4**). Safflower (high-linoleic), grapeseed, sunflower seed (high-linoleic), and soybean oils are rich sources of polyunsaturated FAs.

Essential Concept 6.1 compares certain sources of saturated and unsaturated FAs. **Table 6.1** compares the percentages of saturated FAs, monounsaturated FAs, and polyunsaturated FAs in commonly eaten fats.

saturated fatty acid (saturated FA) fatty acid that only has single bonds holding each carbon in the carbon chain together

monounsaturated fatty acid (monounsaturated FA) fatty acid that has one double bond within the carbon chain

polyunsaturated fatty acid (polyunsaturated FA) fatty acid that has two or more double bonds within the carbon chain

Figure 6.3 Monounsaturated fatty acid.

Figure 6.4 Polyunsaturated fatty acid.

■ *What is the basic structural difference between a polyunsaturated FA and a monounsaturated FA?*

The layer of fat under your skin helps insulate your body against cold temperatures.

Essential Concept

6.1 Comparing Sources of Saturated and Unsaturated FAs

Saturated FAs Comparisons

Beef fat has more **saturated FAs** than corn oil.

Polyunsaturated FAs Comparisons

Corn oil has some **saturated FAs,** but it's a richer source of **polyunsaturated FAs** than beef fat.

Monounsaturated FAs Comparisons

Olive oil has a lot more **monounsaturated FAs** than beef fat or corn oil.

TABLE 6.1 COMPARING FATTY ACID CONTENTS OF FATS AND OILS

Fat/Oil	% Saturated	% Monounsaturated	% Polyunsaturated
Safflower oil (high linoleic)	6.2	14.4	74.6
Canola oil	7.4	64.1	28.5
Walnut oil	9.5	24.0	66.5
Grapeseed oil	10.1	16.8	73.1
Sunflower oil (high linoleic)	10.8	20.4	68.8
Corn oil	13.6	29.0	57.4
Olive oil	14.2	75.0	10.8
Soybean oil	16.3	23.7	60.0
Peanut oil	17.8	48.6	33.6
Chicken fat	31.2	46.9	21.9
Lard (pork fat)	41.0	47.2	11.7
Palm oil	51.6	38.7	9.7
Beef fat	52.1	43.7	4.2
Cocoa butter	62.4	34.4	3.2
Butter fat	68.1	27.9	4.0
Coconut oil	91.9	6.2	1.9

Q Answer This

Based on Table 6.1, which fat or oil has the highest percentage of monounsaturated fatty acids? You can find the answer on the last page of this unit.

Liquid or Solid Fat?

Saturated fatty acid molecules can pack together tightly because they are straighter than unsaturated fatty acids. This structural difference allows animal fats that are rich sources of saturated FAs, such as beef fat and butter fat, to be fairly solid at usual room temperatures. On the other hand, the double bonds of unsaturated fatty acids cause the molecules to have "bends" or kinks in their chemical structures. The "cis" type of kink that's shown in **Figure 6.5** is typical. Such bends prevent the molecules from being arranged tightly together and forming solids. That's why a fat that contains a high proportion of unsaturated fatty acids, such as sunflower seed oil or corn oil, tends to be liquid when it's stored at room temperature.

Figure 6.5 Cis fatty acid. For simplicity, this diagram doesn't show all of the hydrogens within the carbon chain.

■ *How does the cis type of double bond affect the shape of this fatty acid molecule?*

Essential Fatty Acids

The body cannot make two polyunsaturated FAs. These **essential fatty acids** are **alpha-linolenic** (*al-fah lin-o-len'-ik*) **acid** and **linoleic** (*lin'-o-lay'-ik*) **acid**. Alpha-linolenic acid is an **omega-3 fatty acid** (see Fig 6.4). Linoleic acid is an **omega-6 fatty acid** (**Fig. 6.6**). The "3" and "6" in the names identify the position of the first double bond that appears in the fatty acids' carbon chains, when you start counting carbons at the omega end of the molecules.

Figure 6.6 Linoleic acid (an omega-6 fatty acid).

© Wendy Schiff

Cells use alpha-linolenic acid to produce two other omega-3 fatty acids: **eicosapentaenoic** (*eye'-koss-uh-pen'-tah-ee-no'-ik*) **acid** (**EPA**) and **docosahexaenoic** (*doe'-koss-uh-hex'-uh-ee-no'-ik*) **acid** (**DHA**). Cells can convert linoleic acid to another omega-6 fatty acid, **arachidonic** (*a'-rack'-ih-don'-ik*) **acid** (**AA**). **Figure 6.7** shows relationships among the essential fatty acids.

Essential fatty acids are necessary in small amounts for good health. The body uses EPA, DHA, and AA to make several hormone-like substances. These compounds have a variety of important effects, such as regulating blood pressure and the immune system's inflammatory response. Infants require DHA and EPA for nervous system development, and babies don't grow properly when their diets lack essential fatty acids.

essential fatty acids lipids that must be supplied by the diet

alpha-linolenic acid an essential omega-3 fatty acid

linoleic acid an essential omega-6 fatty acid

omega-3 fatty acid type of polyunsaturated fatty acid that has its first double bond at the number 3 carbon

omega-6 fatty acid type of polyunsaturated fatty acid that has its first double bond at the number 6 carbon

eicosapentaenoic acid (EPA) omega-3 fatty acid derived from alpha-linolenic acid

docosahexaenoic acid (DHA) omega-3 fatty acid derived from alpha-linolenic acid

arachidonic acid (AA) omega-6 fat derived from linoleic acid

Figure 6.7 Relationships among essential fatty acids.

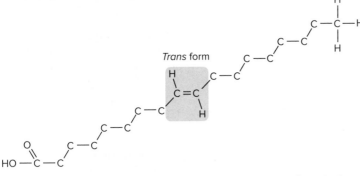
Other signs of essential fatty acid deficiency include scaly skin, hair loss, and poor wound healing. In the United States, essential fatty acid deficiency is uncommon because most Americans eat plenty of fat, especially linoleic acid.

What Are Trans Fats?

Trans fatty acids ("trans fat") are unsaturated fatty acids that have an unusual type of chemical structure (**Fig. 6.8**). This structure enables the carbon chain to be relatively straight, compared to other types of unsaturated fatty acids (see Figure 6.5).

Whole milk and whole milk products, butter, and meat naturally contain small amounts of trans fats. Processed foods, however, contribute the largest share of trans fat in the American diet. Such foods may include

- pies, crackers, cookies, cakes, and other baked goods,
- snack foods,
- frozen pizza,
- fast food,
- vegetable shortenings and stick margarines,
- coffee creamer,
- refrigerated dough products (such as biscuits and cinnamon rolls),
- ready-to-use frostings.[3]

Since 2002, the U.S. Food and Drug Administration (FDA) has required food manufacturers to show their products' trans fat content in the Nutrition Facts panel. For years, partially hydrogenated oils (PHOs) were the major kind of artificial trans fat in processed foods. Medical experts, however, became increasingly concerned about the harmful health effects of eating trans fats, especially PHOs. In response to such safety concerns, many food manufacturers decided to remove PHOs from their products' recipes. According to the FDA, American consumers reduced their trans fat intake by almost 80% between 2003 and 2012.[4]

In 2015, the FDA determined that PHOs posed a health risk, and the agency banned their use in foods.[4] This ban will go into effect in 2018. Keep in mind, however, that trans fat is not likely to disappear completely from your diet because some foods naturally contain small amounts of this type of fat. You can learn how much trans fat is in a serving of most processed foods by reading the ingredient list and Nutrition Facts panel that are on the package's label. According to the 2015 Dietary Guidelines, Americans should keep their trans fat intake as low as possible while eating a healthy diet.[1]

Why were PHOs used by food manufacturers? **Partial hydrogenation** is a process that converts many of an oil's naturally occurring unsaturated cis fatty acids into trans fatty acids and saturated fatty acids. Because the shape of a trans fatty acid is like that of a saturated fat, a partially hydrogenated vegetable oil is more solid at room temperature. This feature enabled food manufacturers to make shortening and sticks of margarine. Furthermore, foods made with PHOs could be stored for longer periods of time than could foods that contained "regular" unsaturated fats. Why? Trans fatty acids are less likely to become rancid. Rancidity results from a chemical process that damages a compound's structure. Rancid food has an unappetizing odor and taste. Regular unsaturated fatty acids, especially polyunsaturated FAs, are very susceptible to rancidity. Food manufacturers, however, can preserve polyunsaturated FAs in foods by adding antioxidants, such as butylated hydroxyanisole (BHA) and butylated hydroxytoluene (BHT), to them.

Why is it important to understand the differences among saturated, unsaturated, and trans fats, and identify foods that contain

trans fatty acids unsaturated fatty acids that have an unusual structure

partial hydrogenation food manufacturing process that adds hydrogen atoms to liquid vegetable oil, forming trans fats and saturated fats

Figure 6.8 Trans fatty acid. For simplicity, this diagram doesn't show all of the hydrogens within the carbon chain.

■ *How does the shape of a trans fatty acid differ from the shape of a cis type of unsaturated fatty acid?*

high amounts of these fats? Populations that consume diets rich in saturated fat and trans fat have higher risk of cardiovascular disease than populations whose diets contain more unsaturated fat.[1] **Cardiovascular disease (CVD)** is a group of diseases that affect the heart and blood vessels. Cardiovascular disease can result in heart attacks, strokes, and kidney failure. In Module 6.3, you'll learn about this disease, and why it's a good idea to limit your intake of certain fats and increase your intake of others.

6.1b Cholesterol

Cholesterol is a sterol. Sterols have carbons arranged in rings (**Fig. 6.9**). Fatty acids and triglycerides don't have carbon rings.

Many people think that cholesterol is unhealthy, so they avoid foods that contain the lipid. Cholesterol, however, is a key nutrient that has a variety of functions in your body. Cholesterol is a component of all your cells' membranes. Your brain cells, in particular, contain high amounts of cholesterol. Although cholesterol isn't metabolized for energy, cells use the lipid to produce a variety of substances, including vitamin D, and steroid hormones such as estrogen and testosterone. Your liver uses cholesterol to make bile salts, which help the small intestine digest lipids.

Although triglycerides are widespread in foods, dietary sources of cholesterol are only in animal foods. Egg yolk, liver, meat, poultry, whole milk, cheese, and ice cream are rich sources of cholesterol (**Table 6.2**). Even if you don't eat animal

Figure 6.9 **Cholesterol.** For simplicity, this diagram just shows the arrangement of cholesterol's carbon atoms. The carbon rings are highlighted.

■ *Why do your cells need cholesterol?*

cardiovascular disease (CVD) group of diseases that affect the heart and blood vessels

cholesterol sterol in animal foods that's made by your body

TABLE 6.2	**APPROXIMATE CHOLESTEROL CONTENT OF SOME FOODS/SERVING**	

Food	Serving Size	Cholesterol (mg)
Liver	3 oz	234
Egg	1 large	186
Egg yolk	1	186
Sardines	3 oz	121
Single-patty cheeseburger	1	111
Beef	3 oz	88
Turkey, ground	3 oz	84
Danish fruit-filled pastry	2½ oz	81
Shrimp	6 large	80
Ham	3 oz	80
Ice cream, soft-serve	½ cup	78
Ground beef, lean (15% fat)	3 oz	77
Salmon	3 oz	75
Turkey, dark meat	3 oz	71
Egg noodles	1 cup	53
Chicken breast	3 oz	49
Hot dog	1	44
Chocolate milkshake	16 oz	43
Whole milk	1 cup	34

Shrimp: © FoodCollection/StockFood RF; Sardines: © Comstock Images/Alamy RF; Salmon: © FoodCollection/StockFood RF; Burger: © McGraw-Hill Education. Mark A. Dierker, photographer

phospholipid type of lipid needed to make cell membranes and for proper functioning of nerve cells

lecithin major phospholipid in food

foods, your body produces all the cholesterol you need, primarily in the liver. If your body makes too much cholesterol, the excess can increase your risk of CVD.

6.1c What Are Phospholipids?

A **phospholipid** is chemically similar to a triglyceride, except that one of the fatty acids is replaced by chemical groups that contain phosphorus and, often, nitrogen. Phospholipids are needed for normal functioning of nerve cells, including those in the brain. Phospholipids are also major structural components of cell membranes. Cell membranes are comprised of a double layer that is mostly phospholipids (**Fig. 6.10**). The phosphate "head" of a phospholipid is water soluble. The fatty acid "tail" of a phospholipid is not water soluble. Thus, phospholipids are soluble in both water and fat. In a cell membrane, the phosphate heads of phospholipids face the watery environments that are inside and outside the cell. The fatty acid tails of phospholipids avoid such watery environments, so they face each other within the membrane (see Figure 6.10). This characteristic enables the membrane to be flexible and allow fat-soluble compounds to move in and out of the cell easily.

Phospholipids are found naturally in plant and animal foods. **Lecithin** (*less'-uh-thin*) is the primary phospholipid in food; egg yolks, liver, wheat germ, peanut butter, and soybeans are rich sources of lecithin.

Figure 6.10 Phospholipids in a cell membrane.

■ *What is the major structural component of cell membranes?*

TASTY **Tidbits**

Eggs with brown shells aren't more nutritious than eggs with white shells; the color of an eggshell is determined by the breed of hen that laid it. Also, "grading" doesn't reflect the nutritional content of an egg. Eggs are given AA, A, and B grades based on certain physical characteristics, such as shell appearance and thickness of egg white, which have nothing to do with an egg's nutrient contents.

Lecithin contains **choline** (*co'-leen*). Nerves use choline to produce acetylcholine (*ah-see'-till-co'-leen*), a chemical that transmits messages between nerve cells.

A healthy adult's body makes phospholipids, so deficiencies among adults are uncommon. Nutritionists, however, classify choline as a vitamin-like nutrient because deficiency symptoms can occur under certain conditions.[5] Unit 8 provides more information about choline.

In foods, phospholipids can serve as an **emulsifier,** a substance that keeps fat-soluble and water-soluble compounds together. Manufacturers may add emulsifiers to foods to keep oily and watery ingredients from separating during storage. Egg yolk naturally contains phospholipids. Eggs are often used to emulsify oil and vinegar when making mayonnaise and mixing oil and milk in cake or pancake batters.

choline vitamin-like compound in lecithin

emulsifier substance that helps fat-soluble and water-soluble compounds mix with each other

Peanut butter

Edamame

Wheat germ

Peanut butter, edamame (fresh soybeans), and wheat germ are rich sources of lecithin.

Module 6.2

What Happens to the Fat and Cholesterol You Eat?

6.2 - Learning Outcomes

After reading Module 6.2, you should be able to

1. Define all of the key terms in this module.

2. Describe what happens to the fat and cholesterol in food as it undergoes digestion and absorption in your intestinal tract.

3. Describe the function of a chylomicron.

© Photodisc/Punchstock RF

6.2a Digesting Lipids

When you eat a cheeseburger and French fries or other foods, the fat in the items undergoes a little digestion in the stomach. However, the small intestine is the primary site of lipid digestion. The pancreas releases enzymes (**lipases**) into the small intestine that digest fats and phospholipids. Because fats don't dissolve well in watery chyme, fat digestion involves the need for an emulsifier (see **Essential Concept 6.2**).

Essential Concept

6.2 Digesting Fat

1 In response to the presence of the fatty chyme in the duodenum, the gallbladder releases bile into the chyme. Bile contains **bile salts**, which emulsify the lipids—that is, keep lipids suspended as small particles in chyme.

| Glycerol
| Free fatty acids
| Monoglycerides
| Triglycerides
| Bile salts

2 The presence of chyme in the small intestine also stimulates the pancreas to secrete **pancreatic lipase**. Pancreatic lipase gains greater access to the fat molecules because of the action of bile salts. As a result, the lipase digests the molecules more easily. Without the presence of bile salts, lipids in chyme would clump together in large fatty globules, making lipid digestion less efficient.

Bile salts in bile

Large fat droplet

Emulsified lipids

Lipase from pancreas

lipases enzymes that break down lipids

bile salts component of bile

pancreatic lipase digestive enzyme that removes two fatty acids from each triglyceride molecule

138

monoglyceride single fatty acid attached to a glycerol backbone

micelle lipid-rich particle that is surrounded by bile salts; transports lipids to absorptive cells

Triglyceride

3 Pancreatic lipase digests fat by removing two fatty acids from each triglyceride molecule. This action converts most fat into monoglycerides and "free" fatty acids. A **monoglyceride** is a lipid that has a single fatty acid attached to the glycerol backbone of the molecule.

Monoglyceride

Pancreatic lipase

4 Glycerol, fatty acids, and monoglycerides are the major products of lipid digestion.

Micelle

Used bile salts

5 Bile salts surround the fatty acids and monoglycerides to form a water-soluble particle called a **micelle**. Micelles transport the lipids to the edge of the absorptive cell. These cells remove the monoglycerides and fatty acids from micelles. The used bile salts that remain can continue to form new micelles.

Absorptive cell of the small intestine

lipoprotein structure that transports lipids through the bloodstream and lymph

very-low-density lipoprotein (VLDL) lipoprotein that transports a high proportion of lipids in the bloodstream

6.2b Absorbing and Transporting Fat and Cholesterol

In the small intestine, absorptive cells remove monoglycerides, fatty acids, glycerol, and cholesterol from chyme. (Cholesterol doesn't undergo digestion.) Under normal conditions, the small intestine digests and absorbs nearly all of the fat in food, but only about 50% of the dietary cholesterol is absorbed. In the absorptive cells, the fatty acids and monoglyceride molecules are reassembled into triglycerides (**Fig. 6.11**).

Lipids aren't very soluble in watery fluids such as lymph and blood. The absorptive cells coat the lipids with a thin layer of protein, phospholipids, and cholesterol to form chylomicrons (see Fig. 6.11). Chylomicrons are a type of **lipoprotein.** A lipoprotein transports lipids through watery environments such as the bloodstream.

Chylomicrons are too large to be absorbed directly into the bloodstream from absorptive cells. However, they can pass through the larger openings of lacteals, lymphatic system vessels in each villus (see Fig. 4.6).

What Happens to Chylomicrons?

Cells in the walls of tiny blood vessels called capillaries release a lipase that breaks down the chylomicron's load of fat into fatty acids and glycerol. Nearby cells can pick up the fatty acids and glycerol, and metabolize them for energy. Ten to 12 hours after a meal, most chylomicrons have been reduced to small, cholesterol-rich particles. The liver clears these particles from the bloodstream and uses their contents to produce various substances, including **very-low-density lipoprotein (VLDL).** VLDL carries a high proportion of lipids in the bloodstream. Module 6.3 provides more details about lipoproteins such as VLDL.

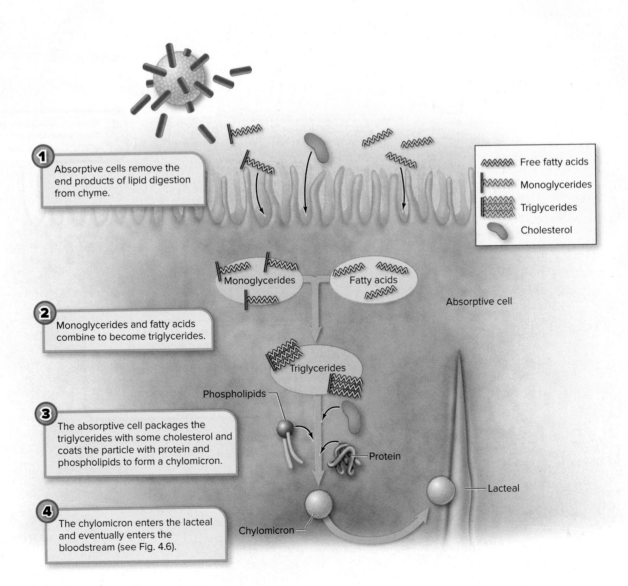

1 Absorptive cells remove the end products of lipid digestion from chyme.

Free fatty acids
Monoglycerides
Triglycerides
Cholesterol

Monoglycerides   Fatty acids

Absorptive cell

2 Monoglycerides and fatty acids combine to become triglycerides.

Triglycerides

Phospholipids

3 The absorptive cell packages the triglycerides with some cholesterol and coats the particle with protein and phospholipids to form a chylomicron.

Protein

Lacteal

4 The chylomicron enters the lacteal and eventually enters the bloodstream (see Fig. 4.6).

Chylomicron

Figure 6.11 **Chylomicron formation.**

6.2c What Happens to the Bile Salts?

After the absorptive cells remove lipids from micelles, the used bile salts remain within the small intestine. **Essential Concept 6.3** explains what happens to the used bile salts.

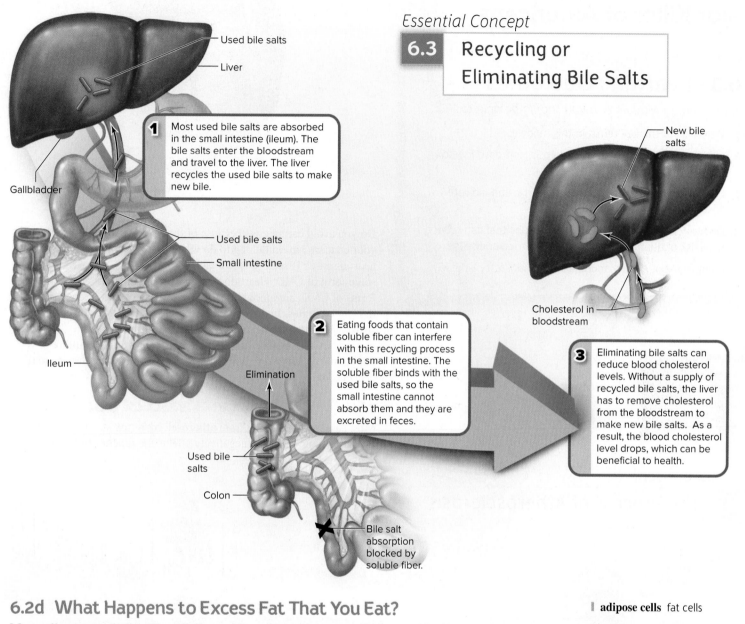

Essential Concept

6.3 Recycling or Eliminating Bile Salts

Used bile salts

Liver

1 Most used bile salts are absorbed in the small intestine (ileum). The bile salts enter the bloodstream and travel to the liver. The liver recycles the used bile salts to make new bile.

Gallbladder

Used bile salts

Small intestine

Ileum

Elimination

2 Eating foods that contain soluble fiber can interfere with this recycling process in the small intestine. The soluble fiber binds with the used bile salts, so the small intestine cannot absorb them and they are excreted in feces.

Used bile salts

Colon

Bile salt absorption blocked by soluble fiber.

New bile salts

Cholesterol in bloodstream

3 Eliminating bile salts can reduce blood cholesterol levels. Without a supply of recycled bile salts, the liver has to remove cholesterol from the bloodstream to make new bile salts. As a result, the blood cholesterol level drops, which can be beneficial to health.

6.2d What Happens to Excess Fat That You Eat?

Most cells can metabolize ("burn") fatty acids to release the energy that's stored in the molecules. Sometimes your body doesn't need the energy from the fat you have just eaten. When this happens, **adipose** (*ad'-eh-pose*) **cells** remove fatty acids and glycerol from the bloodstream and reassemble them into fat for storage.

Adipose cells are commonly called "fat cells" because they are designed to store large amounts of fat (**Fig. 6.12**). When your body needs energy, adipose cells break down some stored triglycerides into fatty acid and glycerol molecules and release these substances into your bloodstream. Muscle and other cells then remove the fatty acids from circulation and metabolize them. The liver clears the glycerol molecules from the bloodstream and converts them into glucose molecules that cells can also use for energy.

Eating too much fat contributes to unwanted weight gain, but consuming too much energy from carbohydrates or protein also increases body fat. Why? The body can convert excess glucose and certain amino acids into fatty acids that are used to make fat. Additionally, the non-nutrient alcohol stimulates fat production, so excess body fat can result from drinking alcohol. For more information about alcohol, see Unit 9.

◗ adipose cells fat cells

Nucleus

Fat droplet

Cell membrane

Figure 6.12 Fat cell.

■ *What is the primary lipid that's stored in fat cells?*

Module 6.3

Cardiovascular Disease: Major Killer of Americans

6.3 - Learning Outcomes

After reading Module 6.3, you should be able to

1. Define all of the key terms in this module.

2. Explain the process of atherosclerosis, and describe how the condition contributes to CVD.

3. List major risk factors for atherosclerosis, and indicate which factors are modifiable.

4. Discuss dietary and other lifestyle actions that can reduce your risk of atherosclerosis and cardiovascular disease.

5. Identify major dietary sources of essential fatty acids.

atherosclerosis long-term disease process in which plaque builds up inside arterial walls, causing hardening of the arteries

Do you avoid eating eggs because of their cholesterol content? Does your concern have anything to do with having a family history of heart disease? If so, you're not alone—one in three Americans has some form of CVD. Heart disease and stroke, the most common forms of CVD, are among the top five leading causes of death in the United States. In 2014, combined deaths from heart disease and stroke accounted for nearly 30% of all deaths in this country.[6] In many instances, CVD begins during adolescence and young adulthood, but people usually don't have signs or symptoms of the disease until decades later.

6.3a The Road to Cardiovascular Disease (CVD)

Most cases of CVD result from **atherosclerosis** (*ath'-er-oh-skler-oh'-sis*), a long-term process that negatively affects the functioning of blood vessels, especially arteries.

Essential Concept

6.4 The Process of Atherosclerosis

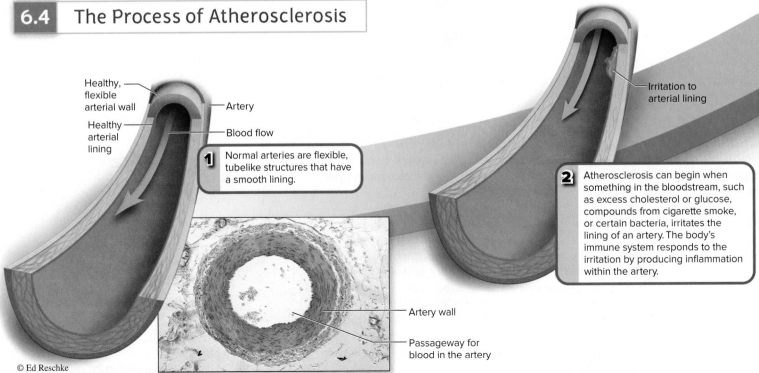

Healthy, flexible arterial wall

Artery

Healthy arterial lining

Blood flow

1 Normal arteries are flexible, tubelike structures that have a smooth lining.

Irritation to arterial lining

2 Atherosclerosis can begin when something in the bloodstream, such as excess cholesterol or glucose, compounds from cigarette smoke, or certain bacteria, irritates the lining of an artery. The body's immune system responds to the irritation by producing inflammation within the artery.

Artery wall

Passageway for blood in the artery

© Ed Reschke

Less flexible arterial wall

Blood clot

Arterial plaque

4 Arterial plaque narrows and may even block the opening through which blood flows in an artery. This process makes arteries less flexible, which causes the heart to work harder to pump blood through the stiff blood vessels. Furthermore, plaque roughens the normally smooth surface of the artery's lining. The rough lining slows blood flow in the area and makes clots more likely to form.

Arterial plaque

3 Inflammation can stimulate healing. In cases of atherosclerosis, inflammation in an artery triggers certain cells within the walls of the blood vessel to deposit cholesterol-rich material under the artery's lining. These deposits are called **arterial plaque** (*plak*).

Passageway for blood in the artery

© Ed Reschke

Plaque

Artery wall

5 Sometimes, a clot breaks away from the fixed mass of clots and travels through the bloodstream. Such clots can lodge in a smaller blood vessel, blocking its blood flow. When the blood flow in an artery is disrupted, the cells supplied by the artery die because they lack oxygen.

Blood flow

Fixed clot

Artery

Clot that travels through the bloodstream

arterial plaque lipid-filled patch that builds up within the wall of an artery

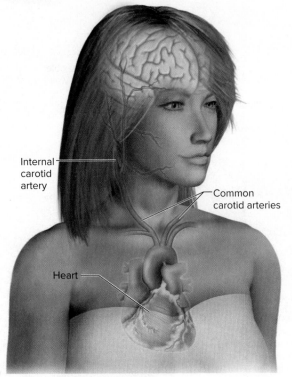

Internal
carotid
artery

Common
carotid arteries

Heart

Figure 6.13 Carotid arteries.

■ *Why are clots that form in the carotid arteries dangerous?*

If a clot or a bunch of clots form in one of the arteries that supplies the heart, they can partially close off the artery. When this happens, the affected section of the heart muscle is unable to receive enough oxygen and nutrients to function properly. As a result, the person with the partially blocked artery typically experiences bouts of chest pain called **angina**. If the plaque or clot completely blocks blood flow to a section of the heart muscle, the tissue dies and a **heart attack** occurs.

A **stroke** ("brain attack") can happen when a clot blocks an artery in the brain, and brain cells that are nourished by the blood vessel die. Plaque can form in the common carotid arteries in the neck (**Fig. 6.13**). Clots that form in those arteries can travel to the brain, causing a stroke.

Atherosclerosis can also develop in arteries that don't carry blood to the heart or brain. This condition is called **peripheral vascular disease** (**PVD**). PVD often affects arteries that carry blood to the kidneys, legs, and arms. When a clot blocks an artery that carries blood to the lower leg, the tissue in the limb dies, causing gangrene to occur. Surgery to remove the gangrenous limb may be necessary to prevent a life-threatening infection.

What's "Hardening of the Arteries"?

Plaques reduce the flexibility of arteries, causing **arteriosclerosis,** a condition that's commonly called "hardening of the arteries." Inflexible arteries contribute to the development of **hypertension**, which is characterized by abnormally high blood pressure levels that persist even when the person is relaxed. For most people, high blood pressure is dangerous if the value remains at or above 140/90 mm Hg. For people who are 20 to 30 years of age, a healthy blood pressure is 120/75.[7]

Hypertension often damages organs, especially the heart, kidneys, brain, and eyes. The heart of a person with hypertension must work harder to circulate blood through abnormally stiff arteries. Furthermore, high blood pressure can tear or burst hardened arteries, causing serious bleeding problems and even sudden death, depending on the artery's size and location. Unit 9 provides more information about hypertension.

Lipoproteins and Atherosclerosis

Lipoproteins transport cholesterol and triglycerides in the bloodstream, so these structures play major roles in the development of atherosclerosis. In addition to chylomicrons, the body makes three major types of lipoprotein (**Fig. 6.14**). Each type carries different proportions of protein, cholesterol, triglycerides, and phospholipids. The protein content of a lipoprotein contributes to its density. A chylomicron, for example, is the largest and least dense of these lipoproteins. Compared to the other types of lipoproteins, chylomicrons carry much more fat and very little protein. HDL is the smallest and densest of these lipoproteins, because it transports more protein and less lipids than the other lipoproteins.

angina chest pain that results from lack of oxygen to heart muscle tissue

heart attack loss of blood flow to a section of the heart muscle, causing the tissue to die

stroke loss of blood flow to a region of the brain, causing the death of brain cells in that area

peripheral vascular disease (PVD) atherosclerosis affecting a blood vessel that doesn't carry blood to the heart or brain

arteriosclerosis ("hardening of the arteries") condition that results from atherosclerosis

hypertension abnormally high blood pressure levels that persist

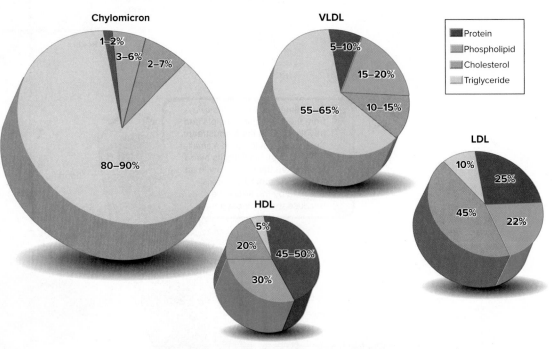

Figure 6.14 Lipoproteins: Composition and size. The composition of a lipoprotein contributes to its size and density.

Essential Concept

6.5 What Happens to Lipoproteins?

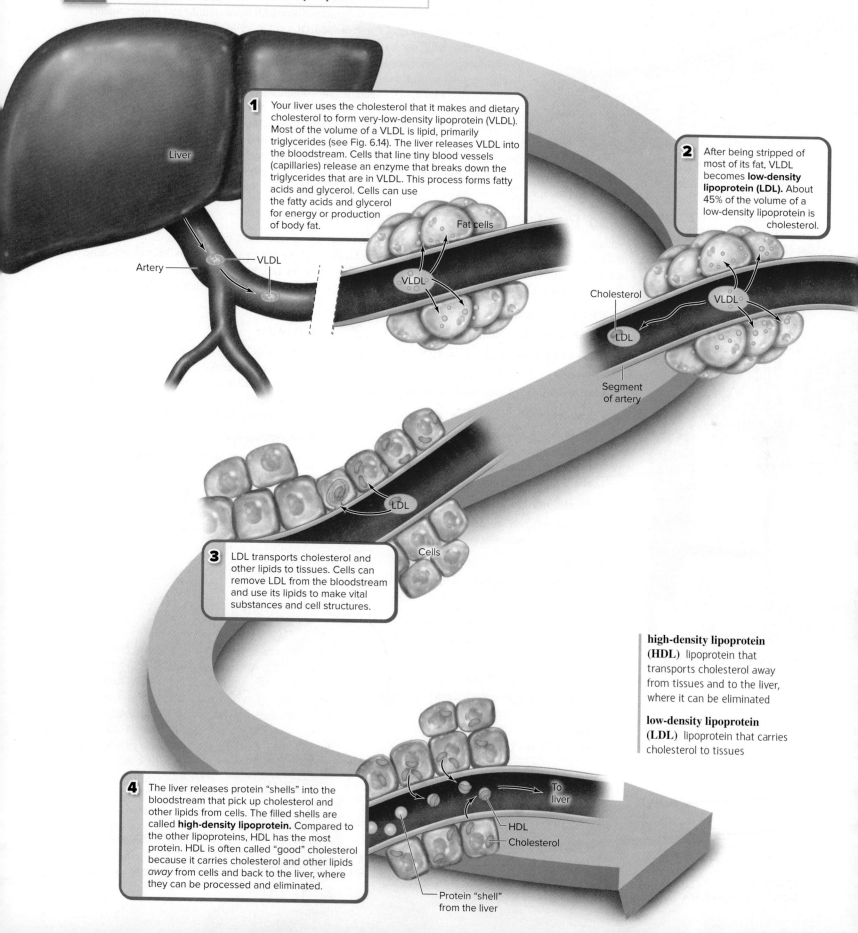

1 Your liver uses the cholesterol that it makes and dietary cholesterol to form very-low-density lipoprotein (VLDL). Most of the volume of a VLDL is lipid, primarily triglycerides (see Fig. 6.14). The liver releases VLDL into the bloodstream. Cells that line tiny blood vessels (capillaries) release an enzyme that breaks down the triglycerides that are in VLDL. This process forms fatty acids and glycerol. Cells can use the fatty acids and glycerol for energy or production of body fat.

2 After being stripped of most of its fat, VLDL becomes **low-density lipoprotein (LDL).** About 45% of the volume of a low-density lipoprotein is cholesterol.

3 LDL transports cholesterol and other lipids to tissues. Cells can remove LDL from the bloodstream and use its lipids to make vital substances and cell structures.

4 The liver releases protein "shells" into the bloodstream that pick up cholesterol and other lipids from cells. The filled shells are called **high-density lipoprotein.** Compared to the other lipoproteins, HDL has the most protein. HDL is often called "good" cholesterol because it carries cholesterol and other lipids *away* from cells and back to the liver, where they can be processed and eliminated.

high-density lipoprotein (HDL) lipoprotein that transports cholesterol away from tissues and to the liver, where it can be eliminated

low-density lipoprotein (LDL) lipoprotein that carries cholesterol to tissues

Liver

Artery

VLDL

Fat cells

VLDL

Cholesterol

VLDL

LDL

Segment of artery

LDL

Cells

To liver

HDL

Cholesterol

Protein "shell" from the liver

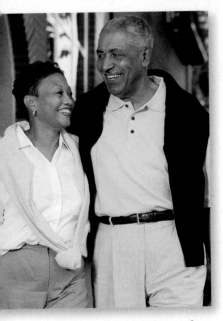

Free radicals
Oxidized LDL cholesterol
LDL
Plaque

Figure 6.15 **Oxidized LDL cholesterol.** Cells that line the artery remove LDL from the bloodstream. This process carries oxidized cholesterol into the cells.

■ *Why is oxidized LDL cholesterol harmful?*

Oxidized LDL Cholesterol

LDL cholesterol is often referred to as "bad" cholesterol because the lipoprotein carries the lipid to cells in the arterial walls that make plaques. However, there are different types of LDL, and not all forms of the lipoprotein are unhealthy. Some LDLs are smaller and denser than others. People with high levels of small dense LDLs are more likely to develop atherosclerosis than are people with low levels of these particular LDLs.[8] Additionally, chemically unstable substances ("free radicals") can damage LDL, especially small dense LDLs. The damage results in *oxidized LDL cholesterol*, which is taken up by the plaque-forming arterial cells (**Fig. 6.15**). Cigarette smoking increases the production of oxidized LDL cholesterol.[9]

Excessive alcohol and refined carbohydrate intakes stimulate VLDL production in the liver. VLDL carries a larger amount of triglycerides than cholesterol (see Fig. 6.14). As blood triglyceride levels increase, concentrations of cholesterol that's carried by HDL (HDL cholesterol) tend to decrease. As a result, high triglyceride levels may contribute to the development of CVD.

6.3b Risk Factors for Atherosclerosis

Although atherosclerosis can begin during adolescence and young adulthood, the disease usually doesn't produce signs or symptoms of CVD until decades later. Medical experts haven't been able to determine a cause of atherosclerosis. However, they have identified risk factors and some health conditions that may increase your risk of the disease.[10] The more risk factors you have, the greater your chances of developing CVD.

The following points are known risk factors for atherosclerosis:

- **Unhealthy blood cholesterol levels**

  High LDL cholesterol and low HDL cholesterol are major risk factors.

- **Hypertension (chronically high blood pressure)**

- **Smoking**

  Exposure to tobacco smoke damages and hardens blood vessels, contributes to hypertension, and raises oxidized LDL cholesterol levels.

- **Insulin resistance**

  If your cells don't respond to insulin normally, your blood glucose levels increase as a result.

- **Diabetes**

  Diabetes often results from insulin resistance.

- **Excess body fat**

  Too much body fat can contribute to insulin resistance, type 2 diabetes, and hypertension.

- **Lack of physical activity**

  Physical inactivity contributes to excess body fat, hypertension, high LDL cholesterol levels, insulin resistance, and type 2 diabetes.

- **Poor diet**

  Diets that supply high amounts of trans fat, saturated fat, added sugars, alcohol, and salt may raise LDL cholesterol levels, lower HDL cholesterol levels, increase insulin resistance, and/or raise blood pressure levels.[10]

- **Increasing age**

  Risk increases after age 45 for men and after age 55 for women.

- **Family history of CVD**

  Risk increases if your father or a brother developed heart disease by age 55 or your mother or a sister developed the disease by age 65.

Age is a major risk factor for CVD.

© David Buffington/Blend Images LLC RF

TASTY Tidbits

Plants contain substances, such as soluble fiber, that interfere with cholesterol and bile salt absorption (see Table 5.5 for common food sources of soluble fiber). Plants also make small amounts of *sterols* and *stanols*, lipids that are chemically related to cholesterol. Plant sterols/stanols block the absorption of dietary cholesterol. Eating manufactured, margarine-like spreads that contain plant sterols or stanols (functional foods) instead of butter or stick margarine may reduce mildly elevated blood cholesterol levels.

© McGraw-Hill Education.
Jill Braaten, photographer

You may have inherited factors that increase your risk of athero-sclerosis. Controlling known risk factors, such as smoking and lack of physical activity, may reduce the possible negative effects of genetics on your cardiovascular health. The following conditions may also be risk factors for atherosclerosis:

- **C-reactive protein**

  High blood levels of C-reactive protein are an indication that inflammation is occurring in your body. Recall that inflammation within arteries is an early step in the process of atherosclerosis.

- **Triglycerides**

  High blood levels of triglycerides may increase your risk, especially if you are a woman.[10]

- **Sleep apnea**

  While asleep, a person with sleep apnea stops breathing intermittently or doesn't breathe deeply. As a result, this person doesn't feel refreshed after sleeping. Untreated sleep apnea may contribute to hypertension, heart attack, and stroke.

- **Emotional stress**

  Emotional stress, particularly anger, may also play a role in the development of atherosclerosis.[10]

- **Alcohol**

  Drinking too much alcohol can damage your heart and worsen some of the other risk factors for atherosclerosis. You can learn more about alcohol in Unit 9.

6.3c Reducing Your Risk of Atherosclerosis and CVD

You may not be able to prevent having a heart attack or stroke some-day, but there's plenty of scientific evidence that suggests you can forestall CVD and live a longer, more satisfying life by reducing or eliminating modifiable risk factors for atherosclerosis. Modifiable risk factors are behaviors you can change.

You can lower your chances of developing atherosclerosis, usually by changing your lifestyle:

- Be more physically active. Regular physical activity can increase your HDL cholesterol level, lower your LDL cholesterol level, and help you lose excess body fat.

- Replace saturated FAs with polyunsaturated FAs, especially the essential fatty acids.

- Quit smoking and avoid exposure to tobacco smoke.

- Limit salt intake.

- Achieve and maintain a healthy weight for height.

- Eat more fiber-rich foods.

- Consume foods that contain antioxidants (see Table 1.4).

- Reduce added-sugar and alcohol intake.

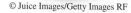

Nancy, the college student featured in the unit opener, should be concerned about her risk of CVD because she may have inherited CVD risk factors from her mother. Based on what you've learned by reading this unit, what lifestyle changes could Nancy make to reduce her risk of CVD?

Stress may be a risk factor for CVD.

© Juice Images/Getty Images RF

Increasing your physical activity level may reduce your risk of CVD.

© Jeff Maloney/Getty Images RF

Focus on Dietary Fats

Although oils, fatty spreads, and salad dressings are obvious sources of dietary fat, much of the fat you eat isn't visible. Saturated fat contributes much of the calories in fatty meats, luncheon meats, sausage, hot dogs, and "full-fat" dairy products such as hard cheeses and whole milk. Populations that consume diets rich in saturated FAs (SFAs) generally have higher rates of heart disease than populations that eat less saturated fat.[11]

You can reduce your risk of CVD by replacing foods that are rich sources of saturated FAs with foods that contain more polyunsaturated FAs.[11] Eating fewer foods that contain trans fats can also lower your risk of CVD.

Following a diet that supplies more monounsaturated FAs than saturated FAs may lower your risk of CVD. More research, however, is needed to support a recommendation to replace foods that are high in saturated FAs with foods that are rich sources of monounsaturated FAs.[11]

TASTY Tidbits

Cooks often use butter to make baked goods such as cookies and pastries. You can substitute vegetable oil for the solid fat in recipes, but use about ¾ as much oil as butter. However, be aware that replacing the solid fat with oil may alter the texture and appearance of the baked product.

Essential Concept

6.6 General Effects of Dietary Fatty Acids on LDL and HDL

Sources of SFAs
Most SFAs increase blood cholesterol levels by raising concentrations of both LDL and HDL cholesterol.

LDL HDL
Blood cholesterol

Sources of trans fatty acids
Trans fats also raise blood cholesterol levels. However, trans fats raise LDL cholesterol while reducing beneficial HDL cholesterol levels.[11]

LDL HDL
Blood cholesterol

Sources of monounsaturated FAs
Monounsaturated FAs generally lower LDL cholesterol and raise HDL cholesterol levels.[11]

LDL HDL
Blood cholesterol

Sources of polyunsaturated FAs
Diets containing more polyunsaturated FAs than saturated FAs may reduce blood levels of total cholesterol and LDL cholesterol. In some individuals, however, polyunsaturated FAs also reduce beneficial HDL cholesterol. Nevertheless, polyunsaturated FAs tend to be good for you because they don't promote atherosclerosis.

LDL HDL (some people)
Blood cholesterol

A healthy eating pattern (see Unit 3) and the traditional Mediterranean Diet are heart healthy diets because they emphasize seafood, unsaturated fats, whole grains, nuts, beans, fruits, and vegetables (see Figure 3.6).[12]

6.3d Assessing Your Risk of Atherosclerosis

To determine your risk of atherosclerosis, it's a good idea to have regular medical checkups. Your physician should measure your blood pressure and listen to blood flow in your carotid arteries to assess whether those particular arteries are becoming blocked. The physician may request a blood test to assess your total blood cholesterol level as well as HDL cholesterol, LDL cholesterol, and triglyceride levels. Ask your physician for a copy of the laboratory results; keep them in your personal "medical file" for future reference.

Table 6.3 presents classifications for healthy and unhealthy blood lipid levels. The desirable range for total cholesterol is less than 200 mg/dl. Do you know what your blood cholesterol level is? Even if it's below 200 mg/dl, you may still have a high risk of atherosclerosis. Why? Although knowing the concentration of cholesterol carried by all lipoproteins is important, the amounts of certain lipoproteins in your blood, particularly LDL and HDL, are more critical risk factors. It's healthier to have higher levels of HDL cholesterol

TASTY Tidbits

Garlic, onions, and chives are sources of sulfur-containing compounds, such as allicin, that have antioxidant properties. Fresh garlic and garlic supplements have been promoted to reduce the risk of heart disease. Many studies don't provide strong scientific support for consuming fresh garlic or garlic supplements to lower elevated blood cholesterol levels.[13] Some studies, however, support the use of garlic supplements to lower blood pressure and slow the progress of atherosclerosis. As is often the case, more research is needed to determine whether eating garlic or taking garlic supplements helps prevent CVD.

© FoodCollection/StockFood RF

than to have higher levels of LDL cholesterol. To calculate your risk of having a future heart attack, use the risk assessment tool at http://cvdrisk.nhlbi.nih.gov/calculator.asp.

TABLE 6.3

CLASSIFICATION OF BLOOD LIPID LEVELS

Total Cholesterol (mg/dl)	Classification
< 200	Desirable
200 to 239	Borderline unhealthy
≥ 240	Unhealthy
LDL cholesterol (mg/dl)	**Classification**
< 100	Optimal for health
100 to 129	Good, but lower is better
130 to 159	Borderline unhealthy
160 to 189	Unhealthy
≥ 190	Very unhealthy
HDL cholesterol (mg/dl)	**Classification**
< 40	Increases risk of heart disease
≥ 60	Protects against heart disease
Triglycerides (mg/dl)	**Classification**
< 150	Acceptable
150 to 199	Borderline unhealthy
≥ 200	Unhealthy

Olives and olive oil are associated with the Mediterranean Diet.

© Image Source/Jupiter Images RF

Source of data: National Institutes of Health, National Heart, Lung, and Blood Institute: *ATP III guidelines at-a-glance quick desk reference.* 2001. http://www.nhlbi.nih.gov/files/docs/guidelines/atglance.pdf Accessed: May 13, 2016

6.3e Recommendations for Fat and Cholesterol Intakes

On average, fat contributes a little more than 36% of adult Americans' daily energy intake from macronutrients (see Fig. 5.2).[14] The Acceptable Macronutrient Distribution Range (AMDR) for fat is 20 to 35% of total calories. The *Dietary Guidelines* recommends that less than 10% of your energy intake should be from saturated FAs. In 2013–2014, American adults consumed an average of about 11.6% of their total daily energy intake from saturated fat.[14] The *Dietary Guidelines* also recommends that you keep your cholesterol and trans fat intakes as low as possible while following a healthy eating pattern. To estimate your average percentage of total energy from fat as well as your saturated fat intake per day, complete the "What's In Your Diet?!" activity at the end of this unit.

How to Increase Your Essential Fat Intake

A "heart healthy" diet, including the Mediterranean Diet (see Fig, 3.6), doesn't recommend eating fatty red meats. Such diets emphasize fruits, vegetables, whole grains, low-fat dairy products, and foods that are rich sources of the essential omega-3 and omega-6 fatty acids. Corn oil, seeds, and nuts are rich sources of the omega-6 fat linoleic acid. Flaxseeds, soybeans, and walnuts are good sources of the omega-3 fat alpha-linolenic acid. You can meet the recommended amounts of essential fatty acids by replacing solid fats with about 5 teaspoons of vegetable oil daily (2000 kcal diet).[1]

Your body can only make small amounts of DHA and EPA. Therefore, it's a good idea to include sources of DHA and EPA, such as fatty, cold-water fish, in your diet. Food sources of omega-3 fats are listed in **Table 6.4**. Shark, swordfish, king mackerel, and tilefish contain high levels of methylmercury, which is toxic, especially for growing bodies. Therefore, pregnant women, breastfeeding women, and young children should avoid those kinds of fish.

To increase your intake of essential fatty acids from dietary sources,

- Eat at least 8 ounces of seafood, especially fatty fish, a week (see Table 6.4). Pregnant or breastfeeding women should limit their seafood intake to 12 ounces per week.[1]

- Bake, grill, or broil fish. Before cooking, marinate fresh fish in soybean oil that has been seasoned with a small amount of garlic, pepper, and lemon juice. The light coating of oil on fish can help keep the food from drying out during cooking.

- Add water-packed canned tuna or salmon to salads, or mix the fish with a little vegetable oil to make a spread for toast or crackers.

- Sprinkle chopped walnuts on salads, yogurt, or cereal, or simply eat the nuts as a snack. However, control your portion sizes because nuts are an energy-dense food.

What About Fish Oil?

What if you don't like to eat fish? Should you take fish oil supplements? The heart healthy benefits of using fish oil supplements haven't been supported by scientific studies.[15] The evidence seems to indicate that eating fish is the best way to obtain omega-3s.

It's a good idea to check with your physician before you decide to increase the omega-3 fatty acid content of your diet by taking fish oil supplements. Taking high doses of omega-3 FAs may cause serious side effects, including reducing the blood's ability to clot and bleeding within the brain.[16]

TABLE 6.4	FOOD SOURCES OF OMEGA-3 FATS			
	Fish/Shellfish (DHA and EPA)	**Oils**	**Nuts and Seeds**	**Other**
	Herring, salmon, sablefish, anchovies, tuna, bluefish, sardines, catfish, striped bass, mackerel, trout, halibut, pollock, flounder, shrimp, mussels, crab	Flaxseed, walnut, canola, soybean	Walnuts, flaxseeds	Algae

6.3f Heart Healthy Food Selection and Preparation Tips

You can change your food selection and preparation practices to reduce the amount of saturated fat, trans fat, salt, and calories in your diet.

- Choose lean cuts of meat such as
  - Round and top round, loin, and top sirloin steaks, as well as chuck and arm roasts.
  - The leanest cuts of pork include pork loin, tenderloin, and center loin.
  - When buying ground beef, consider choosing "extra lean" products. The label on a package of extra lean ground beef should state that the meat is at least 90% lean. To keep the ground beef from tasting "dry," add a small amount of olive or canola oil to the raw meat before shaping it into a meatloaf or hamburger patties.
- Use moist cooking methods for lean cuts of meat:
  - "Pot" roasting, which is adding some water to the meat and covering the pot with a lid or tightly covering the baking dish with foil, helps to tenderize meats without adding fat.
- Reduce the oven temperature from 350°F to less than 325°F. The meat will take longer to cook, but it's less likely to toughen and dry out.
- After cooking, trim away much of the visible fat from the meat.
- Don't use pan drippings to make sauces or gravies.
- Steam meats and vegetables.
- Stir-fry pieces of raw vegetables, lean meat, fish, shellfish, and poultry in small amounts of hot vegetable oil. This method cooks the foods quickly and preserves micronutrients.
- Brown ground beef in a pan, then drain the beef fat before you add other ingredients to the meat. If more fat is needed, add a little vegetable oil to the pan.
- Avoid dipping raw foods in batter or breading and deep-fat frying them. Such coatings absorb the oil.
- Don't add salt while you're preparing meats, fish, and poultry.

Stir-fried vegetables

- If you deep-fat fry foods, place the items on paper towels after cooking them to soak up as much excess fat as possible.

- Peel greasy breading from fried fish before eating it.

- Switch from drinking whole or 2% milk to 1% or fat-free milk. Whole milk is 3.25% fat by volume. Fat-free milk ("skim milk") contains less than 0.5% fat. Switch from using regular cream cheese to reduced-fat cream cheese.

- Use less salad dressing on salads. When in restaurants, order salad dressings "on the side" so you can control the amount that's added. Make your own salad dressing by combining vegetable oil and vinegar with some herbs and spices, such as oregano, basil, and black pepper.

- Substituting tub or diet margarines for butter in recipes is not recommended because such margarine-like spreads have varying water contents. As a result, using a margarine alternative, especially for baked products, can change the texture or quality of the food.

- Eat fewer commercially prepared baked goods, snack foods, and fried fast-food items.

- Purchase brands of microwave popcorn that have little added fat. Buy plain popcorn, and use a small amount of hot oil in a covered saucepan to pop the kernels or use a hot-air machine.

- Replace some fatty foods with reduced-fat or fat-free alternatives.

- Substitute plain, fat-free yogurt in recipes that call for sour cream. Place a spoonful of the yogurt, instead of butter or sour cream, on a baked potato.

Salad dressing "on the side"

What *IS* That? - - - - - - - - - - - - - →

If you need to reduce your cholesterol intake, you can use commercially available egg substitutes to replace whole eggs in recipes. Such products are made from eggs, but they only include the egg whites, which are free of cholesterol and fat. One-fourth cup of an egg substitute replaces one whole egg. If you don't have an egg substitute on hand, you can use two egg whites for each whole egg in a recipe.

© Wendy Schiff

- Replace half or all of the solid fat or oil in recipes for baked goods with unsweetened applesauce. If a recipe, for example, calls for 1 cup butter, you can replace half of the butter with ½ cup of applesauce. Substituting oil for all of the solid fat in a recipe for a baked product is often not recommended. Instead, try replacing up to ¾ of the solid fat with oil.

- To lower the fat content of their products, manufacturers of "lite" spreads may have water as the first ingredient. Therefore, replacing the margarine, butter, oil, or shortening in a recipe with a reduced-fat spread could alter the product's taste, texture, and appearance. It's a good idea to read the reduced-fat spread's label to determine whether the product is suitable to use in recipes.

- Use peanut or soy nut butters instead of cheese or luncheon meat in sandwiches. Some nut butters contain trans fats and added sugars, so read the Nutrition Facts panel and ingredients list before selecting these products.

Appendix I has more tips for reducing the amount of unhealthy solid fats in your favorite recipes.

What If Lifestyle Changes Don't Work?

Some people are unable to lower their risk of CVD by making dietary changes, exercising regularly, and losing excess body fat. If you've made these lifestyle changes and your blood lipids are still too high, it's important to discuss additional treatment options with your physician. Millions of Americans take a class of prescription drugs called statins to reduce their high blood lipid levels. Statins interfere with the liver's metabolism of cholesterol, effectively reducing LDL cholesterol and triglyceride levels as a result. The results of research, however, don't clearly indicate that statins lower the risk of CVD. Statins are relatively safe when taken as directed.

Zetia® is a drug that works differently from a statin. Zetia® inhibits intestinal absorption of cholesterol and, as a result, lowers LDL cholesterol levels. However, questions have been raised about the safety of this medication, particularly when it's taken with other cholesterol-lowering medications.[16]

Nutrition Fact or Fiction?

Eggs are loaded with cholesterol, so you should avoid eating them.

Having too much cholesterol in your blood may increase your risk of heart disease and stroke. Egg yolks are a rich source of cholesterol, but yolks contain more of the "healthy" unsaturated fats than the "unhealthy" saturated fats. Furthermore, whole eggs are nutrient dense and relatively low in cost. If you're healthy, you probably can eat one egg a day without worrying.[17] Why? For most people, the saturated and trans fat contents of a food have more of an effect on their blood cholesterol levels than does the food's cholesterol content. It's wise for healthy people to practice "moderation" when eating all foods, including eggs.

© Pixtal/AGE Fotostock RF

In a **Nutshell**

© McGraw-Hill Education. Mark A. Dierker, photographer

Module 6.1: What Are Lipids?

- The body needs lipids for many functions, including energy, maintaining cell membranes, producing bile and certain hormones, insulating against cold temperatures, regulating blood pressure and inflammation, and cushioning against bumps, blows, and falls. Major lipids are triglycerides, sterols, and phospholipids.

- The fat in food enhances absorption of fat-soluble vitamins and phytochemicals. Dietary lipids also contribute to the appealing flavor, texture, and aroma of foods. Consuming some lipids is essential for health, but high amounts of certain lipids may increase your risk of serious health conditions, particularly heart disease, stroke, and obesity.

- Triglycerides comprise most of the lipid content of your food and body. A triglyceride molecule has three fatty acids in its chemical structure. Fatty acids can be saturated or unsaturated. Unsaturated fatty acids can be either monounsaturated or polyunsaturated.

- The body cannot make the omega-6 fatty acid linoleic acid and the omega-3 fatty acid alpha-linolenic acid; these essential fatty acids must be supplied by the diet. The richest sources of essential fats include canola, soybean, and corn oils and products made with these oils, such as salad dressings. You can also meet your essential fatty acid needs by eating nuts, seeds, whole grains, and, especially, fatty fish.

- Triglycerides usually contain mixtures of unsaturated and saturated fatty acids, but one type of fatty acid tends to predominate. In general, animal fats contain more saturated fatty acids than plant oils. Important exceptions are the highly saturated coconut, palm, and palm kernel oils.

- The partial hydrogenation of unsaturated fats produces saturated fats and trans fats. The trans fats in processed foods are "bad" fats because they're associated with an increased risk of heart disease and stroke.

- Phospholipids are the major structural component of cell membranes and are needed for proper functioning of nerve cells, including those in the brain. Lecithin is the major phospholipid in food. Egg yolks, liver, wheat germ, peanut butter, and soybeans are rich sources of lecithin compound.

- The sterol cholesterol, which is found only in animal foods, is a component of every cell membrane. Cells use cholesterol to make a variety of substances, including vitamin D, bile, and steroid hormones such as estrogen and testosterone. Plants make sterols and stanols that may be beneficial to health because they block cholesterol absorption in the GI tract.

Module 6.2: What Happens to the Fat and Cholesterol You Eat?

- Fat undergoes digestion primarily in the upper part of the small intestine. Cholesterol isn't broken down and is absorbed through the intestinal wall.

- Before leaving the small intestine, triglycerides, cholesterol, and other lipids are formed into chylomicrons. Chylomicrons enter the lymphatic system of the small intestine and eventually reach the bloodstream. The liver removed lipids from chylomicrons to make various lipoproteins—substances that transport lipids in the bloodstream.

- The small intestine absorbs bile components for the liver to recycle to make new bile.

- Triglycerides are major sources of cellular energy. If energy isn't needed, fat cells store the energy in triglycerides. When cells need energy, fat cells break down some stored triglycerides and release glycerol and fatty acids into the bloodstream.

© McGraw-Hill Education. Elite Images, photographer

Module 6.3: Cardiovascular Disease: Major Killer of Americans

- CVD affects the heart and blood vessels. In the United States, heart disease is the leading cause of death; stroke is the fifth-leading cause of death. Atherosclerosis is a long-term process that can result in arteriosclerosis and CVD.

- Numerous risk factors are associated with atherosclerosis; some risk factors are inherited and difficult to modify, but many are related to lifestyle practices that can be altered. Smoking cigarettes, eating certain fats, and being physically inactive are lifestyle practices that can increase your risk of atherosclerosis and CVD.

- Lipoproteins transport much of the lipid content of the blood. Having high blood levels of HDL cholesterol is healthier than having high LDL cholesterol levels. Elevated LDL cholesterol contributes to atherosclerosis, whereas elevated HDL cholesterol reduces the risk of this condition.

- Exercising and replacing saturated and trans fats with unsaturated fats may reduce your LDL cholesterol levels and increase HDL cholesterol levels. On the other hand, physical inactivity and eating high amounts of saturated fat and trans fats can raise LDL cholesterol, increasing your risk of atherosclerosis. Many healthy people, however, do not experience an increase in their blood cholesterol levels when they eat cholesterol in foods.

- Fat contributes 36% of the average American's daily energy intake. The AMDR for fat is 20 to 35% of total calories.

- If you make recommended dietary modifications, lose excess weight, and exercise regularly, and your blood lipid levels still remain high, you should discuss additional treatment options with your physician. Millions of Americans take prescription statin medications to reduce their elevated blood lipid levels.

What's in **Your Diet?!**

1. Refer to the 3-day food log from the "What's In Your Diet?!" feature in Unit 3. List the total number of kilocalories you consumed for each day of recordkeeping. Add the figures to obtain a total, divide the total by 3, then round the figure to the nearest whole number to obtain your average daily energy intake for the 3-day period.

Sample Calculation:

Day 1	2000 kcal
Day 2	1700 kcal
Day 3	2350 kcal
Total kcal	6050 ÷ 3 days = 2017 kcal/day

(average kilocalorie intake, rounded to the nearest whole number)

© Purestock/SuperStock RF

Your Calculation:

Day 1	_____ kcal
Day 2	_____ kcal
Day 3	_____ kcal
Total kcal	_____ ÷ 3 days = _____ kcal/day

(average kilocalorie intake, rounded to the nearest whole number)

2. Add the number of grams of fat eaten each day of the period. Divide the total by 3 and round to the nearest whole number to calculate the average number of grams of fat consumed daily.

Sample Calculation:

Day 1	50 g
Day 2	57 g
Day 3	42 g
Total =	149 g
Total grams	149 ÷ 3 days = 50 g/day (average)

Your Calculation:

Day 1 _____ g

Day 2 _____ g

Day 3 _____ g

Total = _____ g

Total grams _____ ÷ 3 days = _____ g of fat/day

(average, rounded to the nearest whole number)

3. Each gram of fat provides about 9 kcal; therefore, you must multiply the average number of grams of fat that you ate daily (step 2) by 9 to obtain the average number of kilocalories from fat.

Sample Calculation:

50 g/day × 9 kcal/g = 450 kcal from fat

Your Calculation

_____ g/day × 9 kcal/g = _____ kcal from fat

4. To calculate the average percentage of calories that fat contributed to your diet, divide the average number of calories from fat obtained in step 3 by the average total daily calorie intake obtained in step 1, and round to the nearest one-hundredth. Multiply the value by 100, drop the decimal point, and add the percent symbol.

Sample Calculation:

450 kcal ÷ 2017 kcal = 0.22

0.22 × 100 = 22 %

Your Calculation

_____ kcal ÷ _____ kcal = _____

_____ × 100 = _____ %

5. Did your average daily fat intake meet the AMDR of 20 to 35% of total energy?   Yes _____   No _____

6. If your average fat intake was more than 35% of your total energy intake, which foods contributed to your high intake of fats?

Foods: _____

7. Review the log of your 3-day food intake. Calculate your average daily intake of saturated fat by adding the grams of saturated fat consumed over the 3-day period and dividing the total by 3.

Your Calculation:

Day 1 _____ g

Day 2 _____ g

Day 3 _____ g

Total = _____ g

Total g _____ ÷ 3 days = _____ g of saturated fat daily

a. What was your average daily saturated fat intake? _____ g

b. Was your average daily saturated fat intake less than the Dietary Guidelines' recommended limit for a healthy adult (less than 10% of total calories)?

c. If your average saturated fat intake was more than the recommended percentage, list foods that contributed to your high saturated fat intake.

Using Nutrient Labels: Total Fat and Saturated Fat

1. Remove the labels from two different packaged foods that contain fat. Using information from each of the product's Nutrition Facts panel, answer the following questions.

   a. Name of product #1 _____

      Name of product #2 _____

   b. How many kcal are in one serving of each food?

      Product 1 _____ kcal

      Product 2 _____ kcal

   c. How many grams of fat and saturated fat are in a serving?

      Product 1

      _____ grams of fat

      _____ grams of saturated fat

      Product 2

      _____ grams of fat

      _____ grams of saturated fat

© Ingram Publishing RF

   d. Calculate the percentage of total kcal/serving that are from saturated fat. First, multiply the number of grams of saturated fat by 9 (number of kcal per gram of fat). Then, divide the number of kcal contributed by saturated fat by the total number of kcal per serving. (The Nutrition Label uses the term "Calories" for kcal.) To obtain the percentage, move the decimal point two places to the right, remove the decimal point, and insert % symbol.

      Product 1

      _____ grams of saturated fat × 9 kcal = _____ kcal of saturated fat/serving

      _____ % total kcal/serving contributed by saturated fat

      Product 2

      _____ grams of saturated fat × 9 kcal = _____ kcal of saturated fat/serving

      _____ % total kcal/serving contributed by saturated fat

   e. Read the list of ingredients for each product. If the food contained saturated fat, identify ingredients that contributed this type of fat to the product.

      Saturated fat ingredients in Product 1 _____

      Saturated fat ingredients in Product 2 _____

Consider This...

1. Visit the American Heart Association's "Heart attack risk calculator" at www.heart.org. Take the risk calculator. Based on your results, are you concerned about your risk of heart attack? Explain why you are or are not concerned. If you're concerned, discuss steps you can take to reduce your risk of atherosclerosis.

2. Do you avoid fried foods and look for "lite" and "fat-reduced" foods when shopping for groceries? Explain why you do or do not take these actions.

3. Plan a meal that supplies 20 to 35% of energy from fat. The meal should include foods from the major food groups and provide 700 to 900 kcal.

4. Suggest at least four ways you can reduce your intake of saturated fat and increase your intake of unsaturated fat.

5. Develop a lesson for high-school-aged youth that describes atherosclerosis and the role that personal choices (lifestyles) play in the development of the disease.

© FoodCollection/StockFood RF

Test Yourself

Select the best answer.

1. Fats in foods
   a. contribute 7 kcal per gram.
   b. are digested and absorbed in the stomach.
   c. help the body absorb fat-soluble vitamins.
   d. need to be limited to less than 20% of total kcal to have a healthful diet.

2. Liquid fats generally have a high proportion of _____ fatty acids.
   a. unsaturated
   b. saturated
   c. trans
   d. partially hydrogenated

3. A monounsaturated fatty acid has
   a. one double bond within the carbon chain.
   b. two double bonds within the carbon chain.
   c. no double bonds within the carbon chain.
   d. three double bonds within the carbon chain.

4. Which of the following statements is true?
   a. Walnuts are a rich source of PHOs.
   b. Omega-3 fatty acids decrease the risk of cardiovascular disease.
   c. Trans fats are rich sources of omega-3 fatty acids.
   d. The human body converts dietary fiber into omega-3 fatty acids.

© FoodCollection /Stockfood RF

5. Fatty fish
   a. contain too much methylmercury to be eaten.
   b. should be eaten daily, according to the Dietary Guidelines (U.S. version).
   c. are not sources of cholesterol.
   d. are sources of omega-3 fatty acids.

6. Cholesterol is
   a. metabolized for energy.
   b. found only in animal foods.
   c. not made by the human body.
   d. harmful to health.

7. The primary site of fat digestion and absorption is the
   a. stomach.
   b. liver.
   c. small intestine.
   d. gallbladder.

8. Lipoproteins
   a. are made in the kidneys.
   b. transport fat and cholesterol in the bloodstream.
   c. contain oxidized glucose.
   d. are toxic to cells.

9. Major risk factors for atherosclerosis include
   a. educational background.
   b. occupation.
   c. income.
   d. physical inactivity.

10. Atherosclerosis contibutes to
    a. dental decay.
    b. type 2 diabetes.
    c. gallbladder disease.
    d. cardiovascular disease.

A Answer This (Module 6.1a)

Olive oil

References ➡ See Appendix F.

connect

STUDY TIP: Quickly create a customized practice quiz for this chapter by going to your Connect SmartBook "My Reports" section.

Don't have SmartBook and want to learn more? Go to **whysmartbook.com**.

© Radius/SuperStock RF

Proteins
LIFE'S BUILDING BLOCKS

What's on the Menu?

Module 7.1
What Are Proteins?

Module 7.2
What Happens to the Protein You Eat?

Module 7.3
Proteins in Foods

Module 7.4
What's Vegetarianism?

Module 7.5
Proteins and Health

© Wendy Schiff

"I'm very physically active. When I was in high school, I ran cross-country, swam competitively, and played lacrosse. I also did strength and conditioning training. Now that I'm in college, I have to prioritize my time around my class schedule so I can work out and train for half-marathons. This year, I ran a half-marathon and came in second for my age group....I find running is a great stress reliever. I eat more when I'm in training, and my performance suffers when I don't eat the right foods....I have enough 'likes' in each food group; I think my diet is well rounded."

Olivia Coomes

Olivia Coomes is a sophomore, majoring in Accounting, at Auburn University. She is so physically active, she doesn't have to worry about her weight. She says, "I work out and eat healthy." Although she describes herself as a "picky eater," she has become more willing to try new foods since she started college.

Unlike many athletes, Olivia doesn't focus on eating protein-rich foods to ensure her optimal physical performance. Is it necessary for athletes to consume more protein than nonathletes consume? Does eating a high-protein diet help people build muscle tissue?

Many Americans think a meal isn't a meal unless it contains large portions of beef, pork, or poultry. Although it's true that these foods are rich sources of protein, other foods, including those from plants, are often overlooked as sources of protein. Protein is an important nutrient, but it isn't more valuable to your health than other nutrients. Nutrients work together in your body like members of a well-trained lacrosse team on the playing field. Making one player the star while neglecting to develop the other athletes' skills can have disastrous effects on the team's success. Similarly, overemphasizing one class of nutrients in your diet, such as protein, while ignoring other nutrients can lead to nutritional imbalances that result in serious health problems. By reading Unit 7, you'll learn about the roles of proteins in your body and their major food sources. You'll also learn how eating too much or not enough dietary protein can influence your health.

161

Module 7.1

What Are Proteins?

7.1- Learning Outcomes

After reading Module 7.1, you should be able to

1. Define all of the key terms in this module.
2. List the primary functions of proteins in the body.
3. Identify the basic structural unit of proteins.
4. Distinguish between essential and nonessential amino acids.

Proteins are organic nutrients that are chemically similar to lipids and carbohydrates because they contain carbon, hydrogen, and oxygen atoms. Proteins, however, contain nitrogen, the element cells need to make a wide array of important biological compounds. Plants, animals, bacteria, and even viruses contain hundreds of proteins.

7.1a What Roles Do Proteins Play in the Body?

All cells in your body contain proteins. The thousands of different proteins in your body have a wide variety of functions. Your body uses protein to

- *Make, maintain, and repair cells.*

    Cells have proteins in their membranes and other cellular structures. When cells divide, such as during periods of growth, they need protein to form cell membranes and other protein-containing components of the new cells.

- *Build structures.*

    Structural proteins such as *collagen* are in your cartilage, ligaments, and bone tissue. *Keratin* is another structural protein—it's in your hair, nails, and skin. Keratin is tough and resists water, which is why your hair, nails, and skin are water-resistant. Contractile proteins in your muscles enable you to move.

    Your hair contains a protein called keratin.

- *Produce enzymes, lubricants, and clotting compounds.*
    - Nearly all enzymes are proteins. Enzymes speed up the rate of (*catalyze*) chemical reactions without becoming a part of the products. Sucrase, for example, is the enzyme that catalyzes the breakdown of sucrose into glucose and fructose.
    - Lubricants include *mucin*, which is in mucus and saliva.
    - *Fibrin* is a tough protein that forms when a blood clot is needed to stop bleeding.

- *Transport substances.*
    - Transport proteins include hemoglobin, which transports oxygen in red blood cells, and *retinol binding protein*, which carries vitamin A in the bloodstream.
    - Proteins in cell membranes control the movement of substances in and out of cells.

- *Make antibodies.*
    - **Antibodies** are structures in the bloodstream that help prevent and combat infections.

- *Make certain hormones.*

    Many hormones, including insulin and glucagon, are proteins.

- *Maintain proper fluid balance and acid-base balance.*
    - Proteins in blood, such as *albumin*, help maintain the proper distribution of fluids in blood and body tissues. The force of blood pressure moves watery fluid out of the bloodstream and into tissues. Blood proteins help counteract the effects of blood pressure by attracting the fluid, returning it to the bloodstream. When the body's supply of protein is inadequate, the level of protein in blood decreases and, as a result, some water leaks out of the bloodstream and enters spaces between cells. The resulting accumulation of fluid in tissues is called **edema** (*eh-dee´mah*) (**Fig. 7.1**).

Figure 7.1 "Pitting" edema.

■ *How does a protein-deficient diet contribute to edema?*

- Proteins also help maintain **acid-base balance**, the proper concentration of hydrogen ions (H^+), in body fluids. To function properly, blood and tissue fluids need to be slightly basic. If the H^+ concentration of these fluids increases above normal levels, the tissues become too acidic. If the H^+ concentration decreases too much, the blood and tissues become too basic (alkaline). When a particular body fluid becomes too acidic or too basic, cells can have difficulty functioning and may die. A *buffer* helps maintain the proper H^+ concentration of fluids. Proteins can act as buffers because they have acidic and basic components. If cells form an excess of H^+, the basic portions of protein molecules bind to the excess H^+, neutralizing the excess and reducing the concentration of H^+ back to normal.

- *Provide energy.*

  Although cells can use the basic components of proteins for energy, normally they metabolize very little for energy. As a result, cells save protein for other important functions that carbohydrates and lipids are unable to perform.

7.1b What Are Amino Acids?

The basic building blocks of proteins are **amino acids**. Each amino acid has four parts:

- a carbon atom that anchors a hydrogen atom,
- the amino (nitrogen-containing) group,
- the R-group that varies with each type of amino acid, and
- the acid group.

The chemical structure of the amino acid alanine indicates these three groups (**Fig. 7.2**).

When the nitrogen-containing amino group is removed, the R-group, the acid group, and the anchoring carbon atom form the "carbon skeleton" of an amino acid (see Fig. 7.2). The body can convert the carbon skeletons of certain amino acids to glucose and use the simple sugar for energy. Recall from Unit 1 that each gram of protein provides about 4 kcal.

Classifying Amino Acids

The human body contains proteins made from 20 different amino acids. Nutritionists often classify amino acids as either nonessential or essential according to the body's ability to make them. A healthy human body can make 11 of the 20 amino acids. These compounds are the **nonessential amino acids**. The remaining nine amino acids are **essential amino acids** that must be supplied by foods because the body cannot make them or produce enough to meet its needs. **Table 7.1** classifies amino acids as either essential or nonessential.

proteins large, complex organic nutrients made up of amino acids

antibodies proteins that help prevent and fight infection

edema accumulation of fluid in tissues

acid-base balance maintaining the proper hydrogen concentration of body fluids

amino acids nitrogen-containing chemical units that comprise proteins

nonessential amino acids group of amino acids that the body can make

essential amino acids amino acids the body can't make or can't make enough to meet its needs

Carbon skeleton

Figure 7.2 **Components of an amino acid (alanine).**

TABLE 7.1	AMINO ACIDS			
	Essential		**Nonessential**	
	Histidine	Phenylalanine	Alanine	Arginine*
	Isoleucine	Threonine	Aspartic acid	Cysteine*
	Leucine	Tryptophan	Asparagine	Glutamine*
	Lysine	Valine	Glutamic acid	Glycine*
	Methionine		Serine	Proline*
				Tyrosine*

*Under certain conditions, this amino acid can become essential.

Placemat: © McGraw-Hill Education. Mark A. Dierker, photographer

© Pixtal/AGE Fotostock RF

Module 7.2

What Happens to the Protein You Eat?

© Burke/Triolo/Brand X Pictures RF

7.2 - Learning Outcomes

After reading Module 7.2, you should be able to

1. Define all of the key terms in this module.

2. Explain what happens to proteins as they undergo digestion and absorption in the human digestive tract.

3. Explain how cells make proteins.

4. Describe what happens to excess amino acids.

5. Calculate your Recommended Dietary Allowance (RDA) for protein based on your body weight.

7.2a Protein Digestion and Absorption

An amino acid can connect to another amino acid by a **peptide bond,** a chemical attraction between two amino acids. To illustrate how amino acids bind together, we'll use a protein "necklace" that contains amino acid "beads" (**Fig. 7.3**). In our example of the necklace, the string that connects two beads is a peptide bond.

A **polypeptide** forms when two or more amino acids join to form chains (see Fig. 7.3). A dipeptide is a very simple polypeptide that has only two amino acids linked together. A tripeptide is a polypeptide that has only three amino acids bonded together. A protein is a polypeptide that may be comprised of hundreds of amino acids connected to each other by peptide bonds.

When you eat a toasted cheese sandwich for lunch, the large proteins in the bread and cheese must be digested before undergoing absorption. **Essential Concept 7.1** describes what happens to proteins during digestion and absorption.

Amino acid

Amino acids

Peptide bond

peptide bond chemical attraction that connects two amino acids together

polypeptides chains of two or more amino acids

Figure 7.3 Amino acids make up proteins. Human cells use 20 different amino acids to make proteins. In this illustration, amino acids are represented by beads.

Essential Concept

7.1 Digesting and Absorbing Proteins

Inside the stomach

HCl HCl

Inactive pepsin

Pepsin

Shorter polypeptide chains

Inside the small intestine

1 Protein digestion begins in the stomach. Hydrochloric acid (HCl) helps the process by changing the inactive form of pepsin to the active enzyme **pepsin**. HCl also causes proteins to unfold. This action makes it easier for pepsin to break apart the peptide bonds between amino acids. As a result, large protein chains break down into shorter polypeptide chains of several amino acids.

2 When the shortened polypeptide chains enter the small intestine, the pancreas and absorptive cells secrete protein-splitting enzymes called proteases. Proteases digest polypeptides into individual amino acids, dipeptides, and tripeptides.

Pancreas

Proteases from pancreas

Small intestine

Tripeptide

Dipeptide

Intestinal cell enzymes

Microvilli border

Absorptive cell

Tripeptides

3 Enzymes within the microvilli border of absorptive cells digest the di- and tripeptides into amino acids. Thus, amino acids are the end products of protein digestion.

To liver

Bloodstream

pepsin stomach enzyme that breaks down proteins into polypeptides

After being absorbed, the amino acids enter the large vein (hepatic portal vein) that takes absorbed nutrients to the liver. The liver keeps some amino acids for its needs and releases the rest into the general circulation. By the time cells obtain amino acids from blood, they cannot distinguish the ones that were originally in the bread from those that were in the cheese. The cells, however, now have all the amino acids they need to make your body's proteins.

Protein digestion and absorption is very efficient—only a small amount of dietary protein escapes digestion and is eliminated in feces. **Figure 7.4** summarizes protein digestion, absorption, and elimination.

7.2b Using Amino Acids to Build Proteins

To understand how the body uses the 20 different amino acids to make thousands of proteins, let's consider the protein "beaded" necklace that's illustrated in Figure 7.3. Assume that each type of amino acid is represented by a different bead. Alanine, for example, may be a green bead with fine white stripes; methionine might be a red bead with white dots. Each of the other 18 amino acids would have their own colorful pattern. A specific protein, such as insulin or sucrase, can be identified by the kinds of "beads" it contains, the order in which the beads are strung, and the number of beads that are used. The wide variety of proteins in your body reflects the numerous ways your cells can connect amino acids to form proteins.

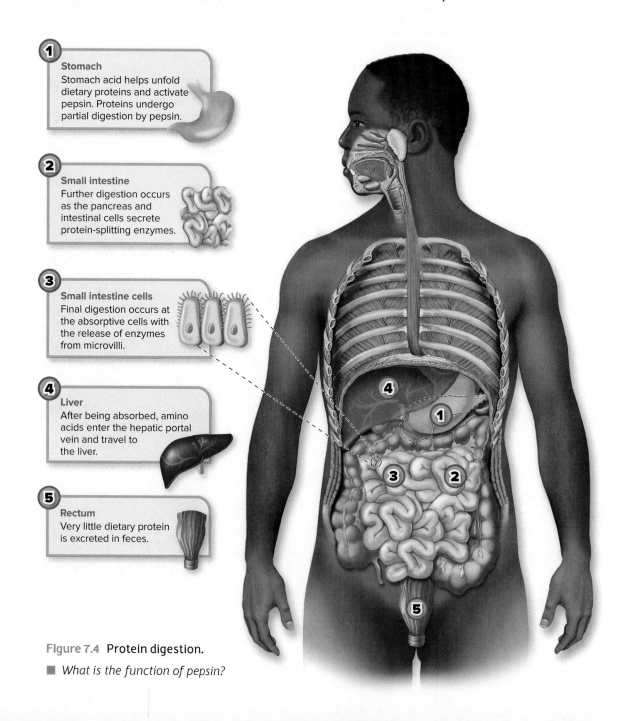

1 **Stomach**
Stomach acid helps unfold dietary proteins and activate pepsin. Proteins undergo partial digestion by pepsin.

2 **Small intestine**
Further digestion occurs as the pancreas and intestinal cells secrete protein-splitting enzymes.

3 **Small intestine cells**
Final digestion occurs at the absorptive cells with the release of enzymes from microvilli.

4 **Liver**
After being absorbed, amino acids enter the hepatic portal vein and travel to the liver.

5 **Rectum**
Very little dietary protein is excreted in feces.

Figure 7.4 **Protein digestion.**

■ *What is the function of pepsin?*

If you have a box of 1000 amino acid "beads," how do you form functional proteins from them? The instructions for making each protein "necklace" are stored in your DNA. **DNA** is often referred to as the cells' master molecule because it contains coded instructions for making proteins. If cells make mistakes and connect the wrong amino acids, they'll produce abnormal proteins that can cause birth defects, chronic health conditions, and even death.

Sickle cell disease is an inherited disorder that primarily affects people with African ancestry. The disease results from a single *mutation* (a change) in the DNA that provides instructions for making a part of hemoglobin, the protein that carries oxygen in your red blood cells (RBCs). As a result of the mutation, the wrong amino acid is added to hemoglobin during its formation. The disease gets its name from the abnormal crescent ("sickle") shape that the RBCs develop when they're in low-oxygen conditions. The sickle-shaped RBCs don't move through tiny blood vessels as easily as normal, round RBCs pass through them. The abnormal cells clump together and block blood flow in the blood vessels, causing tissue damage. In some cases, sickle cell disease is deadly.

DNA master molecule that has the instructions for making proteins

Illustration of a segment of DNA

© Digital Vision/Getty Images RF

7.2c The Fate of Excess Protein

Your body doesn't store excess amino acids in muscle or other tissues. If you consume more protein than you need, what happens to the extra amino acids? **Essential Concept 7.2** illustrates how your body handles the unneeded amino acids. Module 7.5 provides more information about the effects of excess amino acid intakes on the body.

Essential Concept

7.2 What Can Happen to Unneeded Amino Acids?

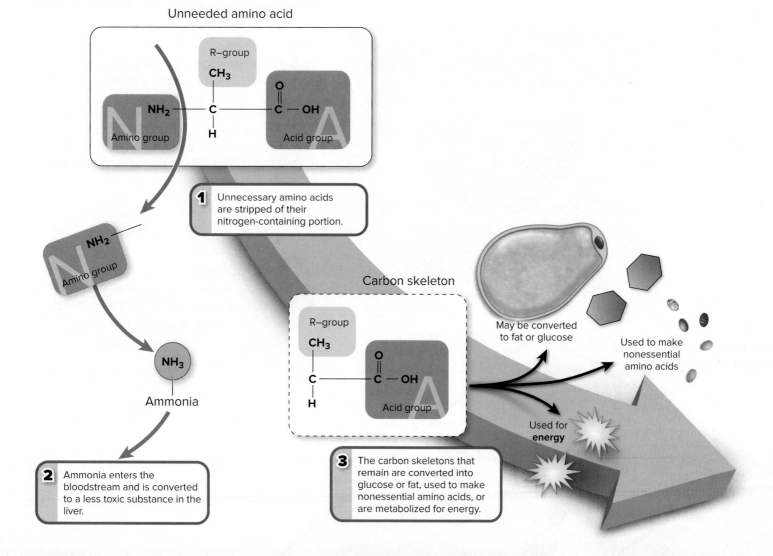

Unneeded amino acid

R–group
CH₃

NH₂ — amino group
C — H
C — OH, acid group, O

1 Unnecessary amino acids are stripped of their nitrogen-containing portion.

NH₂
Amino group

NH₃
Ammonia

2 Ammonia enters the bloodstream and is converted to a less toxic substance in the liver.

Carbon skeleton

R–group
CH₃
C — H
C — OH, Acid group

May be converted to fat or glucose

Used to make nonessential amino acids

Used for **energy**

3 The carbon skeletons that remain are converted into glucose or fat, used to make nonessential amino acids, or are metabolized for energy.

Your body can recycle nitrogen from amino acids to make nonessential amino acids. Each day, however, you lose some protein and the nitrogen it contains from your body. Your urine contains most of the lost nitrogen. Daily nitrogen losses also occur as your nails and hair grow, and when you shed the outermost layer of your skin and cells from your intestinal tract. To be healthy, your body needs amino acids from foods to replace the lost nitrogen.

7.2d How Much Protein Do You Need?

A healthy adult's Recommended Dietary Allowance (RDA) for protein is 0.8 g/kg of body weight. To determine your RDA for protein, first divide your weight in pounds by 2.2 to obtain your weight in kilograms. If, for example, you weigh 145 pounds, you weigh about 66 kg (145 ÷ 2.2). Now, multiply 0.8 g protein times 66 kg body weight. Based on these calculations, you should consume about 53 g of protein daily (66 kg × 0.8 g/kg) to meet your RDA for the nutrient. The body's need for protein increases during pregnancy, when breastfeeding, and in periods of growth, extreme physical exertion, and recovery from serious illnesses, blood losses, and burns. Unit 10 discusses protein needs of athletes.

> Your weight in pounds is _____ lbs.
>
> Now, divide this weight by 2.2 to obtain your weight in kg.
>
> My weight is _____ kg.
>
> Multiply _____ (your weight in kg) by 0.8 g/kg to obtain _____ g.
>
> This amount is your RDA for protein.

How Much Protein Do Americans Eat?

In 2013–2014, adult Americans consumed an average of 83.6 g protein/day.[1] This amount is about 15.6% of this population's total energy intake for a day. For healthy adults, diets that supply this percentage of calories as protein is within the Acceptable Macronutrient Distribution Range (AMDR), which is 10 to 35% of energy from protein. The "What's In Your Diet?!" activity at the end of this unit can help you estimate your daily protein intake.

MyPlate: Recommendations for Protein Intake

Animal foods, including eggs and milk products, supply almost two-thirds of the protein in America's food supply.[2] Animal sources of protein are often rich sources of saturated fat and cholesterol. According to the *Dietary Guidelines for Americans*, you should choose fish and seafood, lean or low-fat meat, and poultry.[3] MyPlate recommends including more plant sources of protein in your diet.

Source: ChooseMyPlate.gov

Your RDA for protein is based on your body weight.

Q Answer This

Josh is a nonathlete who weighs 165 pounds. What is his RDA for protein? You can find the answer on the last page of this unit.

Module 7.3

Proteins in Foods

7.3 - Learning Outcomes

After reading Module 7.3, you should be able to

1. Define all of the key terms in this module.

2. Identify foods that are legumes.

3. Explain the difference between a high-quality protein and a low-quality protein, and identify foods that are rich sources of high-quality proteins.

4. Plan nutritious meals and snacks that reduce animal protein intake.

5. Develop strategies for reducing your intake of animal protein without sacrificing protein quality.

legumes plants that produce pods with a single row of seeds

People often associate animal foods with protein, but beans, nuts, seeds, grains, and certain vegetables are good sources of protein, too. In fact, nearly all foods contain protein, but no naturally occurring food is 100% protein. **Table 7.2** lists some commonly eaten foods and their approximate protein content per serving.

Not all plant foods are good sources of protein. Legumes (*lay'-gumes*), seeds, and tree nuts supply more protein per serving than do servings of fruit or the edible leaves, roots, flowers, and stems of vegetables. **Legumes** are plants that produce pods that have a single row of seeds, such as soybeans, peas, peanuts, lentils, and beans. Tree nuts include walnuts, cashews, and almonds.

TABLE 7.2

APPROXIMATE PROTEIN CONTENT OF SOME COMMONLY EATEN FOODS/PORTION*

Food	Serving Size	Protein g/serving	Food	Serving Size	Protein g/serving
Chicken, breast, roasted, meat only	4 oz	34	Milk, fat-free	1 cup	8
Ham, lean, cooked	4 oz	33	Peanut butter, smooth	2 Tbsp	8
Hamburger, 80% lean, broiled	4 oz	29	Baked beans, vegetarian	½ cup	6
Pepperoni pizza, regular crust, 14" pie	2 slices (200 g)	24	Egg, large, hard cooked	1	6
Tuna, canned, water-packed, drained	4 oz	22	American processed cheese	1 oz	5
Cottage cheese, 2% low-fat	4 oz	13	Vanilla ice cream	1 cup	4
Lasagna with meat sauce	6 oz	12	White rice, cooked	1 cup	4
Tofu, regular	½ cup	10	Peas, green, cooked	½ cup	4
Bagel, plain	1 (3½" diam.)	10	Banana, medium	1	1
Almonds, whole	¼ cup	8			

Source: USDA National Nutrient Database for Standard Reference, Release 25.

Sliced ham on platter: © Ingram Publishing RF; Peas: © FoodCollection/StockFood RF

Nutrition Fact or Fiction?

Red meat is bad for you.

Red meat is a source of saturated fat and cholesterol. However, it's also a good source of B vitamins, zinc, and iron. These minerals are often less easily absorbed from plant foods. Therefore, it's OK to eat *small* portions of lean red meats occasionally. Lean red meats are cuts of beef, pork, and lamb that have "round" or "loin" in their names.

© Burke/Triolo/Brand X Pictures RF

high-quality (complete) protein protein that contains all essential amino acids in amounts that support the deposition of protein in tissues and the growth of a young person

low-quality (incomplete) protein protein that lacks or has inadequate amounts of one or more of the essential amino acids

7.3a Protein Quality

Foods differ not only in the amount of protein they contain but also in their protein quality. A **high-quality, or complete, protein** contains all essential amino acids in amounts that support the health of your muscles and other tissues, as well as a young child's growth. High-quality proteins are well digested and absorbed by your body. Meat, fish, poultry, eggs, milk, and milk products contain high-quality proteins.

A **low-quality, or incomplete, protein** lacks or contains inadequate amounts of one or more of the essential amino acids. Your digestive tract doesn't digest sources of low-quality protein as efficiently as it does foods containing high-quality protein. The essential amino acids that are in relatively low amounts are referred to as *limiting amino acids*. A protein that has limiting amino acids may be unable to provide the amino acids that your cells need to support growth, repair, and maintenance of tissues.

Most plant foods aren't sources of high-quality proteins. Quinoa (*keen'-wa*) and soy protein are exceptions. Quinoa is related to sugar beets and spinach, but the quality and amount of protein in quinoa seeds are superior to those of most other plant sources of protein.[4] Cooked quinoa is often used as a cereal (**Fig. 7.5**). After being processed, the quality of soy protein is comparable to that of most animal proteins. Processed soybeans are used to make a variety of nutritious foods, including soy milk, infant formula, and meat substitutes.

Understanding the concept of protein quality is important. Regardless of how much protein is eaten, a child will fail to grow properly if his or her diet lacks essential amino acids.

TASTY Tidbits

A 3-ounce serving of almonds, dry-roasted peanuts, or sunflower seed kernels supplies about 20 g of protein. Many seeds and nuts are rich sources of "healthy" fats (discussed in Unit 6). Because of their high fat content, seeds and nuts pack a lot of calories. Snack on just 3 ounces of almonds, dry-roasted peanuts, or sunflower seed kernels, and you'll add almost 500 kcal to your diet!

Sunflower seeds

© Royalty-Free/Corbis RF

Figure 7.5 Quinoa.

■ *Why is quinoa a good source of high-quality protein?*

© Wendy Schiff

Combining Complementary Proteins

It's not necessary to consume all essential amino acids during the same meal for your body to use them to make proteins. However, nutrition experts recommend that you consume adequate amounts of the essential amino acids each day. If you eat only plant foods, you need to plan your meals and snacks carefully to be sure your daily diet supplies enough essential amino acids. Certain plant-based recipes ensure that these compounds are eaten together. **Complementary combinations** are mixtures of certain plant foods that provide all essential amino acids without adding animal proteins.

Most plant foods are poor sources of one or more essential amino acids, particularly tryptophan, threonine, lysine, and methionine. Before preparing dishes that contain complementary combinations, it's helpful to know which plant foods are good protein sources and which of these essential amino acids are limiting or low in those plant foods.

Figure 7.6 shows three categories of plant proteins (legumes, grains, and tree nuts and seeds) that make complementary combinations when one or more foods from at least two different groups are mixed together. When menu planning, you can combine a variety of legumes, grains, tree nuts, and seeds with vegetables to prepare dishes that provide adequate mixtures of the essential amino acids. Red beans and rice as well as peanut butter on toast are examples of simple foods comprised of complementary proteins. The Tasty Tidbits feature in Module 7.4 provides other examples.

Most fruits and many kinds of vegetables are poor sources of protein. Therefore, not every mixture of plant foods creates a complementary combination. For example, making a fruit salad by combining apples, grapes, and oranges will not provide a complementary mixture of essential amino acids. Furthermore, combining Boston, iceberg, and romaine varieties of lettuce with carrots and onions makes a tasty salad, but simply mixing leafy greens with other vegetables doesn't make a complementary combination. Why? Leafy vegetables have small amounts of protein that tend to contain low amounts of essential amino acids. However, adding sunflower seed kernels, kidney or black beans, cashews, and bread cubes to the vegetable salad boosts the amount of protein and provides a complete mix of amino acids.

Although fruits and many kinds of vegetables are poor protein sources, these foods add appealing colors and textures as well as vitamins, minerals, and phytochemicals to plant-based meals. Module 7.4 explains how you can obtain a nutritionally adequate diet by reducing your intake of animal foods.

Seeds and Tree Nuts

Primary limiting amino acid:
Lysine

Sesame seeds, sunflower seed kernels, pumpkin seeds
Cashews, pistachios, walnuts, pine nuts, almonds

Grains

Primary limiting amino acid:
Lysine

Wheat and products made from wheat flour
Rice, oats, millet, barley, bulgur
Corn and products made from corn

Legumes

Primary limiting amino acids:
Methionine
Tryptophan

Peas
Peanuts and peanut butter
Soybeans, soy products, and other beans

Figure 7.6 **Complementary combinations.** Combining certain plant foods can result in complementary combinations of essential amino acids.

■ *To improve the protein quality of peas without using animal proteins, you could mix the peas with what food?*

complementary combinations mixing certain plant foods to provide all essential amino acids without adding animal protein

What *IS* That? - - - - - - - - - - - - - - - - - - - →

Tofu is made from pureed soybeans and has the consistency of thick gelatin. Plain tofu has little flavor, so it can be added to a variety of foods, including stir-fried vegetables and vegetable salads.

**Tofu with edamame
(lightly boiled soybeans)**

7.3b Stretching Your Food Dollars

Meat may be among the most expensive items on your grocery list. The following tips can help you keep your food budget under control without sacrificing good nutrition:

- Include only one animal source of protein in a meal and reduce its serving size.

- Replace meat with other high-quality protein sources. Eggs, chicken, fat-free milk, canned sardines and tuna, fat-reduced cheese, and low-fat yogurt are animal sources of high-quality protein that you can substitute for the more expensive meat items in your diet.

- Prepare meals that contain less animal protein and more plant protein. Most animal foods contain enough essential amino acids to extend or "beef up" the lower-quality proteins in peas, beans, cereals, and other grain products.

- Examples include
  - Cereal with milk, pancakes, and waffles;
  - Asian dishes that mix small amounts of chicken, beef, or seafood with large portions of rice;
  - Italian dishes that combine small amounts of cheese or meat sauce with pasta;
  - Macaroni and cheese;
  - Chili con carne;
  - Tuna-noodle casserole; and
  - Tacos or burritos filled with beans and cheese.

See Appendix H for more general information concerning ways to stretch your food dollars.

TASTY Tidbits

Commercially canned beans often have a lot of salt added to them. Consider rinsing the beans to remove much of the salt. Also, consider purchasing canned or frozen beans that have little or no added salt. Dried beans don't have added salt, but to shorten their cooking time, you can soak them in water several hours before cooking and then discard the water. The soaking process also makes the beans more digestible and less likely to contribute to intestinal gas.

Module 7.4

What's Vegetarianism?

Meatless lasagna
© Blue Moon Stock/PunchStock RF

7.4 - Learning Outcomes

After reading Module 7.4, you should be able to

1. Define all of the key terms in this module.
2. Distinguish among the various types of vegetarianism.
3. Discuss the pros and cons of vegetarian diets.

7.4a Vegetarianism

In 2012, about 5% of American adults described themselves as vegetarians; about 2% of adults reported being vegans.[5] **Vegetarians** rely heavily on plant foods and may or may not include some animal foods in their diets. **Vegans** don't eat any animal products. There are different types of vegetarian diets, including some that combine plant foods with certain animal foods:

- A **semivegetarian** (or **flexitarian**) eats eggs, fish, and dairy foods but generally avoids meat.

- A **lactovegetarian** (*lacto* = milk) consumes milk and milk products, including yogurt, cheese, and ice cream, to obtain animal protein.

- An **ovovegetarian** (*ovo* = egg) eats eggs.

- A **lactoovovegetarian** consumes milk products and eggs.

- A **vegan,** or total vegetarian, eats only plant foods.

vegetarians people who eat plant-based diets

semivegetarian or **flexitarian** person who eats eggs, fish, and dairy foods but generally avoids meat

lactovegetarian vegetarian who consumes milk and milk products for animal protein

ovovegetarian vegetarian who eats eggs for animal protein

lactoovovegetarian vegetarian who consumes milk products and eggs for animal protein

vegans vegetarians who eat only plant foods

"My parents are vegetarians, but they eat eggs and dairy products. My dad's parents were strict vegetarians, and after his father died, my dad stopped eating meat and seafood to respect his father's belief. I eat chicken, but I don't eat red meat, because of my religious background and personal preference."

Abby Raghothaman

© McGraw-Hill Education.
Mark A. Dierker, photographer

7.4b Is Vegetarianism a Healthy Lifestyle?

Vegetarian diets are often lower in fat and energy than "Western diets" that contain animal foods, particularly plenty of red meat. Compared to people who eat meat, vegetarians tend to have a lower risk of obesity, type 2 diabetes, hypertension, and certain cancers.[6] Furthermore, vegans tend to be leaner than nonvegans.[6] It's difficult, however, to pinpoint diet as being solely responsible for vegetarians' health status. Why? Vegetarians often adopt other healthy lifestyle practices, such as exercising regularly, practicing relaxation activities such as meditation, and avoiding tobacco products and excess alcohol.

Compared to the typical American diet, vegetarian diets provide more fiber, soy protein, folate (a B vitamin), beta-carotene, vitamins E and C, and the minerals potassium and magnesium.[7] Furthermore, vegetarian diets often supply less saturated fat than do diets that include animal foods.

In general, plant foods add bulk to the diet without adding a lot of calories. Thus, vegetarians may feel "full" soon after eating a meal of plant foods, and they may not consume as much energy and nutrients as they need. Poorly planned plant-based diets may not contain nutritionally adequate amounts of

- omega-3 fatty acids,
- vitamins B-12 and D, and/or
- minerals iron and calcium.[7]

Vegans, even some vegan athletes, can obtain adequate amounts of the essential amino acids by eating processed soybean products and foods that combine complementary plant proteins. Vegetarians who don't consume fish may need to obtain omega-3 fatty acids by eating certain algae or taking supplements that contain the algae. Vegans can obtain vitamin B-12, vitamin D, iron, calcium, and many other micronutrients by consuming fortified foods such as soy and rice beverages. Vegans and other vegetarians can also take a multiple vitamin/mineral supplement to provide an additional source of micronutrients. **Table 7.3** summarizes the nutritional advantages and possible nutritional disadvantages of vegetarian, especially vegan, diets.

TABLE 7.3

VEGETARIAN DIETS: NUTRITIONAL ASPECTS

Advantages	Possible Disadvantages
High:	**Low:**
Vitamins C, E, and folate	Vitamins B-12 and D
Beta-carotene	Iron and calcium
Fiber	Omega-3 fatty acids
Magnesium and potassium	
Low:	
Fat (saturated)	
Cholesterol (particularly, a vegan diet)	

Vegetarian pizza

Placemat: © McGraw-Hill Education. Mark A. Dierker, photographer   © FoodCollection/Superstock RF

Children have higher protein and energy needs per pound of body weight than an adult. Because plant foods add bulk to the diet, vegan children are likely to eat far less food than adult vegans because they become full sooner during meals. Thus, very young vegans may be unable to eat enough plant foods to meet their protein and energy needs. Therefore, it's very important for parents or other caretakers to plan nutritionally adequate diets for vegetarian children and monitor the youngsters' growth rates.

Vegan women who breastfeed their infants may produce milk that's deficient in vitamin B-12, particularly if the mothers' diets lack the vitamin. Such babies have a high risk of developing severe growth and developmental delays associated with nerve damage, especially when breast milk is their only source of vitamin B-12.[8] Vegan mothers who breastfeed their infants may need to provide their babies with a source of vitamin B-12.

With careful planning, vegetarians can overcome the nutritional limitations of a plant-based diet and consume adequate diets.[9] If you're interested in learning more specific details about vegetarian cookery and menu planning, contact a registered dietitian or university extension nutritionist in your area. The MyPlate website (http://www.choosemyplate.gov) also offers suggestions for planning nutritionally adequate meatless meals.

Commercially prepared vegetarian foods that substitute for meat, fish, and poultry items are often available in the frozen food section of supermarkets. These vegetarian products can look and taste like their nonvegetarian counterparts, but they generally don't contain cholesterol and may be lower in saturated fat. Such foods include soy-based sausage patties or links, soy hot dogs, "veggie" burgers, and soy "crumbles" that look like bits of cooked ground beef.

TASTY Tidbits

To reduce your animal protein intake without sacrificing protein quality, try

- black beans and rice;
- vegetable lasagna with layers of pasta, bits of tofu, thinly sliced zucchini, mushrooms, and bell peppers;
- vegetable stir-fry with bits of tofu and cheese;
- grilled vegetable kabobs served over cooked rice and black beans;
- black or red bean burritos; or
- bean and corn tacos.

Black beans and rice

Commercially prepared vegetarian foods are often available in the frozen food section of supermarkets.

Mother measuring son's height: © Dick Lauria/Photodisc/Getty Images RF; Black beans and rice: © Mariano Montero/Alamy RF; Commercially prepared vegetarian foods: © Wendy Schiff

Module 7.5

Proteins and Health

© FoodCollection/StockFood RF

7.5a Excess Protein Intakes

If some protein is essential for proper growth and good health, can eating extra amounts of the nutrient make you extra healthy or physically fit? If your diet contains adequate amounts of protein, then eating more isn't necessary. As mentioned earlier in this unit, the RDA for protein is 0.8 g/kg/day. (This value applies to healthy adults, who are not athletes.) On average, adult Americans consume 83.6 g protein/day. This amount of protein is the RDA for a person who weighs 230 pounds!

© Ingram Publishing/Alamy RF

Recall that the Acceptable Macronutrient Distribution Range (AMDR) for protein is 10 to 35% of total daily calories. Thus, you're eating a high-protein diet if protein supplies more than 35% of your daily energy intake.[10] High-protein diets are generally not recommended for healthy individuals. Excess dietary protein may lead to higher-than-normal urinary losses of the mineral nutrient calcium. However, scientists don't agree on whether this excess contributes to poor bone health.[10,11]

Recall from Essential Concept 7.2 that excess amino acids undergo removal of their nitrogen-containing groups. The reaction forms ammonia, a toxic compound. The liver uses the ammonia to make **urea,** a less toxic substance. The kidneys remove urea from the bloodstream and eliminate it in urine (**Fig. 7.7**). People who have a history of kidney stones, have kidney disease, or are at risk of kidney disease should check with their physician before eating a high-protein diet.[10]

Do Athletes Need More Protein?

About 70% of muscle tissue is water, and only about 22% is protein. An effective way to increase muscle mass safely is to combine a nutritionally adequate diet with a program of muscle-strengthening exercises. During resistance exercise, proteins in working muscles break down. The rebuilding of these proteins occurs during the recovery period that follows.[12] As a result, muscles grow larger and stronger.

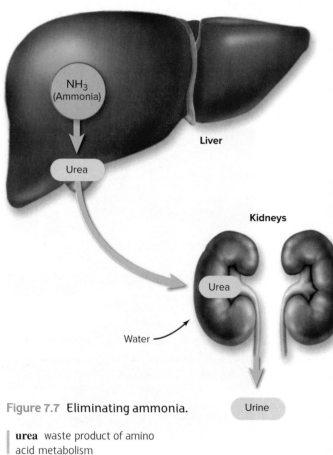

Figure 7.7 Eliminating ammonia.

urea waste product of amino acid metabolism

During high-intensity as well as long-duration physical training, an athlete's diet should supply enough calories to maintain good health and support increased energy needs.[12] Recommended protein intakes for athletes vary from 1.2 to 2.0 g/kg of body weight/day.[12] Healthy people may adapt to protein intakes that are higher than the AMDR for the macronutrient and not experience health problems as a result.

Eating a snack that supplies some high-quality protein before, during, and immediately after exercise is recommended.[13] Nutritious choices include a bowl of cereal, chocolate milk, low-fat cottage cheese and a whole-wheat bagel, or a sandwich made with lean meat or poultry. Unit 10 provides more information about nutrition for physically active people, including protein needs for athletes.

© liquidllibrary/PictureQuest RF

What About Protein Supplements?

Approximately 43% of the protein in an average person's body is in his or her skeletal muscle mass. Not surprisingly, athletes and other people interested in building their muscle mass often eat large portions of animal foods and consume amino acid and protein supplements to boost their protein intakes. However, consuming more protein than the body can use at one time doesn't stimulate increased muscle size and strength.

The use of dietary supplements that contain the milk protein *whey* to help build muscle mass in athletes is controversial.[14] Studies indicate that whey protein supplements can help increase muscle mass. [14]

For thousands of years, people have obtained amino acids directly by eating plants and animals. The use of amino acid and protein supplements as sources of the nutrient is a relatively recent development, and little is known about the long-term safety of using these products.

Olivia, the student featured in the unit opener, often trains for half-marathons. While preparing for competition, Olivia eats rich sources of carbohydrates, such as pasta and "a lot of bananas" to support her performance. After running, she chooses protein-rich foods, including peanut butter and chicken. "I tried protein shakes but didn't see any benefits, so I quit using them," she said.

TASTY Tidbits

Whey is the watery fluid that forms when milk curdles during cheese and yogurt production. The fluid is dried and used to make whey protein powder.

© Wendy Schiff

What About High-Protein Weight-Loss Diets?

Certain popular weight-loss diets, such as the Atkins, Protein Power, and Sugar Busters! diets, promote high intakes of protein. People who follow high-protein diets to lose weight often report decreased feelings of hunger and increased sense of stomach fullness (*satiety*) after meals.[10] This response probably occurs because protein contributes to satiety to a greater extent than does fat or carbohydrate.[10] Unit 10 provides information about the safety and effectiveness of various popular weight-loss diets.

7.5b Protein Deficiency

In the United States, protein deficiency is uncommon. However, certain populations, especially chronically ill, older adults, often have diets that are low in protein. Why? Many older adult Americans have limited incomes and must make difficult choices concerning their expenses. If you were old, on a low fixed income, and taking several prescription medications to control your chronic health problems, what would you think was more important? Would you decide to purchase nutritious foods or the costly medications?

Undernutrition—the lack of food—is often widespread in poor nations where populations endure frequent crop failures or civil wars. In these countries, **protein-energy malnutrition (PEM)** affects people whose diets lack adequate amounts of protein as well as energy. Such diets also result in vitamin and mineral deficiencies.

It's often more difficult for children who live in poor countries to obtain nutritionally adequate diets than for adults to do so. Why? Adults may be able to consume enough plant proteins to meet their protein and energy needs, but children have smaller stomachs and higher energy and protein needs per pound of body weight than adults. They may be unable to eat enough plant foods to meet their relatively high protein and other nutrient requirements.

A peanut butter sandwich is an inexpensive complementary protein source for children who aren't allergic to peanuts.

In children, underweight is often a sign of PEM. According to the World Health Organization (WHO), 16% of children under 5 years of age in developing countries were underweight in 2014.[15] Impoverished children in southern Asia and western Africa are most likely to be underweight, and the effects of undernutrition are especially devastating for the very young. Children whose diets lack sufficient protein and energy don't grow and are very weak, irritable, and vulnerable to dehydration and infections, such as measles, that can kill them. If these children survive, their growth may be permanently stunted. Furthermore, their intelligence may be lower than normal because undernutrition during early childhood can cause permanent brain damage. Unit 11 provides more information about undernutrition and PEM.

7.5c What's a Food Allergy?

Have you ever experienced an allergic reaction after eating certain foods or drinks? A food allergy occurs when the body's immune system reacts to one or more harmless substances (allergens) in the food. In most instances, the allergen is a protein.

Allergic reactions generally occur within a few minutes to a couple of hours after eating the offending food. Some protein in the food doesn't undergo digestion, and the absorptive cells absorb the whole molecule. When this occurs, immune system cells in the small intestine recognize the food protein as a foreign substance. These cells try to protect the body by mounting a defensive response. As a result of the immune response, the person who is allergic to the food typically experiences one or more of the following signs and symptoms:

- Hives—red raised bumps that usually appear on the skin
- Swollen or itchy lips
- Skin flushing
- A scaly skin rash (eczema)
- Difficulty swallowing
- Wheezing and difficulty breathing
- Abdominal pain, vomiting, and diarrhea

Emergency treatment for a severe allergic reaction often involves injecting a medication that prevents or blunts the response. This child is using a special syringe to inject herself with a dose of the medication.

In severe cases, sensitive people who are exposed to food allergens can develop anaphylactic (*an-a-pha-lak'-tic*) shock, a serious drop in blood pressure that affects the whole body. This kind of shock can be deadly, unless emergency treatment is provided.

Although any food protein can cause an allergic reaction in a susceptible person, the most allergenic proteins are in cow's milk, eggs, peanuts and tree nuts, wheat, soybeans, fish, and shellfish.

In the United States, approximately 5% of children and 4% of adults suffer from food allergies.[16] Children tend to outgrow their food allergies by the time they're young adults. Allergies to peanuts and tree nuts, however, usually persist into adulthood.

Accurate diagnosis of a food allergy should be undertaken by a physician who specializes in the diagnosis and treatment of allergies. Skin testing is a reliable way to identify allergens. Although hair analysis, cytotoxic or electrodermal testing, and kinesiology are promoted by alternative medical practitioners to diagnose allergies, these are unproven diagnostic methods.

Treatment of food allergies involves strict avoidance of the offending foods. Food manufacturers must identify potentially allergenic ingredients, such as soy, milk, and peanuts, on product labels (**Fig. 7.8**). Parents or caregivers of young children with food allergies should read food labels carefully to check for allergens listed among ingredients.

Some people have food intolerances, because they experience negative side effects after they consume specific foods, such as milk, aged cheese, or wine. Unlike a food allergy, a **food intolerance** doesn't involve the immune system. Such non-allergic responses to food can mimic the signs and symptoms of food allergies. Lactose intolerance (see Unit 5) is a common type of food intolerance.

For decades, health care providers recommended that parents delay introducing foods that were likely to cause an allergic response (peanuts, for example) to infants. Now, some medical researchers think food allergies can be *prevented* if such foods are given to infants when they can swallow them, which is about 4 to 6 months of age.[17] However, it's a good idea to discuss the timing of food introductions with the infant's health care provider.

Some people experience negative reactions when they consume **sulfites,** a food additive. Sulfites are a group of sulfur-containing compounds that can be found naturally in foods, but the compounds are often added to wines, potatoes, and shrimp as a preservative. People who have asthma often develop breathing difficulties after consuming food treated with sulfites. Other sulfite-sensitive people report skin flushing (redness and warmth), hives, difficulty swallowing, vomiting, diarrhea, and dizziness after consuming foods that contain the compounds. People who have food intolerances often must learn which foods to avoid eating.

Skin patch testing for allergies

This sign on the door of an elementary school classroom lets people know to avoid bringing anything containing peanuts and tree nuts into the room.

Figure 7.8 Allergen labeling.

food intolerance negative physical reactions to eating a food that don't involve the immune system

sulfites group of sulfur-containing compounds in foods and often added to wines, potatoes, and shrimp as a preservative

7.5d What's Gluten?

Gluten is a group of related proteins in wheat, barley, and rye. In the United States, about 1 in 141 people has **celiac** (*see'-lee-ak*) **disease.**[18] People with the disease cannot tolerate foods that contain gluten, a protein in wheat, rye, and barley. Although the tendency to develop celiac disease is probably inherited, environmental factors may trigger the condition.

Celiac disease is an **autoimmune disease,** a chronic disease in which certain immune system cells attack and destroy normal cells in the body. Recall from Unit 5 that type 1 diabetes is also an autoimmune disease. After a person with celiac disease eats something that contains gluten, the protein stimulates an immune response in the small intestine that inflames or destroys villi (see Fig. 4.5 for an illustration of healthy villi). This inflammation results in poor absorption of nutrients from the small intestine. Even though people with celiac disease may follow a nutritionally adequate diet, they often become malnourished because their intestinal tract lacks healthy villi.

The signs and symptoms of celiac disease vary from person to person but usually include abdominal bloating, chronic diarrhea, and weight loss. In some cases, people with celiac disease don't have the usual signs and symptoms, but their long-term health is negatively affected. Serious health problems such as anemia (a blood disorder), osteoporosis, infertility, liver disease, and intestinal cancer can result from untreated celiac disease.

Some people believe they have celiac disease, even though they have not undergone appropriate medical testing. To provide a definite diagnosis, a physician usually orders a blood test and an intestinal biopsy. The biopsy involves removing tiny pieces of tissue from the small intestine. The tissue samples undergo microscopic examination to evaluate the condition of the villi. The presence of damaged villi can help confirm the diagnosis of celiac disease.

There is no cure for celiac disease, but persons with the condition can achieve and maintain good health by carefully following a special gluten-free diet for the rest of their lives. Many supermarkets carry a variety of gluten-free foods. **Table 7.4** lists foods that people with celiac disease must avoid as well as those that are safe for them to consume.

Many Americans have adopted gluten-free diets because they think the diets are healthier than the typical diet. Some people even claim that gluten-free diets helped them lose weight. At this point, there's no evidence that gluten-free diets are useful for people who need to lose weight. Scientific research, however, provides evidence that gluten-containing foods support the growth of "good" bacteria in the large intestine.[19] Gluten may also help lower blood pressure and improve immune function. Unless you have celiac disease, you probably don't need to avoid gluten, and your health may actually benefit from keeping the protein in your diet.

© Wendy Schiff

gluten group of related proteins in wheat, barley, and rye

celiac disease chronic disease characterized by an autoimmune response in the small intestine to the protein gluten

autoimmune disease chronic disease in which certain immune system cells attack and destroy normal cells in the body

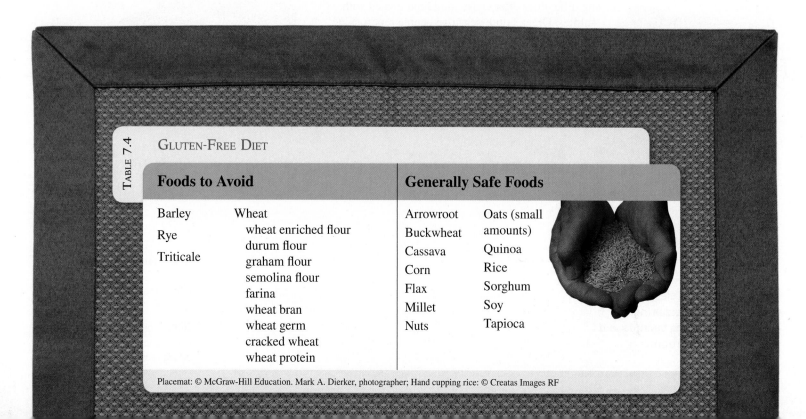

TABLE 7.4	GLUTEN-FREE DIET		
Foods to Avoid		**Generally Safe Foods**	
Barley	Wheat	Arrowroot	Oats (small amounts)
Rye	wheat enriched flour	Buckwheat	Quinoa
Triticale	durum flour	Cassava	Rice
	graham flour	Corn	Sorghum
	semolina flour	Flax	Soy
	farina	Millet	Tapioca
	wheat bran	Nuts	
	wheat germ		
	cracked wheat		
	wheat protein		

Placemat: © McGraw-Hill Education. Mark A. Dierker, photographer; Hand cupping rice: © Creatas Images RF

In a **Nutshell**

© McGraw-Hill Education. Mark A. Dierker, photographer

Module 7.1 What Are Proteins?

- Proteins are organic nutrients that contain nitrogen. Proteins have numerous functions in the body. They're needed for growth, maintenance, and repair of tissues.

- The typical amino acid has a nitrogen-containing or amino group, an acid group, and the R-group.

- Human proteins are comprised of 20 different amino acids arranged in various combinations.

- The diet must supply nine of the amino acids because the body cannot make these essential amino acids or make enough of them to meet its needs. Under normal conditions, cells can produce the remaining amino acids if the raw materials are available.

Module 7.2 What Happens to the Protein You Eat?

- Protein digestion begins in the stomach, where pepsin breaks proteins into shorter polypeptides. In the small intestine, enzymes secreted by the pancreas and absorptive cells digest the polypeptides primarily into peptides with two or three amino acids. The border of the absorptive cell contains enzymes that complete the digestion of the simple polypeptides, converting them into amino acids. The absorptive cells remove the free amino acids from the digestive tract.

- The end products of protein digestion, amino acids, travel to the liver. The liver uses the amino acids or releases them into the general circulation.

- Cells use amino acids to make proteins. Each protein can differ in the kinds of amino acids it contains, the order in which the amino acids are strung, and the number of them that are used. The wide variety of proteins in your body reflects the numerous ways your cells can connect amino acids to form proteins.

- The body conserves nitrogen by recycling amino acids, but each day it loses some protein and nitrogen, primarily in urine. Amino acids from food replace the lost nitrogen.

- The protein requirement increases during pregnancy, breastfeeding, periods of growth, and recovery from serious illnesses, blood losses, and burns.

- The adult RDA for protein is 0.8 g/kg of body weight daily.

- The AMDR for adults is 10 to 35% of energy intake from protein. Excess amino acids are metabolized for energy or converted into body fat.

Module 7.3 Proteins in Foods

- Legumes are plants that produce pods that have a single row of seeds, such as soybeans, peas, peanuts, lentils, and beans.

- Animal foods generally provide more protein than do similar quantities of plant foods.

- High-quality, or complete, protein is well digested and contains all essential amino acids in amounts that will support protein deposition and a young child's growth. In general, meat, fish, poultry, eggs, milk, and milk products contain high-quality proteins.

- Low-quality, or incomplete, protein is low in one or more of the essential amino acids. When compared to animal foods, most plant foods provide low-quality protein.

- Quinoa and foods made from processed soybeans are good plant sources of essential amino acids.

Module 7.4 What's Vegetarianism?

- Vegetarian diets are based on plant foods and limit animal foods to some extent. Although vegetarians are generally healthier than people who eat Western diets, it's difficult to pinpoint diet as being solely responsible for vegetarians' better health.

- If not properly planned, plant-based diets may not contain enough omega-3 fatty acids, vitamins B-12 and D, iron, and calcium to meet a person's nutritional needs, especially children's needs.

Module 7.5 Proteins and Health

- An effective way to increase muscle mass safely is to combine a nutritionally adequate diet with a program of muscle-strengthening exercises. During high-intensity as well as long-duration physical training, an athlete's diet should supply enough calories to support good health and energy needs for increased physical activity. Recommended protein intakes for athletes vary from 1.2 to 2.0 g/kg of body weight per day. High-protein diets are generally safe for healthy people.

- PEM affects people whose diets lack sufficient protein as well as energy, but children are more likely to be affected by PEM than adults. In impoverished developing countries, PEM is a major cause of childhood deaths. Severely undernourished children don't grow and are very weak, irritable, and vulnerable to dehydration and life-threatening infections. Undernutrition during early childhood can cause permanent brain damage.

- A food allergy occurs when the body's immune system reacts to allergens in the food. Food allergens usually are proteins. The most allergenic proteins are in cow's milk, eggs, peanuts and other nuts, wheat, soybeans, fish, and shellfish. A food intolerance isn't the same condition as a food allergy. People with celiac disease must avoid foods that contain gluten.

© Pixtal/AGE Fotostock RF

What's in **Your Diet?!**

1. Refer to the 3-day food log from the "What's in Your Diet?!" feature in Unit 3. Calculate your average protein intake by adding the grams of protein eaten each day, dividing the total by 3, and rounding the figure to the nearest whole number.

Sample Calculation:

Day 1	76 g
Day 2	55 g
Day 3	103 g
Total grams	234 g ÷ 3 days = 78 g of protein/day

Your Calculation:

Day 1	_____ g
Day 2	_____ g
Day 3	_____ g
Total grams	_____ ÷ 3 days = _____ g/day

My average daily protein intake was _____ g.

2. The RDA for protein is based on body weight. Using the RDA of 0.8 g of protein/kg of body weight, calculate the amount of protein that you need to consume daily to meet the recommendation. To determine your body weight in kilograms, divide your weight (pounds) by 2.2, then multiply this number by 0.8 to obtain your RDA for protein. Then round the figure to the nearest whole number.

My weight in pounds _____ ÷ 2.2 = _____ kg

My weight in kg _____ × 0.8 = _____ g   My RDA for protein = _____ g

a. Did your average intake of protein meet or exceed your RDA level that was calculated in step 1?

_____ yes _____ no

b. If your answer to 2a is "yes," which foods contributed the most to your protein intake?

3. Review the log of your 3-day food intake. Calculate the average number of kilocalories that protein contributed to your diet each day during the 3-day period.

a. Each gram of protein provides about 4 kcal; therefore, you must multiply the average number of grams of protein obtained in step 1 by 4 kcal to obtain the average number of kcal from protein.

Sample Calculation:

78 g/day × 4 kcal/g = 312 kcal from protein

Your Calculation:

_____ g/day × 4 kcal/g = _____ average number of kcal from protein

4. Determine your average energy intake over the 3-day period by adding the kilocalories for each day and dividing the sum by 3, and round to the nearest whole number.

Sample Calculation:

Day 1	2500 kcal
Day 2	3200 kcal
Day 3	2750 kcal
Total kcal	8450 ÷ 3 days = 2817 kcal/day (average caloric intake)

Your Calculation:

Day 1	_____ kcal
Day 2	_____ kcal
Day 3	_____ kcal
Total kcal	_____ ÷ 3 days = _____ kcal/day (average)

5. Determine the average percentage of energy that protein contributed to your diet by dividing the average kilocalories from protein obtained in step 3 by the average total daily energy intake obtained in step 4. Then round this figure to the nearest one-hundredth. Multiply this value by 100, move the decimal point two places to the right, drop the decimal point, and add a percent symbol.

Sample Calculation:

312 kcal from protein ÷ 2817 kcal intake = 0.11 (rounded)

0.11 × 100 = 11%

Your Calculation:

_____ kcal from protein ÷ _____ kcal intake = _____

_____ × 100 = _____ %

6. Did your average intake of protein meet the recommendation of 10 to 35% of total calories? If your average protein intake was below 10%, list at least five foods you could eat that would boost your intake.

Consider This...

1. Does a recipe that combines apples and oranges with peanuts provide a complementary mixture of proteins? Explain why or why not.

2. A recipe mixes cereals made from wheat, rice, and corn. What plant foods could you add to this combination of cereals to make the recipe a source of high-quality protein?

3. Are you a vegetarian? If so, describe your dietary practices (e.g., vegan or semivegetarian) and explain why you decided to become vegetarian. If you're not a vegetarian, explain why you would or would not consider this lifestyle.

4. Using only plant foods, plan a day's meals and snacks for a healthy 154-pound (70 kg) adult vegan male. The menu should supply at least 2200 kcal, follow the recommendations of the MyPlate plan, and include foods from the major food groups (except for the dairy group, unless calcium-fortified soy milk is used).

5. A recipe for bean salad has the following main ingredients:

   1 cup kidney beans

   1 cup green beans

   1 cup lima beans

   1 cup black beans

   1½ cups wine vinegar

   ⅓ cup canola oil

   ¼ cup chopped onion

   Explain why this recipe isn't a complementary mixture of plant proteins. What plant foods could you add to the recipe to make it a complementary mixture?

© Image Source/Getty Images RF

Test Yourself

Select the best answer.

1. Which of the following nutrients has nitrogen in its chemical structure?

   a. Protein

   b. Cholesterol

   c. Glucose

   d. Glycogen

2. Which of the following statements is false?

   a. Proteins are the building blocks of triglycerides.

   b. Nearly all enzymes are proteins.

   c. Cells use amino acids to make proteins.

   d. The body uses amino acids to make antibodies.

3. Which of the following foods generally provides the least amount of protein per serving?

   a. Sunflower seeds

   b. Fat-free milk

   c. Almonds

   d. Apples

4. Which of the following foods is not a source of complete protein?

   a. Milk

   b. Broccoli

   c. Fish

   d. Eggs

© FoodCollection /Stockfood RF

5. What's the RDA for protein of a healthy adult woman who weighs 71 kg?

   a. 36.8 g

   b. 46.8 g

   c. 56.8 g

   d. 66.8 g

6. Which of the following foods isn't a source of complementary protein?

   a. Red beans and rice

   b. Macaroni and cheese

   c. Soy nut butter on a bagel

   d. Split pea soup with noodles

7. A person following a lactoovovegetarian diet wouldn't eat
   a. eggs.
   b. cheese.
   c. nuts.
   d. fish.

8. Which of the following nutrients is most likely to be lacking in a vegan's diet?
   a. Magnesium
   b. Folate
   c. Calcium
   d. Vitamin C

9. People with celiac disease should
   a. take amino acid supplements.
   b. limit their protein intake to 20 g per day.
   c. avoid foods that contain gluten.
   d. eliminate protein from plant sources.

10. Which of the following substances is needed to digest proteins?
    a. Bile
    b. Pepsin
    c. Sucrase
    d. Alanine

11. Amino acids can bind together to form
    a. polypeptides.
    b. triglycerides.
    c. ketones.
    d. starches.

12. Annie experiences diarrhea and abdominal discomfort a few hours after she eats wheat bread, barley cereal, and rye crackers. Based on this information, she should obtain medical testing that can diagnose
    a. lactose intolerance.
    b. gallstones.
    c. PEM.
    d. celiac disease.

© Justin Minns/Getty Images RF

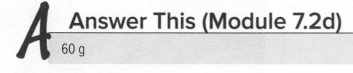

Answer This (Module 7.2d)

60 g

References ➡ See Appendix F.

STUDY TIP: Quickly create a customized practice quiz for this chapter by going to your Connect SmartBook "My Reports" section.

Don't have SmartBook and want to learn more? Go to **whysmartbook.com.**

Unit 8

Vitamins
NUTRIENTS THAT MULTITASK

What's on the Menu?

Module 8.1
Introducing Vitamins

Module 8.2
Fat-Soluble Vitamins

Module 8.3
Water-Soluble Vitamins

Module 8.4
Vitamins and Cancer

"I'm taking a prescription dose of vitamin D because my family doctor tested my blood and found out that I didn't have enough of the vitamin in my body. She told me that people need sunlight to make vitamin D, but she said she wasn't surprised that I'm deficient, since I have red hair. I told her that I try to avoid being out in the sun for more than 30 minutes, because I 'crisp' when I get exposed to sun. My skin is so light, I even got a sunburn in Kansas in the middle of October because I was outside for a couple hours! Anyway, I don't notice that much of a difference now that I'm on the medication."

Amanda Croker

Amanda Croker, a junior majoring in East Asian Language and Culture at the University of Kansas, routinely tried to limit her sun exposure to avoid sunburn and the possibility of skin cancer in the future. She was unaware that her efforts to protect her skin were also limiting her body's ability to make vitamin D, "the sunshine vitamin." If her doctor hadn't discovered that Amanda was vitamin D-deficient, her bones eventually may have become soft and weak.

Rickets, the vitamin D deficiency disease in children, is characterized by weak and deformed bones. Several decades before vitamin D's discovery in the early 1920s, scientists knew that exposure to sunlight could cure as well as prevent rickets, but they didn't know why. They also learned that cod liver oil contained a factor that prevented and cured the disease. In the mid-1930s, scientists extracted vitamin D from the oil and confirmed that it was the factor that prevented rickets.

This unit provides information about vitamin D, the 12 other vitamins, and the vitamin-like nutrient choline. By reading this unit, you'll learn what can happen when your intake of vitamins is too low or too high. The last section of this unit focuses on cancer, including the role of diet in the development of the disease and whether vitamin supplements can prevent cancer.

Sunflowers are the state flower of Kansas.

Module 8.1

Introducing Vitamins

© Brand X Pictures/PunchStock RF

8.1a What's a Vitamin?

A **vitamin** is an organic micronutrient that

- regulates certain processes in your body;

- isn't made by your body, or it's not made in amounts your body needs for good health;

- occurs naturally in commonly eaten foods; and

- prevents a specific deficiency disorder when consumed in adequate amounts.

Foods generally contain much smaller amounts of vitamins than of macronutrients. Furthermore, your body requires vitamins in very small amounts (milligram or microgram quantities), but it needs grams of macronutrients.

A few vitamins have **precursors** (**provitamins, previtamins**). These are substances in foods or your body that don't function as vitamins until your cells convert them into the active forms.

Vitamin Deficiencies

You're at risk of a vitamin deficiency disorder when your diet doesn't supply enough of the micronutrient to meet your needs. Additionally, diseases that reduce your intestinal tract's ability to absorb nutrients can increase your body's losses of vitamins and result in deficiencies of these micronutrients.

If your usual diet is nutritionally adequate but you occasionally have low intakes of vitamins, you're unlikely to develop most vitamin deficiency diseases. Why? Your cells store vitamins to some extent. However, the likelihood of developing a deficiency disease increases when your diet consistently lacks a particular vitamin. When this happens, your body's tissue levels of the vitamin become depleted, and the signs and symptoms of the nutrient's deficiency disease begin to occur. To estimate your intakes of certain vitamins, complete the "What's in Your Diet?" activity at the end of this unit.

vitamin precursors (provitamins, previtamins) substances in food or the body that cells can convert into active vitamins

Vitamin Toxicities

When your cells have enough vitamins to meet their needs, you're more likely to experience good health. However, supplying your body with amounts of vitamins that are much higher than required doesn't mean you'll become super healthy as a result. Vitamin excesses can lead to toxicity signs and symptoms. This is because vitamins can have druglike or toxic effects on your body when you take them in large amounts.

Most commonly eaten foods don't contain toxic levels of vitamins. Vitamin toxicity is most likely to occur in people who take megadoses of vitamin supplements or consume large amounts of vitamin-fortified foods regularly. Recall from Unit 3 that a megadose of a vitamin is an amount that greatly exceeds the recommended amount of the nutrient.

8.1b Classifying Vitamins

Vitamins A, D, E, and K are **fat-soluble vitamins.** These vitamins are in fats, oils, and the fatty portions of foods and tend to associate with fats in your body. Vitamin C and the "B vitamins" (thiamin, riboflavin, niacin, vitamin B-6, pantothenic acid, folate, biotin, and vitamin B-12) are **water-soluble vitamins.** Water-soluble vitamins dissolve in the watery components of food and your body. The vitamin-like nutrient choline is also water soluble. **Table 8.1** presents the vitamins and provides some other names that are sometimes used to identify them.

Why is it important to know the difference between fat- and water-soluble vitamins? Your body stores excess fat-soluble vitamins because these nutrients don't dissolve in watery substances such as urine. Over time, these vitamins can accumulate in body fat or the liver and cause toxicity. Water-soluble vitamins are generally not as toxic as fat-soluble vitamins. Why? Your body stores only limited amounts of most water-soluble vitamins. Furthermore, your kidneys can remove excess water-soluble vitamins from your bloodstream and eliminate them in urine.

TABLE 8.1

CLASSIFYING VITAMINS

Fat-Soluble Vitamins	Water-Soluble Vitamins	Vitamin-Like
A (retinol)	Thiamin (thiamine, B-1)	Choline
D	Riboflavin (B-2)	
E (alpha-tocopherol)	Niacin (B-3, nicotina-mide, nicotinic acid)	
K	B-6 (pyridoxine)	
	B-12 (cobalamin, cobalamine)	
	Biotin (H)	
	Pantothenic acid (B-5)	
	Folate, folic acid	
	C (ascorbic acid)	

Placemat: © McGraw-Hill Education. Mark A. Dierker, photographer

To maximize your vitamin intakes from fresh produce, consider buying locally grown fruits and vegetables.

Source: USDA Photo by Bill Tarpening

fat-soluble vitamins vitamins A, D, E, and K

water-soluble vitamins thiamin, riboflavin, niacin, vitamin B-6, pantothenic acid, folate, biotin, vitamin B-12, and vitamin C

8.1c Vitamins: Digestion and Absorption

Vitamins don't undergo digestion because they would lose their ability to function as a result. The small intestine absorbs vitamins, but it doesn't absorb 100% of the vitamins in food. Vitamin absorption tends to increase when needs for the micronutrients increase, such as during periods of growth and pregnancy.

Bile enhances lipid as well as fat-soluble vitamin absorption (see Unit 6). Therefore, adding a small amount of fat to low-fat foods, such as tossing raw vegetables with some salad dressing, adding a pat of soft margarine to steamed carrots, or stir-frying green beans in peanut oil, can enhance your intestinal tract's ability to absorb the fat-soluble vitamins in these foods. Diseases that interfere with fat absorption, such as cystic fibrosis, can lead to deficiencies of fat-soluble vitamins.

People who are unable to absorb vitamins may need to take large oral doses of vitamin supplements just to enable small amounts of the vitamins to be absorbed. In other cases, physicians inject vitamins into their patients' bodies, completely bypassing the need for the intestine to absorb the micronutrients. To review lipid digestion, see Unit 6.

Vitamin needs generally increase during periods of growth, such as pregnancy.

8.1d Retaining the Vitamin Content of Foods

Exposure to air, excessive heat, alkaline conditions, and light can destroy certain vitamins. The following tips can help you conserve much of the vitamins in your food.

- Purchase fresh produce when it's in season or at local farmers' markets. Fresh produce loses some vitamin content, especially if it has to be shipped hundreds of miles to reach your supermarket.

- Eat fruits and vegetables when they are fresh—cooking can reduce their vitamin content.

- Cook fresh or frozen vegetables by microwaving, steaming, or stir-frying.

Steaming vegetables can preserve their vitamin content.

Cooking them in water increases the loss of water-soluble vitamins. Vegetables generally have high water content; therefore, add no water or just a small amount when microwaving vegetables.

- Don't overcook vegetables, and minimize reheating—prolonged heating can reduce vitamin content.

- When cooking vegetables in water, don't add baking soda. Baking soda makes the water more alkaline, which destroys certain vitamins.

- Don't add fat to vegetables during cooking. Fat-soluble vitamins and phytochemicals in the food may enter the fat and be discarded when the vegetables are drained before serving. Add some fat, such as olive oil or liquid margarine, to vegetables after they're cooked.

- Store canned foods in a cool place. Canned foods can vary in the amount of nutrients they contain, largely because of differences in storage times and temperatures. If the can has been on the shelf for a year or more, the food's vitamin content may be reduced. To get maximal nutritive value from canned vegetables, drain the liquid that's packed with the food and use it as a base for soups, sauces, or gravies. If the liquid is too salty, discard it.

Adding some healthy fats, such as olive oil, to foods enhances the absorption of the fat-soluble vitamins in them.

Bone Health

Vitamin A
Vitamin D
Vitamin K
Vitamin C

Growth and Development

Vitamin A
Vitamin D
Choline

Energy Metabolism

Thiamin
Riboflavin
Niacin
Pantothenic acid
Biotin
Vitamin B-12
Vitamin B-6

Red Blood Cell Formation

Vitamin B-6
Vitamin B-12
Folate
Riboflavin (indirect)

Immune Function

Vitamin A
Vitamin C
Vitamin D
Vitamin E

Blood Clotting

Vitamin K

Amino Acid Metabolism

Vitamin B-6
Folate
Vitamin B-12
Vitamin C
Choline

Antioxidant Defense

Vitamin E
Vitamin C (likely)
Certain carotenoids

Figure 8.1 Major functions of vitamins and related compounds.
© Purestock/SuperStock RF

8.1e General Roles of Vitamins

Vitamins play numerous roles in your body, and each of these micronutrients generally has more than one function (**Fig. 8.1**). Advertisements for vitamin supplements often promote the notion that the micronutrients can "give" you energy. Vitamins, however, aren't a source of energy because cells don't metabolize them for energy. Although your body doesn't use vitamins directly for energy, certain B vitamins participate in the chemical reactions that release energy from glucose, fatty acids, and amino acids.

© Wendy Schiff

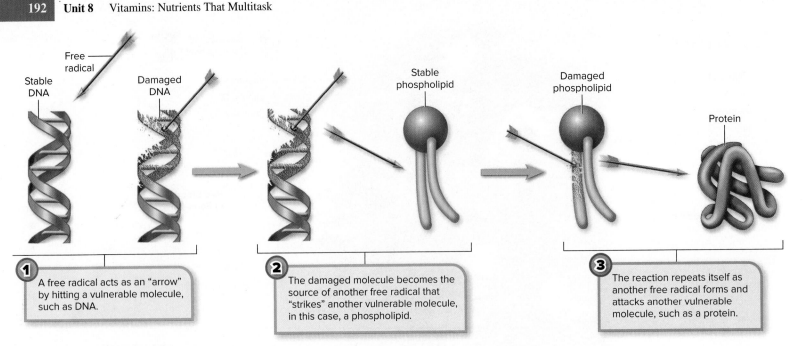

1. A free radical acts as an "arrow" by hitting a vulnerable molecule, such as DNA.

2. The damaged molecule becomes the source of another free radical that "strikes" another vulnerable molecule, in this case, a phospholipid.

3. The reaction repeats itself as another free radical forms and attacks another vulnerable molecule, such as a protein.

Figure 8.2 Free radical damage.

■ *Why is it important to reduce the damaging effects of free radicals?*

What's an Antioxidant?

Many chemical reactions that occur in your body result in the removal of tiny particles (*electrons*) from atoms or molecules. This chemical change can form free radicals, which are highly unstable substances. Free radicals can remove electrons from more stable molecules, such as proteins, fatty acids, and DNA (**Fig. 8.2**). As a result, free radicals can damage or destroy these molecules. Free radical damage may be responsible for promoting chemical changes in cells that ultimately lead to heart attack, stroke, cancer, Alzheimer's disease, and even the aging process.

Vitamins C and E, and beta-carotene, a plant pigment that is a vitamin A precursor, function as antioxidants. Antioxidants protect cells by giving up electrons to free radicals. When the chemically unstable substance accepts an electron, it can form a more stable structure that doesn't pull an electron away from another compound. By sacrificing electrons, antioxidants protect molecules such as polyunsaturated fatty acids or DNA from being damaged by free radicals (**Fig. 8.3**).

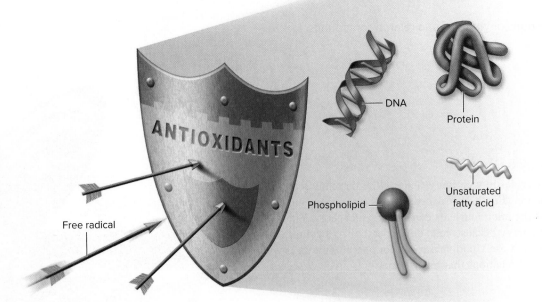

Figure 8.3 Antioxidants protect DNA and other body compounds from being harmed by free radicals.

■ *How do antioxidants reduce the damaging effects of free radicals?*

Module 8.2

Fat-Soluble Vitamins

8.2 – Learning Outcomes

After reading Module 8.2, you should be able to

1. Define all of the key terms in this module.

2. Identify the fat-soluble vitamins and foods that are rich sources of these micronutrients.

3. Explain a major function of each fat-soluble vitamin in the body.

4. Describe major deficiency and/or toxicity signs and symptoms for each fat-soluble vitamin.

This module of Unit 8 focuses on fat-soluble vitamins. At the end of each section that discusses a particular vitamin, you'll find a table that summarizes the information about the vitamin. **Figure 8.4** indicates food groups of MyPlate that are good sources of fat-soluble vitamins.

Oils
- Vitamin E
- Vitamin D (cod liver oil)
- Vitamin A (butter)
- Vitamin K (soybean oil)

Fruits
- Vitamin A precursors
- Vitamin E (mangoes)

Vegetables
- Vitamin A precursors
- Vitamin K
- Vitamin E

Dairy
- Vitamins A and D (if fortified)

Grains
- Vitamin E (wheat germ, whole grains, whole-grain or fortified ready-to-eat cereals)

Protein
- Vitamin E (nuts and seeds, sardines)
- Vitamin A (liver and eggs)
- Vitamin D (salmon, egg yolk, liver)

Figure 8.4   MyPlate and fat-soluble vitamins.

8.2a Vitamin A

Vitamin A is actually a family of compounds that includes **retinol**, which may be called **preformed vitamin A.** Although retinol is only in animal foods, plants contain yellow-orange pigments called **carotenoids.** The body can convert a few kinds of carotenoids, particularly **beta-carotene,** into retinol. We sometimes refer to these carotenoids as "**provitamin A.**"

Why Does My Body Need Vitamin A?

Do you associate vitamin A with eating carrots and good vision? It's true that vitamin A is involved in the visual process and carrots contain lots of beta-carotene. However, vitamin A can multitask, that is, the micronutrient has numerous functions in the body. Vitamin A participates in the processes of cell production, growth, and development. Vitamin A is also needed for building strong bones, regulating immune system activity, and maintaining epithelial cells. **Epithelial cells** form protective tissues that include your skin and linings of the respiratory, reproductive, and intestinal tracts. Some epithelial cells secrete mucus. Mucus keeps tissues moist and forms a sticky barrier against many environmental pollutants and infectious agents.

Food Sources of Vitamin A

Animal foods such as liver, butter, fish liver oils, and eggs are good sources of preformed vitamin A. Other important sources of the vitamin include

retinol (preformed vitamin A) form of vitamin A that's in animal sources of food

carotenoids yellow-orange pigments in fruits and vegetables

beta-carotene carotenoid that the body can convert to vitamin A

provitamin A carotenoids that the body converts to vitamin A

epithelial cells cells that form protective linings of the body

vitamin A-fortified milk, yogurt, margarine, and cereals. A fruit or vegetable's color is usually an indication of its provitamin A content. To maximize your provitamin A intake, choose produce with dark green, orange, or yellow-orange colors.

In addition to the antioxidant beta-carotene, common carotenoids include lutein (*loo-tee-en*), zeaxanthin (*zee-ah-zan-thin*), and lycopene (*lie-ko-peen*). Green, leafy vegetables, such as spinach and kale, have high concentrations of lutein and zeaxanthin. Tomato juice and other tomato products, including pizza sauce, contain considerable amounts of lycopene. Although lutein, zeaxanthin, and lycopene are carotenoids, the body doesn't convert them to vitamin A. Nevertheless, these plant pigments may function as beneficial antioxidants in the body.

Cantaloupe, Fruit and vegetable display: © C Squared Studios/Getty Images RF; Vitamin D3: © Wendy Schiff

Fruits and vegetables generally are good sources of antioxidants, including carotenoids such as beta-carotene and lycopene.

What *IS* That?

Kale is a leafy, green, cruciferous (*krew-siff'-er-rus*) vegetable that's related to cabbage and broccoli. Cruciferous vegetables contain antioxidants that may protect against cancer. Kale is a rich source of beta-carotene, fiber, and vitamins B-6 and C.

The raw vegetable has a strong flavor, so tear raw kale leaves into small pieces and add them to salad greens. Cooking small pieces of the leaves in soups or stews adds nutrients and fiber to the meals.

Table 8.2 lists some foods that are sources of vitamin A or provitamin A carotenoids. Amounts of vitamin A in food are often reported as micrograms of *retinol activity equivalents* (*RAEs*). One RAE is approximately 1 mcg of retinol. Americans who are 2 years of age and older consume diets that provide, on average, a little less than the RDA for vitamin A.[1]

Vitamin A Deficiency

Epithelial cells are among the first to become affected by a deficiency of vitamin A. When mucus-secreting epithelial cells lack the vitamin, they no longer produce mucus, and the cells lose their effectiveness in preventing infections. Thus, vitamin A-deficient people are at greater risk of infections than are those with adequate levels of the vitamin in their bodies.

TASTY Tidbits

Dark yellow and orange fruits and vegetables usually contain more beta-carotene and other provitamin A carotenoids than does lightly colored produce. Dark green fruits and vegetables also contain provitamin A, but their green pigment hides the yellow-orange pigments. So, don't discard the dark green leaves of cabbage, lettuce, or broccoli when preparing food. Use them in salads and soups or on sandwiches.

TABLE 8.2

VITAMIN A CONTENT OF SELECTED FOODS

Food	mcg RAE
Beef liver, cooked, 3 oz	6970
Papaya, 1 fruit (5 oz)	1492
Sweet potato, baked, ½ cup	961
Butternut squash, cooked, cubed, ½ cup	572
Carrots, raw, chopped, ½ cup	534
Mustard greens, frozen, boiled, drained, ½ cup	266
Mixed vegetables, frozen, boiled, drained, ½ cup	195
Eggs, hard-cooked, large, 2	149
Cantaloupe, ½ cup	135
Lettuce, romaine, shredded, ½ cup	104
Fat-free milk with vitamin A, ½ cup	78
Spinach, raw, ½ cup	70
Green peas, cooked, drained, ½ cup	32

RDA for adult women = 700 mcg/day
RDA for adult men = 900 mcg/day
Source: USDA National nutrient database for standard reference, release 25.

Kale: © Stockdisc/PunchStock RF; Cabbage, Sweet potato: © FoodCollection/StockFood RF;
Bowl of cooked vegetables: © Royalty-Free/Corbis RF

What Is Night Blindness?

Have you ever walked from a brightly lit theater lobby into the darkened movie auditorium and felt blinded for a few seconds? This is a normal visual response to the sudden and dramatic reduction in light intensity. The *retina*, the light-sensitive area inside each eye, contains rods and cones, which are specialized nerve cells that are essential for vision (**Fig. 8.5**). Rods and cones need vitamin A, particularly retinol, to function properly. *Night blindness*, the inability to see in dim light, occurs if retinol is unavailable. Night blindness is an early sign of vitamin A deficiency.

What Is Dry Eye?

The **cornea** is the clear covering that enables light to enter your eye, which is necessary for vision (see Fig. 8.5). The epithelial cells that line the inner eyelids secrete mucus, which helps keep the cornea moist and clean. In a person suffering from vitamin A deficiency, these cells harden and stop producing mucus. This condition causes the corneas to become dry and easily damaged by dirt and bacteria. Unless the affected person receives vitamin A, he or she will become blind.

Each year, an estimated 250,000 to 500,000 children in developing nations become blind because of severe vitamin A deficiency.[2] Worldwide, vitamin A deficiency is the primary cause of preventable blindness among children. Vitamin A deficiency also reduces the effectiveness of the immune system, so many vitamin A-deficient children die from infections such as measles. In developing countries, efforts to improve people's health and prevent blindness include

- promoting the production of foods that are rich in beta-carotene,

- fortifying foods with vitamin A, and

- providing dietary supplements that contain vitamin A to members of the population who are most at risk.[2]

Figure 8.5 **Vitamin A and vision.** Rods and cones need vitamin A to function properly.

Retina
Macula
Cornea
Iris
Optic nerve
Rod
Cone

cornea clear covering over the front of eyeball

carotenemia yellowing of the skin that results from excess beta-carotene in the body

teratogen agent that causes birth defects

TASTY Tidbits

Tomatoes are a good source of certain carotenoids, particularly beta-carotene and lycopene. Exposure to heat can break down plant cells, and as a result, the cells release carotenoids. Thus, cooking tomatoes can improve the intestinal tract's ability to absorb carotenoids in the food.

© Ingram Publishing/Alamy RF

TASTY Tidbits

Carotenemia (*kar′-et-eh-ne′-me-ah*) is a condition characterized by yellowing of the skin that can result from eating too much beta-carotene–rich produce. This condition occasionally develops in infants who eat a lot of baby foods that contain carrots, apricots, winter squash, or green beans. Carotenemia is usually harmless.[3] The skin's natural color eventually returns when the carotenoid-rich foods are no longer eaten.

© McGraw-Hill Education. Mark Steinmetz, photographer

Can Vitamin A Be Toxic?

Compared to other vitamins, vitamin A is very toxic. Toxicity signs and symptoms include

- headache,
- nausea and vomiting,
- visual disturbances,
- hair loss, and
- bone pain and fractures.

When taken during pregnancy, excess vitamin A is a **teratogen,** an agent that causes birth defects. Medications that are chemically similar to vitamin A, such as tretinoin (Retin-A), may be prescribed to treat severe acne. Although these medications are less toxic than natural vitamin A, there's a lack of information concerning whether they're safe to use during pregnancy. If you're using such medications, check with your physician if you're planning a pregnancy.

Q Answer This

A young man who's been a vegan for several years doesn't take a dietary supplement that contains vitamin A. Why doesn't he have night blindness or become blind? You can find the answer on the last page of this unit.

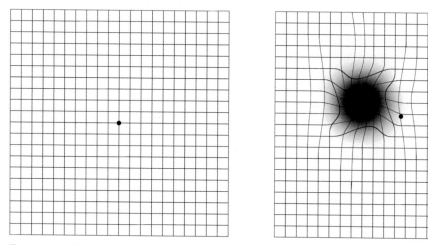

Figure 8.6 **Simple screening test for macular degeneration.** When people who don't have AMD look at the center of the grid on the left, they will see straight grid lines. If people who have AMD look at the center of that grid, they will see a distorted image, such as the grid on the right.

What's Macular Degeneration?

Results of studies suggest an association between eating diets that are rich in fruits and vegetables and lower risk of *age-related macular degeneration (AMD)*. Such diets provide plenty of beta-carotene and other anti-oxidant carotenoids. Should you take dietary supplements that contain carotenoids to prevent AMD?

AMD is a leading cause of blindness in the United States. People with AMD have damaged maculas. The macula is the region within the eye that provides the most detailed central vision (see Fig. 8.5). When the macula is damaged, objects appear to be distorted, as in the grid shown in **Figure 8.6** (right side). Major risk factors for AMD are genetics, smoking, and advanced age, but diet also plays a role in the development of the condition.

In the Age-Related Eye Disease Study (AREDS), patients who already had AMD took dietary supplements that contained relatively high amounts of beta-carotene, vitamins C and E, and the minerals zinc and copper.[4] The combination of these substances appeared to slow the progression of vision loss associated with macular degeneration. In later studies, scientists determined that beta-carotene was not an effective ingredient in the formula of dietary supplements that were given to subjects with AMD.

Vitamin A: Reviewing the Basics

Table 8.3 provides a summary of basic information about vitamin A, including Dietary Reference Intake (DRI) recommendations, and major signs and symptoms of the vitamin's deficiency and toxicity disorders.

Mango is a rich source of beta-carotene.

TABLE 8.3 VITAMIN A SUMMARY

Major Functions in the Body	Adult RDA	Major Dietary Sources	Major Deficiency Signs and Symptoms	Major Toxicity Signs and Symptoms
Normal vision and reproduction, cellular growth, and immune system function	700–900 mcg RAE	Preformed: liver, milk, fortified cereals Provitamin: yellow-orange and dark green fruits and vegetables	Night blindness, dry eye, poor growth, dry skin, reduced immune system functioning	Adult Upper Limit (UL) = 3,000 mcg/day Nausea and vomiting, headaches, bone pain and fractures, hair loss, liver damage, interference with vitamin K absorption

8.2b Vitamin D

In 1922, scientists discovered a fat-soluble substance in cod liver oil that people needed for proper bone health and to prevent rickets. As mentioned in the unit opener, children with **rickets** have bones that are soft and can become misshapen. Leg bones, for example, bow under the weight of carrying the upper part of the body (**Fig. 8.7**). Children with rickets can also develop other bone deformities and may complain of muscle pain. The scientists named the substance that cured rickets *vitamin D*.

Today, the fat-soluble substance that cured rickets is still called a vitamin because rickets can be prevented or treated by taking vitamin D supplements or eating vitamin D-rich foods. Vitamin D, however, is a hormone as well as a nutrient. **Essential Concept 8.1** shows how your body can make vitamin D when your skin is exposed to sunlight.

rickets vitamin D deficiency disorder in children

previtamin D inactive form of vitamin D

Figure 8.7 Rickets.

■ *Why does a child with rickets have weak leg bones?*

© Biophoto Associates/Science Source

Essential Concept

8.1   How Your Body Makes Vitamin D

Ultraviolet light (UVB)

Skin

1 Your body can make vitamin D when your skin is exposed to the sun's ultraviolet (UV) radiation. The radiation converts a substance in skin that's derived from cholesterol into **previtamin D.** This explains why the nutrient is often called the "sunshine vitamin."

Previtamin D

2 Previtamin D is unable to function in your body until it's activated. The previtamin circulates to the liver and then to the kidneys where it's converted to the active form of vitamin D. The liver and kidneys are critical for the activation of vitamin D.

Liver

Kidneys

Active Vitamin D

Why Does My Body Need Vitamin D?

Vitamin D's most well-known role is in the production and maintenance of healthy bones. The minerals calcium and phosphorus are essential for strong bones. Vitamin D stimulates bone cells to form *calcium phosphate*, the hard major mineral compound in bone tissue. Without adequate vitamin D, bone cells can't deposit enough calcium phosphate to produce strong bones (**Fig. 8.8**). The vitamin also enhances the absorption of calcium and phosphorus by the small intestine and reduces the elimination of calcium by the kidneys.

Vitamin D has other roles in the body, including regulating muscular and immune function and reducing inflammation.[5] Vitamin D is also involved in controlling cell growth and, as a result, the micronutrient may reduce the risk of certain cancers. However, more research is needed to clarify the vitamin's role in immune function and disease prevention.

Figure 8.8 Vitamin D actions.

Food Sources of Vitamin D

Fish liver oils and fatty fish, especially salmon, sardines, and tuna, are among the few foods that naturally contain vitamin D. Milk is routinely fortified with vitamin D, and some brands of ready-to-eat cereals, orange juice, and margarine also have the vitamin added to them. **Table 8.4** lists some food sources of vitamin D. Food composition tables often list the vitamin D content of foods in International Units; 1 mcg of vitamin D equals 40 IU.

TASTY **Tidbits**

Vitamin D has two major forms—D_2 and D_3. Mushrooms and some plants produce vitamin D_2; animals make vitamin D_3. Your body generally uses both forms of the vitamin effectively.[5]

Mushrooms: © FoodCollection/StockFood RF; Glass of milk: © McGraw-Hill Education. Ken Carp, photographer; Fish: © Digital Vision/Getty Images RF; Placemat: © McGraw-Hill Education. Mark A. Dierker, photographer

TABLE 8.4

VITAMIN D CONTENT OF SELECTED FOODS

Food	Vitamin D (mcg)
Cod liver oil, 1 Tbsp	34
Salmon, pink, canned, 3 oz	12
Sardines, Atlantic, canned in oil, 3 oz	4
Milk, fat-free, vitamin D-fortified, 1 cup	3
Tuna, canned in water, drained, 3 oz	2
Egg, whole, hard-cooked, 1 large	1

RDA for adults = 15–20 mcg/day

Source: USDA National nutrient database for standard reference, release 25.

Amanda, the student featured in the opener of this unit, took a high-dose supplement of vitamin D that was prescribed by her doctor. As a result of the treatment, her blood level of the vitamin became normal within a few weeks. Because few foods are good sources of vitamin D, she'll need to take a daily supplement of the micronutrient that's available without a prescription for the rest of her life. By taking the supplement, she should be able to maintain a healthy blood level of vitamin D.

TASTY Tidbits

Too much sun exposure may lead to skin cancer. Therefore, physicians who treat skin disorders often advise people to apply sunscreens consistently before going outdoors. When properly applied, a sunscreen with a sun protection factor (SPF) of 8 or more blocks sunlight that's needed to form vitamin D_3.[5] To allow your body to make some vitamin D, you can expose your skin to the sun for 5 to 30 minutes twice a week *before* applying a commercial sunscreen.

© Purestock/SuperStock RF

Vitamin D and Sunlight

osteomalacia adult rickets; condition characterized by poorly mineralized (soft) bones

Because vitamin D isn't widespread in food, you can't count on eating enough vitamin D-rich foods to meet your needs. Therefore, your body must make up the difference, and sunlight is the key. If you are outdoors exposing your skin to the sun for about 5 to 30 minutes twice a week, you may obtain enough sun exposure during the summer to make adequate amounts of vitamin D.[5] The amount of vitamin D your body makes depends on many factors, including your age, skin color, location, and the time of year.[6] Older adults don't make as much vitamin D as they did when they were younger. Darker skin contains higher amounts of the pigment *melanin*, which may reduce the skin's ability to produce vitamin D_3 from sunlight. Clouds, shade, window glass, air pollution, and clothing are environmental factors that can limit the amount of UV radiation that reaches your skin.

If you live in the Northern Hemisphere, north of the 33rd parallel, the angle of the winter sun is such that the sun's rays must pass through more of the atmosphere than at other times of the year (**Fig. 8.9**). As a result, your skin cannot make sufficient amounts of vitamin D_3 during the winter.[6] Therefore, you may need to take a supplement that contains 100% of the adult Daily Value for vitamin D (400 IU or 10 mcg), especially from November through February.

Vitamin D Deficiency

Many Americans don't consume enough vitamin D to meet the RDA.[1] Although rickets isn't a widespread health problem in the United States, medical experts are concerned that many Americans don't have enough vitamin D in their bodies for optimal health. Thus, vitamin D is a nutrient of public health concern, according to the Dietary Guidelines for Americans.

Breast milk doesn't contain enough vitamin D to prevent rickets. Infants who are most likely to develop rickets are breastfed, and they have dark skin, minimal sunlight exposure, and little or no vitamin D intake.[5] Therefore, most breastfed infants should consume a daily vitamin D supplement soon after birth.

The adult form of rickets is called **osteomalacia** (*ahs-tee-o-mah-lay-she-a*). The bones of people with osteomalacia are soft and break easily because they contain less-than-normal amounts of calcium. Muscle weakness is a symptom of osteomalacia.

The following people are at risk of osteomalacia and may need to take a vitamin D supplement:

33rd parallel

Figure 8.9 Vitamin D and geography.

■ *To form the most vitamin D throughout the year, where would be the best place in the United States for you to live?*

- Older adults: As a person ages, production of previtamin D in skin declines.
- People who have liver or intestinal diseases because these conditions may reduce both vitamin D_3 production and calcium absorption.
- Adults who stay indoors or are almost fully covered during the day.[5]

TABLE 8.5

VITAMIN D SUMMARY

Major Functions in the Body	Adult RDA	Major Dietary Sources	Major Deficiency Signs and Symptoms	Major Toxicity Signs and Symptoms
Absorption of calcium and phosphorus, maintenance of normal blood calcium, calcification of bone, maintenance of muscular and immune function	15–20 mcg (600–800 IU)	Vitamin D-fortified milk, fortified cereals, fish liver oils, fatty fish	Rickets in children, osteomalacia in adults: soft bones, muscular weakness, and reduced immune system functioning	Adult UL = 100 mcg/day (4000 IU) Loss of appetite, calcium deposits in soft tissues

© FoodCollection/StockFood RF

People with osteomalacia may also have *osteoporosis*, a condition characterized by loss of bone mass that usually occurs with aging. Although osteoporosis is usually associated with low calcium intakes, a long-term vitamin D deficiency contributes to the condition because lack of the vitamin reduces calcium absorption.[5] The calcium section of Unit 9 provides more information about osteoporosis.

Can Vitamin D Be Toxic?

Your body stores vitamin D. Taking vitamin D supplements that supply 10,000 to 40,000 IU/day over a long period of time can cause the vitamin to accumulate in your body and produce toxicity.[5] The excess vitamin D stimulates your small intestine to absorb too much calcium from foods. When this occurs, calcium deposits form in your soft tissues, including the kidneys, heart, and blood vessels. The calcium deposits can interfere with cells' ability to function and cause their death. Other signs and symptoms of vitamin D toxicity include kidney stones. You don't have to be concerned about your body making toxic levels of vitamin D when exposed to sunlight because skin limits its production of previtamin D.

Vitamin D: Reviewing the Basics

Table 8.5 provides a summary of basic information about vitamin D, including Dietary Reference Intake (DRI) recommendations, and major signs and symptoms of the vitamin's deficiency and toxicity disorders.

8.2c Vitamin E

There are different forms of vitamin E, but your body only uses the **alpha-tocopherol** (*al-´fah toe-kof ´-eh-roll*) form.[7] Alpha-tocopherol is an antioxidant that protects polyunsaturated fatty acids in cell membranes from being damaged by free radicals (**Fig. 8.10**). Preventing free radical damage may lower your risk of atherosclerosis, cancer, and premature cellular aging and death. Other roles for vitamin E include maintaining healthy nervous tissue and immune system function.

alpha-tocopherol vitamin E

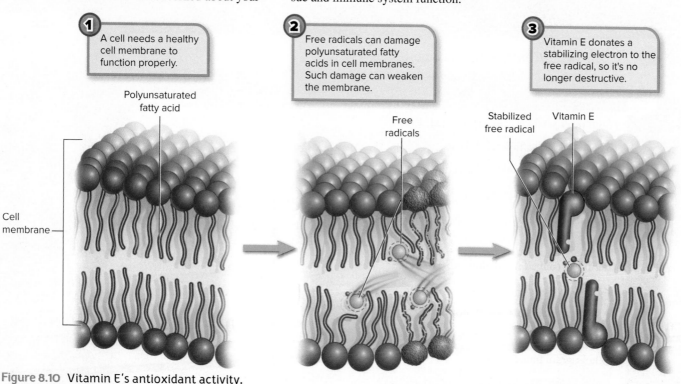

1 A cell needs a healthy cell membrane to function properly.

2 Free radicals can damage polyunsaturated fatty acids in cell membranes. Such damage can weaken the membrane.

3 Vitamin E donates a stabilizing electron to the free radical, so it's no longer destructive.

Polyunsaturated fatty acid

Free radicals

Stabilized free radical

Vitamin E

Cell membrane

Figure 8.10 Vitamin E's antioxidant activity.

Food Sources of Vitamin E

Rich food sources of vitamin E include sunflower seeds, almonds, and plant oils, especially sunflower, safflower, and olive oils. Products made from vitamin E-rich plant oils—margarine and salad dressings—also supply the micronutrient. Meats, processed grain products, and dairy products generally don't contain much vitamin E. **Table 8.6** lists some common foods that are sources of vitamin E.

Harvesting, processing, storage, and cooking methods can reduce amounts of vitamin E in food. During the milling process, most of the vitamin E that's in whole grains is lost, and it's not restored by enrichment. Furthermore, exposure to oxygen, metals, light, and high cooking temperatures can destroy much of the vitamin E in food before it reaches your table.

Vitamin E Deficiency

Americans, on average, don't consume enough vitamin E to meet the RDA for the nutrient.[1] However, vitamin E deficiency rarely occurs in healthy adults.[7] High-risk populations include people who have intestinal diseases that interfere with vitamin E absorption. Common signs and symptoms of the deficiency are nerve damage, difficulty walking, and reduced immune function.

Can Vitamin E Be Toxic?

Unlike vitamins A and D, vitamin E has low toxicity.[7] However, taking dietary supplements that supply excessive amounts of vitamin E may interfere with vitamin K's role in blood clotting and lead to uncontrolled bleeding. Therefore, people who take medications that interfere with blood clotting ("blood thinners") should check with their physicians before using vitamin E supplements.

Vitamin E Supplements and Chronic Diseases

According to the results of several large population studies, taking vitamin E supplements is not likely to reduce your risk of cardiovascular diseases, including heart disease and cancer.[7]

Furthermore, studies generally don't provide evidence that vitamin E helps people with signs of *mild cognitive impairment,* a condition characterized by declining thought-processing abilities that can progress to Alzheimer's disease.[7] Despite these findings, scientists continue to conduct research to determine whether taking vitamin E alone or with other antioxidant nutrients can reduce the risk of heart disease, cancer, and AMD.

TABLE 8.6

VITAMIN E CONTENT OF SELECTED FOODS

Food	Alpha-tocopherol (mg)
Sunflower seed kernels, dry-roasted, 1 oz	7.4
Vegetable oil (safflower), 1 Tbsp	4.6
Spinach, frozen, cooked, drained, ½ cup	3.4
Mango, 1 raw	3.0
Peanuts, dry roasted, 1 oz (approx. 28)	2.2
Olive oil, 1 Tbsp	2.0
Sardines, canned in oil, drained, 3 oz	1.7
Red pepper, sweet, raw, chopped, ½ cup	1.2
Asparagus, frozen, cooked, drained, ½ cup	1.1
Broccoli, cooked, chopped, ½ cup	1.1
Whole-grain bread, 1 slice	0.2

RDA for adults = 15 mg/day

Source: USDA National nutrient database for standard reference, release 25.

TABLE 8.7	VITAMIN E SUMMARY				
	Major Functions in the Body	**Adult RDA**	**Major Dietary Sources**	**Major Deficiency Signs and Symptoms**	**Major Toxicity Signs and Symptoms**
	Antioxidant	15 mg (22.5 IU)	Vegetable oils and products made from these oils, certain fruits and vegetables, nuts and seeds, fortified cereals	Loss of muscular coordination, reduced immune function	Adult UL = 1000 mg/day Excessive bleeding as a result of interfering with vitamin K

Vitamin E: Reviewing the Basics

Table 8.7 provides a summary of basic information about vitamin E, including Dietary Reference Intake (DRI) recommendations, and major signs and symptoms of the vitamin's deficiency and toxicity disorders.

8.2d Vitamin K

Your liver needs vitamin K to produce four blood clotting factors. When a blood vessel is cut, the blood in the area of the injury needs to form a clot to stop the bleeding (**Fig. 8.11**). If your body lacks vitamin K, you may experience excessive bleeding because all the blood clotting factors aren't available. Some people take the prescribed medication *warfarin* because their blood clots too easily. Warfarin decreases vitamin K's ability to form blood clots. Vitamin K can interfere with warfarin's "blood-thinning" activity, so people who take the medication should not use vitamin K supplements.

Vitamin K also helps bone-building cells produce a protein that's needed for healthy bones. Low blood levels of vitamin K are associated with the risk of the bone disorder osteoporosis, but more research is needed to clarify the vitamin's role in bone health.

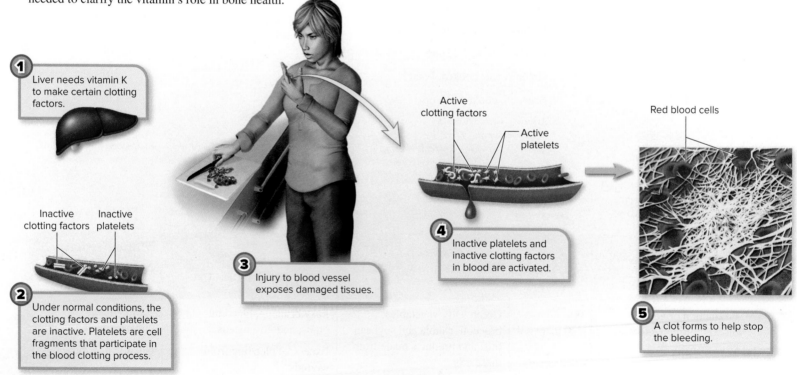

1. Liver needs vitamin K to make certain clotting factors.

Inactive clotting factors   Inactive platelets

2. Under normal conditions, the clotting factors and platelets are inactive. Platelets are cell fragments that participate in the blood clotting process.

3. Injury to blood vessel exposes damaged tissues.

Active clotting factors   Active platelets

4. Inactive platelets and inactive clotting factors in blood are activated.

Red blood cells

5. A clot forms to help stop the bleeding.

Figure 8.11 Vitamin K and blood clotting.

Sunflower seeds, Fibrin: © Royalty-Free/Corbis RF; Sardines: © IT Stock/PunchStock RF

Sources of Vitamin K

Major food sources of vitamin K are green leafy vegetables such as kale, turnip greens, salad greens, cabbage, and spinach. Other reliable sources of the vitamin are soybean and canola oils, and products made from these oils, such as salad dressing. **Table 8.8** lists some foods that are sources of the vitamin. Vitamin K is very stable and resists being destroyed by usual cooking methods.

Vitamin K Deficiency

Your body stores very little vitamin K, but you're unlikely to become vitamin K-deficient because bacteria that normally live in your large intestine make vitamin K. The intestine may absorb some of the vitamin.[8] Vitamin K deficiency, however, can develop in people who have liver diseases or conditions that impair fat absorption, such as cystic fibrosis. Additionally, long-term antibiotic therapy can reduce the number of bacteria that make vitamin K and, as a result, contribute to a deficiency of the nutrient. The most reliable sign of vitamin K deficiency is an increase in the time it takes for blood to clot.

Infants are born with low amounts of vitamin K in their bodies. Therefore, babies can develop a deficiency of the vitamin soon after birth. Vitamin K-deficient infants are at risk of serious bleeding that can be deadly. To prevent vitamin K deficiency from developing during infancy, newborns generally receive a single injection of vitamin K.

Vitamin K: Reviewing the Basics

Table 8.9 provides a summary of basic information about vitamin K, including Dietary Reference Intake (DRI) recommendations, and major signs and symptoms of the vitamin's deficiency and toxicity disorders.

TABLE 8.8

VITAMIN K CONTENT OF SELECTED FOODS

Food	Vitamin K (mcg)
Kale, cooked, ½ cup	531
Spinach, cooked, ½ cup	514
Beet greens, cooked, ½ cup	348
Turnip greens, cooked, ½ cup	265
Brussels sprouts, cooked, ½ cup	109
Spinach, raw, ½ cup	72
Asparagus, frozen, cooked, ½ cup	46
Cabbage, raw, shredded, ½ cup	27
Soybean oil, 1 Tbsp	25
Lettuce, romaine, shredded, ½ cup	24
Blueberries, raw, ½ cup	14
Green beans, cooked, ½ cup	10
Broccoli, cooked, ½ cup	8

AI for adult men = 120 mcg/day
AI for adult women = 90 mcg/day
Source: U.S. Department of Agriculture, Agricultural Research Service: *USDA National nutrient database for standard reference, release 25,* 2012.

TABLE 8.9

VITAMIN K

Major Functions in the Body	Adult AI	Major Dietary Sources	Major Deficiency Signs and Symptoms	Major Toxicity Signs and Symptoms
Production of active blood-clotting factors, bone growth	90– 120 mcg	Green leafy vegetables, broccoli, canola and soybean oils, and products made from these oils	Easy bruising, bleeding gums, and nosebleeds Excessive bleeding from wounds	Adult UL = undetermined Unknown

Module 8.3

Water-Soluble Vitamins

8.3 - Learning Outcomes

After reading Module 8.3, you should be able to

1. Define all of the key terms in this module.

2. Explain how most B vitamins function as coenzymes.

3. List major functions and food sources for each water-soluble vitamin.

4. Describe major deficiency and/or toxicity signs and symptoms for each water-soluble vitamin.

© McGraw-Hill Education. Mark A. Dierker, photographer

Recall that the water-soluble vitamins are thiamin, riboflavin, niacin, folate, B-6, B-12, pantothenic acid, biotin, and vitamin C. Most water-soluble vitamins have no function unless they're in a coenzyme. **Essential Concept 8.2** describes a coenzyme and how it activates an enzyme.

coenzyme ion or small molecule that interacts with enzymes, enabling the enzymes to function

Essential Concept

8.2 What's a Coenzyme, and How Does It Function?

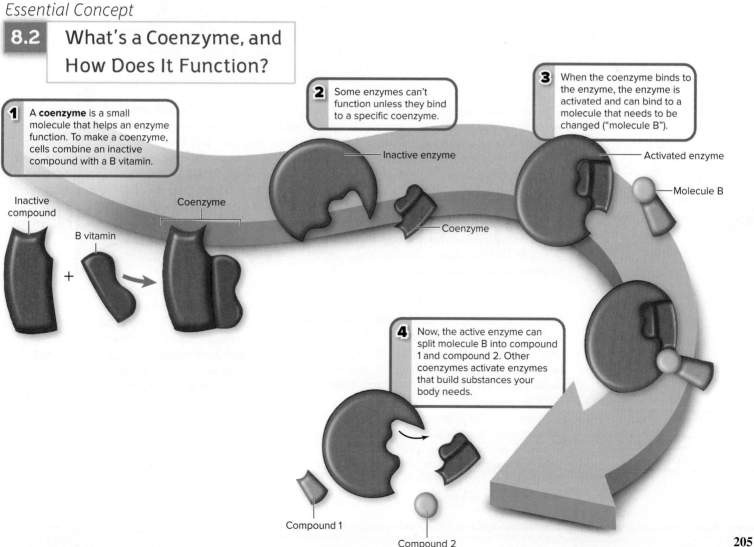

1 A **coenzyme** is a small molecule that helps an enzyme function. To make a coenzyme, cells combine an inactive compound with a B vitamin.

2 Some enzymes can't function unless they bind to a specific coenzyme.

3 When the coenzyme binds to the enzyme, the enzyme is activated and can bind to a molecule that needs to be changed ("molecule B").

4 Now, the active enzyme can split molecule B into compound 1 and compound 2. Other coenzymes activate enzymes that build substances your body needs.

Inactive compound

B vitamin

Coenzyme

Inactive enzyme

Coenzyme

Activated enzyme

Molecule B

Compound 1

Compound 2

Dairy
- Riboflavin
- Choline
- Vitamin B-12
- Pantothenic acid

Grains
- Thiamin
- Folic acid
- Riboflavin
- Other B vitamins (whole-grain and fortified cereals)
- Niacin

Fruits
- Folate
- Vitamin C

Vegetables
- Folate
- Vitamin C

Protein
- Thiamin
- Vitamin B-6
- Riboflavin
- Vitamin B-12
- Niacin
- Choline
- Biotin
- Pantothenic acid

Figure 8.12 MyPlate, water-soluble vitamins, and choline.

Foods usually contain B vitamins in their coenzyme forms. Health-food stores often sell dietary supplements that contain coenzymes, but buying these products is a waste of money. In your small intestine, coenzymes in food and dietary supplements undergo digestion to release their B-vitamin components. The small intestine absorbs the freed B vitamins, and the micronutrients eventually enter the general circulation. Your cells then remove the vitamins from the bloodstream and use them to make coenzymes. If you consume more coenzymes or water-soluble vitamins than you need, your kidneys filter the excess from your blood and eliminate them in urine. Vitamin B-12 is an exception; the liver stores excesses of this micronutrient.

Figure 8.12 indicates MyPlate food groups that are good sources of water-soluble vitamins. This section of Unit 8 focuses on the eight water-soluble vitamins and the vitamin-like nutrient, choline.

8.3a The Power Player Vitamins

Thiamin, riboflavin, and niacin are B vitamins that we refer to as "power players." Why? Your cells need these micronutrients to make coenzymes that help release energy from glucose, fat, and amino acids. Therefore, you'll feel tired if your body lacks the power players.

In the early 1900s, power player vitamin deficiencies were common in the United States. The thiamin deficiency disease is called **beriberi**; **ariboflavinosis** is the riboflavin deficiency disorder; the niacin deficiency disease is **pellagra** (*peh-lah-́gra* or *peh-lay-́gra*).

beriberi thiamin deficiency disease

ariboflavinosis riboflavin deficiency disease

pellagra niacin deficiency disease

TASTY Tidbits

Physicians may prescribe megadoses of niacin (nicotinic acid) to treat high blood cholesterol levels. Such large doses of nicotinic acid can reduce blood cholesterol. However, patients receiving this treatment may experience facial flushing (redness) and more serious side effects such as liver damage. The niacinamide form of the B vitamin usually doesn't cause serious problems, but it doesn't lower blood cholesterol.[9]

People suffering from beriberi are very weak, and they have poor muscular coordination. Ariboflavinosis causes muscle weakness and inflamed eyes and mouth. The classic signs and symptoms of severe pellagra are *dermatitis* (scaly, reddened skin), *diarrhea*, *dementia* (loss of normal thinking abilities), and *death*—the "4 Ds of pellagra" (**Fig. 8.13**). In the 1940s, the introduction of the enrichment program, which added these vitamins to grains, greatly reduced the number of people suffering from beriberi, ariboflavinosis, and pellagra in the United States.

Food Sources of Power Player Vitamins

Whole-grain and enriched breads and cereals are among the best sources of the power player vitamins. Milk, yogurt, and other milk products are among the best sources of riboflavin. Exposure to light causes the vitamin to break down rapidly. Therefore, riboflavin-rich foods, such as milk and milk products, shouldn't be kept in clear glass containers. Niacin is very heat stable, so food retains much of its niacin content during usual preparation and cooking methods. **Tables 8.10, 8.11,** and **8.12** list rich sources of thiamin, riboflavin, and niacin, respectively.

Figure 8.13 Pellagra.

■ *What are the "4 Ds of pellagra"?*

TABLE 8.10

THIAMIN CONTENT OF SELECTED FOODS

Food	Thiamin (mg)
Canadian bacon, grilled, 3 oz	.58
Canned lean ham, 3 oz	.53
Flour tortilla, 12″, 1	.35
Cooked green peas, frozen, boiled, drained, ½ cup	.27
White bread, enriched, 1 slice	.15
Wheat germ, 1 Tbsp	.14
Baked beans, canned, ½ cup	.12
Orange juice, frozen, unsweetened, diluted, ½ cup	.10
Whole-wheat bread, enriched, 1 slice	.07

RDA for adult women = 1.1 mg/day
RDA for adult men = 1.2 mg/day
Source: U.S. Department of Agriculture, Agricultural Research Service: *USDA National nutrient database for standard reference, release 25,* 2012.

TABLE 8.11

RIBOFLAVIN CONTENT OF SELECTED FOODS

Food	Riboflavin (mg)
Beef liver, cooked, 3 oz	3.1
Chicken liver, cooked, 3 oz	2.0
Whole-grain Total cereal, ¾ cup	1.7
Wheaties cereal, ¾ cup	0.8
All-Bran cereal, ½ cup	0.8
Yogurt, plain, fat-free, 8 oz	0.5
Cottage cheese, 2% fat, 1 cup	0.4
Milk, fat-free or 1%, 1 cup	0.4
Chicken, cooked, 3 oz	0.2
Mushrooms, cooked, drained, sliced, ½ cup	0.2
Spinach, frozen, cooked, and drained, ½ cup	0.2

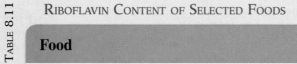

RDA for adult women = 1.1 mg/day
RDA for adult men = 1.3 mg/day
Source: U.S. Department of Agriculture, Agricultural Research Service: *USDA National nutrient database for standard reference, release 25,* 2012.

TABLE 8.12

NIACIN CONTENT OF SELECTED FOODS

Food	Niacin (mg)
Whole-grain Total, ready-to-eat cereal, ¾ cup	20.00
Beef liver, cooked, 3 oz	15.77
Chicken, breast, cooked, 3 oz	12.34
Tuna, canned in water, 3 oz	11.30
Raisin bran, ready-to-eat cereal, ¾ cup	6.48
Pork loin, roasted, 3 oz	6.19
Turkey roast, meat only, cooked, 3 oz	4.90
White rice, enriched, cooked, ½ cup	3.88
Peanuts, dry roasted, 1 oz	3.83
Potato, baked with skin, 6 oz	2.45
Mushrooms, canned, drained, ½ cup	1.24
Macaroni, enriched, elbow, cooked, ½ cup	1.18
Wheaties, ready-to-eat cereal, ¾ cup	1.00

RDA for adult women = 14 mg/day, RDA for adult men = 16 mg/day
Source: U.S. Department of Agriculture, Agricultural Research Service: *USDA National nutrient database for standard reference, release 25,* 2012.

TASTY Tidbits

Corn contains niacin, but the B vitamin is tightly bound to a protein that resists digestion. Thus, people who eat corn as their staple food are likely to develop pellagra. The Mexican practice of soaking corn kernels in lime water before using them to prepare tortillas helps free the niacin, enhancing its ability to be absorbed. In the United States, corn products such as hominy and grits are sources of niacin because they've been treated with lime before cooking.

heme iron-containing portion of hemoglobin

hemoglobin protein in red blood cells that transports oxygen

homocysteine a toxic amino acid

Reviewing the Basics: Power Player Vitamins

Table 8.13 summarizes information about the power player vitamins. The table includes Dietary Reference Intake (DRI) recommendations and major signs and symptoms of the vitamins' deficiency and toxicity disorders.

TABLE 8.13

THIAMIN, RIBOFLAVIN, AND NIACIN: THE POWER PLAYER VITAMINS

Vitamin	Major Functions in the Body	Adult RDA	Major Dietary Sources	Major Deficiency Signs and Symptoms	Major Toxicity Signs and Symptoms
Thiamin	Part of coenzyme needed for energy metabolism	1.1–1.2 mg	Pork, wheat germ, enriched breads and cereals	Beriberi	None (upper limit [UL] not determined)
Riboflavin	Part of coenzymes needed for energy metabolism	1.1–1.3 mg	Milk and other milk products; enriched breads and cereals; liver	Ariboflavinosis	None (UL not determined)
Niacin	Part of coenzymes needed for energy metabolism	14–16 mg	Enriched breads and cereals, beef, liver, tuna, poultry, pork, mushrooms	Pellagra	Adult UL = 35 mg/day Flushing of facial skin, liver damage

8.3b Vitamin B-6: Amino Acid Manager

Your body needs vitamin B-6 to make a coenzyme that's involved in amino acid metabolism. The coenzyme is needed to

- make nonessential amino acids;
- make glucose from certain amino acids;
- produce **heme**, the iron-containing portion of hemoglobin. **Hemoglobin** is the protein in red blood cells that transports oxygen;
- make proteins that transmit messages between nerves; and
- convert a toxic amino acid **homocysteine** to a nonessential amino acid. If the body lacks vitamin B-6, homocysteine can accumulate in blood. High homocysteine levels may contribute to cardiovascular disease.

TABLE 8.14

VITAMIN B-6 CONTENT OF SELECTED FOODS

Food	Vitamin B-6 (mg)
All-Bran, ready-to-eat cereal, ½ cup	3.72
Beef liver, cooked, 3 oz	.92
Pork loin, cooked, 3 oz	.61
Chicken, cooked, 3 oz	.54
Potato, white, baked, flesh and skin, 6 oz	.38
Hamburger patty, broiled, 3 oz	.37
Sweet potato, canned, mashed, ½ cup	.30
Tuna, light, canned in water, 3 oz	.30
Banana, raw, sliced, ½ cup	.28
Pinto beans, boiled, drained, ½ cup	.20
Broccoli, cooked, ½ cup	.16
Salmon, canned sockeye, 3 oz	.10

RDA for adult women = 1.3 mg/day, RDA for adult men = 1.7 mg/day

Source: U.S. Department of Agriculture, Agricultural Research Service: *USDA National nutrient database for standard reference, release 25,* 2012.

TASTY **Tidbits**

Unlike most B vitamins, taking too much vitamin B-6 can be harmful.[10] Vitamin B-6 causes severe nerve damage when taken in doses that exceed the UL (100 mg/day) for extended periods. Signs and symptoms of vitamin B-6 toxicity include walking difficulties and numbness of the hands and feet. The nerve damage usually resolves when the affected person stops taking vitamin B-6 supplements.

Food Sources of Vitamin B-6

Liver, meat, fish, and poultry are among the best dietary sources of vitamin B-6. Additionally, potatoes, bananas, spinach, and broccoli are good sources of the vitamin. During the refining process, the vitamin B-6 that's naturally in grains is lost, and the nutrient isn't added back to the grain products during enrichment. However, many ready-to-eat and cooked cereals have been fortified with the vitamin. **Table 8.14** lists some foods that are major sources of vitamin B-6. During cooking, excessive heat can cause major losses of the vitamin.

Reviewing the Basics: Vitamin B-6

Table 8.15 summarizes information about vitamin B-6. The table includes Dietary Reference Intake (DRI) recommendations, major food sources, and major signs and symptoms of the vitamin's deficiency and toxicity disorders.

TABLE 8.15

VITAMIN B-6

Major Functions in the Body	Adult RDA	Major Dietary Sources	Major Deficiency Signs and Symptoms	Major Toxicity Signs and Symptoms
Part of coenzyme needed for amino acid metabolism and production of heme and chemicals that nerves use to transmit information	1.3–1.7 mg	Meat, fish, and poultry; potatoes, bananas, spinach, broccoli, fortified ready-to-eat cereals	Dermatitis, anemia, depression and confusion, swollen tongue	Adult UL = 100 mg/day Nerve destruction, skin sores, nausea, and heartburn

8.3c Folate and Vitamin B-12: DNA Duo

Certain roles of folate and vitamin B-12 are interrelated, but these B vitamins also have unique functions in your body. *Folate* refers to a family of related compounds that includes naturally occurring **food folate** and **folic acid**. Folic acid is the form of folate that's in dietary supplements, and it's used to fortify foods.

Your cells need folate to make coenzymes involved in DNA production. Before a cell can divide, it needs to make enough DNA for the new cell that's produced. Thus, a person's requirements for folate and vitamin B-12 are high during periods of rapid growth, such as before birth, and in pregnancy, infancy, and childhood.

Initially, folate and vitamin B-12 deficiencies affect cells that rapidly divide, such as red blood cells (RBCs). Mature RBCs don't have nuclei, and they live for only about 4 months. Thus, your body must replace old or worn-out RBCs constantly. To keep up with their rapid rate of cell division, the cells that mature into RBCs (RBC precursors) must make DNA. Without vitamin B-12 and folate, RBC precursor cells that are in your bone marrow enlarge, but they cannot divide normally because they're unable to form new DNA. The bone

marrow releases some of the abnormal RBCs into your bloodstream before they mature (**Fig. 8.14**). This condition, called **megaloblastic** (*mega* = large; blast = immature cell) **anemia**, is characterized by large, immature RBCs (megaloblasts) that still have nuclei and don't carry normal amounts of oxygen (see Fig. 8.14).

Another important function of folate and vitamin B-12 is related to amino acid metabolism. The two B vitamins work together to make the amino acid methionine from the toxic amino acid homocysteine. Recall that vitamin B-6 also helps convert homocysteine to methionine.

Cells need vitamin B-12 to convert a toxic compound to a substance the body needs. When cells lack the vitamin, the toxic compound can build up in the body and damage nerves.[11]

© Banana Stock/PunchStock RF

folic acid and **food folate** forms of folate

megaloblastic anemia condition characterized by fewer and abnormal red blood cells

Figure 8.14 Folate and B-12 for red blood cell production.

Food Sources of Folate and Vitamin B-12

Enriched grain products and fortified cereals are among the richest sources of folate in the American diet. **Table 8.16** lists some foods and their folate contents, which are reported as micrograms of dietary folate equivalents (DFEs).

Plants don't make vitamin B-12, so we rely almost entirely on animal foods to supply the vitamin naturally. Major sources of vitamin B-12 in the typical American's diet are meat, milk and milk products, poultry, fish, shellfish, and eggs. Although liver isn't a popular food, it's one of the richest sources of vitamin B-12. Many soy products, such as soy milk, and ready-to-eat cereals are fortified with vitamin B-12. **Table 8.17** lists some foods that are good sources of this micronutrient.

TABLE 8.16

FOLATE CONTENT OF SELECTED FOODS

Food	Folate (mcg DFE)
Whole-grain Total, ready-to-eat cereal, ¾ cup	676
Chicken liver, cooked, 3 oz	520
Pinto beans, cooked, ½ cup	147
Asparagus (frozen), cooked, drained, ½ cup	134
Turnip greens, boiled, drained, ½ cup	85
Papaya, raw, mashed, 1 cup	85
Broccoli, chopped, boiled, drained, ½ cup	84
White rice, long-grain, cooked, enriched, ½ cup	77
English muffin, plain, toasted, enriched, 1	75
Spinach, raw, 1 cup	58
Orange juice, frozen, unsweetened, diluted, ½ cup	55

RDA for adults = 400 mcg (DFE)/day

Source: U.S. Department of Agriculture, Agricultural Research Service: *USDA National nutrient database for standard reference, release 25,* 2012. Nutrient Data Laboratory Home Page.

TABLE 8.17

VITAMIN B-12 CONTENT OF SELECTED FOODS

Food	Vitamin B-12 (mcg)
Beef liver, cooked, 3 oz	63.52
Chicken liver, cooked, 3 oz	15.17
Sardines, canned in oil, drained, 3 oz	7.60
Special K, ready-to-eat cereal, 1 cup	6.01
Salmon, sockeye, canned, 3 oz	4.68
Wheaties, ready-to-eat cereal, 1 cup	4.00
Ground beef patty, 80% lean, cooked, 3 oz	2.55
Tuna, light, canned in water, drained, 3 oz	2.54
Soy milk, fortified, 1 cup	2.07
Milk, fat-free, 1 cup	1.22
Cottage cheese, 2% fat, 1 cup	1.02

RDA for adults = 2.4 mcg/day

Source: U.S. Department of Agriculture, Agricultural Research Service: *USDA National nutrient database for standard reference, release 25,* 2012.

Beef liver

Absorbing Vitamin B-12

Absorbing the vitamin B-12 that's naturally in foods requires a complex series of steps that are unique for a vitamin (see **Essential Concept 8.3**).

Essential Concept

8.3 Absorbing the Vitamin B-12 in Your Food

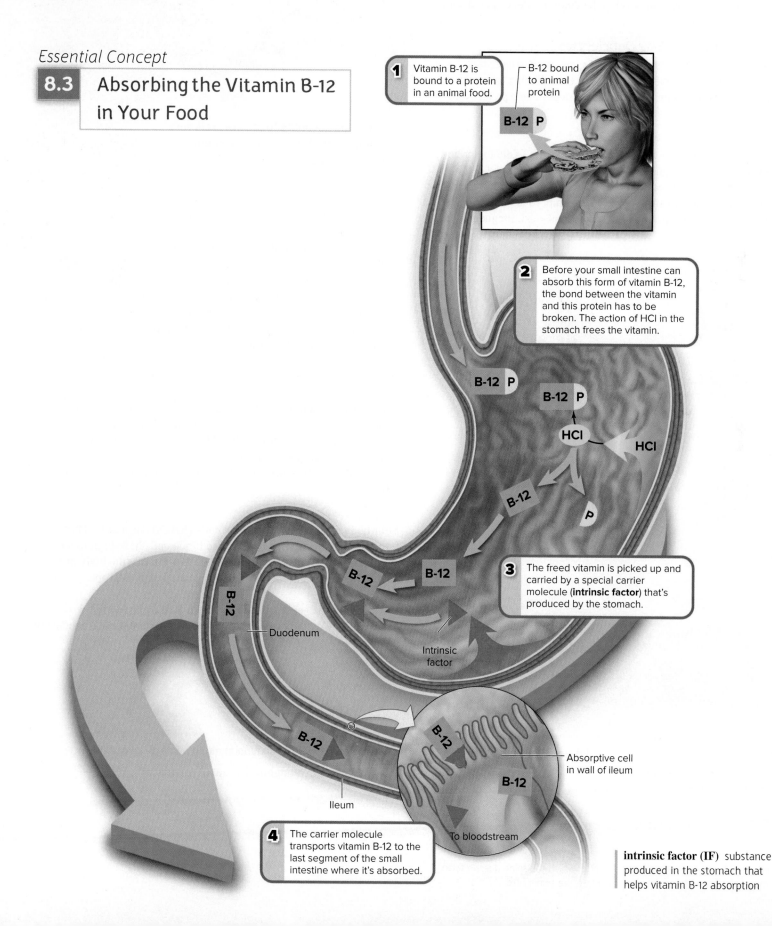

1 Vitamin B-12 is bound to a protein in an animal food.

B-12 bound to animal protein

2 Before your small intestine can absorb this form of vitamin B-12, the bond between the vitamin and this protein has to be broken. The action of HCl in the stomach frees the vitamin.

3 The freed vitamin is picked up and carried by a special carrier molecule (**intrinsic factor**) that's produced by the stomach.

Duodenum

Intrinsic factor

Absorptive cell in wall of ileum

Ileum

To bloodstream

4 The carrier molecule transports vitamin B-12 to the last segment of the small intestine where it's absorbed.

intrinsic factor (IF) substance produced in the stomach that helps vitamin B-12 absorption

Unlike the other B vitamins, the liver stores excesses of vitamin B-12. A healthy liver has enough vitamin B-12 reserves to last 5 to 10 years.[12] Therefore, a person who follows a diet that completely lacks vitamin B-12 may not develop the vitamin's deficiency disorder for as long as 10 years.

Folate and Vitamin B-12 Deficiencies

If you develop megaloblastic anemia, it's important to determine whether you have a deficiency of folate or B-12. Taking folic acid supplements for a vitamin B-12 deficiency doesn't help protect your nerves.

What Are Neural Tube Defects?

It's very important for a woman to have adequate folate in her body when she becomes pregnant. An embryo undergoes rapid cell division, so it has a high need for folate. During the first few weeks after conception, the **neural tube** forms in the embryo (**Fig. 8.15**). The neural tube develops into the brain and spinal cord. Pregnant women

Having adequate folate status is very important for pregnant women.

© Brand X Pictures/Jupiter Images RF

who are deficient in folate have a high risk of giving birth to infants with neural tube defects, such as **spina bifida** (*spy´-na bif´-eh-dah*). Spina bifida occurs when the embryo's spine doesn't form properly and the bones fail to enclose the spinal cord. Infants with severe spina bifida can have a section of their spinal cord bulging through an opening in their backs (see Fig. 8.15). Often, people with severe spina bifida are unable to walk independently. Each year, about 1500 babies are born with spina bifida in the United States.[13] The good news: Cases of spina bifida have declined sharply since enrichment of foods with folic acid began in 1999.

Because women of childbearing age may become pregnant at some point, they need to be aware of the link between neural tube defects and the lack of folate. In addition to including folate-rich foods in their diets, women can prepare for pregnancy by taking a daily multivitamin supplement that contains 400 mcg of synthetic folic acid.

Megaloblastic Anemia

Your body replaces old red blood cells (RBCs) constantly. Therefore, the cells that divide to form red blood cells have high folate and vitamin B-12 needs. Without these B vitamins, the body produces large, immature RBCs that don't carry oxygen properly (see Fig. 8.14).

Megaloblastic anemia is a sign of both folate and vitamin B-12 deficiencies. Common signs and symptoms of vitamin B-12 deficiency include

- muscle weakness,
- sore mouth,
- smooth and shiny tongue,
- memory loss and confusion,
- difficulty walking and maintaining balance, and
- numbness and tingling sensations, particularly in legs and feet.

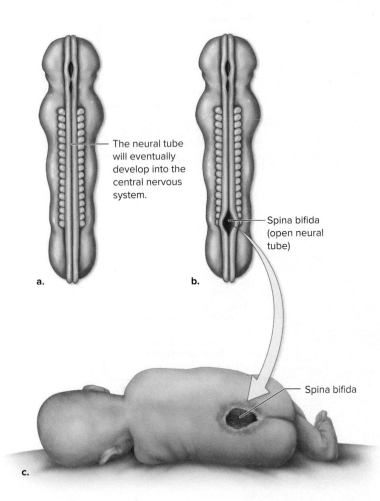

The neural tube will eventually develop into the central nervous system.

Spina bifida (open neural tube)

Spina bifida

a. **b.** **c.**

Figure 8.15 **Neural tube formation. (a)** Normal neural tube in a human embryo. **(b)** Open neural tube. **(c)** Newborn with severe spina bifida.

neural tube embryonic structure that eventually develops into the brain and spinal cord

spina bifida type of neural tube defect in which the spine doesn't form properly before birth and it fails to enclose the spinal cord

What's Pernicious Anemia?

One to 2% of people who are over 60 years of age have an *autoimmune* disorder that causes inflammation and destruction of the cells in the stomach that produce intrinsic factor, the special vitamin B-12 carrier molecule.[11] (An autoimmune disorder results when a person's immune system attacks his or her own cells.) In these cases, diets may supply adequate amounts of vitamin B-12, but there's no carrier molecule to help the intestine absorb the micronutrient. Eventually, a person with this condition develops **pernicious** ("deadly") **anemia**, a form of anemia that features megaloblastic red blood cells and nerve damage. As its name implies, pernicious anemia can be deadly. Treatment involves bypassing the need for intestinal absorption, usually by providing routine vitamin B-12 injections.

Family history is a risk factor for pernicious anemia. Therefore, consider having your blood tested for signs of vitamin B-12 deficiency as you grow older, especially if you have a close relative with pernicious anemia.

Older adults have a higher risk of vitamin B-12 deficiency than do younger persons.

Vitamin B-12 Deficiency in Older Adults

Vitamin B-12 deficiency usually occurs in older adults and results from conditions that interfere with intestinal absorption of the vitamin in foods and not from inadequate intakes.[11] As people age, the production of hydrochloric acid (HCl) in the stomach declines. Thus, many older adults are unable to release vitamin B-12 from the protein to which it's bound in food. People with this condition develop vitamin B-12 deficiency despite consuming diets that contain the vitamin. In addition to advanced age, alcoholism, gastric bypass surgeries for weight reduction, and medications that reduce stomach acid production can contribute to a deficiency of the vitamin. Older adults with reduced stomach acid can take dietary supplements that contain synthetic vitamin B-12 because this form of the vitamin doesn't require the action of stomach acid. Vegans should also be concerned about the need for vitamin B-12 because plant foods aren't natural sources of the vitamin. For more information about vitamin B-12 and vegetarians, see the "What's Vegetarianism?" section of Unit 7.

Reviewing the Basics: DNA Duo

Table 8.18 summarizes information about folate and vitamin B-12. The table includes Dietary Reference Intake (DRI) recommendations, major food sources, and major signs and symptoms of the vitamins' deficiency and toxicity disorders.

pernicious anemia condition caused by the lack of intrinsic factor

---

TABLE 8.18

FOLATE AND VITAMIN B-12

Major Functions in the Body	Adult RDA	Major Dietary Sources	Major Deficiency Signs and Symptoms	Major Toxicity Signs and Symptoms
Folate Part of coenzyme needed for DNA metabolism, preventing homocysteine accumulation	400 mcg DFE	Dark green, leafy vegetables, liver, legumes, asparagus, broccoli, orange juice, enriched breads and cereals (folic acid)	Megaloblastic anemia, neural tube defects in embryos	Adult UL = 1000 mcg/day May stimulate cancer cell growth
Vitamin B-12 Part of coenzymes needed for various cellular processes, including folate metabolism and maintenance of myelin sheaths	2.4 mcg	Animal foods, fortified cereals, fortified soy milk	Pernicious anemia: megaloblastic anemia and nerve damage resulting in paralysis and death	None (UL not determined)

TABLE 8.19

PANTOTHENIC ACID, BIOTIN, AND CHOLINE

Vitamin	Major Functions in the Body	Adult RDA/AI	Major Dietary Sources	Major Deficiency Signs and Symptoms	Major Toxicity Signs and Symptoms
Pantothenic Acid	Part of the coenzyme needed for making fat and releasing energy from macronutrients	5 mg	Beef and chicken liver, sunflower seeds, mushrooms, yogurt, soy milk, fortified cereals	Rarely occurs	Unknown (UL not determined)
Biotin	Needed for enzymes involved in glucose and fatty acid production	30 mcg	Liver, eggs, peanuts, salmon, and pork; bacterial production in large intestine	Rarely occurs: skin rash, hair loss, convulsions, developmental delays in infants	Unknown (UL not determined)
Choline	Production of chemicals that transmit messages between nerves and phospholipids; methionine (an amino acid) metabolism	425–550 mg	Liver, wheat germ, eggs; cellular production	Liver damage	Fishy body odor and reduced blood pressure

8.3d Pantothenic Acid, Biotin, and Choline

Pantothenic acid, biotin, and the vitamin-like nutrient choline are in a wide variety of foods. Therefore, deficiencies of these micronutrients are uncommon, especially among healthy adults who eat items from all food groups regularly. Furthermore, bacteria that normally live in the human large intestine make biotin, and the intestine may absorb some of the vitamin. **Table 8.19** summarizes basic information about pantothenic acid, biotin, and choline.

TASTY Tidbits

Avidin is a protein in raw egg whites that binds to biotin, making the vitamin resist digestion. If you eat raw eggs regularly, you may develop a skin rash and other signs of biotin deficiency. Cooking eggs destroys avidin, making biotin available for absorption.

Nutrition Fact or Fiction?

Taking vitamin C protects you against infection by cold viruses.

Results of several scientific studies indicate that routine vitamin C supplementation (200 mg or more of the vitamin daily) doesn't prevent colds in the general population.[14] However, taking such large doses of the vitamin may reduce the duration of cold symptoms by a day or so. Additionally, vitamin C may reduce the severity of cold symptoms because the micronutrient acts like an antihistamine when taken in very large doses.[15]

© McGraw-Hill Education. John Flournoy, photographer

8.3e Vitamin C: Collagen Connector

Vitamin C (**ascorbic acid**) enables many enzymes to work, but the vitamin doesn't function as part of a coenzyme as do most B vitamins. Your body uses vitamin C to form and maintain **collagen**, the protein that gives strength to connective tissue. Connective tissues, such as bone, cartilage, and tendons, connect and support other structures in your body. If vitamin C is unavailable, your body forms weak connective tissue and is unable to maintain existing collagen. Weak collagen can allow teeth to loosen and fall out of their sockets and scars to break down.

In addition to forming and maintaining collagen, your body needs vitamin C to

- maintain the immune system,
- produce bile,
- make certain chemicals that transmit messages between nerves, and
- produce various hormones, including the "stress hormone" cortisol.

Vitamin C also serves as an antioxidant by donating electrons to stabilize free radicals. Vitamin C can give an electron to another antioxidant—vitamin E. Thus, vitamin C recycles vitamin E, enabling it to regain its antioxidant function. *Calcium ascorbate* and *sodium ascorbate* are forms of vitamin C that are often added to packaged foods to protect against free radical damage. Such antioxidants increase a food's shelf life.

TASTY **Tidbits**

Most animals don't need dietary sources of vitamin C because they can make all the vitamin they need. Humans and guinea pigs are among the few animals that are unable to make vitamin C. For these animals, the micronutrient is essential.

© G.K. & Vikki Hart/Getty Images RF

ascorbic acid vitamin C

collagen fibrous protein that gives strength to connective tissue

What *IS* That? - - - - - - - - - - - →

Guava is a tropical fruit that's available in many varieties. Although guavas can be eaten fresh, the fruit is often used to make sauces, jellies, and juices. Guavas are an excellent source of fiber and vitamin C.

Three ounces of the fruit contain about 125 g vitamin C, which is almost four times the vitamin C that's in the same amount of fresh orange slices.

Food Sources of Vitamin C

Table 8.20 lists some common foods and their vitamin C contents. Note that plant foods are among the best dietary sources of vitamin C. Most animal foods aren't sources of the micronutrient. By including vitamin C-rich fruits and vegetables in your diet each day, you can obtain adequate amounts of vitamin C.

Vitamin C is very unstable in the presence of heat, oxygen, light, alkaline conditions, and the minerals iron and copper. Storing vitamin C-rich foods in cool conditions, such as in the refrigerator, will help preserve the micronutrient. Because vitamin C is water soluble and destroyed by heat, it's easily lost when you use large amounts of water and high heat to cook foods. Therefore, avoid overcooking vegetables, use a minimum amount of cooking water, and eat raw fruits and vegetables whenever possible.

TABLE 8.20

VITAMIN C CONTENT OF SELECTED FOODS

Food	Vitamin C (mg)
Kiwifruit, raw, green, ½ cup	83
Papaya, raw, mashed, ½ cup	70
Green pepper, sweet, raw, chopped, 1 cup	60
Red peppers, sweet, raw, sliced, ½ cup	59
Broccoli, cooked, drained, chopped, ½ cup	51
Strawberries, raw, sliced, ½ cup	49
Orange juice, from concentrate, ½ cup	48
Brussels sprouts, cooked, drained, ½ cup	48
Cantaloupe, raw, cubed, ½ cup	29
Cabbage, cooked, shredded, drained, ½ cup	28
Potato, white, baked with skin, approx. 6 oz	21
Peas, edible pods, cooked, drained, ½ cup	18
French fries, frozen, oven-heated, 10 strips	18

RDA for adult women (nonsmokers) = 75 mg/day; RDA for adult men (nonsmokers) = 90 mg/day
Source: USDA National nutrient database for standard reference, release 25, 2012.

Figure 8.16 Sign of scurvy.

What's Scurvy?

Scurvy is the vitamin C deficiency disease. Signs of scurvy include swollen gums that bleed easily, teeth that loosen and fall out, skin that bruises easily, and old scars that open. These signs result from poorly formed and maintained collagen (**Fig. 8.16**).

Even if you don't regularly eat foods that contain the vitamin or take a vitamin C supplement, you're unlikely to develop scurvy. Why? Most people require less than 10 mg of the vitamin daily to prevent scurvy.[15] A 6-ounce serving of fresh orange juice provides about 60 mg of vitamin C—well beyond the requirement. Additionally, Americans rarely develop scurvy because vitamin C is added to many popular processed foods, including fruit and sports drinks, ready-to-eat cereals, and nutrition or power bars.

scurvy vitamin C deficiency disease

Can Vitamin C Be Toxic?

When adults exceed the UL of the vitamin (2000 mg/day), gastrointestinal upsets, including diarrhea, often occur.[15] Taking megadoses of vitamin C supplements is wasteful because your small intestine reduces absorption of the micronutrient when intakes of the vitamin are more than 200 mg/day. Furthermore, when your cells contain all the vitamin C they can hold, the excess vitamin and *oxalate*, a by-product of breaking down vitamin C, circulate in your bloodstream. Your kidneys filter and eliminate these unnecessary substances in urine. Excess oxalate in the kidneys may raise your risk of kidney stones.[15] Therefore, consider avoiding vitamin C supplements, especially if you have a history of kidney stones.

Reviewing the Basics: Vitamin C

Table 8.21 summarizes information about vitamin C. The table includes Dietary Reference Intake (DRI) recommendations, and major signs and symptoms of the vitamin's deficiency and toxicity disorders.

TABLE 8.21

VITAMIN C

Major Functions in the Body	Adult RDA	Major Dietary Sources	Major Deficiency Signs and Symptoms	Major Toxicity Signs and Symptoms
Antioxidant; connective tissue production and maintenance; production of chemicals that transmit messages between nerves; production of certain hormones; immune system functioning	75–90 mg (nonsmokers) 110–125 mg (smokers)	Peppers, citrus fruits, papaya, broccoli, cabbage, berries	Scurvy: Poor wound healing, pinpoint bleeding, bleeding gums, bruises, depression	Adult UL = 2000 mg/day Diarrhea and GI tract discomfort

Module 8.4

Vitamins and Cancer

© Science Photo Library RF/Getty Images RF

Group of cancer cells

8.4 - Learning Outcomes

After reading Module 8.4, you should be able to

1. Define all of the key terms in this module.

2. Identify lifestyle practices associated with increased risk of certain cancers.

3. Identify foods that may increase your risk of cancer.

4. Explain why it may not be useful to take dietary supplements for cancer prevention.

carcinogen agent that causes cancer

cancer group of diseases characterized by abnormal cell behavior

Are you among the millions of Americans who take vitamin supplements? If your answer is "yes," why do you use them? Vitamin supplements are effective for treating people with specific vitamin deficiency diseases, disorders that increase vitamin requirements, and a few other medical conditions. However, scientific evidence generally doesn't support claims that megadoses of vitamins can prevent or treat serious chronic diseases, including cancer. This module of Unit 8 takes a closer look at cancer and the role that diet may play in the prevention and treatment of the disease.

8.4a What's Cancer?

As mentioned in Unit 7, DNA is the material in cells that contains the instructions for protein production. Sometimes, the parts of DNA (genes) that regulate a cell's growth, reproduction, and death become damaged. In many cases, a specific **carcinogen** such as a virus or toxic chemical harms the DNA. When the damage leads to rapid cell growth and unchecked cell division, cancer can result. **Cancer** refers to a group of chronic diseases characterized by abnormal cells that are "out of control."

Cancer cells are *malignant* because they divide repeatedly and frequently, and they don't die (**Fig. 8.17**). When a cell becomes malignant, it doesn't perform the specialized functions of the cells from which it was derived. A cancerous liver cell, for example, doesn't remove toxins from the bloodstream or store nutrients properly.

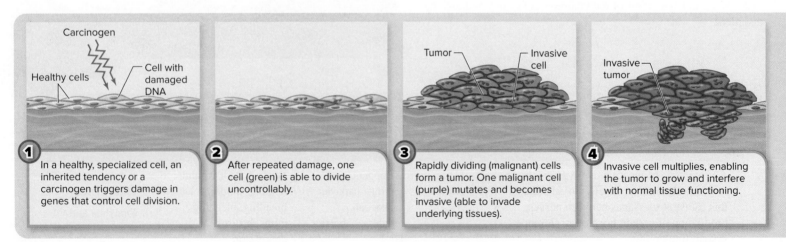

1 In a healthy, specialized cell, an inherited tendency or a carcinogen triggers damage in genes that control cell division.

2 After repeated damage, one cell (green) is able to divide uncontrollably.

3 Rapidly dividing (malignant) cells form a tumor. One malignant cell (purple) mutates and becomes invasive (able to invade underlying tissues).

4 Invasive cell multiplies, enabling the tumor to grow and interfere with normal tissue functioning.

Figure 8.17 Cancer progression.

As a result of their rapid growth rate, many types of cancer cells form masses, called malignant tumors. Malignant cells often break away from the tumor. These cells can move to and invade other parts of the body. When cancer spreads to other tissues, the disease has *metastasized* (*meh-tass´-tah-sized*).

Because of their rapid growth and frequent cell divisions, malignant cells require more nutrients than do normal cells. To supply enough nutrients to meet their needs, cancerous tumors stimulate the body to form blood vessels that divert blood away from healthy cells and into the tumor (see Figure 8.17). Eventually, healthy tissues are unable to obtain adequate supplies of nutrients, and they die.

What Are Risk Factors for Cancer?

Medical researchers have discovered several risk factors for many forms of cancer. These factors include

- age (half of cancers occur in people over 66 years of age),
- family history of cancer,
- tobacco use,
- exposure to some forms of radiation,
- exposure to certain environmental substances,
- chronic inflammation,
- history of certain viral or bacterial infections,
- high levels of certain hormones,
- diet,
- alcohol use, and
- excess body fat.[16]

Cancer causation is a complex process. Therefore, it may be impossible to pinpoint a single cause of a patient's cancer. Individuals differ widely in their genetic makeups, lifestyle practices, environmental exposures, and nutritional states. Some medical experts estimate that over 50% of cancer deaths among Americans can be prevented if people adopt healthier lifestyles, including their diets.[17]

8.4b The Role of Obesity and Diet in Cancer Development

Obesity is a risk factor for certain cancers, particularly breast cancer (after menopause) and cancers of the esophagus, lining of the uterus, colon and rectum, kidney, pancreas, thyroid, and gallbladder.[16] Medical researchers don't fully understand why obesity increases the risk of these forms of cancer. One possible explanation has to do with fat tissue's production of the female hormone estrogen. High levels of estrogen are associated with the risk of breast, uterine, and some other types of cancer. Obesity can also increase blood insulin levels, which may promote cancer development.

Some foods and beverages contain carcinogens. Alcohol, for example, is a carcinogen.[18] People who consume two or more alcoholic drinks daily have higher risks of cancers of the mouth, throat, esophagus, voice box, liver, colon, rectum, and breast.[18] The higher the alcohol intake, the greater the risk of these cancers. Furthermore, the chances of developing cancers of the mouth, throat, or voice box increase sharply when cigarette smoking is combined with drinking. To reduce your risk of cancer, it's wise to limit your consumption of alcohol or avoid the drug altogether. If you drink, do so in moderation—no more than one standard drink per day for women and no more than two standard drinks per day for men. (A standard alcoholic drink is 1.5 oz of liquor, 12 oz of regular beer, or 5 oz of wine.)

Advanced age, obesity, and lack of physical activity are risk factors for cancer.

© Photodisc/Getty Images RF

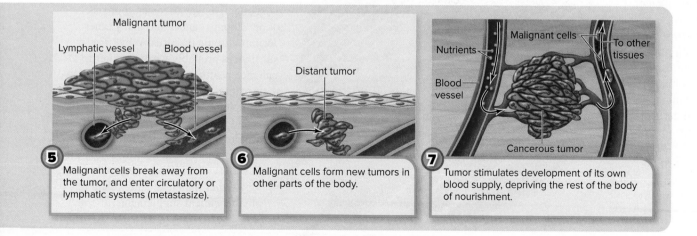

5 Malignant cells break away from the tumor, and enter circulatory or lymphatic systems (metastasize).

Malignant tumor
Lymphatic vessel
Blood vessel

6 Malignant cells form new tumors in other parts of the body.

Distant tumor

7 Tumor stimulates development of its own blood supply, depriving the rest of the body of nourishment.

Malignant cells
To other tissues
Nutrients
Blood vessel
Cancerous tumor

TABLE 8.22

POSSIBLE DIET-RELATED CARCINOGENS[19,20]

Possibly Carcinogenic	Common Dietary Sources	Possible or Known Action
Aflatoxin	Moldy nuts and grains	Increases risk of liver cancer
Arsenic	Natural contaminant in drinking water	May increase risk of bladder cancer
Alcohol	Alcoholic beverages	Unclear, but may increase certain hormone levels or the body's breakdown of alcohol may result in carcinogens
Benzene	Contaminated water	Known carcinogen
Fried, grilled, smoked, pickled, or salted meat and poultry	Foods exposed to salt or high temperatures, especially grilled meat that has charred areas	May increase risk of throat, stomach, and colorectal cancers
Processed meats and poultry	Deli meats	
Salted fish	Chinese-style fish; Pickled herring	Increased risk of stomach cancer

Table 8.22 lists dietary factors that may be associated with increased risk of various cancers. Currently, there's no scientific evidence that consuming artificial sweeteners such as aspartame, coffee, foods made from genetically modified organisms (GMOs), or foods preserved by radiation causes cancer.[20]

TASTY Tidbits

High temperatures used to cook meat may cause charring of the meat and the formation of a group of carcinogens called heterocyclic (het´-eh-ro-si´-klic) amines. Therefore, you may be able to reduce your risk of certain cancers by limiting your intake of grilled meats and avoiding charred parts of charcoal-grilled meats. Also, covering the grate with aluminum foil, poking a few holes in the foil, and placing the meat on top of it will reduce charring of the meat.

Diet and Cancer Risk Reduction

You can reduce your risk of cancer by

- avoiding exposure to tobacco smoke,
- achieving and maintaining a healthy weight,
- adopting a physically active lifestyle, and
- eating a healthy diet that limits intakes of red and processed meats and emphasizes intakes of plant foods, including fruits, vegetables, and whole grains.

Although research is ongoing, results of scientific studies generally don't provide evidence that taking dietary supplements that contain antioxidants reduces the risk of cancer.[19]

Consuming a wide variety of vitamins and phytochemicals in their natural states and concentrations (in foods) may be the most effective way to lower your risk of developing cancer and many other serious chronic diseases. Why? These substances probably work together to enhance health, and isolating them from their natural sources and making them into supplements may reduce their usefulness and increase their risk of toxicity. Therefore, registered dietitian nutritionists recommend that healthy adults eat a variety of fruits and vegetables each day rather than take antioxidant or phytochemical supplements.

In a **Nutshell**

© McGraw-Hill Education. Mark A. Dierker, photographer

Module 8.1 Introducing Vitamins

- Vitamins are organic micronutrients that the body cannot make or make enough of to maintain good health; that naturally occur in commonly eaten foods; that cause deficiency disease when they're missing from diets; and that restore good health when added back to the diet. Foods generally contain much smaller amounts of vitamins than of macronutrients.

- Vitamins play numerous roles in your body, and each vitamin generally has more than one function. In general, vitamins regulate a variety of body processes, including those involved in cell division and development as well as the growth and maintenance of tissues. Vitamins, however, aren't a source of energy because cells don't metabolize them for energy.

- Certain chemical reactions can form free radicals. A free radical is a chemically unstable substance because it is missing an electron. Free radicals can damage or destroy molecules by removing electrons from them. Many medical researchers suspect excess free radical damage in the body ultimately leads to heart attack, stroke, cancer, Alzheimer's disease, and even the aging process. Cells normally regulate free radical formation by using antioxidants such as vitamin E.

- Vitamins A, D, E, and K are fat-soluble vitamins; thiamin, riboflavin, niacin, vitamin B-6, pantothenic acid, folate, biotin, vitamin B-12, and vitamin C are water-soluble vitamins. (The vitamin-like substance choline is water soluble.) Your body has more difficulty eliminating excess fat-soluble vitamins than water-soluble vitamins. As a result, your body stores extra fat-soluble vitamins. Over time, these vitamins can accumulate and cause toxicity. Water-soluble vitamins are generally not as toxic as fat-soluble vitamins.

- The enrichment program specifies amounts of thiamin, riboflavin, niacin, folic acid, and the mineral iron that manufacturers must add to their refined flour and other milled grain products. However, enrichment doesn't replace vitamin B-6, vitamin E, and other nutrients that were naturally in the unrefined grains.

- Vitamin deficiency disorders generally result from inadequate diets or conditions that increase the body's requirements for vitamins or reduce the intestinal tract's ability to absorb nutrients. Your chances of developing a vitamin deficiency disease increase when your diet consistently lacks the micronutrient and levels of the nutrient in your body become too low.

- Most commonly eaten foods don't contain toxic levels of vitamins. Vitamin toxicity is most likely to occur in people who take megadoses of vitamin supplements or consume large amounts of vitamin-fortified foods regularly.

Module 8.2 Fat-Soluble Vitamins

- Vitamin A is involved in vision, immune function, and cell development. The vitamin A provitamin, beta-carotene, functions as an antioxidant. Dietary sources of preformed vitamin A include liver and fortified milk; provitamin A carotenoids are especially plentiful in dark green and orange fruits and vegetables. Excess vitamin A can be quite toxic and can cause birth defects when taken during pregnancy.

- Vitamin D is both a hormone and a vitamin. Exposure to sunlight enables human skin to make a previtamin vitamin D from a cholesterol-like substance. The body can convert this substance to the active form of the vitamin. A few foods, including fatty fish and fortified milk, are dietary sources of the vitamin. Vitamin D helps regulate the level of blood calcium by increasing calcium absorption from the intestine. Vitamin D also stimulates bone cells to form calcium phosphate, the hard major mineral compound in bone tissue. Infants and children who don't obtain enough vitamin D may develop rickets. Adults with inadequate amounts of the vitamin in their bodies may develop osteomalacia. Older adults and breastfed infants often need a supplemental source of the vitamin. Excess intakes of vitamin D can cause the body to deposit calcium in soft tissues.

© Digital Vision/Getty Images RF

- Vitamin E functions primarily as an antioxidant. By donating electrons to free radicals, vitamin E stabilizes them. This effect shields DNA, proteins, phospholipids, and unsaturated fatty acids from destruction. Plant oils and products made from these oils are generally rich sources of vitamin E.

Module 8.3 Water-Soluble Vitamins

- Thiamin, riboflavin, and niacin play key roles as part of coenzymes in energy-yielding reactions. These water-soluble vitamins help cells metabolize carbohydrates, fats, and proteins. Whole-grain and enriched grain products are common sources of all three of the vitamins. Beriberi is the severe thiamin deficiency disease; ariboflavinosis results from the lack of riboflavin; pellagra results from a severe lack of niacin. Excess intakes of niacin can cause toxicity.

- Vitamin B-6 is involved in the production of nonessential amino acids. The vitamin also participates in the production of chemicals that transmit messages between nerves and the metabolism of homocysteine. High doses of vitamin B-6 should be avoided because the vitamin can cause nerve damage.

- Folate plays important roles in DNA production and homocysteine metabolism. Rich food sources of folate are leafy vegetables, organ meats, and orange juice. Signs of folate deficiency include megaloblastic anemia. Pregnancy increases the body's needs for folate; a deficiency during the first month of pregnancy can result in neural tube defects in offspring. Women of childbearing age can meet the RDA for the vitamin by taking dietary supplements that contain folic acid.

- The body needs vitamin B-12 to metabolize folate and homocysteine, and maintain nerves. Although vitamin B-12 doesn't occur naturally in plant foods, the vitamin is in animal foods and products that have been fortified with the micronutrient. Vitamin B-12 deficiency is more common in older adults. As people age, their stomachs produce less HCl. This condition can result in B-12 deficiency even though adequate amounts of the micronutrient are consumed in foods. Furthermore, a vitamin B-12 deficiency and a condition called pernicious anemia result if the stomach is unable to produce the vitamin B-12 carrier protein.

- The body uses vitamin C to make and maintain collagen, a major protein in connective tissue. Vitamin C also functions as an antioxidant. Fresh fruits and vegetables, especially citrus fruits, are generally good sources of the micronutrient. Because vitamin C is easily lost in cooking, diets should emphasize raw or lightly cooked fruits and vegetables. Smoking increases the body's requirement for vitamin C. Scurvy is the vitamin C deficiency disease. Excess vitamin C may cause diarrhea and increase the risk of kidney stones in some people.

Module 8.4 Vitamins and Cancer

- Cancer occurs when DNA undergoes changes that affect a cell's growth, reproduction, and death. Such changes result in abnormal cell development, rapid cell growth, and unchecked cell division.

- Maintaining a healthy body weight, exercising regularly, consuming diets that supply plenty of fruits and vegetables, limiting intakes of red and/or processed meats, and avoiding tobacco smoke and excess alcohol may reduce the risk of cancer.

What's in Your Diet?!

Using the DRIs

© Wendy Schiff

1. Refer to your 1- or 3-day food log from the "What's in Your Diet?!" feature in Unit 3.

   a. Find the RDA values for vitamins under your life stage/sex group category in the DRI tables (see Appendix G). Write those values under the "My RDA" column in the table at the bottom of the page.

   b. Review your personal dietary assessment. Find your 3-day average intakes of vitamins A, E, C, D, folate, B-12, thiamin, riboflavin, and niacin. Write those values under the "My Average Intake" column of the table.

   c. Calculate the percentage of the RDA you consumed for each vitamin by dividing your intake by the RDA amount and multiplying the figure you obtain by 100. For example, if your average intake of vitamin C was 100 mg/day and your RDA for the vitamin was 75 mg/day, you would divide 100 mg by 75 mg to obtain 1.25. To multiply this figure by 100, simply move the decimal point two places to the right, and replace the decimal point with a percentage sign (125%). Thus, your average daily intake of vitamin C was 125% of the RDA. Place the percentages for each vitamin under the "% of My RDA" column.

   d. Under the ">, <, =" column, indicate whether your average daily intake was greater than (>), less than (<), or equal to (=) the RDA.

2. Use the information you calculated in the first part of this activity to answer the following questions:

   a. Which of your average vitamin intakes equaled or exceeded the RDA value?

   b. Which of your average vitamin intakes was below the RDA value?

   c. What foods would you eat to increase your intake of the vitamins that were less than the RDA levels? (Review sources of certain vitamins in Unit 8.)

   d. Turn in your completed table and answers to your instructor.

What's in Your Diet?

Vitamin	My RDA	My Average Intake	% of My RDA	>, <, or =
A				
E				
C				
D				
Folate				
B-12				
Thiamin				
Riboflavin				

© Royalty-Free/Corbis RF

Consider **This...**

1. Choose a vitamin and type the nutrient's name in the search box of an Internet browser. Locate three sites that sell products containing the vitamin. Review the pages of each site, making notes about claims, prices, and the kinds of links provided. Then write a three- to five-page report that describes and compares the information you found at the sites. In your paper, discuss any claims made on behalf of these products that you consider false or misleading. Include the URLs for the sites in your report.

2. Nick complains of having no energy and feeling tired most of the time. He's thinking about taking high doses of dietary supplements that contain thiamin, riboflavin, and niacin to boost his energy level. What would you tell Nick about these vitamins that might influence his decision to use the supplements?

3. While watching an infomercial on TV, you hear a so-called nutrition expert make claims for a substance that he or she claims to be a vitamin. What questions would you ask the expert to ascertain whether the substance truly is a vitamin?

4. One of your friends takes megadoses of vitamins A, C, B-6, and E because she thinks they help her stay healthy. What would you tell her about taking such large doses of these vitamins?

5. Consider your current lifestyle and the recommendations for reducing cancer risk that are provided in this unit. Which recommendations are you unlikely to follow? Explain why you are not likely to follow those recommendations.

Salted herring is a popular menu item among northern Europeans. The salt helps keep the fish from spoiling and is often the first step in "pickling" fish. People who eat salted fish regularly are more likely to develop stomach cancer than people who don't eat such fish.
© lynx/iconotec.com/Glow images

Test **Yourself**

Select the best answer.

1. Vitamin toxicities generally occur as a result of
   a. taking megadoses of dietary supplements.
   b. consuming a wide variety of foods.
   c. eating enriched breads and cereal products.
   d. having diseases that interfere with intestinal absorption.

2. Vitamins
   a. don't provide any calories.
   b. occur in gram amounts in foods.
   c. aren't organic molecules.
   d. are macronutrients.

3. People who are unable to absorb fat are likely to develop a _____ deficiency.
   a. vitamin B-12
   b. folate
   c. vitamin D
   d. riboflavin

4. Enriched grain products have specific amounts of _____ added during processing.
   a. pantothenic acid
   b. riboflavin
   c. biotin
   d. vitamin D

5. Which of the following foods is not a rich source of provitamin A?
   a. Green beans
   b. Carrots
   c. Chicken
   d. Sweet potato

© FoodCollection/StockFood RF

6. During pregnancy, excess _____ intake is known to be teratogenic.
   a. pantothenic acid
   b. vitamin A
   c. vitamin K
   d. choline

7. Vitamin K can be produced by

a. skin exposure to ultraviolet radiation.

b. hydrolysis of seawater.

c. red blood cell synthesis.

d. intestinal bacteria.

8. To reduce the likelihood of giving birth to babies with neural tube defects, women of childbearing age should obtain adequate

a. vitamin K.

b. biotin.

c. folic acid.

d. niacin.

9. Major food sources of vitamin B-12 include

a. enriched grain products.

b. meat and dairy products.

c. fruit and vegetables.

d. nuts and seeds.

10. Which of the following statements is true?

a. The stomach can easily absorb vitamin B-12.

b. Vitamin B-12 deficiency is common among older adults.

c. Patients with pernicious anemia are treated with high doses of folic acid.

d. Vitamin B-12 is absorbed in the lower segment of the large intestine.

11. Which of the following foods is a rich source of vitamin C?

a. Whole milk

b. Egg white

c. Guava

d. Egg yolk

12. Which of the following practices may reduce your risk of cancer?

a. Consuming salted fish

b. Eating grilled meats regularly

c. Smoking no more than 10 cigarettes daily

d. Eating fruits and vegetables

© C Squared Studios/Getty Images RF

A Answer This (Module 8.2a)

The young man consumes plenty of vitamin A precursors in plant foods.

References ➡ See Appendix F.

STUDY TIP: Quickly create a customized practice quiz for this chapter by going to your Connect SmartBook "My Reports" section.

Don't have SmartBook and want to learn more? Go to **whysmartbook.com**.

Key Minerals, Water, and the Nonnutrient Alcohol

What's on the Menu?

Module 9.1
Minerals for Life

Module 9.2
Key Minerals and Your Health

Module 9.3
Water: Liquid of Life

Module 9.4
Drink to Your Health?

© Purestock/SuperStock RF

"When I was in middle school, I found out that I developed lactose intolerance. I could drink small amounts of milk and eat a little ice cream, though I'd find myself with stomach problems later if I ate as much as my friends. I tried taking [lactase] tablets when I consumed dairy products, but I got tired of using them. They seemed to become less effective over time as well. For a little while, I tried other kinds of milk, like coconut milk. I couldn't get used to the taste. I also have soy, nut, and fish allergies, so soy and almond milk aren't viable alternatives. Now, I eat cheese and drink Lactaid® milk, so hopefully I get enough calcium in my diet."

Damian Nguyen

Damian Nguyen is a sophomore, majoring in Music Composition and Instrumental Music Education, at the Bob Cole Conservatory of Music, California State University-Long Beach. Should Damian be concerned about his calcium intake? Yes, because men as well as women can develop weak bones as a result of low intakes of the mineral.

Minerals, such as calcium, are elements in Earth's rocks, soils, and natural water sources, especially the ocean. Plants, animals, and other living things cannot make minerals. Plants obtain the minerals they need to grow and survive from soil or fertilizer. You obtain the minerals that you require when you eat plants and animals or substances that contain these elements.

The functions of many minerals in your body involve water. Although alcohol isn't a nutrient, the chemical affects your body's contents of water, minerals, and other nutrients. This unit focuses on some key mineral nutrients, water, and the nonnutrient alcohol.

minerals elements in the Earth's rocks, soils, and natural water sources

Module 9.1

Minerals for Life

9.1- Learning Outcomes

After reading Module 9.1, you should be able to

1. Define all of the key terms in this module.
2. Classify a mineral nutrient as a major or trace mineral.
3. Describe general functions of mineral nutrients.
4. Discuss practical ways of retaining the mineral contents of foods.
5. Discuss factors that influence the body's ability to absorb and use minerals.

Minerals are naturally in your environment.

In their natural state, most foods contain small amounts of minerals. **Figure 9.1** indicates food groups from MyPlate that are generally rich sources of various minerals.

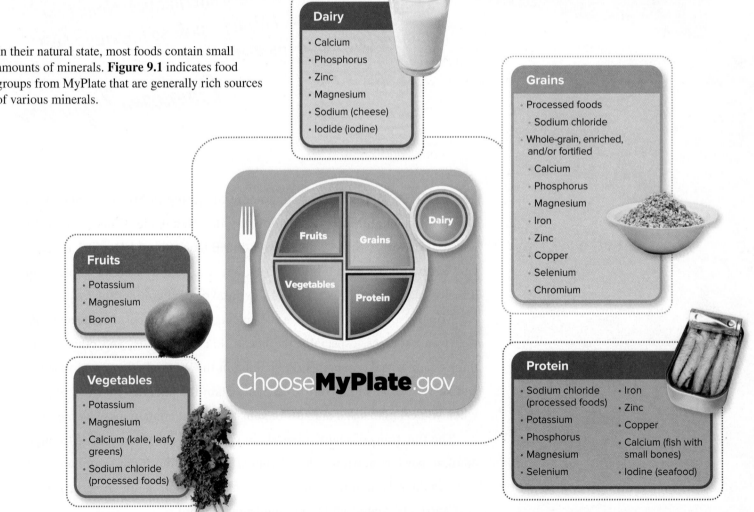

Dairy
- Calcium
- Phosphorus
- Zinc
- Magnesium
- Sodium (cheese)
- Iodide (iodine)

Grains
- Processed foods
  - Sodium chloride
- Whole-grain, enriched, and/or fortified
  - Calcium
  - Phosphorus
  - Magnesium
  - Iron
  - Zinc
  - Copper
  - Selenium
  - Chromium

Fruits
- Potassium
- Magnesium
- Boron

Vegetables
- Potassium
- Magnesium
- Calcium (kale, leafy greens)
- Sodium chloride (processed foods)

Protein
- Sodium chloride (processed foods)
- Potassium
- Phosphorus
- Magnesium
- Selenium
- Iron
- Zinc
- Copper
- Calcium (fish with small bones)
- Iodine (seafood)

ChooseMyPlate.gov

Fruits Grains Vegetables Protein Dairy

Figure 9.1 MyPlate major food sources of mineral nutrients.

9.1a Water as a Source of Minerals

In addition to foods, the tap water in your community may be a source of minerals that can add to your daily intake. "Hard" water naturally contains a variety of minerals, including calcium, magnesium, sulfur, iron, and zinc. Fluoride is often added to public water supplies. Although fluoride isn't an essential nutrient, the mineral strengthens bones and teeth (see Section 9.2a).

9.1b Major Mineral or Trace Mineral?

About 15 mineral elements have known functions in your body and are necessary for health (**Table 9.1**). Your body requires mineral nutrients in milligram or microgram amounts. The essential minerals are classified into two groups: major minerals and trace minerals. If a person requires 100 mg or more of a mineral per day, the mineral is classified as a **major mineral;** otherwise, the micronutrient is a **trace mineral.**

Your body also contains very small amounts of other minerals, such as nickel and arsenic. This particular group of minerals may have roles in the body that have yet to be determined (see Table 9.1). Some minerals, including lead, cadmium, and mercury, may be in the human body, but they're environmental contaminants that have no known functions and are toxic.

As with vitamins, cells don't obtain any calories from minerals. Unlike vitamins, minerals cannot be destroyed. Thus, heating a food or exposing it to most other environmental conditions will not affect the food's mineral content. However, minerals are water soluble, and they can leach out of a food and into cooking water. By using the cooking water to make soups or sauces, you can obtain minerals from the food that would otherwise be discarded.

TASTY **Tidbits**

Water with high mineral content often tastes and smells unpleasant. Water "softening" is a process that removes "hard" minerals from household water supplies. However, many water softening systems replace the minerals with sodium chloride ("salt"). It's unhealthy to consume too much sodium, so avoid drinking water that has been softened with salt.

TABLE 9.1

MINERALS WITH KNOWN OR POSSIBLE ROLES IN THE BODY*

Major Mineral	**Trace Mineral**	**Possible Essential Mineral**
Calcium (Ca)	Chromium (Cr)	Arsenic (As)
Chloride (Cl⁻)	Copper (Cu)	Boron (B)
Magnesium (Mg)	Fluoride (F⁻)	Lithium (Li)
Phosphorus (P)	Iodine (I)	Nickel (Ni)
Potassium (K)	Iron (Fe)	Silicon (Si)
Sodium (Na)	Manganese (Mn)	Vanadium (V)
Sulfur (S)	Molybdenum (Mo)	
	Selenium (Se)	
	Zinc (Zn)	

*Chemical symbol is shown in parentheses next to mineral's name.

Faucet running: © Comstock Images/PictureQuest RF; Cheese: © Wendy Schiff; Placemat: © McGraw-Hill Education. Mark A. Dierker, photographer

major minerals essential mineral elements required in amounts of 100 mg or more per day

trace minerals essential mineral elements required in amounts that are less than 100 mg per day

9.1c Why Are Minerals Necessary?

Each mineral nutrient has more than one function in your body (**Fig. 9.2**). Some minerals form inorganic structural components of tissues, such as calcium and phosphorus in your bones and teeth. Many minerals are components of various substances, including enzymes, hormones, or other organic molecules. For example, cobalt is in vitamin B-12, iron is in red blood cells (RBCs), and sulfur is in the amino acids methionine and cysteine. Although cells cannot metabolize minerals for energy, certain minerals are involved in chemical reactions that release energy from macronutrients.

Many minerals also function as electrolytes (*ions*). **Electrolytes** are minerals that have positive ($^+$) or negative ($^-$) electrical charges when they're dissolved in water. Electrolytes include

- sodium (Na^+),
- calcium (Ca^{2+}),
- potassium (K^+),
- magnesium (Mg^{2+}), and
- chloride (Cl^-).

Electrolytes perform a variety of functions in your body. Calcium ions, for example, are needed for blood clotting and muscle contraction. Sodium, potassium, and chloride ions participate in fluid and acid-base balance. Nerves also use sodium and chloride ions to send messages to other cells. Certain ions, such as magnesium and copper are cofactors. A **cofactor** is an ion or small molecule that helps an enzyme function.

Red blood cells

electrolytes minerals that have electrical charges when dissolved in water; ions

cofactor ion or small molecule that helps an enzyme function

Bone Health
Calcium
Phosphorus
Iron
Zinc
Copper
Manganese
Fluoride
Magnesium

Transmission of Nerve Impulses
Sodium
Potassium
Chloride
Calcium

Red Blood Cell Formation
Iron
Copper

Muscle Contraction and Relaxation
Sodium chloride
Potassium
Calcium
Magnesium

Fluid Balance
Sodium
Potassium
Chloride
Phosphorus
Magnesium

Blood Clotting
Calcium

Cellular Metabolism
Iron
Calcium
Phosphorus
Magnesium
Zinc
Chromium
Iodine
Copper
Manganese

Antioxidant Defense
Selenium
Zinc
Copper
Manganese

Growth and Development
Calcium
Phosphorus
Zinc

Figure 9.2 Major functions of minerals in your body.

9.1d Factors That Affect Mineral Absorption and Use

Your digestive tract doesn't absorb 100% of the minerals in foods or dietary supplements. The tract's ability to absorb and use mineral nutrients (**bioavailability**) depends on many factors.

bioavailability body's ability to absorb and use a nutrient

- *Need for the mineral*: In general, mineral requirements increase during periods of growth, such as during infancy, puberty, and pregnancy, and when producing milk for breastfeeding. Furthermore, you're likely to absorb more of a mineral nutrient if your body lacks it.

- *Sources of minerals*: Compared to plant foods, animal foods tend to be more reliable sources of minerals, such as iron and calcium. Why? Animal products often have higher concentrations of these minerals. Additionally, plant foods can contain substances that reduce the intestinal tract's ability to absorb certain minerals, particularly calcium, zinc, and iron. On the other hand, plant foods supply more magnesium and manganese than do animal foods. By eating a balanced diet that includes a variety of plant and animal foods, you can enhance your body's ability to absorb minerals.

- *Food processing*: In general, the more processing a plant food undergoes, the lower its natural mineral content. Cereal grains, for example, naturally contain selenium, zinc, copper, and some other minerals. When grains are refined, they can lose a lot of their natural mineral contents. Iron is the only mineral added to grains if they undergo enrichment.

© Wendy Schiff

If your digestive tract absorbs more minerals than your body needs, the excess is excreted, primarily in urine or feces. In some instances, however, your body stores the extra minerals in the liver, bones, or other tissues. When the need arises, your body releases minerals from storage so they can be used by all cells. Toxicity signs and symptoms occur when minerals accumulate in the body to such an extent that they interfere with the functioning of cells. The summary table for each mineral that's featured in this unit and Table 9.18 provide signs and symptoms of mineral toxicity disorders.

Should You Take Mineral Supplements?

A daily multiple vitamin and mineral supplement is generally safe for healthy people because a dose of this type of supplement doesn't provide high amounts of minerals. However, you need to be careful when taking dietary supplements that contain individual minerals, such as iron or selenium. Many minerals have a narrow range of safe intake; therefore, it's easy to consume a toxic amount, especially by taking supplements that contain only a particular mineral. Additionally, an excess of one mineral can interfere with your body's ability to absorb and use other minerals. For example, having high amounts of zinc in your intestinal tract decreases copper absorption. Single-mineral supplements are usually unnecessary unless they're prescribed to treat a specific medical condition, such as iron deficiency.

© McGraw-Hill Education. John Flournoy, photographer

Module 9.2

Key Minerals and Your Health

Seafood, including shrimp and octopus, is a rich source of many minerals.

© Ingram Publishing RF

This module focuses primarily on calcium, fluoride, magnesium, sodium, potassium, iron, copper, iodine, selenium, zinc, and chromium. For basic information about some other mineral nutrients, see Table 9.18 at the end of this module.

9.2a Hard Tissue Builders: Calcium and Fluoride

The major mineral calcium (Ca) is the most plentiful mineral element in the human body. Your body needs calcium to build and maintain strong bones and teeth. The mineral is also needed for other important functions, including blood clotting, blood vessel function, and muscle contraction.

Regulating Your Blood's Calcium Level

Your body maintains its level of calcium in blood carefully. A group of hormones that includes vitamin D helps regulate blood calcium levels. Recall from Unit 8 that vitamin D signals the small intestine to absorb calcium. In response to falling blood calcium levels, the parathyroid glands secrete **parathyroid hormone (PTH)**, which signals special bone cells to tear down bone tissue (**Fig. 9.3**). This process releases calcium from bones so the mineral can enter the bloodstream. PTH also works with vitamin D to increase intestinal calcium absorption and reduce calcium elimination in urine.

When the level of calcium in blood is too high, the thyroid gland secretes the hormone **calcitonin** (*cal'-sih-toe'-nin*). The thyroid gland is shown in Figure 9.3. Calcitonin signals another type of bone cell to remove excess calcium from blood and rebuild bone tissue. As a result of these responses, your body can maintain your blood calcium level within the normal range.

Sources of Calcium

On average, Americans who are 2 years of age and over consume about 980 mg of calcium daily.[2] This amount is less than the RDAs for some groups of people (see the DRI tables in Appendix G). According to the Dietary Guidelines for Americans, calcium is a nutrient of public health concern.

Healthy adults absorb about 30% of the calcium in foods, but this percentage varies, depending on the type of food.[3] During early stages of life when the body needs extra calcium—such as infancy and childhood—absorption can be as high as 60%. Older people, especially aging women, don't absorb calcium as well as do younger people. Other factors that reduce calcium absorption include being deficient in vitamin D and taking too many dietary supplements that contain calcium at one time.

TASTY Tidbits

Bone remodeling occurs throughout life, and as a result of this process, most of your skeleton is replaced about every 10 years.[1]

parathyroid hormone (PTH) hormone secreted by parathyroid glands when blood calcium levels are too low

calcitonin hormone secreted by the thyroid gland when blood calcium levels are too high

© Comstock/Alamy RF

234

Figure 9.3 Parathyroid glands and the thyroid gland.

■ *What effect does parathyroid hormone have on bone cells?*

Back of thyroid gland

Parathyroid glands

Esophagus

Trachea "windpipe"

Posterior (back) view

Larynx "voice box"

Thyroid gland

Trachea "windpipe"

Anterior (front) view

Dairy foods are reliable sources of calcium. Each of the foods shown in **Figure 9.4** contains about the same amount of calcium that's in 1 cup of fat-free milk (approximately 300 mg):

- 1¼ cups low-fat (2% milk) cottage cheese
- 1 oz processed cheese (American cheese)
- 2/3 cup plain, fat-free yogurt
- 1.5 oz natural cheese (e.g., Cheddar or Swiss)
- 1 cup calcium-fortified soy milk

TASTY Tidbits

Canned fish with edible soft bones, such as sardines and salmon, are good calcium sources. When making salmon patties using canned fish, mash up the bones along with the salmon. The bones are so soft, you won't notice them in the cooked product.

© Burke/Triolo Productions/Getty Images RF

American processed cheese
1 oz, 100 kcal

Plain, fat-free yogurt
2/3 cup, 84 kcal

Low-fat cottage cheese (2% milk)
1.25 cups, 230 kcal

Natural cheese
1.5 oz, 170 kcal

Soy milk, calcium fortified
1 cup, 100 kcal

Figure 9.4 Calcium-rich food equivalents from dairy foods group.
© Wendy Schiff

What *IS* That? - - - - - - - - - - - - →

Bok choy is a vegetable that's related to cabbage and broccoli. The leaves and stalks are steamed or sautéed with other vegetables. The vegetable can also be shredded and added to salads. Bok choy is a good source of minerals, especially iron, calcium, and potassium; the vegetable also contains high amounts of vitamin C and beneficial phytochemicals.

Not all products made from milk are rich sources of calcium. Cottage cheese, for example, doesn't supply as much calcium as the milk from which it's made. Why? Milk loses more than half of its calcium content when it's processed to make cottage cheese. **Table 9.2** includes some foods that are among the richest sources of calcium.

Chinese cabbage (bok choy), kale, and broccoli are good plant sources of calcium. However, the calcium in other plant foods is generally not as bioavailable as the calcium in dairy foods. Why? Plant foods such as spinach, collard greens, and sweet potatoes contain calcium, but the foods also contain oxalic (*awk-sal'-ik*) acid. Oxalic acid binds to calcium, interfering with its absorption as a result. If you eat foods that contain oxalic acid as part of a varied diet and meet the RDA for calcium, you're unlikely to become deficient in the mineral.[3]

Calcium is added to a variety of foods, including ready-to-eat breakfast cereals, fortified orange juice, margarine, soy milk, and breakfast bars. Another source of calcium is soybean curd (tofu) that's made with calcium sulfate. **Figure 9.5** indicates food groups from MyPlate that are good sources of calcium.

TASTY **Tidbits**

Rhubarb leaves are toxic because they contain high amounts of oxalic acid. Although rhubarb stalks contain less oxalic acid than the leaves of the plant, the amounts aren't toxic. One-half cup of cooked, sugar-sweetened rhubarb supplies about 140 kcal, 2.4 g fiber, 175 mg calcium, and 4 mg vitamin C.

The following tips can help add more calcium to your diet.

- Sprinkle grated low-fat cheeses on top of salads, bean or pasta dishes, and cooked vegetables.

- Add shredded bok choy to salads or soups.

- If you don't like the taste of plain fat-free milk or plain yogurt, try blending it with one half of a banana or some strawberries. Consider drinking soy milk as a substitute for cows' milk.

- For a snack, melt a slice of low-fat cheese on half a whole-wheat bagel, whole-wheat crackers, or a slice of rye bread.

- If a recipe calls for water, substitute fat-free milk for water if it's appropriate. For example, use fat-free milk or plain soy milk when making cooked oatmeal or pancake batter.

- Add ¼ cup nonfat milk powder to 1 pound of raw ground meat when preparing hamburgers, meatballs, or meatloaf.

- Make homemade smoothies by blending plain low-fat yogurt with fresh or frozen fruit and fat-reduced ice cream or sherbet.

TABLE 9.2

CALCIUM CONTENT OF SELECTED FOODS

Food	Calcium (mg)
Whole-grain Total cereal, ¾ cup	1000
Yogurt, plain, low-fat, 1 cup	448
Sardines, canned, with bones, 3 oz	325
Yogurt, soy, plain, 1 cup	300
Milk, fat-free, fluid, 1 cup	299
American cheese, pasteurized process, 1 oz	296
Swiss cheese, 1 oz	224
Cottage cheese, 2% fat, 1 cup	206
Kale, frozen, boiled, drained, chopped, 1 cup	179
Tofu, firm, made with calcium sulfate, 3 oz	100
Ice cream, vanilla, light, ½ cup	122
Baked beans, canned, plain, 1 cup	86
Bok choy, raw, shredded, 1 cup	74

RDA for adults = 1000–1200 mg/day
Source: Data from *USDA National nutrient database for standard reference, release 25.*

Figure 9.5 MyPlate: Good food sources of calcium.

Should You Take a Calcium Supplement?

Dietary supplements that contain calcium generally provide calcium carbonate or calcium citrate.[3] Calcium carbonate is 40% elemental calcium by weight, whereas calcium citrate is 21% elemental calcium by weight. (Check the Supplement Facts panel on the product's label for information about the milligrams of elemental calcium in each pill.) The calcium in calcium carbonate is absorbed most efficiently when taken with food, because this form of the mineral relies on stomach acid for absorption. Calcium citrate can be taken with or without food.

Your intestinal tract absorbs a higher percentage of calcium from a dietary supplement when your dose is less than 500 mg. If, for example, you want to maximize the amount of calcium obtained from a calcium supplement pill that contains 1000 mg/day of calcium, consider splitting the pill in half to take a 500 mg dose twice a day.

Taking calcium supplements that contain calcium and vitamin D is a common practice, especially among older adults. This practice may increase the risk of heart attack.[3] More research, however, is needed to clarify whether taking calcium-containing dietary supplements can have negative effects on heart health.[3] Therefore, consider improving your intake of foods that are naturally rich sources of calcium before using a dietary supplement to boost your intake of the mineral.

What's Osteoporosis?

Osteoporosis is a chronic disease characterized by a loss of normal bone mass (**Fig. 9.6**). People with osteoporosis have weak bones that fracture easily. More than 40 million Americans either have osteoporosis or a high risk of the disease because they have reduced bone mass.[3] About half of all women and up to one in four men older than 50 years of age will break a bone because of osteoporosis.[4] Fractures of the hip, wrist, or vertebra (bone of the spine) are common among people in this age group. At least 20% of older adults who break a hip die within one year because they developed serious health problems associated with the fracture or its surgical repair.[5] Of those who recover, many are unable to live independently and require costly long-term health care.

osteoporosis chronic disease characterized by bones with low mass and reduced structure

Figure 9.6 **Bone tissue.** Compare the appearance of healthy bone tissue (left photo) with that of bone tissue taken from a person with osteoporosis (right photo).

■ *What is osteoporosis?*

Damian, the young man featured in the unit opener, has Asian ancestry, which places him at risk for osteoporosis later in life. He now drinks lactase-treated milk, a rich source of calcium and vitamin D, micronutrients that can help keep his bones healthy. While he's young, he should consider adding foods to his diet that have been fortified with the mineral, such as certain brands of orange juice and ready-to-eat cereals.

Many people don't realize their bones are becoming weaker and they have osteoporosis until they experience a fracture. Osteoporosis-related fractures often involve the upper spine. In severe cases, bones in the upper spine fracture and then heal in an abnormally curved position, giving the obvious "widow's ("dowager's") hump" appearance associated with osteoporosis (**Fig. 9.7**). Osteoporosis is a major cause of pain and disability among older adults.

What Causes Osteoporosis?

You're more likely to develop osteoporosis if you didn't reach optimal peak bone mass by the end of your bone-building years. During your childhood and teenage years, your body added new bone tissue faster than it removed old bone tissue. As a result, your bones became larger and denser. Girls achieve as much as 90% of their total bone mass by the time they're 18 years of age; boys reach up to 90% of their "peak" bone mass when they're 20 years of age.[6] By around 30 years of age, a person has maximized his or her bone mass. Bone loss is slow and steady beginning around age 30. In women, however, the rate of bone loss increases significantly after *menopause*—that is, after menstrual cycles have ceased. At this time of life, women have the highest risk of osteoporosis. Why? The hormone estrogen is needed for normal bone development and maintenance. After menopause, a woman's ovaries produce considerably less estrogen than when she

Figure 9.7 Older adult woman with osteoporosis.

■ *What are some major risk factors for osteoporosis?*

© Yoav Levy/Phototake.com

was in her childbearing years. Eventually, her ovaries stop making the hormone. As a result, her rate of bone loss exceeds the rate of bone replacement during this stage of life.

Several factors contribute to bone loss and osteoporosis. Major risk factors are

- growing older and being a *postmenopausal* woman,
- having white or Asian ancestry,
- having a family history of osteoporosis,
- having a small body frame,
- having low estrogen levels in women and low testosterone levels in men,
- following diets that contain inadequate amounts of calcium and vitamin D,
- being physically inactive,
- smoking cigarettes,
- consuming excessive alcohol, and
- having anorexia nervosa (an eating disorder).[7]

Efforts to reduce the risk of osteoporosis should begin early in life. Proper diet and regular exercise are especially important from early childhood through late adolescence because the body actively builds bone during these life stages. By following the recommendations of MyPlate, you can obtain adequate amounts of calcium from foods. Exposing skin to sunlight can stimulate your body's ability to form vitamin D, but you may need to take vitamin D supplements.

Exercise, especially weight-bearing activities, increases bone mass because contracting muscles keep tension on bones.[7] Such tension stimulates bones to become stronger. Weight-bearing activities include

- dancing;
- playing basketball;
- walking, jogging, and hiking;
- jumping rope;
- stair climbing; and
- strength training with weights.

Table 9.3 summarizes basic information about calcium. RDA values are for adults, excluding pregnant or breastfeeding women.

TASTY Tidbits

Certain brands of antacids contain calcium carbonate and magnesium. An antacid pill that contains 750 mg of calcium carbonate provides 300 mg of elemental calcium. However, using antacids that contain calcium carbonate and magnesium to boost your calcium intake can increase the likelihood of toxicity.[8] Bone pain is a symptom of long-term calcium carbonate and magnesium toxicity. Such toxicity is likely to occur if you take more of the antacids than the recommended amount. Kidney stones can also result from obtaining excess calcium from nonfood sources, such as dietary supplements.[3] Therefore, you should avoid taking too many antacids as well as too many dietary supplements that contain calcium.

© Wendy Schiff

2b The Fluid Balancers: Potassium and Sodium

Major minerals potassium and sodium play a vital role in maintaining normal body fluid balance. The typical American diet supplies far more sodium than potassium. This mineral imbalance may lead to high blood pressure, a serious long-term health problem. However, you can help reduce the risk that excess sodium poses to your health, by consuming more foods that supply potassium.[10]

Potassium

Potassium (K) is the major positively charged ion in the fluid that's inside cells. Fresh fruits, fruit juice, and vegetables are good dietary sources of potassium. Milk, whole grains, dried beans, and meats are also major contributors of potassium to American diets.

On average, Americans who were 2 years of age or older consumed only about 2540 mg of potassium per day in 2013–2014.[2] This amount is much lower than the Adequate Intake amount (4700 mg). According to the *Dietary Guidelines for Americans,* potassium is a nutrient of public health concern. You can raise your potassium intake by eating more fruits, vegetables, whole-grain breads and cereals, and low-fat and fat-free dairy foods. **Table 9.4** provides information about the potassium content of a few selected foods. **Figure 9.9** indicates food groups that are naturally good sources of potassium.

People who experience excessive body fluid losses through sweating, vomiting, or diarrhea are at risk for electrolyte depletion. Symptoms of low blood potassium levels generally include muscle cramps, confusion, and constipation. In severe cases, the lack of potassium causes muscular weakness and abnormal heartbeat. Therefore, it's important to seek medical treatment when potassium depletion is suspected.

TABLE 9.4

POTASSIUM CONTENT OF SELECTED FOODS

Food	Potassium (mg)
Beet greens, boiled, drained, 1 cup	1309
Baked potato, including skin, 6 oz	963
Spinach, cooked, drained, 1 cup	839
Coconut water, 1 cup	600
Kiwi, sliced, 1 cup	562
Banana, sliced, 1 cup	537
Sweet potato, canned, mashed, 1 cup	536
Orange juice, frozen, reconstituted, 1 cup	473
Cantaloupe, cubes, 1 cup	427
Papaya, raw, mashed, 1 cup	419
Milk, fluid, 1% fat, 1 cup	366
Salmon, sockeye, cooked, 3 oz	347
Peaches, raw, sliced, 1 cup	293
Grapes, raw, red, 1 cup	288
Yogurt, low-fat, plain, 8 oz	264
Corn, canned yellow, 1 cup	226
Tuna, canned in water, drained, 3 oz	202

AI for adults = 4700 mg/day

Source: USDA National nutrient database for standard reference, release 25.

Figure 9.9 MyPlate: Good food sources of potassium.

Fruits
- Pears
- Prunes
- Peaches
- Avocados
- Cantaloupes
- Bananas

Dairy
- Milk
- Yogurt
- Cottage cheese
- Ricotta cheese

Grains
- Whole-wheat bread
- Whole-grain products

Vegetables
- Spinach
- Squash
- Potatoes
- Tomatoes
- Lettuce
- Lima beans

Protein
- Meat
- Chicken
- Fish
- Shrimp
- Beans

ChooseMyPlate.gov

Key Minerals a...

240

9

To ...
of flu...
childre...
a "pea-s...
of toothp...

Fluoride and Health

Although fluoride (F⁻) isn't an essential nutrient, the mineral strengthens bones and teeth when ingested in small amounts. In some parts of the United States, well water contains high amounts of the trace mineral. To ensure that people living in other sections of the country obtain healthful amounts of fluoride, the mineral is often added to public water supplies (fluoridation), toothpastes, and dental rinses. Tea naturally contains fluoride.

Long-term consumption of too much fluoride can cause *fluorosis*. In cases of skeletal fluorosis, excess fluoride builds up in bones, causing joint stiffness and bone pain. Skeletal fluorosis rarely occurs in the United States. Dental fluorosis often affects young children who drink well water that contains high amounts of fluoride, but it also can occur in children who routinely swallow toothpaste and dental rinses. Children with severe fluorosis develop permanently stained teeth that don't resist decay as do healthy teeth (**Figure 9.8**). Parents should teach their children to place a "pea-sized" amount of toothpaste on their brush, rinse with water, and spit out the excess fluid. Table 9.3 summarizes information about fluoride.

Figure 9.8 Stained teeth due to dental fluorosis.

TASTY Tidbits

In 2014, almost 75% of the U.S. population served by community water systems had access to drinking water that contained optimal fluoride levels.[9] Some Americans oppose fluoridation for a variety of reasons, including the belief that the practice is a form of involuntary medication. Other people oppose fluoridation because they're concerned about long-term risks of drinking the treated water. For more information about fluoridation, visit www.cdc.gov/Fluoridation/.

TABLE 9.3 CALCIUM AND FLUORIDE: SUMMARY OF BASIC NUTRITION INFORMATION

Mineral	Major Functions in the Body	Adult RDA/AI	Major Dietary Sources	Major Deficiency Signs and Symptoms	Major Toxicity Signs and Symptoms
Calcium (Ca)	Structural component of bones and teeth Blood clotting Transmission of nerve impulses Muscle contraction Regulation of metabolism	1000–1200 mg	Dairy foods, canned fish, tofu made with calcium sulfate, leafy vegetables, calcium-fortified foods such as orange juice	Increased risk of osteoporosis May increase risk of hypertension	UL = 2.0 to 2.5 g/day Intakes > 2.5 g/day: Bone pain, headaches, constipation, abdominal discomfort; kidney stones (excess dietary supplements)
Fluoride (F⁻)	Increases resistance of tooth enamel to cavity formation Stimulates bone formation	Men: 4 mg Women: 3 mg	Fluoridated water, tea, seaweed	No true deficiency but increased risk of tooth decay	UL = 10 mg/day Stomach upset, fluorosis, bone deterioration

Sodium

Sodium (Na) is the major positively charged ion in the fluid that surrounds cells. Most uncooked vegetables, raw meats, and grain products are naturally low in sodium. Table salt is sodium chloride, a compound comprised of two minerals, sodium and chloride.

Manufacturers often add salt to food during processing, and you may add more salt when you prepare or eat the food. Processed foods, however, are the primary sources of sodium in American diets. Salted snack foods, French fries, canned and dried soups, sauces and gravies, hot dogs and "deli" meats, cheeses, and pickled foods are high in sodium. **Table 9.5** lists some selected foods and their sodium contents.

TASTY Tidbits

Salt substitutes often contain a type of salt called potassium chloride. People who have kidney disease may accumulate toxic levels of potassium in their blood. Therefore, kidney disease patients should consult their physicians before using salt substitutes made with potassium chloride.[11] To increase your potassium intake safely, consider adding more fruits, vegetables, whole grains, and low-fat dairy foods to your diet.

TABLE 9.5

SODIUM CONTENT OF SELECTED FOODS/FOOD ADDITIVES

Food	Sodium (mg)
Fast food: biscuit with egg, cheese, and sausage	1440
Tomato sauce, canned, 1 cup	1284
Sauerkraut, canned, solids and liquid, 1 cup	939
Chicken noodle soup, canned, prepared, 1 cup	866
Luncheon meat, oven-roasted turkey breast, 3 oz	811
Ham, cured, cooked, 3 oz	810
Cottage cheese, 2% milk, 1 cup	746
Miso (soybean paste), 1 Tbsp	634
Baking soda, ½ tsp	629
Hot dog, 1.5 oz	504
Soy sauce, 1 tsp	341
Dill pickle, 1 spear, approx. 1 oz	306
Tortilla chips, nacho-flavored, 1 oz	284
Cheddar cheese, 1 oz	174
Catsup, 1 Tbsp	167

AI for young adults = 1500 mg/day
Source: USDA National nutrient database for standard reference, release 25.

What's Hypertension?

Hypertension is a condition characterized by chronic high blood pressure. Compared to people with normal blood pressure, hypertensive individuals have greater risk of cardiovascular disease (CVD), especially heart disease and stroke, as well as kidney failure and damage to other organs. In the United States, hypertension is a widespread disease. Approximately 33% of adult Americans have hypertension.[12]

Hypertension is often called the "silent killer" because high blood pressure generally doesn't cause symptoms until the affected person's organs and blood vessels have been damaged. The best way to detect hypertension is to have regular blood pressure screenings. When you have your blood pressure determined, two measurements are actually taken. The first measurement is the **systolic pressure,** which is the maximum blood pressure

within an artery. This value occurs when the heart's pumping chambers contract. The second measurement is the **diastolic pressure,** which measures the pressure in an artery when the heart relaxes between contractions. The systolic value is always higher than the diastolic value.

Table 9.6 presents the three categories for blood pressure levels in adults. For adults, healthy blood pressure readings are less than 120/80 millimeters of mercury (mm Hg). People with **prehypertension** are more likely to develop hypertension than are people with normal blood pressure.

Even if your blood pressure is normal now, it's important to have regular blood pressure checks as you grow older because the risk of hypertension increases with age. In the United States, approximately 70% of women who are 65 to 74 years of age and 64% of men in this age group have hypertension.[12] When was the last time you had your blood pressure measured? What were the systolic and diastolic values? Every time you have your blood pressure measured, ask the clinician for your systolic and diastolic readings and keep a record of the values.

hypertension condition characterized by persistently elevated blood pressure

systolic pressure maximum blood pressure within an artery that occurs when the heart contracts

diastolic pressure pressure in an artery that occurs when the heart relaxes between contractions

prehypertension persistent systolic blood pressure readings of 120 mm Hg to 139 mm Hg and diastolic readings of 80 mm Hg to 89 mm Hg

What Causes Hypertension?

Most cases of hypertension don't have simple causes, but major risk factors for the condition are

- family history,
- advanced age,
- African-American ancestry,
- obesity and physical inactivity,
- consuming excess sodium,
- smoking and drinking excess alcohol, and
- type 2 diabetes.[13]

TABLE 9.6

BLOOD PRESSURE LEVELS (ADULTS)

	Systolic mm Hg	Diastolic mm Hg
Normal	< 120	< 80
Prehypertension	120 to 139	80 to 89
Hypertension	≥ 140	≥ 90

Key: < is "less than," ≥ is "more than or equal to."
Source: Centers for Disease Control and Prevention: *Measuring blood pressure.* Last updated November 2014. http://www.cdc.gov/bloodpressure/measure.htm Accessed: May 22, 2016.

Sodium Intake and Hypertension Risk

High sodium intakes are strongly associated with the development of hypertension.[14] Thus, health experts generally recommend that you limit your sodium consumption. Take the **"Sodium Intake Assessment"** in this module to evaluate your sodium intake habits.

On average, Americans who were 2 years of age or older consumed more than 3400 mg of sodium per day in 2013–2014.[2] According to the *Dietary Guidelines for Americans,* healthy people should consume less than 2300 mg of sodium daily.[15] That's the amount of sodium in about 1 teaspoon of table salt. According to the American Heart Association, Americans should limit their intake of sodium to 1500 mg per day.[14]

Treating the "Silent Killer"

Treatment for hypertension usually includes taking certain medications, following dietary modifications, and making some other lifestyle changes. You can counteract high sodium intakes by consuming foods naturally rich in potassium and low in sodium, such as fruits and vegetables (without added salt). Research indicates that you may be able to lower your blood pressure and risk of CVD by losing excess body fat, increasing physical activity, and following a diet that is low in sodium and high in fruits, vegetables, and low-fat dairy foods. The DASH diet is a healthy eating plan that includes more fruits and vegetables than the typical American diet. For more information about the DASH diet, visit http://www.nhlbi.nih.gov/ and search for "DASH eating plan."

To reduce your sodium intake, consider taking these actions:

- Limit your intake of processed foods that contain salt.
- Don't add salt while preparing foods, even though instructions tell you to "add salt."
- Taste your food before salting it and don't keep a salt shaker on your table.
- When ordering items in restaurants, request that no salt be added to your food while it's being prepared.

Nutrition Facts

28 servings per container

Serving size   **3 flatbreads (28g)**

Amount Per Serving

Calories   110

	% Daily Values*
Total Fat 3g	5%
Saturated Fat 1g	5%
Trans Fat 0g	
Cholesterol 0mg	0%
Sodium 170mg	7%
Total Carbohydrate 19g	6%
Dietary Fiber 1g	4%
Total Sugars 1g	
Includes 0g Added Sugars	0%
Protein 3g	6%
Vitamin D 0IU	0%
Calcium 0mg	0%
Iron 1.44mg	8%
Potassium 0mg	0%

* The % Daily Value (DV) tells you how much a nutrient in a serving of food contributes to a daily diet. 2,000 calories a day is used for general nutrition advice.

INGREDIENTS:
SPROUTED WHEAT FLOUR, VEGETABLE OIL

To learn about a serving of food's sodium content, read the Nutrition Facts panel.

TASTY **Tidbits**

Try using garlic, citrus juice, and herbs and spices instead of salt to enhance the taste of foods. Furthermore, consider avoiding seasonings with added salt, such as "garlic salt" or "onion salt." Check the ingredients list to purchase seasonings without added salt (garlic powder or onion powder) instead.

Tarragon

Nutrition Facts panel: © Wendy Schiff; Blood pressure monitor: © Ilene McDonald/Alamy RF; Tarragon: © FoodCollection/StockFood RF

SODIUM INTAKE ASSESSMENT

For each question, place a check in the column that best describes your sodium intake habits.

How Often Do You...	Rarely	Often	Daily
1. Eat cured or processed meats ("deli" meats), such as bacon, sausage, hot dogs, ham, and other luncheon meats?			
2. Eat canned vegetables?			
3. Eat commercially prepared meals or soups?			
4. Eat processed cheeses, such as cheese spreads?			
5. Eat salted nuts, popcorn, pretzels, corn chips, or potato chips?			
6. Add salt to cooking water for vegetables, rice, or pasta?			
7. Add salt, seasoning mixes, or condiments—such as soy sauce, steak sauce, pickles, and catsup—to foods during preparation?			
8. Salt your food before tasting it?			
9. Ignore the Nutrition Facts panel for sodium content when buying foods?			
10. Choose salty menu items when dining out?			

Scoring: The more checks you put in the "often" or "daily" columns, the higher your sodium intake is.

Adapted from: USDA: *Home and Garden Bulletin*, No. 232–6, April 1986.

Table 9.7 summarizes basic information about potassium and sodium, including major food sources of the minerals.

© Brand X Pictures/Getty Images RF

TABLE 9.7

POTASSIUM AND SODIUM: SUMMARY OF BASIC NUTRITION INFORMATION

Mineral	Major Functions in the Body	Adult AI	Major Dietary Sources	Major Deficiency Signs and Symptoms	Major Toxicity Signs and Symptoms
Potassium (K)	Maintenance of proper fluid balance Transmission of nerve impulses Maintenance of acid-base balance	4700 mg	Fruits, vegetables, milk, meat, legumes, whole grains	Irregular heartbeat Muscle cramps Muscle weakness	No UL has been determined. Slowing of heart rate that can result in death
Sodium (Na)	Maintenance of proper fluid balance Transmission of nerve impulses Muscle contraction Transport of certain substances into cells	1500 mg (19–50 years of age)	Processed foods, luncheon meats; pretzels, chips, and other snack foods; condiments; sauces	Muscle cramps	UL = 2300 mg/day Contributes to hypertension in susceptible individuals Increases urinary calcium losses

© Siede Preis/Getty Images RF

Nutrition Fact or Fiction?

Children should eat spinach because it's a rich source of iron.

The cartoon character Popeye may have inspired some children to eat spinach, especially those hoping to become instantly strong. However, naturally occurring substances in spinach bind to iron, reducing the intestinal tract's ability to absorb the mineral. Although spinach isn't a good source of iron, the leafy green vegetable is a rich source of folate, beta-carotene, magnesium, potassium, and dietary fiber.[16]

9.2c Iron and Magnesium: Power Minerals

Although minerals don't provide any calories (energy), magnesium and iron are involved in chemical reactions that release energy from macronutrients. The major mineral magnesium is a cofactor that helps regulate energy metabolism. The trace mineral iron helps release energy from macronutrients and transport oxygen in red blood cells (RBCs). Oxygen is critical for energy metabolism. Without a source of oxygen, cells can't obtain much energy and die.

Iron

Iron (Fe) is a component of hemoglobin and myoglobin (*my'-o-glow-bin*). **Hemoglobin** is the iron-containing protein in RBCs that transports oxygen to tissues. **Myoglobin** is the iron-containing protein in muscle cells that controls their removal of oxygen from RBCs. Cells also have a group of iron-containing proteins that are necessary for the release of energy from macronutrients. If the body doesn't have enough iron to make hemoglobin, myoglobin, and the energy-releasing proteins, muscle and other cells cannot obtain the energy they need to perform work. Thus, feeling tired is a major symptom of iron deficiency. Iron also plays roles in immune system function and brain development.

Dietary Sources

On average, American males who are 2 years of age and older obtained adequate amounts of iron in 2013–2014.[2] However, the typical diet of American females, especially those who were of childbearing age, provided less than recommended amounts of the mineral. Meat is the major source of iron in the typical American diet. Other important sources of iron are fortified cereals and products made from enriched flour, such as breads and rolls. Dairy foods are poor sources of iron.

The two major forms of iron in food are heme and nonheme iron. Your body absorbs more **heme iron** than **nonheme iron.** Beef, fish, and poultry ("meat") contain heme and nonheme iron. However, plant foods and eggs contain only nonheme iron.

Some plant foods, such as spinach, are good sources of nonheme iron, but other substances that are naturally in spinach bind to the mineral, reducing its absorption. Phytic acid in whole grains and tannins in tea are other naturally occurring compounds that reduce nonheme iron absorption.

Consuming foods that contain vitamin C (ascorbic acid) can boost your body's absorption of nonheme iron.[17] For example, adding orange slices or lemon juice to a spinach salad can enhance the absorption of the iron in the leafy vegetable. You can also drink orange juice with an iron-fortified breakfast cereal to improve the absorption of iron in the cereal. Another way to increase your body's ability to absorb the nonheme iron in foods is by including some sources of heme iron to menu items. For example, add cooked chicken cubes to a salad that contains spinach and raisins or eat a hamburger with baked beans or peas to increase your body's absorption of the nonheme iron in the plant foods.

Table 9.8 lists some foods that are sources of iron. **Figure 9.10** indicates MyPlate food groups that are good sources of iron.

hemoglobin iron-containing protein in red blood cells that transports oxygen to tissues

myoglobin iron-containing protein in muscle cells that controls oxygen uptake from red blood cells

heme iron form of iron that's well absorbed

nonheme iron form of iron in vegetables, grains, meats, and supplements

TASTY Tidbits

Accidental ingestion of iron supplements is a leading cause of poisoning among preschool children.[17] Children's vitamin and/or mineral supplements often look and taste like candy, which makes them very appealing to preschoolers. Parents and guardians should keep iron-containing and other dietary supplements out of young children's reach.

Can of spinach, Iron supplement warning label: © Wendy Schiff; Woman on treadmill: © Stockbyte/PunchStock RF

TABLE 9.8

IRON CONTENT OF SELECTED FOODS

Food	Iron (mg)
Whole-grain Total, ready-to-eat cereal, ¾ cup	18.00
Product 19, ready-to-eat cereal, ¾ cup	13.57
Oysters, breaded, fried, 3 oz	5.91
Beef liver, cooked, 3 oz	5.89
Beef round, cooked, 3 oz	2.30
Pumpkin seeds, roasted, 1 oz	2.29
Clams, canned, drained, 3 oz	2.28
Kidney beans, canned, drained, ½ cup	2.00
Turkey, roasted, 3 oz	1.60
Peas, edible pods, frozen, boiled, drained, ½ cup	1.58
Baked beans, canned, plain, ½ cup	1.51
White enriched rice, cooked, ½ cup	0.95
Raisins, seedless, ¼ cup	0.78
Mushrooms, canned, drained, ½ cup	0.62

RDA for women 19–50 years of age = 18 mg/day; >50 years of age = 8 mg/day
RDA for adult men = 8 mg/day
Source: Data from *USDA National nutrient database for standard reference, release 25.*

Fruits
- Peaches
- Prune juice
- Dried apricots

Grains
- Whole grains
- Enriched grains
- Wheat germ
- Oatmeal

Vegetables
- Spinach
- Peas
- Potatoes
- Green beans
- Broccoli

Protein
- Beef
- Tofu
- Beans
- Seafood
- Organ meats

ChooseMyPlate.gov

Figure 9.10 MyPlate: Good food sources of iron.

Figure 9.11 Red blood cells. (a) Normal red blood cells; (b) red blood cells of a person with iron deficiency anemia.

■ *What is the connection between iron and red blood cells?*

Iron Deficiency–Related Disorders

In cases of iron deficiency, the body's iron stores are low but not low enough to cause severe health problems. Nevertheless, iron deficiency can cause fatigue (tiredness) and interfere with the ability to perform physical and mental tasks. Iron deficiency can lead to iron deficiency anemia. Recall that anemias are conditions characterized by unhealthy RBCs or RBCs with low hemoglobin levels.

In cases of **iron deficiency anemia,** RBCs don't contain enough hemoglobin (**Fig. 9.11**). As a result of the anemia, oxygen transport in blood is impaired. When cells lack oxygen, they can't release much energy from macronutrients. Iron deficiency is the leading cause of anemia.[18]

Common signs and symptoms of iron deficiency anemia are

- pale skin,
- fatigue,
- irritability,
- sore tongue,

- brittle, spoon-shaped nails,[17]
- inability to concentrate on tasks, and
- headache.[19]

> **iron deficiency anemia** condition characterized by red blood cells that don't contain enough hemoglobin

Women with heavy menstrual blood losses are especially prone to iron deficiency anemia. Although pregnant women don't experience menstrual blood losses, they still should be concerned about their iron intake. A woman's RDA for iron increases dramatically during pregnancy. She requires the extra iron to meet her body's needs as well as those of her developing fetus. Iron deficiency during pregnancy can result in giving birth to a low-birth-weight baby or a baby that's born too early (premature birth). According to the Dietary Guidelines for Americans, iron is a nutrient of public health concern for pregnant women.

Children with anemia often experience poor physical growth and abnormal mental functioning. Treatment for iron deficiency anemia generally includes iron supplements and the addition of iron-rich foods to the diet.

TASTY Tidbits

Iron cookware may be a source of dietary iron. When you cook acidic foods, such as tomato sauce, in a cast-iron skillet, some iron leaves the cookware and enters the food. This unusual dietary source of iron can add to your overall iron intake. Replacing the iron cookware with lighter stainless steel and aluminum pots and pans can reduce the amount of iron in your diet.

Increasing Your Iron Intake

To add more iron to your diet or increase your body's ability to absorb iron, consider

- eating lean meat, poultry, or fish with plant sources of iron;
- combining soybeans with tomatoes or tomato sauce;
- adding orange segments or chopped tomatoes to spinach salads or cooked spinach;
- adding chopped onions and green peppers to peas or beans;
- serving sweet potatoes with fresh orange segments or dried apricots;
- adding raspberries, strawberries, raisins, or dried apricots to cereal;
- drinking orange juice when eating peanut butter or soy nut butter sandwiches; and
- eating watermelon, dried plums, dried apricots, or raisins for snacks.

Table 9.10 summarizes basic information about iron. RDA values are for adults, excluding pregnant or breastfeeding women.

TASTY Tidbits

Donating 1 pint of blood represents a loss of 200 to 250 mg of iron. Your body generally needs several weeks to replace the iron that was in the donated blood. According to the American Red Cross, healthy people can give whole blood every 56 days.[20] Young women, however, may need to donate blood less often, especially if they have heavy menstrual losses of blood.

Magnesium

Your body needs magnesium (Mg) for energy metabolism, enzyme activity, and bone health. Magnesium also helps maintain normal blood sugar and blood pressure levels. More research is needed, but dietary supplements that contain the mineral may be useful in preventing or controlling hypertension and cardiovascular disease.[21]

Magnesium is in chlorophyll, the green pigment in plants. Therefore, plant foods, such as spinach, green leafy vegetables, whole grains, beans, nuts, seeds, and chocolate, are among the richest sources of magnesium. Animal products, such as milk and meats, also supply some magnesium. Refined grains are generally low in magnesium because the magnesium-rich bran and germ are removed during processing. **Table 9.9** lists some commonly eaten foods that supply magnesium. **Figure 9.12** indicates MyPlate food groups that are naturally good sources of magnesium.

In 2013–2014, most Americans didn't consume recommended amounts of magnesium.[2] Magnesium intake is generally low among older adults in every racial and ethnic group. However, cases of magnesium deficiency rarely occur among healthy members of the population.[21] Alcoholics, people with poorly controlled diabetes, or persons who use certain medications that increase urinary losses of the mineral have high risk of magnesium deficiency. Older adults are also at risk of magnesium deficiency because their bodies absorb less of the mineral and urinary losses increase with advancing age. Magnesium toxicity rarely occurs in healthy people who don't use dietary supplements or medications that contain a lot of magnesium, such as milk of magnesia. **Table 9.10** summarizes basic information about magnesium, including signs and symptoms of magnesium deficiency and toxicity.

TABLE 9.9

MAGNESIUM CONTENT OF SELECTED FOODS

Food	Magnesium (mg)
All-Bran, ready-to-eat cereal, ½ cup	112
Almonds, 1 oz	76
Pumpkin seeds, roasted, 1 oz	74
Black beans, cooked, ½ cup	60
Chocolate chips, semisweet, ¼ cup	52
Cheerios, ready-to-eat cereal, 1 cup	40
Kidney beans, canned, drained, ½ cup	40
Baked beans, canned, plain, 1 cup	34
Sweet potato, canned, mashed, ½ cup	31
Baked potato, flesh and skin, approx. 3 oz	27
Fish, halibut, cooked, 3 oz	24
Spinach, raw, 1 cup	24
Brown rice, long grain, cooked, ½ cup	24
Peas, edible pods, frozen, cooked, 1 cup	22

RDA for women, 19–30 years of age = 310 mg/day; >30 years of age = 320 mg/day
RDA for men, 19–30 years of age = 400 mg/day; >30 years of age = 420 mg/day
Source: Data from *USDA National nutrient database for standard reference, release 25.*

Figure 9.12 MyPlate: Good food sources of magnesium.

TABLE 9.10

IRON AND MAGNESIUM: SUMMARY OF BASIC NUTRITION INFORMATION

Mineral	Major Functions in the Body	Adult RDA	Major Dietary Sources	Major Deficiency Signs and Symptoms	Major Toxicity Signs and Symptoms
Iron (Fe)	Component of hemoglobin and myoglobin that carries oxygen Energy generation Immune system function	Women (of childbearing age): 18 mg Men: 8 mg	Meat and other animal foods, except milk; whole-grain and enriched breads and cereals; fortified cereals	Fatigue upon exertion Small, pale red blood cells Low hemoglobin levels Poor immune system function Growth and developmental retardation in infants	UL = 45 mg/day Intestinal upset Organ damage Death
Magnesium (Mg)	Strengthens bone Cofactor for certain enzymes Heart and nerve functioning	Men: 400–420 mg Women: 310–320 mg	Wheat bran, green vegetables, nuts, chocolate, legumes	Muscle weakness and pain Poor heart function	UL = 350 mg/day (when intake is from medications only) Diarrhea

9.2d Selenium and Copper: Free Radical Fighters

Selenium and copper are trace minerals that play many important roles in your body. These minerals are components of hundreds of enzymes, many of which act as antioxidants. Recall from Unit 8 that antioxidants protect your body's cells from being damaged by free radicals. **Table 9.13** summarizes the basic information about selenium and copper.

Selenium

Your body uses selenium (Se) to make a group of proteins that act as major antioxidants. The mineral also assists iodine in the production of thyroid hormone.

Organ meats, such as liver, and seafood are excellent sources of selenium.[22] Nuts, whole-grain products, turkey, and meat are also rich sources of the trace mineral (**Table 9.11**). Because Brazil nuts can have very high selenium contents, consume them in moderation.

In the United States, selenium deficiency is uncommon, but the condition may occur in people who have serious digestive tract conditions that interfere with the mineral's absorption. In parts of China where the soil lacks selenium and the population consumes locally produced foods, diets typically contain inadequate amounts of selenium. A form of arthritis is common in these areas of China. Over the past 25 years, scientists conducted several human studies to determine whether taking selenium supplements could reduce the risk of heart disease and certain cancers. The results of these studies generally found that the supplements didn't help prevent heart disease or cancer.[22]

Selenium toxicity is rare in the United States. The condition, however, can occur from drinking well water that naturally contains too much selenium or from taking megadoses of dietary supplements that contain the trace mineral. In humans, signs and symptoms of long-term selenium toxicity include brittle fingernails, loss of hair and nails, garlicky body odor, nausea, diarrhea, and fatigue.

Brazil nuts are rich sources of selenium.

© Wendy Schiff

TABLE 9.11

SELENIUM CONTENT OF SELECTED FOODS

Food	Selenium (mg)
Brazil nuts, 1 oz (6–8 nuts)	544
Fish, orange roughy, baked, 3 oz	75
Fish, tuna, canned in oil, drained, 3 oz	65
Oysters, breaded, fried, 3 oz	57
Egg noodles, cooked, 1 cup	38
Sunflower seeds, roasted, ¼ cup	25
Soy milk, 1 cup	12

RDA = 55 mcg for adults

Source: Data from U.S. Department of Agriculture, Agricultural Research Service: Selenium, Se (µg) Content of Selected Foods per Common Measure. *National nutrient database for standard reference, release 25,* 2012.

Placemat: © McGraw-Hill Education. Mark A. Dierker, photographer

Copper

Your body uses the trace mineral copper (Cu) to make several enzymes that act as antioxidants. The mineral is also involved in iron metabolism, immune function, and collagen production (see Unit 8).

A wide variety of foods contain copper, but the foods listed in **Table 9.12** are among the richest sources of the micronutrient. Healthy people rarely develop copper deficiency or copper toxicity. High doses of iron and zinc can interfere with the intestinal tract's ability to absorb copper, so taking these supplements may cause copper deficiency. People with chronic digestive system diseases may also develop copper deficiency because their bodies' ability to absorb the mineral is depressed.

TABLE 9.12

COPPER CONTENT OF SELECTED FOODS

Food	Copper (mg)
Beef liver, cooked, 3 oz	12.40
Crab meat, canned, ½ cup	1.10
Cashews, dry roasted, 1 oz	0.63
Mushrooms, white, cooked, drained, ½ cup	0.40
Soybeans, mature, boiled, drained, ½ cup	0.35
Chocolate, semisweet, ¼ cup	0.30
Baked beans, canned, with pork and tomato sauce, ½ cup	0.27
Sunflower seeds, dry roasted, 1 oz	0.26

RDA adults = 0.9 mg/day

Source: Data from U.S. Department of Agriculture, Agricultural Research Service: Copper, Cu (mg) Content of Selected Foods per Common Measure. *National nutrient database for standard reference, release 25,* 2012.

© C Squared Studios/Getty Images RF

TABLE 9.13

SELENIUM AND COPPER: SUMMARY OF BASIC NUTRITION INFORMATION

Mineral	Major Functions in the Body	Adult RDA	Major Dietary Sources	Major Deficiency Signs and Symptoms	Major Toxicity Signs and Symptoms
Selenium (Se)	Component of an antioxidant system	55 mcg	Meat, eggs, fish, seafood, whole grains	Joint pain Form of heart disease	UL = 400 mcg/day Nausea Diarrhea Hair loss Weakness Kidney failure, heart failure, and death
Copper (Cu)	Promotes iron metabolism Component of antioxidant enzymes Component of enzymes involved in connective tissue formation	0.9 mg	Liver, cocoa, legumes, whole grains, shellfish	Anemia Reduced immune system function Poor growth and development	UL = 10 mg/day Vomiting Abnormal nervous system function Liver damage

© Nancy R. Cohen/Getty Images RF

9.2e Iodine, Zinc, and Chromium: Metabolism Regulators

Many minerals, including iodine, zinc, and chromium, are involved in the regulation of energy metabolism. This section provides some basic information about these trace minerals, including good food sources. **Table 9.17** summarizes the information about the three trace minerals.

Why Is Iodine Necessary?

Your thyroid gland traps iodine (in the form of *iodide*) from your bloodstream and uses the mineral for the production of **thyroid hormone** (see Figure 9.3). Thyroid hormone controls the rate of cell metabolism, that is, the rate at which your cells obtain energy. The lack of thyroid hormone can cause your thyroid gland to enlarge and metabolism rate to slow. It's important to note that an enlarged thyroid gland can also be a sign of an "overactive" thyroid gland that makes too much thyroid hormone and some conditions that aren't related to iodine intake.

During World War I, physicians noted that men drafted into the U.S. military from the Great Lakes region were far more likely to have **goiter** (*goy'-ter*) than men from some other areas of the country. Goiter is enlargement of the thyroid gland that's not the result of cancer (**Fig. 9.13**). Goiters often occur among populations living in areas that have iodine-depleted soil. In general, these regions are inland and far from an ocean. If people in these communities limit their diets to locally produced foods, they might not have enough iodine in their diets to prevent goiter.

In 1924, iodine was added to table salt in the United States, and as a result, cases of goiter caused by iodine deficiency rarely occur in this country. Today, the use of iodized salt is the major method of preventing iodine deficiencies in developed nations, but inadequate iodine intake and goiters are still common in central Asia and central Africa.

© Biophoto Associates/Science Source

Figure 9.13 Goiter.

goiter enlargement of thyroid gland

thyroid hormone hormone that regulates the body's metabolic rate

Food Sources of Iodine

Major dietary sources of iodine include saltwater fish; seafood; seaweed; some plants, especially the leaves of plants grown near oceans; and iodized salt. Iodine fortification of salt is voluntary in the United States, so not all salt has the trace mineral added to it. Other dietary sources of iodine include food additives that contain the mineral, such as certain dough conditioners and food dyes. **Table 9.14** lists some foods that are good sources of iodine.

Dietary Adequacy

Most Americans have adequate iodine intakes.[23] As many Americans try to reduce their risk of hypertension by using less salt, iodine intakes may decline to marginal or inadequate levels.

Iodine-deficient people generally have low metabolic rates and elevated blood cholesterol levels. Other signs and symptoms of iodine deficiency include fatigue, difficulty concentrating on mental tasks, weight gain, intolerance of cold temperatures, constipation, and dry skin.

TASTY Tidbits

In the United States, manufacturers often add iodine to table salt to make "iodized salt." The sea salt that's usually sold in supermarkets isn't a good source of iodine because it hasn't been fortified with the mineral.[24] It's wise to avoid excess sodium from all sources, including sea salt.

© Wendy Schiff

Q Answer This

People who must restrict their sodium intake could have a higher than normal risk of _____ deficiency. You can find the answer on the last page of this unit.

TABLE 9.14

IODINE CONTENT OF SELECTED FOODS

Food	Iodine (mcg)
Seaweed, dried, ¼ oz	Varies but may be greater than 4500 mcg
Iodized salt, ½ tsp	231
Codfish, 3 oz	99
Milk (cow's), 8 fluid oz	99
Potato, baked with peel, 1 medium	60
Shrimp, 3 oz	35
Egg, hard-cooked, 1 large	12

RDA = 150 mcg for adults

Source: Data from Higdon J: *Iodine.* Micronutrient Information Center, Linus Pauling Institute, Oregon State University, Updated 2015. http://lpi.oregonstate.edu/infocenter/minerals/iodine/. Accessed: July 25, 2016.

Throughout the world, millions of people are at risk of iodine deficiency. It's very important for pregnant women to have adequate iodine intakes. Pregnant women who are iodine deficient have a high risk of giving birth to a dead infant, a low-birth-weight baby, or a baby that has **cretinism** (*krē'-tin-ih-zim*). Babies with cretinism have permanent brain damage, reduced intellectual functioning, and growth retardation.

Worldwide, iodine deficiency is the most common cause of preventable intellectual disability.[23] Pregnant women can reduce the risk of giving birth to infants with cretinism by consuming adequate amounts of iodine throughout pregnancy.

Over time, consuming very high amounts of iodine can cause thyroid gland enlargement and reduced production of thyroid hormone. These side effects are the same as those that occur when diets are deficient in iodine. Excess iodine is also associated with an increased risk of a form of thyroid cancer.[23]

cretinism condition that affects babies born to iodine-deficient women

Zinc

Zinc (Zn) is needed for a wide variety of functions in your body. The trace mineral is a component of about a hundred enzymes, many of which are involved in the metabolism of protein, carbohydrate, and fat.[25] Zinc is essential for growth and development during pregnancy, childhood, and adolescence. The micronutrient is also necessary for wound healing, the sense of taste and smell, DNA production, and proper functioning of the immune system.

Food Sources of Zinc

Zinc is widespread in foods (**Table 9.15**). Oysters are among the richest sources of zinc, but red meat, poultry products, and fortified cereals supply most of the zinc in the typical American's diet. **Figure 9.14** indicates MyPlate food groups that have foods that are good sources of zinc.

The average adult American consumes adequate amounts of zinc.[2] Thus, zinc deficiency is not a widespread problem in the United States. However, alcoholics have a high risk of zinc deficiency, because alcohol reduces zinc absorption and increases excretion of the mineral in urine. People with chronic diarrhea or digestive tract diseases can also develop zinc deficiency. Furthermore, vegetarians need more zinc than people who eat meat because the digestive tract does not absorb zinc from plant foods as well as from animal foods.[25] In children and adolescents, zinc deficiency can cause growth retardation and delayed sexual maturation. Other signs of zinc deficiency include loss of appetite, diarrhea, hair loss, dermatitis, poor wound healing, impaired sense of taste, and mental slowness.[25]

Ingesting more than 150 mg of zinc per day can depress beneficial HDL cholesterol levels and can result in diarrhea, cramps, nausea, vomiting, and depressed immune system function. Additionally, megadoses of zinc may interfere with copper absorption and metabolism. Therefore, you should avoid high intakes of zinc unless you are under a physician's supervision.

TASTY Tidbits

Results of studies provide evidence that zinc, when taken in the form of lozenges and syrups, helps reduce the severity or duration of colds.[25] Using zinc-containing nasal gels or sprays, however, may harm a person's sense of smell.

Raw oyster

TABLE 9.15	ZINC CONTENT OF SELECTED FOODS	
	Food	**Zinc (mg)**
	Oysters, breaded, fried, 3 oz	74.0
	Whole-grain Total, ready-to-eat cereal, ¾ cup	15.0
	Wheaties, ready-to-eat cereal, 1 cup	8.34
	Beef, chuck roast, cooked, 3 oz	7.0
	Baked beans, canned with pork and tomato sauce, ½ cup	6.9
	Ground beef, 80% lean, broiled patty, 3 oz	5.3
	Yogurt, plain, low-fat, 8 oz	2.2
	Sunflower seed kernels, dry roasted, ¼ cup	1.7

RDA for women = 8 mg/day; RDA for men = 11 mg/day

Source: Data from U.S. Department of Agriculture, Agricultural Research Service: Zinc, Zn (mg sorted by nutrient content) Content of Selected Foods per Common Measure. *National nutrient database for standard reference, release 25*, 2012.

Zinc lozenges, Oyster: © Wendy Schiff; Sunflower seeds: © McGraw-Hill Education. Jacques Cornell, photographer

Figure 9.14 MyPlate: Good food sources of zinc.

Chromium

The trace mineral chromium (Cr) plays an important role in maintaining proper carbohydrate and lipid metabolism. Chromium appears to promote energy metabolism by working with the hormone insulin to allow glucose to enter cells. Chromium may enhance insulin's action on cell membranes and, in a way, help to "hold the door open" for glucose's entry into the cells. Some people take chromium supplements to improve their blood glucose levels, but studies don't provide consistent evidence that the supplements are helpful for people with diabetes. Scientists continue to explore chromium's effects on metabolism.

Sources of Chromium

Chromium is widely distributed in foods, but most foods contain less than 2 mcg of the mineral per serving.[26] In general, meat, whole-grain products, yeast, fruits, and vegetables are good sources of chromium (**Table 9.16**). The average American adult consumes a diet that provides adequate amounts of chromium.[26] In the past, a few cases of chromium deficiency were reported in people maintained on special-formula diets that did not contain chromium. The major sign of chromium deficiency is an elevated blood glucose level.

Amounts of chromium that are naturally in foods generally don't cause toxicity. However, the safety of taking various chromium supplements is unknown. Medical researchers are studying the safety and usefulness of supplemental forms of chromium. Until more is known about the safety of such products, consumers should check with their physician before taking them.[26]

Other Important Minerals

Table 9.18 provides basic information about some mineral nutrients that aren't covered in this unit because most Americans consume adequate amounts of them. It's important to note that most of these minerals can be toxic if taken in large amounts.

TABLE 9.16	**CHROMIUM CONTENT OF SELECTED FOODS**	

Food	Chromium (mcg)
Broccoli, ½ cup	11
English muffin, whole-wheat, 1	4
Potatoes, mashed, 1 cup	3
Garlic powder, 1 teaspoon	3
Beef, 3 ounces	2
Orange juice, 1 cup	2
Turkey breast, 3 ounces	2
Whole-wheat bread, 1 slice	1

AI = 30–35 mcg for men; 20–25 mcg for women

Source: Data from Office of Dietary Supplements, National Institutes of Health: *Dietary supplement fact sheet: Chromium.* Updated 2013. http://ods.od.nih.gov/factsheets/Chromium-HealthProfessional/. Accessed: July 25, 2016.

TABLE 9.17

IODINE, ZINC, AND CHROMIUM: SUMMARY OF BASIC NUTRITION INFORMATION

Mineral	Major Functions in the Body	Adult RDA/AI	Major Dietary Sources	Major Deficiency Signs and Symptoms	Major Toxicity Signs and Symptoms
Iodine (I)	Component of thyroid hormone	150 mcg	Iodized salt, saltwater fish, dairy foods	Enlargement of thyroid gland (goiter) Cretinism	UL = 1100 mcg/day Reduced thyroid gland function
Chromium (Cr)	Enhances insulin action	Men: 30–35 mcg Women: 20–25 mcg	Egg yolks, whole grains, pork, nuts, mushrooms	Blood glucose level remains elevated after meals.	Unknown but currently under scientific investigation May interact with certain medications
Zinc (Zn)	Component of numerous enzymes	Men: 11 mg Women: 8 mg	Seafood, meat, whole grains	Skin rash Diarrhea Depressed sense of taste and smell Hair loss Poor growth and physical development	UL = 40 mg/day Intestinal upset Depressed immune system function Supplement use can reduce copper absorption.

TABLE 9.18

SOME OTHER MINERAL NUTRIENTS: BASIC NUTRITION INFORMATION

Mineral	Major Functions in the Body	Adult RDA/AI	Major Dietary Sources	Major Deficiency Signs and Symptoms	Major Toxicity Signs and Symptoms
Phosphorus (P)	Structural component of bones and teeth Maintenance of acid-base balance Component of DNA, phospholipids, and other organic compounds	700 mg	Dairy foods, processed foods, soft drinks, fish, baked goods, meat	None reported	UL = 4 g/day Poor bone mineralization
Chloride (Cl^-)	Maintenance of proper fluid balance Production of stomach acid Transmission of nerve impulses Maintenance of acid-base balance	2300 mg (19–50 years of age)	Processed foods, including salty snacks, table salt	Convulsions (observed in infants)	UL = 3600 mg/day Hypertension (because of the association with sodium in sodium chloride [table salt])
Sulfur (S)	Component of sulfur-containing amino acids	None has been established.	Dried fruit, tap water, beer, wine	Doesn't occur in healthy people	UL (none) Diarrhea
Manganese (Mn)	Component of several enzymes	AI = 1.8 mg for women; 2.3 mg for men	Tea, coffee, whole-grain cereals, nuts, legumes, blueberries	Not known	UL = 11 mg/day Irritability and lack of physical coordination

Module 9.3

Water: Liquid of Life

Compared to other nutrients, water is so important, it's in a class of nutrients by itself. Your body has many kinds of watery fluids, including blood, lymph, and urine. Water is also a major component of many foods and beverages (**Table 9.19**). Fat-free milk is about 91% water; romaine lettuce is almost 95% water; and a slice of whole-grain bread is about 37% water by weight. Water is such a simple molecule, it doesn't need to be digested before it's absorbed.

We often take water for granted, but this molecule is highly essential. You can survive for weeks, even months, if your diet lacks carbohydrates, lipids, proteins, and vitamins. But if you don't have any water from beverages and foods, your life will end within a week or two. This module focuses on the importance of water in your body.

TABLE 9.19

How Much Water Is in That Food or Beverage?

Food	Water % by Weight
Lettuce	95
Tomato	95
Watermelon	91
Milk, 1% fat	90
Apple, with skin	86
Avocado	79
Potato, white, baked with skin	75
Chicken, white meat, roasted	65
Bread, whole-wheat	37
Butter	16
Crackers, saltines	5
Vegetable oil	0

Source: Data from U.S. Department of Agriculture, Agricultural Research Service, USDA Nutrient Data Laboratory: *USDA National nutrient database for standard reference, release 25.*

9.3a What Water Does in Your Body

As a major component of body fluids, water has many functions in your body. Water

- is a **solvent** (water-soluble substances dissolve in it);
- is a major component of blood, saliva, sweat, tears, mucus, and joint fluid;
- removes wastes;
- helps transport substances;
- helps lubricate tissues;
- regulates body temperature;
- helps digest foods;
- participates in many chemical reactions; and
- helps maintain proper blood chemistry.

Although water has numerous functions in the body, this unique nutrient doesn't provide energy.

9.3b Your Body's Fluid Compartments

Depending on your age, sex, and body composition, 50 to 75% of your body is water weight (see Fig. 1.3). Lean muscle tissue contains more water (about 73%) than is present in fat tissue (about 20%). On average, young adult men have more lean tissue than young women. Approximately 55 to 60% of an average young man's body weight is water. The average young adult woman's body has more fat and, therefore, slightly less water than an average young man's body. Your percentage of body weight that's water declines from birth to old age. Water may comprise only 45% of a typical older adult's weight.[27]

One reason why water is such a vital nutrient is its role in helping cells obtain materials from their environment and eliminate wastes. Each cell has a membrane that defines the area of the cell and controls the passage of material into and out of the cell.

To survive, your cells must maintain proper **hydration**, that is, adequate water status. Proper hydration requires a balance between the body's two major fluid compartments: **intracellular water** and **extracellular water** (**Fig. 9.15**). Intracellular water is the fluid inside cells. Extracellular water surrounds cells (tissue fluid) or is the fluid portion of blood (plasma).

© Royalty-Free/Corbis RF

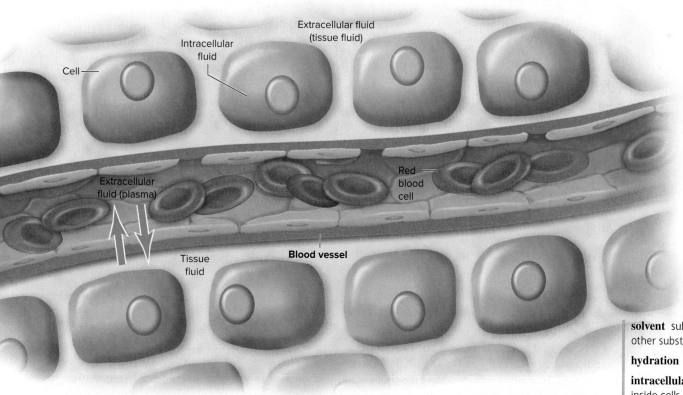

Figure 9.15 Fluid compartments. Your body must maintain a balance between the extracellular fluid and intracellular fluid. If too much plasma leaves a blood vessel and enters tissue fluid, the tissue swells (edema).

solvent substance in which other substances dissolve

hydration water status

intracellular water fluid that's inside cells

extracellular water fluid that surrounds cells or is in blood

How Do Electrolytes Influence Hydration?

Cells maintain proper hydration primarily by controlling amounts of electrolytes in each compartment. Water is attracted to electrolytes. Overall, where these ions go, water follows. As a result, changes in normal electrolyte levels can cause water to shift out of one compartment and move into the other. Recall from Unit 7 that edema occurs when an excessive amount of water moves into the space surrounding cells (extracellular fluid). **Essential Concept 9.1** illustrates what can happen to your cells when there's an imbalance in the concentration of ions in intracellular fluid or extracellular fluid.

Essential Concept

9.1 Why Your Body Must Maintain Fluid Balance

1 Sodium (Na⁺), for example, is a major extracellular ion. If extracellular fluid has fewer-than-normal sodium ions, water (H_2O) moves from the extracellular compartments into cells. When this occurs, the cells swell and can burst.

2 On the other hand, if extracellular fluid has an excess of sodium ions, water moves out of cells. As a result, the cells shrink and die because they lack enough extracellular fluid to function.

Na⁺ ion

Cell

H_2O

H_2O

H_2O

Dilute solution
Low concentration of Na⁺

H_2O

H_2O

H_2O

Concentrated solution
High concentration of Na⁺

9.3c The Essential Balancing Act

An average healthy adult's water intake from foods and beverages is about 2.3 quarts per day.[27] Depending on your physical activity level, your body also forms about 1 cup of water daily as a result of energy metabolism. Such water (*metabolic water*) also contributes to the body's fluid balance. **Total water intake** refers to water obtained from all sources, including metabolic water, and amounts to about 2.5 quarts per day (**Fig. 9.16**).[27]

Your body loses about 2.5 quarts of water in urine, exhaled air, feces, and sweat (perspiration) each day (see Fig. 9.16). Thus, your average daily total water intake is approximately equal to your average daily losses (output). To maintain good health, it's very important for your body to balance water intake with water output.

total water intake refers to water obtained from metabolic and external sources

Figure 9.16 Daily water balance. To maintain proper hydration, your water intake should equal your water output.

■ *What happens to the excess water you drink?*

How Much Water Do You Need?

How much water is necessary to drink for good health? Contrary to popular belief, there's no "rule of thumb" recommendation for how many glasses of water you must consume each day.[28] The Adequate Intake (AI) for total water intake is approximately 11 cups for young women and approximately 15.5 cups for young men.[29] Factors such as environmental temperatures and your health, physical activities, and dietary choices influence your body's water requirements. Thus, total water intakes vary widely among individuals.

Water Losses

Your kidneys are the major regulator of your body's water content and ion concentrations. The kidneys remove excess ions from blood. When the kidneys remove ions such as sodium, water follows and becomes the main component of urine.

© JGI/Blend Images LLC RF

The amount of urine you produce is determined primarily by your total water intake. A healthy person produces about 1.5 quarts of urine per day.[27] If you drink more watery fluids than your body needs, your kidneys excrete the excess water in urine. Healthy kidneys become less able to filter blood when water intakes are less than about 2 cups per day.

Your body loses water and electrolytes, including sodium, potassium, and chloride, when you have vomiting, diarrhea, a fever, or a runny nose. That's why you're often reminded to drink plenty of fluids, such as clear soups or sports drinks, when you're sick. Environmental factors such as temperature, humidity, and altitude also affect body water losses. When you're in a hot environment, for example, you perspire heavily. Perspiration is body water that reaches the skin's surface and evaporates into the air. This process causes water losses, but it helps cool the body. Water is also lost when you breathe because warm, moist air leaves your lungs. Physical activity, especially when it's intense and performed in warm conditions, causes the body to sweat more heavily. Therefore, athletes and other people who work or exercise outdoors, especially in hot conditions, need to stay properly hydrated.

TASTY Tidbits

Have you ever noticed that your weight increases by a few pounds after you have eaten a lot of salty foods and then consumed beverages? The weight gain is due to a temporary increase in body water volume. If you resume eating foods that supply your usual intake of sodium, your kidneys will eliminate the excess sodium and water in urine within a day. As your body regains its normal fluid balance, your weight also returns to normal.

© Comstock Images/Getty Images RF

Dehydration

When you're hot and sweating heavily, you become mildly dehydrated and your kidneys try to conserve water. Your mouth becomes dry and you feel uncomfortable. What do you do? You find something to drink! Most healthy people meet their AI for water by letting thirst be their guide.[29] Feeling thirsty is the brain's way of signaling you to drink watery fluids to avoid severe dehydration.

Dehydration occurs when your body's water content is too low. Dehydration can be a life-threatening condition. Rapid weight loss is a sign of dehydration. Every 16 ounces of water that the body loses represents a pound of body weight. If you lose 1 to 2% of your usual body weight in fluids, you will feel fatigued and thirsty. If you weigh 150 pounds, for example, and your weight drops 3 pounds after exercising in hot conditions, you've lost 2% of your body weight, primarily as water weight.

As the loss of body water approaches 4% of your weight, your muscles lose a lot of strength. By the time your body weight is reduced by 7 to 10% because of body fluid losses, severe weakness results. At a 20% reduction of body weight, you're likely to lose consciousness and die. Older adults do not sense thirst as accurately as do younger adults.[30] Furthermore, older adults may be more susceptible to develop dehydration than younger persons because as kidneys age, they become less able to conserve water when fluid intakes are low. Therefore, it may be necessary to remind older adults to drink more watery fluids, especially when they're physically active or in warm conditions.

What Are Diuretics?

A **diuretic** (*die'-uh-reh'-tic*) is a substance that stimulates kidneys to form urine. Caffeine is a mild diuretic. Coffee, tea, energy drinks, and soft drinks often contain caffeine or caffeine-related compounds. However, the water consumed in caffeinated beverages isn't completely lost in urine, so drinking these fluids still contributes to meeting your water needs.[29]

Alcohol is also a diuretic. Alcohol interferes with the kidneys' ability to conserve water, so the kidneys eliminate more urine than normal. Alcohol consumption actually results in urinary water losses that are greater than the volume of water consumed in the beverages. This explains why drinking alcohol increases the need to urinate and contributes to dehydration.

A "hangover" is the headache and overall discomfort that occurs a few hours after drinking too much alcohol. Dehydration, the body's immune response, a drop in blood glucose levels, and *congeners* may be responsible for a hangover.[31] Congeners are substances in alcoholic drinks that contribute to the taste and color of the beverages. Alcoholic drinks with high congener contents (brandy and whiskey, for example) tend to produce more severe hangovers than drinks with lower amounts of these substances, such as gin and vodka.

Can Too Much Water Be Toxic?

There's no Upper Limit (UL) for water. **Water intoxication**, however, can occur when an excessive amount of water is consumed in a short time period or when the kidneys have difficulty filtering water from blood. The excess water dilutes the sodium level of blood, upsetting the blood's water balance. As a result of the imbalance, too much water moves into cells, including brain cells. Signs and symptoms of water intoxication may include nausea and vomiting, headache, confusion, muscle spasms and weakness, and seizures.[32] If the condition isn't detected early and treated effectively, loss of consciousness and death can result.

Healthy people rarely drink enough water to become intoxicated. Water intoxication, however, can develop in people with disorders that interfere with the kidneys' ability to excrete water normally. Furthermore, marathon runners who consume large amounts of plain water in an effort to keep hydrated during competition may be at risk of water intoxication. Unit 10 provides more information about dehydration.

How Much Water Is Enough?

The simplest way to determine if you're consuming enough water is to note the volume of your urine. If you consume more fluid than needed, your kidneys will eliminate the excess, and you will produce plenty of urine. On the other hand, if you limit your fluid intake or have high fluid losses such as in sweat, you will produce small amounts of urine.

In addition to urine volume, the color of urine may be a useful sign of hydration status. Light yellow urine can indicate adequate hydration, whereas dark-colored urine may be a sign of dehydration. However, the color of urine isn't always a reliable guide for judging hydration status.[28] Having urinary tract infections or ingesting certain medications, foods, and dietary supplements, especially those containing the B-vitamin riboflavin, can alter urine's color.

---

dehydration condition characterized by inadequate body water

diuretic substance that increases urine production

water intoxication condition that occurs when too much water is consumed in a short time period or the kidneys have difficulty filtering water from blood

9.3d From the Tap or Bottle?

Many people drink bottled water as a substitute for tap water because they think bottled water tastes better and it's safer. In fact, the water in some bottled water products actually comes from a municipal water supply. For most Americans, drinking bottled water is usually unnecessary and expensive. However, when public water supplies are disrupted by water main breaks, natural disasters, or environmental contaminants, drinking bottled water may be your only safe option.

The Environmental Protection Agency (EPA) regulates the sanitation of public water supplies in the United States. Safety standards for bottled water are similar to those established by the EPA for tap water. Therefore, most Americans can trust the safety of their tap water because the vast majority of municipal water systems in the United States are regulated by the Safe Drinking Water Act. As a result of this law, most tap water undergoes a purification process and is constantly tested for safety. If such testing indicates the local water supply poses a threat to consumers, a "boil order"—a requirement to boil water for 10 minutes to kill harmful microorganisms—may be issued for the public to follow.

The Food and Drug Administration (FDA) regulates bottled water products that are marketed for interstate commerce. According to FDA regulations, bottled water manufacturers are responsible for producing safe products. Bottled water must be sealed in containers and have no added ingredients other than a substance that prevents the growth of microbes, such as bacteria. Bottled water may have the tooth- and bone-strengthening mineral fluoride added, but amounts must meet FDA guidelines. If bottled water manufacturers add flavorings or other ingredients to their products, the name of the product must indicate the added ingredients—"Bottled Water with Cherry Flavor," for example. These drinks are often called "flavored water beverages." A growing number of flavored waters also have added nutrients, such as vitamins, sodium, potassium, and amino acids. The beverage's label must identify the additives in the list of ingredients.

Although bottled water is safe to drink, the plastic used to contain it may contain harmful substances. Bisphenol A (*biss'-feen-ol*) (BPA) is a chemical used to make polycarbonate plastics and epoxy resins. Polycarbonate plastics are in many consumer products that come in contact with foods and beverages, including some water bottles. The epoxy resin that contains BPA is used to coat the inside of certain food cans. The coating prevents the can's metal from coming in contact with and being damaged by the food (**Fig. 9.17**). However, BPA can leach from polycarbonate plastic containers or epoxy resin-coated cans and enter the food or beverage stored within them.

In 2012, the FDA banned the use of BPA in plastic baby bottles and sipping cups that babies use to prepare for drinking out of cups. Concern over the safety of BPA has encouraged many plastic bottle manufacturers to discontinue using the chemical in their products.

To reduce exposure to BPA, consider taking the following actions:

- Avoid buying used plastic baby bottles and "sipping" cups, because they may have been made before the FDA baned the use of BPA in such plastic products;

- Use water bottles and plastic containers that are not made with BPA, as indicated on the label;

- Don't wash polycarbonate containers in the dishwasher or with harsh detergents;

- Reduce your intake of canned foods that are in epoxy resin-coated containers;

- Cook or store foods and beverages in glass, porcelain, or stainless steel containers; and

- Avoid using polycarbonate dishware, cups, or eating utensils for serving foods (especially hot foods or liquids).

© Wendy Schiff

© Wendy Schiff

Figure 9.17 BPA and epoxy resins.

■ *Why do some cans have an epoxy coating on their insides?*

Module 9.4

Drink to Your Health?

9.4 - Learning Outcomes

After reading Module 9.4, you should be able to

1. Define all of the key terms in this module.

2. Describe the amounts of beer, malt liquor, liquor, and wine that represent a standard drink.

3. Discuss how alcohol affects your body.

4. Identify factors that influence the blood alcohol concentration.

5. Discuss how your alcohol use can affect others.

Alcohol (ethanol) is a mind-altering depressant drug that's often classified as a food. When consumed in moderation, alcoholic beverages can make social situations more enjoyable. Many people, however, experience serious social and physical problems as a result of their drinking habits. This module focuses on alcohol, including its effects on the body.

9.4a What's Alcohol?

Alcohol (ethanol) is a simple nonnutrient that supplies energy but is poisonous to cells. Alcohol dissolves in water (it's water soluble), and alcoholic beverages generally contain a lot of water.

- Beers are typically 3 to 6% alcohol.

- Wines are 8 to 14% alcohol.

- Malt liquors are about 7% alcohol by volume.

- Hard liquors (for example, whiskey, bourbon, and vodka) are generally 40 to 50% alcohol.

TASTY **Tidbits**

You can determine the percentage of alcohol in hard liquor by dividing the "proof" declaration on the label by two. Gin, for example, is "80 proof," or 40% alcohol.

Figure 9.18 What's a standard drink?

Although alcohol is a nonnutrient, each gram of the substance provides 7 kcal. Beer and wine contain simple carbohydrates and small amounts of certain minerals and B vitamins. Distilled spirits have essentially no nutritional value other than water; preparing "cocktails" by adding mixers to spirits provides small amounts of nutrients to the drinks. A *standard drink* is approximately 12 ounces of beer, 8 to 9 ounces of malt liquor, 5 ounces of wine, or 1½ ounces of liquor. Each standard drink contains 13 to 14 grams of alcohol (**Fig. 9.18**).

9.4b Classifying Drinkers

People who drink alcohol can be classified according to their usual intake patterns. **Table 9.20** indicates this classification scheme, which includes binge drinkers. Binge drinking is a serious public health concern. More than 50% of the alcohol consumed by American adults is in the form of binge drinks.[33]

Binge drinking is often associated with driving while drunk. Furthermore, the practice may increase a person's later risk of alcoholism and can result in death. If you drink alcohol, which type of drinker are you?

alcohol (ethanol) a mind-altering depressant drug that's often classified as a food

blood alcohol concentration (BAC) estimated percentage of alcohol in blood

TABLE 9.20 CLASSIFYING DRINKERS		
	Amount of Standard Alcoholic Drinks Consumed	
Level	**Males**	**Females**
Moderate	Up to 2 drinks/day	Up to 1 drink/day
Heavy	15 or more drinks/week	8 drinks or more/week
Binge drinker	5 or more drinks/occasion (2-hour period)	4 or more drinks/occasion (2-hour period)

Source: Centers for Disease Control and Prevention: *Frequently asked questions.* February 2016. http://www.cdc.gov/alcohol/faqs .htm#heavyDrinking.

© Ingram Publishing/AGE Fotostock RF

9.4c How Your Body Processes Alcohol

Alcohol requires no digestion and readily passes into the bloodstream through the tissues lining the inside of your mouth, esophagus, stomach, and small intestine. When alcohol is consumed with meals, food delays its absorption from the stomach and slows the rate in which the drug enters the bloodstream.

Detoxification converts alcohol to less damaging compounds. Detoxification begins in the stomach, where a specific enzyme metabolizes up to 20% of the alcohol. In the small intestine, the absorptive cells remove nearly all of the remaining alcohol. After entering the bloodstream, the alcohol circulates to the liver. The liver is the primary site for metabolizing the substance. In the liver, alcohol can be metabolized completely to form carbon dioxide (CO_2) and water (H_2O), or the molecule can be used to make fatty acids.

What's Blood Alcohol Concentration?

Until the liver can detoxify all the alcohol that has been consumed, the toxic chemical circulates in the bloodstream and passes into the watery fluids within and surrounding cells. The lungs eliminate some of the alcohol; that's why you can smell alcohol on the breath of someone who's been drinking. Law enforcement officials use special devices to analyze the alcohol in blood, urine, or expired air to estimate a person's **blood alcohol concentration (BAC)**. BAC is the estimated percentage of alcohol in the bloodstream.

Table 9.21 indicates typical nervous system effects when BAC reaches various levels. At present, a BAC of 0.08% is the legal limit for intoxication for motor vehicle operators. Some officials want to reduce the limit to 0.05%. To estimate your BAC after consuming one or more standard drinks, use the "0.08 BAC law in Wisconsin" estimator at Wisconsin's Department of Transportation's website http://wisconsindot.gov/Documents/safety/education/drunk -drv/08law.pdf.

© INSADCO Photography/Alamy

TABLE 9.21 TYPICAL NERVOUS SYSTEM EFFECTS OF ALCOHOL AT VARIOUS BAC LEVELS (ADULTS)	
BAC	**Typical Effects***
0.05	Reduced inhibitions
0.10	Slurred speech
0.20	Markedly elevated mood, loss of motor control
0.30	Confusion
0.40	Stupor
0.50 to 0.60	Coma, respiratory paralysis, and death

*Effects may vary among adults. Moderate to heavy drinkers may not display these effects until higher BACs are reached.

Adapted from: National Institutes of Health, U.S. National Library of Medicine: Alcohol use and safe drinking. *MedlinePlus,* Last updated May 3, 2016. https://www.nlm.nih.gov/ medlineplus/ency/article/001944.htm. Accessed: May 23, 2016.

Nutrition Fact or Fiction?

Drinking strong coffee, running around the block, or taking cold showers can help you sober up quickly.

Drinking caffeinated beverages, exercising, taking cold showers, and following other popular recommendations for sobering up aren't useful. Why? These actions don't increase your body's rate of alcohol detoxification. To sober up, you must stop consuming alcohol and give your liver time to metabolize the chemical.

© Don Farrall/Photodisc/Getty Images

Factors That Influence BAC

You may have noticed that a few of your friends who drink can "hold their liquor" better than others. Why? Many factors influence the rate at which a person becomes noticeably affected by his or her alcohol consumption.

- *Amount and timing of alcohol consumption*

  A person who drinks six beers in an hour will become noticeably more intoxicated than if he or she drinks one beer in an hour.

- *Body size and composition*

  The average man is larger than the average woman. Larger people have bigger livers that detoxify more alcohol at a time.

- *Sex*

  Women tend to have more body fat than men. Alcohol doesn't move easily into fatty tissues, so the chemical circulates in the bloodstream longer in women (**Fig. 9.19**).

  Compared to men, women generally make lower amounts of the enzyme that's needed to metabolize alcohol.

- *Eating food along with the alcohol*

- *Prior drinking history*

  People who drink alcohol regularly develop tolerance to the substance.

Figure 9.19 Alcohol consumption and approximate BAC.

■ *How does a person's sex influence his or her ability to metabolize alcohol?*

Male 170 lbs.	Blood Alcohol Concentration (percentage)	Female 140 lbs.
	.10	
	.09	
	.08 Legal limit (May 2013)	
	.07	
	.06	
	.05	
	.04	
	.03	
	.02	
	.01	

Tolerance occurs when the liver adjusts to the usual amount of alcohol that's been consumed and metabolizes it more quickly. As a result of tolerance, a regular drinker eventually needs to consume more alcohol to achieve the same mind-altering effects as in the past. Tolerance can lead to alcohol dependence (alcoholism).

What's Alcohol Poisoning?

On March 15, 2004, Jason Reinhardt was living in a fraternity house at Minnesota State University, Moorhead. While celebrating his twenty-first birthday with friends in a bar, Jason rapidly drank 16 shots of alcohol. Although he managed to return to the fraternity house and go to bed, his lifeless body was discovered a few hours later. The young man's BAC was 0.361, close to the deadly range. What makes binge drinking so dangerous?

Binge drinking increases a person's BAC rapidly and to a point at which signs of alcohol poisoning occur. An individual suffering from alcohol poisoning

- is confused,
- "passes out" and cannot be aroused,
- breathes slowly and irregularly, and
- has pale or bluish skin.

The heart rate of a person with alcohol poisoning slows and becomes irregular. If a "passed out" person vomits, his or her stomach contents can enter the lungs, causing the person to choke to death. Additionally, the lungs of the person who has alcohol poisoning can stop functioning, resulting in death. Jason died in his sleep from the effects of alcohol poisoning. It's important to recognize that alcohol poisoning is a life-threatening condition. If you suspect someone has consumed a deadly amount of alcohol, call 911 immediately.

Alcohol Use Disorders

When a person's drinking behavior creates serious problems for him- or herself, the condition may be classified as an alcohol use disorder. An **alcohol abuser** experiences problems at home, work, and school that are associated with his or her drinking habits.

An **alcoholic** is a person who is dependent on alcohol (addicted) and experiences *withdrawal* signs and symptoms, such as shakiness, when he or she hasn't consumed the substance. Both abusers and alcoholics engage in behaviors that place themselves and others in danger, such as drinking and driving. **Table 9.22** lists possible signs of alcohol use disorder that follows. For more information about alcoholism and to take the "Am I Alcoholic Self Test" quiz, visit https://www.ncadd.org/get-help/take-the-test/am-i-alcoholic-self-test.

tolerance state that occurs when the liver adjusts to the usual amount of alcohol that's been consumed and metabolizes it more quickly

alcohol abuser person who experiences problems at home, work, and school that are associated with his or her drinking habits

alcoholic person who is dependent on alcohol and experiences withdrawal signs and symptoms when he or she hasn't consumed the drug

TABLE 9.22

POSSIBLE SIGNS OF ALCOHOL USE DISORDER

Not everyone who drinks alcohol regularly abuses the drug, but you might be abusing alcohol. Have you

- Had times when you drank more than you intended?
- Wanted to reduce or stop drinking, or you tried to but couldn't?
- Had a strong need or urge to drink?
- Felt that drinking or its effects interfered with your ability to take care of your personal responsibilities, do your job, or keep up with school work?
- Continued to drink even though it was causing trouble with your family or friends?
- Gotten into situations while or after drinking that increased your chances of being harmed, such as driving, swimming, using machinery, walking in a dangerous area, or having unsafe sex?
- Continued to drink even though it was making you feel depressed or anxious, or was causing other health problems?
- Continued to drink even after having a memory blackout?
- Found that when the effects of alcohol were wearing off, you had withdrawal symptoms, such as trouble sleeping, shakiness, irritability, anxiety, depression, restlessness, nausea, or sweating?

If you've had one or more of these signs, your alcohol use may already be a concern for you and others. Seek professional help.

Adapted from: National Institutes of Health, National Institute of Alcohol Abuse and Alcoholism: *Alcohol use disorder*. ND. http://www.niaaa.nih.gov/alcohol-health/overviewalcohol-consumption/alcohol-use-disorders Accessed: May 24, 2016.

© Stockbyte/Getty Images RF

9.4d Alcohol and Health

Alcohol is a central nervous system depressant. Thus, mild alcohol intoxication often produces pleasant sensations and relaxed inhibitions. Consuming large amounts, however, depresses the ability to control thought processes and muscular movements, including those needed for safe driving. Excessive alcohol use is responsible for 1 in 10 deaths of Americans who are of working age.[33] Alcohol is often involved in motor vehicle accidents, falls, and drownings, as well as acts of violence and abuse. An estimated 88,000 Americans die each year as a result of excessive alcohol use.[34] Thousands of other people suffer physical injuries and have damaged interpersonal relationships related to excess alcohol consumption.

Alcohol affects every cell in the body, and when consumed in excess, the drug damages every system in the body, particularly the digestive, nervous, and cardiovascular systems.

Some Serious Effects of Alcohol on the Body

If you have consumed distilled spirits without adding mixers, you probably felt a burning sensation as the alcohol entered your throat and stomach. This sensation is an indication of alcohol's irritating effects on the lining of your gastrointestinal tract. Not surprisingly, chronic drinking contributes to intestinal ulcer formation, particularly in the esophagus and stomach.

Alcohol's effects on the brain appear within a few minutes of having a drink. Alcohol acts as a depressant, which means it's a drug that slows the transmission of messages between nerve cells (neurons). Long-term consumption of excessive amounts of alcohol can cause the brain's neurons to shrink, and the organ develops other structural abnormalities. Confusion and memory loss are common signs of the extensive brain damage that occurs in a chronic heavy drinker.

In addition to harming the brain, alcohol can damage the liver. After a heavy drinking episode, the liver makes an excess of fatty acids that accumulate in liver cells, causing a condition called "fatty liver." Fatty liver is reversible; if the affected person avoids alcohol for an extended period, the liver metabolizes the fat, and the organ eventually heals itself. If the person continues to drink, the buildup of fat destroys his or her liver cells, and tough scar tissue replaces them. This irreversible condition is called liver cirrhosis or hardening of the liver. Liver cirrhosis can cause the organ to fail. Alcoholics are also prone to develop a form of **hepatitis**, inflammation of the liver. Hepatitis can cause **cirrhosis** and increases the risk of liver cancer. People who consume alcohol have an increased risk of other cancers, including mouth, throat, esophagus, breast (women), colorectal, and, possibly, pancreatic cancers.[35]

When consumed in moderate intakes (1 to 2 drinks/day), alcohol may reduce the risk of heart disease. Excess consumption, however, can damage heart muscle and elevate blood pressure to dangerous levels. As a result, chronic alcoholics often have enlarged but weakened hearts and suffer strokes. **Figure 9.20** summarizes the major damaging effects of alcohol on the body.

Alcohol and Body Water

Billboard and media advertisements for alcoholic beverages often show sweaty, physically active young adults gulping down beer or liquor to relieve their thirst. These ads are misleading. Alcohol is not a good thirst quencher because it's a diuretic that causes the kidneys to produce more urine, and the body loses water and certain vitamins and minerals along with it. If a dehydrated drinker consumes even more alcohol to relieve thirst, this response only increases his or her water losses. Drinking water and other nonalcoholic drinks is the best way to keep the body well hydrated.

Alcohol's Effects on Your Nutritional Status

When consumed in moderation, alcohol stimulates the appetite. Alcohol, however, lowers blood glucose levels and raises blood triglycerides. Alcohol also interferes with the absorption, metabolism, and storage of various vitamins and minerals, and increases the excretion of other nutrients, particularly magnesium.

Many alcoholics consume a considerable portion of their energy intake as alcohol. As a result, alcoholic beverages often displace nutrient-dense foods from alcoholics' diets. Chronic excessive alcohol intake contributes to malnutrition. Deficiencies of magnesium, vitamin A, vitamin C, and the B vitamins thiamin and folate are common among alcoholics.

hepatitis inflammation of the liver

cirrhosis hardening of tissues

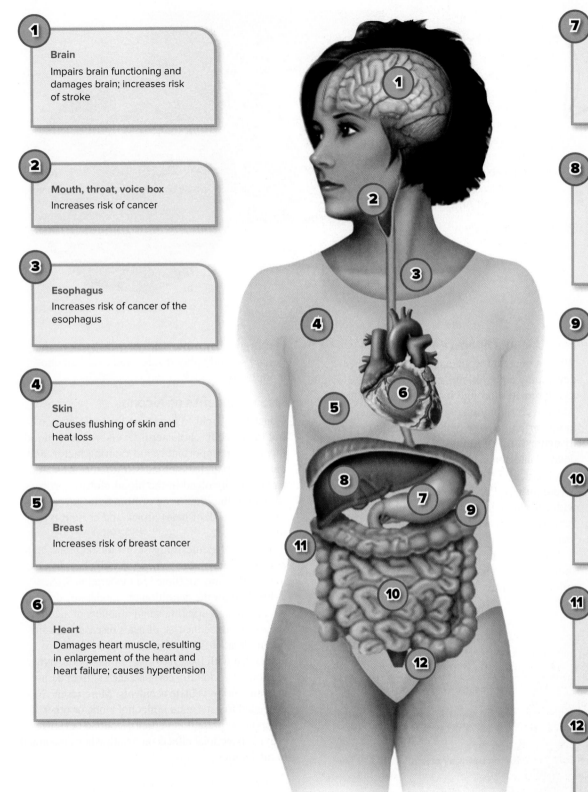

1 Brain
Impairs brain functioning and damages brain; increases risk of stroke

2 Mouth, throat, voice box
Increases risk of cancer

3 Esophagus
Increases risk of cancer of the esophagus

4 Skin
Causes flushing of skin and heat loss

5 Breast
Increases risk of breast cancer

6 Heart
Damages heart muscle, resulting in enlargement of the heart and heart failure; causes hypertension

7 Stomach
Irritates stomach lining and increases risk of stomach cancer

8 Liver
Causes liver cells to fill with fat, eventually resulting in hepatitis, cirrhosis, and liver failure; increases risk of liver cancer

9 Pancreas
Impairs pancreatic function, can cause inflammation of the pancreas and increases risk of pancreatic cancer

10 Small intestine
Interferes with nutrient absorption

11 Abdomen
Increases fat deposits in abdominal region

12 Colon and rectum
Increases risk of colon and rectal cancer

Figure 9.20 Some effects that alcohol can have on your body.

TASTY **Tidbits**

People who abuse alcohol are prone to develop hepatitis. Hepatitis can cause cirrhosis of the liver and increases the risk of liver cancer. Chronic alcohol abuse is a major cause of liver failure among adult Americans.

a.
Normal liver (a); liver damaged by cirrhosis (b)

b.

© Arthur Glauberman/Photo Researchers, Inc.

fetal alcohol spectrum disorder (FASD) condition characterized by abnormal physical and intellectual development that affects newborns of women who consumed alcohol during pregnancy

Fetal Alcohol Spectrum Disorder

When a pregnant woman drinks alcohol, her developing embryo/fetus is exposed to the alcohol as it circulates through its mother's bloodstream. Alcohol consumption during pregnancy can result in the birth of a baby with **fetal alcohol spectrum disorder** (**FASD**). Babies with FASD experience delayed and abnormal physical and intellectual development. Fetal alcohol syndrome (FAS) is a severe form of FASD. A child with FAS is born with certain facial and heart defects as well as irreversible nervous system damage that causes intellectual disability (**Fig. 9.21**).

The amount of alcohol that can be safely consumed by a pregnant woman has not been determined. Therefore, if you or someone you know is trying to conceive or is pregnant, you or that person should "play it safe" and avoid alcohol completely.

Health Benefits of Alcohol

Consuming light to moderate amounts of alcohol raises HDL cholesterol levels, reduces blood levels of an important blood-clotting factor, and decreases platelet stickiness. *Platelets* are cell fragments involved in the blood-clotting process. Reducing the likelihood of blood clot formation lowers the risk of heart attack and certain types of strokes.

Results of studies suggest that all alcoholic beverages provide the same heart-healthy benefits, as long as they are consumed in moderation.[36] (See Table 9.20 for the definition of "moderate" drinkers.) Although drinking small amounts of alcohol seems to reduce the risk of heart disease, consuming moderate to excessive amounts of alcohol is associated with increased risks of addiction, hypertension, heart failure, certain cancers, liver damage, and motor vehicle accidents. More research is needed to determine if alcohol alone or other compounds present in certain alcoholic beverages provide beneficial effects on health when consumed in moderation.

9.4e Where to Get Help for Alcohol Abuse or Dependence

If you think you are abusing alcohol or are dependent on the substance, seek help from your personal physician. For information about alcohol abuse, you can contact the Substance Abuse and Mental Health Services Administration's National Helpline at 1-800-662-HELP. You can also visit the websites of Alcoholics Anonymous (www.aa.org/) or Al-Anon /Alateen (www.al-anon.alateen.org/).

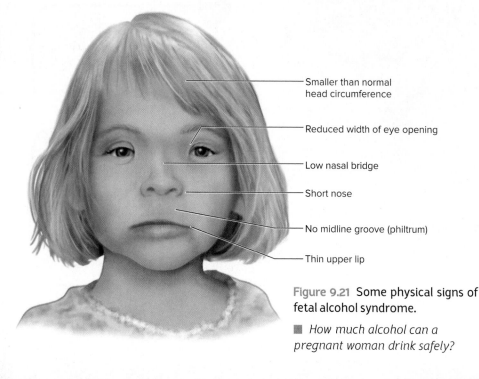

Smaller than normal head circumference

Reduced width of eye opening

Low nasal bridge

Short nose

No midline groove (philtrum)

Thin upper lip

Figure 9.21 **Some physical signs of fetal alcohol syndrome.**

■ *How much alcohol can a pregnant woman drink safely?*

In a Nutshell

© McGraw-Hill Education. Mark A. Dierker, photographer

Module 9.1 Minerals for Life

- Minerals are a group of elements in Earth's rocks, soils, and natural water sources. About 15 mineral elements have known functions in the body and are necessary for your health. The two primary groups of dietary minerals are major minerals and trace minerals.

- Most minerals have more than one function in your body. Some minerals function as inorganic ions or structural components of tissues; other minerals are components of various enzymes, hormones, or other organic molecules. Cells cannot metabolize minerals for energy. The body, however, needs certain minerals as cofactors to speed up the rate of some chemical reactions that release energy from macronutrients. Lack of energy is often a symptom of these particular mineral deficiency disorders. Excessive amounts of minerals in the body can disrupt normal cell functioning, causing toxicity.

Module 9.2 Key Minerals and Your Health

- Calcium is a major structural component of bones and teeth, and the mineral is necessary for blood clotting, muscle contraction, and nerve function. Calcium absorption depends on vitamin D. Most dairy foods are rich calcium sources. Although people, especially women, are at risk of developing osteoporosis as they age, various lifestyle modifications help reduce this risk. Fluoride works with calcium to strengthen bones and teeth.

- Potassium, the major positively charged ion found inside cells, is vital for maintaining normal fluid balance and nerve functioning. The typical American diet doesn't supply enough potassium. Plant foods, meat, and milk are good sources of potassium.

- Sodium, the major positively charged ion found outside cells, has some functions that are similar to those of potassium. The typical American diet provides high amounts of sodium, primarily from processed foods. Diets high in sodium are associated with increased risk of hypertension.

- Hypertensive individuals have greater risk of CVD, kidney failure, and damage to other organs than people with normal blood pressures. Advanced age, African-American ancestry, obesity, physical inactivity, cigarette smoking, and excess alcohol and sodium intakes are major risk factors for hypertension. Treatment for hypertension usually includes following dietary modifications and making some other lifestyle changes.

- Iron is a critical component of hemoglobin, myoglobin, and a group of proteins that help release energy from macronutrients. Hemoglobin in RBCs transports oxygen from the lungs to the tissues.

- Iron deficiency can result in iron deficiency anemia, a condition characterized by low hemoglobin levels. People suffering from anemia become fatigued easily and lack interest in activities. Iron deficiency during pregnancy can result in giving birth to a premature baby or low-birth-weight baby. In children, anemia interferes with normal growth and development.

- Iron absorption depends on the body's need for the mineral and the form of iron in food. Heme iron is better absorbed than nonheme iron. Meat and liver are among the best sources of dietary iron. Women of childbearing age often have higher needs for iron than men because of menstrual blood loss. Iron deficiency is the leading cause of anemia.

- Magnesium is a cofactor for numerous chemical reactions and is needed for energy metabolism, and nerve and heart function. Cases of magnesium deficiency rarely occur among healthy members of the population. Plant foods are good sources of magnesium.

- In your body, selenium and copper help reduce free radical damage. Iodine, zinc, and chromium function as regulators of energy metabolism. Iodine deficiency can cause goiter and cretinism.

© McGraw-Hill Education. Ken Karp, photographer

Module 9.3 Water: Liquid of Life

- In the body, water is a major component of body fluids. Water is a solvent that often participates directly in chemical reactions. Water's other physiological roles include transporting substances, removing waste products, lubricating tissues, and regulating body temperature and acid-base balance. Water doesn't provide energy for the body. Depending on a person's age, sex, and body composition, about 45 to 75% of his or her body is water.

- The body maintains a balance between intracellular and extracellular fluids primarily by controlling concentrations of electrolytes (ions) in each fluid compartment. If the normal concentrations of these ions change too much, water shifts out of a compartment, and cells shrink or swell as a result.

- Total water intake includes water from beverages and foods. About 80% of a person's total water intake is from beverages. Metabolic water is another source of water for the body.

- A healthy body loses water in urine, sweat, exhaled air, and feces. A healthy person's average daily total water input equals his or her average output. Environmental factors, physical condition, and lifestyle practices can alter your body's fluid balance.

- The kidneys are the major regulator of the body's water content and ion concentrations. In a healthy person, the kidneys maintain proper hydration by filtering excess ions from blood. When the kidneys remove ions such as sodium, water follows and becomes the main component of urine.

Bottle: © Photodisc/Getty Images RF; Glass of water: © John A. Rizzo/Getty Images RF

- To avoid overheating, your body must release the excess heat into the environment, primarily by perspiration. When water evaporates from your skin, it takes some heat along with it, cooling your body.

- Thirst is the primary regulator of fluid intake. The majority of healthy people meet their AI for water by letting thirst be their guide. Under certain conditions, however, older adults, sick persons, and people who work or exercise outdoors, especially in hot conditions, are at risk of dehydration.

- In the United States, bottled water is often derived from a municipal water supply. When public water supplies are disrupted, drinking bottled water may be the only option. The EPA regulates the sanitation of public water supplies in the United States. The FDA regulates bottled water products that are marketed for interstate commerce. Bottled water may have fluoride added, but amounts must meet FDA guidelines. If bottled water manufacturers add flavorings or other ingredients to a product, the name of the product must indicate the added ingredients, and the beverage's label must identify the additives in the list of ingredients.

Module 9.4 Drink to Your Health?

- Alcohol is a simple nonnutrient substance that supplies energy but is toxic to cells. Beers are typically 3 to 6% alcohol, wines contain about 8 to 14% alcohol, and malt liquors are about 7% alcohol by volume. Each gram of alcohol provides 7 kcal, but alcohol isn't a nutrient; it's a mind-altering drug.

- A standard drink (approximately 12 ounces of beer, 5 ounces of wine, 8 to 9 ounces of malt liquor, or 1½ ounces of liquor) contains 13 to 14 grams of alcohol.

- Alcohol requires no digestion and readily passes through the tissues lining the inside of the mouth, esophagus, stomach, and small intestine. The body detoxifies alcohol by converting the chemical into less-damaging compounds. Until the liver has had enough time to metabolize all the alcohol that has been consumed, the amount of the substance that remains circulates in the bloodstream.

- Binge drinking is a major public health problem in the United States.

- Although drinking small amounts of alcohol raises HDL cholesterol, excessive amounts of the substance damage every system in the body, particularly the gastrointestinal, nervous, and cardiovascular systems. Alcohol has especially devastating effects on an embryo. Infants born with fetal alcohol syndrome have certain facial and heart defects as well as extensive, irreversible nervous system damage that causes intellectual disability. Therefore, pregnant women should not drink alcohol.

© McGraw-Hill Education.
Jill Braaten, photographer

What's in **Your Diet?!**

Using the DRIs

1. Refer to your 3-day food log from the "What's in Your Diet?!" feature in Unit 3.

   a. Find the RDA/AI or other DRI for electrolyte values for minerals under your life stage/sex group category in the DRI tables (see Appendix G). Write those values under the "My DRIs" column in the table below.

   b. Review your personal dietary assessment. Find your 3-day average intakes of potassium, sodium, calcium, magnesium, iron, and zinc. Write those values under the "My Average Intake" column of the table.

   c. Calculate the percentage of the DRI you consumed for each mineral by dividing your intake by the DRI amount and multiplying the figure you obtain by 100. For example, if your average intake of iron was 9 mg/day, and your RDA for the mineral is 18 mg/day, you would divide 18 mg by 9 mg to obtain .50. To multiply this figure by 100, simply move the decimal point two places to the right, and replace the decimal point with a percentage sign (50%). Thus, your average daily intake of iron was 50% of the RDA. Place the percentages for each mineral under the "% of My DRI" column.

   d. Under the ">, <, =" column, indicate whether your average daily intake was greater than (>), less than (<), or equal to (=) the DRI.

2. Use the information you calculated in the first part of this activity to answer the following questions:

   a. Which of your average mineral intakes equaled or exceeded the DRI value?

   b. Which of your average mineral intakes was below the DRI value?

   c. What foods would you eat to increase your intake of the minerals that were less than the DRI levels? (Review food sources of the minerals in Unit 9, including those listed in tables.)

   d. Turn in your completed table and answers to your instructor.

© D. Hurst/Alamy RF

Personal Dietary Analysis: Minerals				
Mineral	My DRI	My Average Intake	% of My DRI	>, <, or =
Iron				
Calcium				
Zinc				
Sodium				
Potassium				

© Wendy Schiff

Consider This...

1. A friend of yours refuses to drink her community's tap water because it has been fluoridated. She's heard that fluoride is toxic. She drinks only bottled water. What advice about fluoride and bottled water would you tell your friend?

2. Paul is a total vegetarian (vegan), and he doesn't like soy-based foods. Based on this information, identify at least three minerals that are likely to be lacking in his diet.

3. Consider your family history and lifestyle to determine whether you're at risk of osteoporosis. If you're at risk, what steps can you take at this point in your life to reduce your chances of developing this disease?

4. Consider your family history and lifestyle to determine whether you're at risk of hypertension. If you're at risk, what steps can you take at this point in your life to reduce your chances of developing this disease?

5. In a televised interview, a person claiming to be a doctor recommends taking megadoses of chromium and selenium supplements to enhance muscular strength and endurance. Discuss why you would or wouldn't follow this person's advice.

6. If you drink alcohol, consider assessing your alcohol use habits in the assessment in Module 9.4c. According to the assessments, are you at risk for alcoholism? If your answer is "yes" to either classification, what can you do to obtain help?

© Burke/Triolo Productions /Getty Images RF

Test Yourself

Select the best answer.

1. Which of the following statements is false?
   a. Lean tissue contains more water than fat tissue.
   b. Water is a major solvent.
   c. Generally, young women have more body water than do young men.
   d. Water doesn't provide energy.

2. If the extracellular fluid has an excess of sodium ions,
   a. sodium ions move into cells.
   b. intracellular fluid moves to the outside of cells.
   c. phosphate and calcium ions are eliminated in feces.
   d. blood levels of arsenic and oxalate increase.

3. Which of the following foods has the lowest percentage of water?
   a. Tomatoes
   b. Oranges
   c. Whole-grain bread
   d. Vegetable oil

4. In the United States, table salt is often fortified with
   a. iron.
   b. selenium.
   c. potassium.
   d. iodine.

5. Which of the following foods isn't a good source of calcium?
   a. Butter
   b. Cheddar cheese
   c. Canned sardines
   d. Kale

© FoodCollection /Stockfood RF

6. Henry is concerned about his risk of osteoporosis. Which of the following characteristics is a known risk factor for this chronic condition?
   a. Occupation
   b. Racial/ethnic background
   c. Vitamin B-12 intake
   d. Iron exposure

7. The primary source of sodium in the typical American's diet is
   a. bottled water.
   b. processed food.
   c. fruit.
   d. milk.

8. Which of the following populations has the highest risk of hypertension?

   a. People with African-American ancestry

   b. Young, physically active Asian men

   c. Hispanic women who don't drink alcohol

   d. Young adults who consume high amounts of fruit

9. Sources of heme iron include

   a. fortified grain products.

   b. beef.

   c. spinach.

   d. cast-iron cookware.

10. In the United States, the most common cause of anemia is _____ deficiency.

    a. iodine

    b. cobalt

    c. iron

    d. calcium

11. Cretinism is caused by a deficiency of ____ during pregnancy.

    a. iron

    b. sodium

    c. copper

    d. iodine

12. Which of the following statements is true?

    a. Safety standards for bottled water are similar to those for tap water.

    b. Most brands of water bottled in the United States contain unsafe amounts of arsenic and lead.

    c. The EPA inspects and certifies water bottling facilities at least three times a year.

    d. The majority of Americans should drink bottled water because water from municipal systems is unsafe.

13. Many Americans have low intakes of

    a. potassium.

    b. chloride.

    c. phosphorus.

    d. manganese.

A Answer This (Module 9.2e)

Iodine

References → See Appendix F.

© Hannah Johnston/Getty Images

Nutrition for a Healthy Weight and Fit Body

What's on the Menu?

Module 10.1
Overweight or Obese?

Module 10.2
Factors That Influence Your Body Weight

Module 10.3
Managing Your Weight Safely

Module 10.4
Disordered Eating and Eating Disorders

Module 10.5
Get Moving; Get Healthy!

"I started gaining weight just before I started college, and by the end of my freshman year, I weighed 30 pounds more than I weighed in high school. I didn't feel good about myself. When I broke the buttons on two pairs of jeans because they were too tight, I realized it was time for me to change. The first thing I did was eliminate 'pop' [soft drinks]. That was definitely hard to do, but I lost 15 pounds in 6 weeks. I made other changes, too. I started cutting back on my portion sizes and stopped going to the cafeteria. I avoided hamburgers and French fries, drank more water, and ate more fruits, vegetables, and salads. I also began to eat breakfast every day. . . . I feel great."

McKenzie Frey

© Wendy Schiff

© Pixtal/AGE Fotostock RF

McKenzie Frey realized that she had gained too much weight when she noticed that her jeans didn't fit. McKenzie identified foods and beverages that contributed to the unwanted weight. Then she made the effort to change and improve her eating habits. If she's able to continue her new dietary practices, she's likely to maintain the weight loss.

This unit provides practical tips for helping you achieve or maintain a healthy body weight through sensible eating practices as well as increased physical activity. By reading Unit 10, you'll also learn about the major factors that contribute to excess body fat and health consequences linked to having too much or too little body fat. Unreasonable concern about body size and poor self-image can result in disordered eating practices. Unit 10 also includes information about eating disorders, focusing primarily on anorexia nervosa and bulimia nervosa.

Module 10.1

Overweight or Obese?

© Stockbyte/Getty Images RF

10.1 - Learning Outcomes

After reading Module 10.1, you should be able to

1. Define all of the key terms in this module.

2. List major health risks associated with excess body fat.

3. Explain why the distribution of body fat may be more important to health than the percentage of body fat.

4. Calculate your BMI and use the value to determine whether your weight is healthy.

5. Describe practical ways to measure body composition.

What's the difference between "overweight" and "obese"? According to the National Heart Lung and Blood Institute, a person who's **overweight** has extra body weight that's contributed by bone, muscle, body fat, and/or body water.[1] A professional football player, for example, may be "overweight" by this definition because of his muscular body build. Nevertheless, this particular athlete is healthy because he has less body fat and is more physically active than the average man who's his age. Many people, however, have too much body fat (**"overfat"**). **Obesity** is a condition characterized by excessive and unhealthy amounts of body fat. Unless otherwise noted, we'll use the term *overweight* when referring to people who are overfat but not obese. Overweight and obese people have greater risk of developing serious chronic diseases, including type 2 diabetes, hypertension, and cardiovascular disease (CVD) than people who aren't overweight or obese.[1]

Obesity is a *prevalent* (common) nutritional disorder in the United States. In 2013–2014, almost 38% of Americans who were 20 years of age and older were obese (**Table 10.1**).[2] Compared to non-Hispanic white adults, obesity is more common among non-Hispanic black and Mexican-American adults, particularly among non-Hispanic black women. In 2013–2014, 57% of non-Hispanic black women were obese.[2] According to experts at the Centers for Disease Control and Prevention (CDC), cultural, behavioral, and environmental factors may be largely responsible for racial/ethnic differences in obesity rates.

In the United States, obesity has reached epidemic proportions (**Fig. 10.1**). An epidemic is a widespread health problem. Between 1988–1994 and 2013–2014, the percentage of obese adult Americans rose by almost 66% (see Table 10.1).[2] Public health experts are also concerned about childhood obesity. In 2011–2014, 17% of children who were 2 to 19 years of age were obese.[3]

overweight having extra weight from bone, muscle, body fat, and/or body water

overfat having too much body fat

obesity condition characterized by an excessive and unhealthy amount of body fat

TABLE 10.1	AGE-ADJUSTED PREVALENCE OF OVERWEIGHT AND OBESITY AMONG U.S. ADULTS AGED 20 AND OVER		
	Weight Status	**1988–1994**	**2013–2014**
	Overweight	33.1%	32.7%
	Obese	22.9%	37.9%

Source of data: Fryar CD and others: *Prevalence of overweight, obesity, and extreme obesity among adults aged 20 and over: United States, 1960–1962 through 2013–2014.* July 18, 2016. http://www.cdc.gov/nchs/data/hestat/obesity_adult_13_14/obesity_adult_13_14.htm Accessed: July 18, 2016

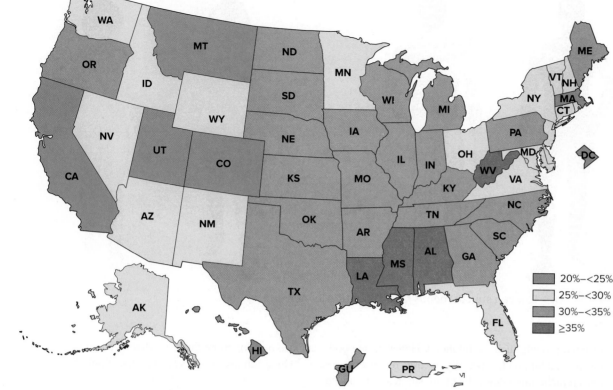

Figure 10.1 Obesity Map of the United States (2015)

Source: Centers for Disease Control and Prevention.

	20%–<25%
	25%–<30%
	30%–<35%
	≥35%

Rates of overweight and obesity are also increasing rapidly throughout the world ("globesity"). The World Health Organization (WHO) estimated that worldwide, more than 1.3 *billon* adults were overweight and 600 million adults were obese in 2014.[4] In most countries, overweight and obesity are responsible for more deaths than the number caused by being underweight.

10.1a Body Composition and Adipose Tissue

Your body is composed of two major compartments: **fat-free mass** (lean tissues) and **total body fat.** Fat-free mass is comprised of body water, mineral-rich tissues such as bones and teeth, and protein-rich tissues, including muscles and organs.

Total body fat includes "essential fat" and fat tissue. Essential fat is vital for your survival—every cell in your body contains some essential fat in its cell membrane. Furthermore, essential fat is also in certain bones and nervous tissue. Fat tissue contains **adipose** ("fat") **cells** that are specialized for storing energy in the form of triglycerides (**Fig. 10.2**). In addition to storing and releasing energy as fat, adipose cells secrete numerous proteins, some of which have roles in regulating food intake, glucose metabolism, and immune responses. Some body fat is needed for good health, but overweight and obese people have excessive amounts of fat tissue.

Adipose Cells

When food is plentiful, your fat cells remove excess triglycerides from the bloodstream for storage. As the amount of fat stored in your adipose cells increases, the size of each cell expands, and your body gains weight. At one time, scientists thought the human body could only produce fat cells during periods

Figure 10.2 Fat (adipose) cells.

© McGraw-Hill Education. Dennis Strete, photographer

fat-free mass lean tissues

total body fat essential fat and storage fat tissue

adipose cells specialized cells that store fat

Many children don't "grow out of" obesity.

© Ingram Publishing/SuperStock RF

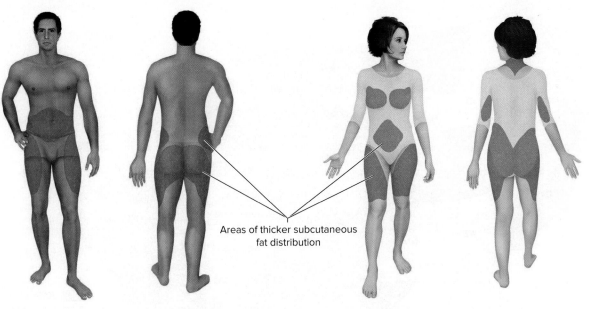

Figure 10.3   Uneven subcutaneous fat distribution in men and women.

of rapid growth, such as childhood. However, the body can also develop more fat cells when overeating occurs in adulthood, especially in cases of extreme obesity.[5] Once adipose cells form, scientists think the cells remain, unless they die or are surgically removed.

When your body needs energy, your adipose cells release fat into the bloodstream for other cells to use as fuel. As each adipose cell loses some fat, it shrinks. Your body eventually loses weight, and you appear slimmer as a result.

Subcutaneous Fat and Visceral Fat

Subcutaneous (*sub-qu-tay'-nee-us*) tissue holds skin in place over underlying tissues such as muscles. Subcutaneous tissue also contains fat cells. When subcutaneous tissue has more fat cells than other kinds of cells, it's referred to as **subcutaneous fat**.[6] Subcutaneous fat helps insulate your body against cold temperatures and protects muscles and bones from bumps and bruises. This layer of fat is thicker in certain regions of men's and women's bodies, especially in the abdominal area, thighs, and buttocks (**Fig. 10.3**).

Your body also has **visceral** (*viss'-eh-rol*) **fat**. Visceral fat is adipose tissue that's under your abdominal muscles and hangs over your stomach and intestines like a protective apron (**Fig. 10.4**). Women generally have more subcutaneous fat than men, whereas men tend to have more visceral fat than women.[7] Excessive visceral fat and/or subcutaneous abdominal fat result in what's commonly called a "beer belly" or the "middle-age spread." The following section of this module explains why having too much visceral fat can be unhealthy.

Pinching subcutaneous fat
© Stockbyte/Getty Images RF

subcutaneous fat layer of tissue that's under the skin and has more fat cells than other kinds of cells

visceral fat adipose tissue that's under the abdominal muscles, which forms a protective apron over the stomach and intestines

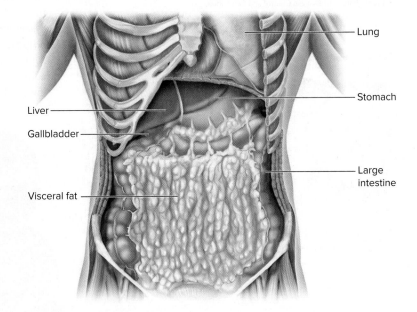

Figure 10.4   Visceral fat.

■ *Why is it unhealthy to have too much visceral fat?*

Nutrition Fact or Fiction?

Cellulite is toxic wastes trapped under the skin.

This statement is false because the body doesn't store toxic wastes under the skin. Whenever possible, your body detoxifies poisonous substances or eliminates them. Scientists don't fully understand why cellulite occurs, but it may simply be subcutaneous fat held in place by irregular bands of connective tissue. Despite claims by cosmetic manufacturers that their products eliminate cellulite, there are no effective ways to permanently smooth the skin's dimpled appearance.[8]

© Caro/Alamy

10.1b Health Effects of Excess Fat

Several chronic health problems that affect millions of Americans are associated with excessive body fat. Obese people have increased risks of

- heart disease,
- type 2 diabetes,
- certain cancers (uterine, breast, liver, kidney, gallbladder, and colon),
- hypertension (high blood pressure),
- high total cholesterol or high triglyceride levels,
- stroke,
- liver and gallbladder disease,
- sleep apnea and other breathing problems,
- osteoarthritis (breakdown of joint tissues), and
- all causes of death (mortality).[9]

central-body obesity condition characterized by having a large amount of visceral fat and an "apple" shape

A person's mental health and self-esteem can be negatively affected by his or her "weight problem." Many Americans admire people with slim and muscular body builds. Thus, overweight and obese people often suffer from poor self-images because they think their bodies are unattractive. The general public tends to view obesity as a condition that results from lack of willpower and the inability to "push oneself away from the table." People who aren't overfat or obese often characterize obese persons as lazy, lacking in willpower, and not intelligent.[10] Thus, many obese people must deal with the negative attitude that slimmer people have toward them.

Body Fat Distribution: Effects on Health

The distribution of a person's excess body fat is closely associated with the risk of obesity-related diseases. Central-body obesity is characterized by a large amount of visceral fat ("spare tire") that causes the waistline to spread beyond the buttocks and thighs. A person with **central-body obesity** is sometimes described as having an "apple" body shape (see **Fig. 10.5a**). People with central-body obesity have higher risks of CVD and type 2 diabetes than people who have waists that don't extend beyond their hips.[11] Fat cells, particularly visceral fat, make substances that cause inflammation in the body. These inflammatory factors may increase risks of type 2 diabetes and CVD.

Some people, especially women, tend to store extra subcutaneous fat below the waist, primarily in the buttocks and thighs (see **Fig. 10.5b**). Having a "pear shape" pattern of fat distribution adds stress to hip and knee joints that must carry the extra weight, which can lead to osteoarthritis (breakdown of joint tissues). This particular type of body fat distribution, however, isn't associated with increased risk of more serious chronic diseases such as type 2 diabetes.

a. Central-body fat distribution (apple shape)

b. Lower-body fat distribution (pear shape)

Figure 10.5 Body fat distribution: Typical sex differences.

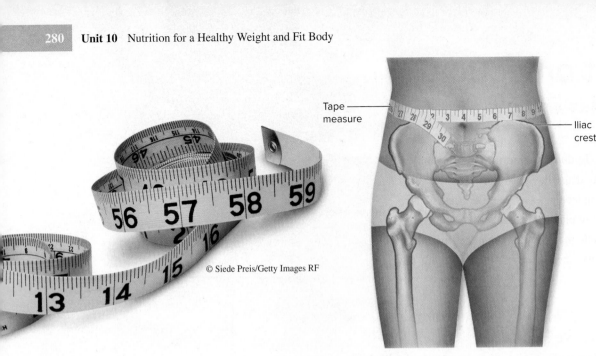

© Siede Preis/Getty Images RF

Figure 10.6 **Measuring waist circumference.**

■ *What is the waist circumference of a man who has central body obesity? What is the waist circumference of a woman with central-body obesity?*

A quick and easy method to determine whether you have an unhealthy amount of visceral fat is to measure your waist circumference. **Figure 10.6** shows the recommended placement of the tape measure. Note the positioning of a measuring tape at the top of the hip bones and not necessarily at the narrowest point.[12] A person with central-body obesity has a waist circumference that's greater than 40 inches (men) and greater than 35 inches (women).[12]

How can you determine whether your weight is within the healthy range for your height? How much body fat is unhealthy? The following sections of this module answer these questions.

10.1c What's Body Mass Index?

body mass index (BMI)
numerical value of relationship between body weight and risk of chronic health problems associated with excess body fat

At one time, people referred to height/weight tables to determine whether their body weights were "ideal" or "desirable." Today, medical experts use the **body mass index** (**BMI**) to judge whether an adult's weight is healthy. BMI is a numerical value based on the relationship between body weight and risk of chronic health problems associated with excess body fat.

How to Calculate Your BMI

To calculate your BMI, you can use the following formula:

$$\text{weight (lb)} \div [\text{height (in)}]^2 \times 703$$

For example, let's calculate the BMI of a person who weighs 140 pounds and is 5'3" (63"). Fill these numbers into the formula: $[140 \div (63)^2] \times 703$

Do the math:

Step 1: 63^2 is 63×63, which $= 3969$

Step 2: $[140 \div 3969] = 0.03527$

Step 3: $0.03527 \times 703 = 24.8$

This person's BMI is 24.8. To determine your BMI, replace the numbers in the formula with your height and weight values. You can also use the BMI calculator at http://www.nhlbi.nih.gov/health /educational/lose_wt/BMI/bmicalc.htm. What's your BMI?

Q Answer This

Calculate the BMI of a person who weighs 157 pounds and is 5' 6". You can find the answer on the last page of this unit.

BMI Categories

Table 10.2 presents adult weight classifications based on BMI ranges. Note that healthy BMIs range from 18.5 to 24.9. The "overweight" BMI category includes people who are overfat as well as people who have extra muscle and/or bone.

As BMI increases, the risks of heart disease, hypertension, type 2 diabetes, gallstones, certain cancers, and breathing problems increase. Thus, obese and *extremely* obese people are far more likely to develop the serious chronic diseases associated with excess body fat and to die prematurely than are people who have BMIs that range from 18.5 to 30.0. Extremely obese adults have BMIs that are 40.0 and higher. In 2011–2012, 6.4% of adult Americans were extremely obese.[3] This percentage is about 125% higher than the percentage of adults who were extremely obese in 1988 to 1994.

Limitations of the BMI

Muscle is denser than fat. Therefore, a muscular person whose BMI is in the overweight range may actually have a healthy percentage of body fat. For example, a college athlete with a BMI of 25.5 is more likely to be healthy than a nonathletic college student who also has a BMI of 25.5. The BMI may underestimate body fat in people who have lost muscle tissue as a result of aging or illness.[13] Therefore, BMIs should be used with caution when assessing the health of highly muscular individuals, people who are elderly, or chronically ill persons. However, people with BMIs of 30 or higher generally have excess body fat.

Your BMI doesn't provide the entire picture regarding your chances of developing diseases that are associated with having excess body fat. You should also consider whether you have major risk factors for cardiovascular disease, such as high blood pressure, a large waistline, and an inactive lifestyle.[13]

10.1d Measuring Body Fat

How is body fat measured? There are several scientific methods of measuring body fat, but most involve large and expensive equipment. Let's take a closer look at some less costly and more practical ways to estimate your level of body fat.

Bioelectrical Impedance

Bioelectrical impedance is a quick way to estimate body fat content. This method is based on the principle that water and electrolytes, such as sodium ions, conduct electricity. Fat tissue contains less water and electrolytes than does lean tissue. Therefore, body fat resists the flow of electricity more than lean tissue does.

The bioelectrical impedance device sends a painless, low-energy electrical current through a person's body via wires connected to electrodes placed on the subject's skin (**Fig. 10.7**). The device converts information about the body's resistance to the electrical current into an estimate of total body water. This information is used to predict the percentage of fat tissue in the body. The method is fairly accurate, as long as the subject's hydration status is normal. For home use, you can purchase a bioelectrical impedance device that resembles a bathroom scale, but scientific data about the machine's accuracy are lacking.

TABLE 10.2

ADULT WEIGHT STATUS CATEGORIES (BMI)	
BMI	**Weight Status**
Below 18.5	Underweight
18.5 to 24.9	Healthy
25.0 to 29.9	Overweight
30.0 to 39.9	Obese
40 and above	Extremely obese

Source: National Institutes of Health, National Heart Lung and Blood Institute: Classification of overweight and obesity by BMI, waist circumference, and associated disease risks. ND. http://www.nhlbi.nih.gov/health/educational/lose_wt/BMI/bmi_dis .htm Accessed: May 24, 2016.

Figure 10.7 Measuring bioelectrical impedance.

bioelectrical impedance
technique of estimating body composition in which a device measures the conduction of a weak electrical current through the body

Obese woman: © McGraw-Hill Education. Lars A. Niki, photographer; Bioelectrical impedance analysis device: RJL Systems

Skinfold Thickness

A commonly used technique for estimating total body fat involves taking **skinfold thickness measurements** at multiple body sites, including the triceps muscle of the arm (**Fig. 10.8**). The width of a skinfold indicates the depth of the subcutaneous fat at that site. To perform the measurements, a trained person pinches a section of the subject's skin, gently pulls it away from underlying muscle tissue, and uses special calipers to measure the thickness of the fat. After taking the measurements, the values are incorporated into a mathematical formula that provides a fairly accurate estimate of the subject's amount of body fat.

Skinfold thickness measurements are relatively easy and inexpensive to perform, but the method's accuracy largely depends on the number of sites that are measured and skill of the person performing the measurements. Also, the technique may underestimate total body fat when used on obese subjects. However, by combining the information collected from skinfold, waist and hip circumference, and body frame measurements, researchers can obtain more reliable estimates of an individual's total body fat.[14]

Figure 10.8 Measuring skinfold thickness.
© FotoSearch Stock Photography RF

skinfold thickness measurements
technique of estimating body composition in which calipers are used to measure the width of skinfolds at multiple body sites

10.1e How Much Body Fat Is Healthy?

Some body fat is essential for good health, but too much fat tissue can interfere with your body's ability to function normally. What percentage of body fat is too much for good health? **Table 10.3** classifies people into weight categories according to their percentage of body fat. A man is overweight when his body is 22 to 25% fat; a woman is overweight when her body is 32 to 37% fat.[15] A man is obese when fat comprises 26% or more of his body; a woman is obese when fat makes up 38% or more of her body. The average healthy young woman has more body fat than the average healthy young man because she needs the extra fat for reproductive purposes.

Adults tend to gain fat tissue as they age, but for older adults, some additional fat doesn't necessarily contribute to serious health problems. The extra fat may actually provide some health benefits, such as providing an energy reserve for a very ill person who cannot eat. Furthermore, the extra padding of fat may protect a person from being injured by falling.

TABLE 10.3

ADULT BODY WEIGHT CLASSIFICATION BY PERCENTAGE OF BODY FAT

Classification	Body Fat (%)	
	Men	**Women**
Healthy	13 to 21%	23 to 31%
Overweight	22 to 25%	32 to 37%
Obese	26 to 31%	38 to 42%
Extremely obese	32% or more	43% or more

Source: Adapted from: Food and Nutrition Board: *Dietary Reference Intakes for energy, carbohydrate, fiber, fat, fatty acids, cholesterol, protein, and amino acids (macronutrients).* Table 5.5, page 126, 2005. www.nap.edu/openbook/0309085373/html/126.html.

Women need more body fat than men for reproductive purposes.
© Jack Hollingsworth/Blend Images LLC RF

Module 10.2

Factors That Influence Your Body Weight

© Brand X Pictures/PunchStock RF

10.2 - Learning Outcomes

After reading Module 10.2, you should be able to

1. Define all of the key terms in this module.
2. Describe the uses of energy by the body, and explain the concept of energy balance.
3. Identify factors that influence the development of excess body weight.

10.2a Calories In; Calories Out

Just as a car engine uses a mixture of gasoline, ethanol, and oxygen to run properly, your body uses a mixture of biological fuels and oxygen to do its work. Biological fuels are foods and beverages that contain macronutrients (**energy intake**). Under normal conditions, our cells metabolize primarily glucose and fatty acids, but small amounts of amino acids are also used for energy.

Energy output (energy expenditure) refers to the energy (calories) cells use to carry out their activities. For example, your muscle cells need energy to contract, liver cells use energy to convert toxic compounds to safer substances, and intestinal cells need energy to absorb certain nutrients. The following sections discuss the major ways your body uses food energy.

Metabolic Energy Needs

Metabolism refers to all chemical changes, or reactions, that constantly occur in living cells. **Anabolic reactions** require energy to occur; **catabolic reactions** release energy. **Basal metabolism** is the minimal number of calories the body uses for vital activities after fasting and resting for 12 hours. Vital metabolic processes include breathing, circulating blood, and maintaining constant liver, brain, and kidney functions. Generally, basal metabolism accounts for most of the body's total energy use.[16]

Thyroid hormone, secreted by the thyroid gland, regulates the **metabolic rate,** that is, the rate at which cells use energy for their metabolic activities (see Fig. 9.3). A person who has an overactive thyroid gland produces too much thyroid hormone. This person has a higher-than-normal metabolic rate and loses weight as a result of this disease. Many overweight or obese people have thyroid hormone levels that are within the normal range. However, an individual who secretes slightly less thyroid hormone than other persons may have lower caloric needs and be more likely to become obese as a result.[17]

What Influences the Metabolic Rate?

In addition to thyroid hormone, numerous factors can increase or decrease basal metabolic rates:

- *Body composition:* Lean body mass is the major factor that influences the metabolic rate.[15] Muscle tissue, a component of lean body mass, is more metabolically active than fat tissue. In general, a person who has more muscle mass will have a higher metabolic rate than someone with less muscle tissue.

- *Sex:* Males generally have higher metabolic rates than women because they tend to have more lean body mass.

© Purestock/SuperStock RF

energy intake calories from foods and beverages that contain macronutrients and alcohol

energy output calories cells use to carry out their activities

anabolic reactions chemical changes in cells that require energy to occur

catabolic reactions chemical changes in cells that release energy

basal metabolism the minimal number of calories the body uses for vital activities after fasting and resting for 12 hours

metabolic rate body's rate of energy use a few hours after resting and eating

The metabolic rate declines as people grow older.

© Steve Mason/Getty Images RF

- *Age:* Basal metabolism declines as one grows older, primarily due to the loss of fat-free tissues such as muscle. As many adults grow older, they think their muscles have "turned into" fat. A muscle cell, however, cannot transform itself into a fat cell. During the aging process, lean tissue mass shrinks, as cells from muscle, bone, and organs die and aren't replaced. Fat cells, however, can continue to develop throughout life, especially when a person overeats consistently. When fat tissue expands in size, it can fill in the spaces formerly occupied by muscle and organ tissues. Regular exercise helps build and preserve lean body mass, so to some extent, you can reduce the decline in the metabolic rate by being physically active as you grow older.

- *Calorie intake:* Calorie intake also affects the metabolic rate. The body conserves energy when calorie intakes are very low or lacking altogether. Because following a very-low-calorie diet (fewer than 800 kcal/day) can reduce the metabolic rate, such diets aren't generally recommended for weight loss.

Calculating Metabolic Energy Needs

Your basal metabolic rate is fairly constant from day to day.[18] Thus, you can estimate your daily metabolic rate by following a "rule of thumb" formula:

$$\text{Formula for men} = 1.0 \text{ kcal/kg/hr}$$

$$\text{Formula for women} = 0.9 \text{ kcal/kg/hr}$$

To estimate the number of kcal you need for your basal metabolism, first convert your weight in pounds to kilograms by dividing your weight by 2.2. (A kilogram is approximately 2.2 pounds.)

$$\underline{\qquad} \text{ lb} \div 2.2 \text{ lb} = \underline{\qquad} \text{ kg}$$

Then, depending on your sex, use one of the following formulas:

$$\underline{\qquad} \text{ kg} \times 0.9 \text{ (women)} = \underline{\qquad} \text{ kcal/hr}$$

$$\underline{\qquad} \text{ kg} \times 1.0 \text{ (men)} = \underline{\qquad} \text{ kcal/hr}$$

Finally, use this hourly basal metabolic rate to estimate your basal metabolic rate for an entire day by multiplying the hourly value by 24.

$$\underline{\qquad} \text{ kcal/hr} \times 24 \text{ hr} = \underline{\qquad} \text{ kcal/day}$$

These calculations only provide an estimate of your daily metabolic rate. To estimate your Estimated Energy Requirement (EER) for a 24-hour period, you need to add kilocalories used for physical and other activities to your BMR figure.

Energy for Physical Activity

Physical activity increases energy output above basal metabolic needs. The number of kilocalories expended for a particular physical activity depends largely on the type of activity, how long it's performed (duration), the degree of effort used while performing the activity, and the weight of the person. A heavy person expends more kilocalories when performing the same activity, for the same duration, and at the same intensity than a lighter person. Why? The muscles of the heavier person must work harder to move the larger body.

Table 10.4 lists various physical activities and the approximate number of kilocalories an individual who weighs 150 pounds expends while performing each activity for a minute. For example, a 150-pound person who walks for 30 minutes (3.5 mph) burns approximately 153 kcal during the walk (30 × 5.1). The number of kilocalories you need for physical activity can vary widely, depending on how active you are each day. Because you can control the type, intensity, and duration of your physical activities, you can manipulate your energy output to increase, decrease, or maintain your weight. When you are sedentary, you don't burn as many calories as when you are moderately or vigorously active. To estimate your daily calorie expenditures for physical activity, visit https://www.supertracker.usda.gov/ and use the "Physical Activity Tracker" feature.

© Digital Vision/PunchStock RF

Nonexercise Activity Thermogenesis (NEAT)

Nonexercise activity thermogenesis (**NEAT**) refers to physical activity that a person doesn't consciously control. NEAT activities include

- shivering,
- fidgeting,

- maintaining muscle tone, and
- maintaining body posture when not lying down.

Some individuals may resist weight gain from overeating because they have higher-than-average energy expenditures for NEAT. Nevertheless, NEAT's contribution to overall calorie needs is minor for most people.

Thermic Effect of Food (TEF)

The body needs a relatively small amount of energy to digest foods and beverages as well as to absorb and further process the macronutrients. The energy used for these tasks, generally 5 to 10% of total caloric intake, is referred to as the **thermic effect of food** (**TEF**). For example, if your energy intake was 3000 kcal/day, TEF would account for 150 to 300 kcal.

nonexercise activity thermogenesis (NEAT) involuntary skeletal muscular activities such as fidgeting

thermic effect of food (TEF) energy used to digest foods and beverages as well as absorb and further process the macronutrients

TABLE 10.4

APPROXIMATE CALORIC OUTPUT/MINUTE OF SELECTED PHYSICAL ACTIVITIES (150-POUND PERSON)

Physical Activity	Approximate kcal/min.
Sitting and sewing	2
Canoeing (4 mph)	4
Dancing (fox trot)	4
Weight training	5
Bowling	6
Walking (3.5 mph)	6
Bicycling (10–12 mph)	10
Walking (4.5 mph)	10
Tennis (singles, recreational)	12
Hiking (with pack, 3 mph)	12
Touch football (vigorous)	12
Swimming (vigorous breaststroke)	15
Running/jogging, steady pace (6 mph)	15
Bicycling (15 mph)	15
Karate and other martial arts	15

Source: https://supertracker.usda.gov/physicalactivitytracker.aspx Accessed: June 1, 2016.

Figure 10.9   Energy balance. In addition to macronutrients, energy intake includes alcohol consumption.

■ *What will happen to your weight if your energy intake is consistently greater than your energy output?*

10.2b Energy Balance

Understanding the concept of energy balance is critical to understanding why people gain, lose, or maintain weight. Your body is in a state of **energy balance** when your calorie intake from food and beverages equals your calorie output for basal metabolism, physical activity, and TEF (**Fig. 10.9**). By maintaining a balanced energy state, your weight will remain relatively stable over time.

If your calorie intake is lower than your calorie output, you're in a **negative energy state**. Your body needs more calories to carry out its activities than your diet is supplying. Therefore, your body metabolizes more stored fat than usual for energy. Weight loss results from being in a negative energy state. Over time, you'll notice your clothes have become baggy as your fat tissue shrinks.

If your calorie intake is greater than your calorie output, you're in a **positive energy state**. Your body stores excess dietary fat in adipose cells. Additionally, your body converts surplus dietary carbohydrate and protein to fat and stores that fat in adipose cells. Weight gain results from being in a positive energy state, and eventually, you notice that your clothes seem to have shrunk.

One pound of body fat represents about 3500 kcal. This fact is often used to estimate how much you should reduce or increase your calorie intake to lose or gain a pound within a week or month. According to the "3500-kcal rule-of-thumb," you'll lose approximately 52 pounds of weight in a year if you reduce your usual caloric intake by 500 kcal/day (500 kcal/day × 365 days = 182,500 kcal; 182,500 kcal ÷ 3500 kcal/pound = ~52 pounds). Scientific studies, however, don't support using the 3500-kcal rule-of-thumb for predicting weight change over the long term.[19] Losing or gaining weight over time involves more factors (current weight, height, age, and physical activity level, for example) than simply cutting calories. Scientists developed a new formula that takes into account these factors. To estimate your caloric intake to achieve weight change by using this formula, visit https://www.nih.gov/ and type "body weight planner" in the search box.

Maintenance of energy balance—matching calorie intake to calorie output over the long term—is critical for controlling

energy balance calorie intake equals calorie output

negative energy state calorie intake is less than calorie output

positive energy state calorie intake is greater than calorie output

hunger uncomfortable feeling that drives a person to consume food

satiety sense that enough food or beverages have been consumed to satisfy hunger

ghrelin protein that stimulates eating behavior

Figure 10.10 Your body's possible energy states.

body weight (**Fig. 10.10**). To lose weight, you need to create a negative energy state by eating significantly fewer calories, expending more calories than the amount consumed, or taking both actions. If you're like many people, however, it isn't easy to make major changes to your calorie input and output and maintain the new lifestyle.

Putting It All Together

To estimate your daily energy expenditure, add the kilocalories you burned for basal metabolism, physical activity, and TEF in a day. An easier way to estimate your "calories in and calories out" is to visit the MyPlate web site (http://www.choosemyplate.gov) and access "Super-Tracker." By using the tools developed for the site, you can track and analyze your daily food intake and physical activity level.

10.2c Factors That Influence Weight Gain

Does your mood influence your eating behavior? Many people eat not because they are hungry but because they are bored, anxious, angry, or depressed. Other factors, including biological and environmental forces, also influence your calorie intake and output.

Biological Factors

Hunger and satiety are key sensations that regulate eating behavior. **Hunger** is an uncomfortable feeling that drives a person to consume food. **Satiety** is the sense that enough food or beverages have been consumed to satisfy hunger. A small area of the brain helps control hunger and satiety.

The size of your stomach also influences satiety. During meals, your stomach stretches as it fills. The sensation that the stomach has reached its capacity can make you stop eating. Nevertheless, many overfat persons don't recognize the sensation of stomach fullness, and as a result, they may eat even when they shouldn't be hungry.

The stomach, intestines, and fat tissue produce certain proteins that stimulate nerve cells involved in the regulation of hunger and satiety. **Ghrelin** (*greh'-lin*), a hormone secreted mainly by the stomach, stimulates eating behavior. Some scientists think that reducing

TASTY Tidbits

Results of scientific studies suggest that watching television is associated with obesity among children and adults.[20,21] Television programming is a sedentary activity that may include food advertisements. Additionally, people often eat high-fat foods while they watch TV. Health experts recommend that you limit your nonwork-related screen time (including activities involving computers and video games) to no more than 2 hours/day.[22]

© BananaStock/PunchStock RF

leptin hormone that reduces hunger and inhibits fat storage in the body

set-point theory scientific notion that body fat content is genetically predetermined

appetite desire to eat appealing food

ghrelin production or activity is the key to helping people lose or maintain their weight. Fat cells secrete **leptin**, a hormone that reduces hunger and inhibits fat storage in the body. Studies involving humans generally find that obese people produce high amounts of leptin, but their bodies resist the hormone's hunger-suppressing action.[23]

Genetic Factors

Several genes contribute to human fatness. Researchers are interested in developing medications that regulate these genes. If such medications are safe and effective, they could help people manage their weight over the long term.

If you gain weight easily, you may have inherited a *thrifty metabolism*. A person with a thrifty metabolism has a body that's more efficient at storing excess energy as fat than a person who doesn't have such a metabolism. An energy "thrifty" person

is more likely to survive periods of starvation than other persons. In the United States, however, high-calorie "convenience" foods are available 24 hours a day and starvation is unlikely. Therefore, having a thrifty metabolism is not beneficial for most Americans because depositing excess body fat often results in serious health problems.

According to the **set-point theory,** the body's fat content is genetically predetermined. The set point acts like a home thermostat, except that it regulates body weight instead of temperature. For example, a person infected with an intestinal virus may lose a pound or two because he or she has no interest in eating for a few days. During and after recovery, the person generally regains the lost weight. This may explain why the majority of people who intentionally lose weight regain the weight over time.

Environmental Influences

Appetite is the desire to eat appealing food. If you often eat when you're not hungry, then you're probably aware of the effect your environment can have on your appetite. For example, do you get the urge to eat when you see an open bag of candy or a clock that indicates it's "lunch time"?

Food advertising is an aspect of the environment that has a powerful influence on your food choices. To entice you to buy their products, food manufacturers usually appeal to your senses, emphasizing the appearance and taste of food, in particular. How do you respond when you see food advertisements on television? Do the ads make you hungry or eager to try a new food product?

Food advertisers also try to appeal to your emotions. You may choose to purchase "supersized" portions of foods because you like the idea of getting more for your money. In many instances, however, "more" means more fat and calories per serving. According to some nutrition experts, the increased consumption of oversized portions of many popular restaurant foods contributes to the widespread obesity problem in the United States.[24]

Your environment also affects whether you choose to be physically inactive (*sedentary*) or physically active. At home, you may rely on a variety of "energy-saving" devices such as floor-hugging automatic vacuum sweepers, TV remote controls, and garage door openers to work for you. Outside your home, you may use cars, elevators, escalators, and other motorized devices, instead of your feet, to move from place to place. With the help of machines, your life is considerably easier, but you may not be burning enough calories every day as a result.

Environmental factors, including the 24-hour-a-day availability of high-calorie foods, can contribute to overeating.

© McGraw-Hill Education. Andrew Resnick, photographer

Module 10.3

Managing Your Weight Safely

© Mike Kemp/Getty Images RF

10.3 - Learning Outcomes

After reading Module 10.3, you should be able to

1. Define all of the key terms in this module.
2. Evaluate weight-reduction diets for safety and long-term effectiveness.
3. Identify medical options for overweight and obesity.
4. Identify key factors for successful weight loss and maintenance.
5. Plan a long-term weight-loss regimen that's safe and effective.
6. Discuss ways to gain weight safely and sensibly.

McKenzie, the young woman featured in the unit opener, lowered her intake of total calories by reducing her consumption of added sugars and fats.

An overweight or obese person doesn't have to shed a lot of weight to reduce risk factors associated with CVD, stroke, and type 2 diabetes. Just losing 5 to 10% of excess body fat can increase beneficial high-density lipoprotein levels (HDL cholesterol), reduce elevated blood pressure, and lower blood glucose and triglyceride levels.[13]

10.3a Features of Medically Sound Weight-Loss Plans

Despite claims made in Internet advertisements and TV infomercials, there are no quick cures for overweight and obesity. No particular diet or food has a "metabolic advantage" by promoting greater calorie burning by the body. A dieter's goal should be reducing total calorie intake while obtaining all essential nutrients.

A sound weight-loss plan

- is safe and effective;
- meets nutritional, psychological, and social needs;
- incorporates a variety of common foods from all food groups;
- doesn't require costly devices or diet books;
- accommodates family and restaurant meals, parties and special occasions, ethnic foods, and food likes;
- doesn't make you feel deprived;
- emphasizes readily available nutritious foods;
- promotes changing habits that encourage overeating;
- encourages regular physical activity;
- provides suggestions for obtaining social support; and
- can be followed for a lifetime.

© Wendy Schiff

289

10.3b Weight Loss: Key Factors for Success

The motivation to lose weight and keep it off requires an overfat person to recognize that there's a need to change his or her behaviors. Furthermore, the person is committed to making those changes permanent. For some people, this recognition occurs when they are diagnosed with a serious health disorder that's associated with excess body fat. The commitment to lose weight, maintain the lost weight, and enjoy better health must become far more important than the desire to overeat.

Successful weight-loss treatments and long-term weight maintenance often include making lifestyle changes and changing behaviors.[25] The following sections provide some basic information and practical tips for achieving and maintaining a healthy weight.

Setting Goals

For many overfat people, the first step to losing excess body fat is to set a realistic weight-loss goal.[25] Overfat adults should strive to lose at least 5 to 10% of their current weight over a 6-month period. How much weight an overfat person loses during this period depends on many factors, including the person's starting weight and the degree of calorie restriction.

Making Lifestyle Changes

Lifestyle includes diet and physical activity. To make your lifestyle healthier, you need to identify what needs to change. What or how much do you eat? How do your food choices contribute to your excess body fat? During a typical day, how physically active are you? For example, are your portion sizes too generous, do you eat fast foods and/or drink sugary soft drinks too often, or do you sit too much?

Calorie Reduction

A reasonable rate of weight loss for an overweight or obese person is 1 to 2 pounds per week.[25] People who have excess body fat can usually accomplish this rate of loss by reducing their calorie intake or increasing their physical activity (energy output). Although many overweight and obese people would like to shed more than 2 pounds per week, registered dietitians recommend a slow and steady rate.

In general, the more weight a person needs to lose, the faster he or she will lose weight when following a calorie-restricted diet. However, an obese dieter's rate of weight loss tends to slow down as his or her weight reaches a healthier level.

Certain diets severely limit food intake and provide fewer than 800 kcal/day. Such very-low-calorie diets aren't recommended for most overfat persons.[26] Such diets generally require a physician's supervision. Patients (especially women) who follow a very-low-calorie diet and lose weight rapidly often develop gallstones. It is not unusual for obese people to lose a lot of weight during the first few months of following a very-low-calorie diet. However, they are likely to regain the weight quickly after they "go off" the diet and return to their former eating and physical activity habits.

Physical Activity

When combined with reduced calorie intake, regular physical activity is critical for weight loss and maintenance. The more physically active you are, the more calories you'll burn. Module 10.5 focuses on physical activity, including the health benefits of a physically active lifestyle.

TASTY Tidbits

Regular exercise, such as walking, can shrink abdominal fat, but it isn't possible to "spot-reduce" by exercising a fatty body part intensely.[16] The energy needed to fuel muscle activity comes from fatty deposits within muscle tissue and the rest of the body. Exercise, however, can improve muscle tone, so that fat tissue appears less flabby.

© Fancy Collection/SuperStock RF

Changing Your Food- and Exercise-Related Practices

Consider the following suggestions, which may help you lose excess weight as well as maintain a lower, healthier body weight.

- **Planning Menus**
  1. Plan meals and snacks to cover three or more days, then use the plan to prepare grocery lists.
  2. When menu planning, include sources of protein, unsaturated fat, and complex carbohydrates in meals and snacks.
  3. Avoid labeling certain foods as "off limits." Depriving yourself of such items can result in bingeing on the "forbidden" food. Analyze why you have difficulty controlling your intake of these foods. Then develop strategies to learn how to reduce your intake of them.

- **Shopping Carefully**
  1. To reduce the likelihood of making impulsive food choices, shop for food after eating.
  2. Shop from a grocery list. If a food isn't on your list, ask yourself if you really need to buy it and if it will hinder or help your weight-loss efforts.
  3. Read food labels to compare calorie and saturated fat contents per serving.

- **Preparing and Serving Your Food**
  1. Reduce the use of solid fat in cooking; bake, broil, or roast meats instead of frying them.
  2. Add less solid fat to foods such as cooked vegetables before serving or eating them.
  3. If you sample foods while preparing them, consider the amounts you ate, and at mealtimes reduce your portion sizes accordingly.
  4. Prepare only enough food to provide one limited-size portion for yourself. Using measuring cups and a small scale for weighing food can be helpful.

  5. Take your usual-size portion and return one-third to one-half of it to the serving dish or container.
  6. Remove serving dishes from the table. Keeping foods or their containers in sight can encourage overeating.

- **Eating Smart**
  1. Keep nutrient-dense, low-calorie snack foods, such as fresh fruits and vegetables, on hand.
  2. Eat meals and snacks at scheduled times; don't skip meals, especially breakfast.
  3. Eat all food in a "dining" area; avoid eating while engaged in other activities, such as when reading a book or watching television.

TASTY Tidbits

According to limited data, approximately 20% of overweight and obese people who intentionally lose weight can avoid regaining most of the weight for at least 5 years.[27]

  4. Slow down the pace of meals by putting eating utensils down between mouthfuls and eating more slowly.
  5. Leave some food on your plate.
  6. Become a "defensive eater." Practice ways to refuse food graciously or request smaller portions. Be aware of people, especially relatives and friends, who sabotage your weight-loss efforts. Examples of such sabotage include a person who repeatedly offers calorie-dense foods to you, even though you have turned down the food and this person knows you're trying to lose weight.

- **Preparing for Holidays and Parties**
  1. Before you go, think about what you'll eat and drink while attending the meal or event.
  2. Consider limiting your food intake earlier in the day of the special occasion to avoid consuming too many calories at the event.
  3. Eat a low-calorie snack about an hour before the occasion.
  4. Drink fewer alcoholic and sugar-sweetened beverages. Replace such beverages with ice water.

- **Using Caution at Restaurants**
  1. Avoid eating regularly at fast-food outlets.
  2. Choose pasta with red sauce instead of white sauce.
  3. Request salad dressing "on the side" so you can control the amount.
  4. Think "small." Order an entrée and share it with another person.
  5. Don't be a member of the "clean plate club." Ask your server for a carryout box when he or she brings your order to the table. Then divide the food in half, and place one-half in the container. Be sure to refrigerate the leftovers within 2 hours after the meal, and eat them for a meal the following day.
  6. If you choose a dessert item, share it with others.
  7. Avoid fried menu items or those made with butter, gravy, or cream sauce.
  8. When at fast-food outlets, make substitutions:
     - salad instead of a fried fish sandwich,
     - regular hamburger instead of a specialty burger,
     - roasted chicken sandwich instead of a breaded and fried chicken sandwich,
     - plain water instead of a regular soft drink, and
     - baked potato instead of fries, if possible.

Woman looking at food label: © McGraw-Hill Education. Andrew Resnick, photographer; Small food scale: © Wendy Schiff; Man on scales: © Digital Vision/Getty Images RF

© liquidllibrary/PictureQuest RF

- *Self-Monitoring*

   1. Set reasonable weight-loss goals, for example, losing 1 to 4 pounds in 1 month. When you achieve that goal, set another reasonable goal, and continue with this process until the goal weight is achieved.

   2. Keep a special notebook to use as a food and exercise diary where you can see it—near the kitchen table or refrigerator, for example.

   3. In the diary, note the time and place of eating as well as the type and amount of food eaten. Also record your mood when you ate meals and snacks. Use the diary to identify your food-related problem areas, such as eating when bored or depressed.

   4. In the exercise section of the diary, record the form of moderate-intensity exercise you performed and the number of minutes you spent engaging in that activity each day.

   5. Measure your waistline weekly and record the measurements in the diary.

   6. Weigh yourself several times a week, preferably at the same time and without clothing. However, don't rely only on your weight as an indication of your progress. Regular exercise often increases muscle mass that can result in weight gain or failure to lose weight. Still, adding muscle mass is healthier than maintaining too much body fat.

- *Obtaining Social Support*

   1. Consider joining a group weight-loss program. You may make new friends and benefit from others' experiences and support as a result.

   2. Encourage family and friends to provide praise and encouragement for your efforts to manage your weight. Let family, friends, and associates know that you're trying to lose weight and you would appreciate their help and support.

- *Changing Negative Thought Patterns*

   1. Don't get discouraged by occasional setbacks—relapses can be expected when changing behaviors. For example, instead of thinking, "I can't lose weight. I'm a failure," say to yourself, "OK, so I lost control and had too much to eat at the wedding. I just need to get back on track. I'll pull in the reins on my eating for the next day and exercise more."

   2. Think positively about progress. "I didn't lose any weight this week, but I didn't gain any either. I must be losing fat and getting trimmer—those jeans fit better than they did 2 months ago."

   3. Counter negative thoughts with positive statements. "This afternoon, I'll just have to walk a little longer and harder to burn off those extra calories."

Successful Dieters— How Do They Manage Their Weight?

The National Weight Control Registry tracks a group of over 10,000 adult Americans, mostly women, who have lost an average of 66 pounds and maintained the weight loss for at least 5.5 years.[28] Registry members tend to

- eat a low-calorie, low-fat diet;

- exercise, on average, for about an hour daily;

- eat breakfast daily;

- watch less than 10 hours of television per week; and

- weigh themselves at least once a week.

© Wendy Schiff

Overfat people may find it easier to lose weight by eating regular meals, including breakfast.

10.3c Medical Treatments for Obesity

Obese patients are often unsatisfied with the amount of weight they lose while following fad as well as conventional diets. The frustration of repeated dieting leads some obese persons to turn to physicians for medications and even surgical procedures to help lose weight.

Weight-Loss Medications

In 2015, the only medications approved by the FDA for long-term use for weight loss were orlistat ("Alli"), Contrave, Saxenda, Belviq, and Qsymia.[29] Orlistat reduces some fat absorption by the small intestine; Belviq and Qsymia suppress hunger. These medicines can aid weight-loss efforts, but they don't replace the need to reduce calorie intake and increase physical activity.

Surgical Procedures

Bariatric (*bar-ee-a'-tric*) **medicine** is the medical specialty that focuses on the treatment of obesity. Such surgical procedures drastically reduce the size of an obese person's stomach, markedly limiting food intake. Bariatric surgeries result in weight loss partly because the stomach pouch fills quickly with food; patients experience satiety sooner than they did prior to surgery. Moreover, overeating causes discomfort or vomiting. Thus, people who undergo such surgical procedures must make major lifestyle changes, such as learning to plan and consume frequent, small meals.

Patients often achieve normal blood pressure, glucose levels, and triglyceride levels after surgery. Furthermore, overall death rates may be lower for extremely obese people who lose weight after undergoing bariatric surgery.[30] Such surgeries are relatively safe; fewer than 1% of patients die as a result of a bariatric surgical procedure.[31]

In the United States, bariatric surgery is commonly used to treat extreme obesity. **Figure 10.11a** illustrates the appearance of the stomach and intestine after the *Roux-en-Y* operation. This procedure involves using surgical staples to reduce the obese patient's stomach capacity to about 1.5 oz, which is approximately the volume of one egg. Additionally, the surgeon cuts the small intestine and attaches the lower end of it to the newly formed stomach pouch (see Fig. 10.11a). The "bypassed" section of the intestine doesn't receive food, so digestion and absorption are reduced as a result of the surgery.

Sleeve gastrectomy also reduces the stomach's size (**Fig. 10.11b**). During this procedure, the surgeon staples the stomach to form a banana-shaped pouch that holds about 2 to 5 ounces of food. The surgery doesn't involve bypassing a section of the small intestine, so nutrient absorption isn't reduced. These patients lose weight because they aren't as hungry as they were before having the surgery. Why? The portion of the stomach that secretes ghrelin is removed during surgery, and as a result, hunger sensations are reduced (see Fig. 10.11b). Sleeve gastrectomy surgery is irreversible because the unused portion of the stomach is removed.

Complications often associated with gastric bypass surgery include intestinal blockage and bleeding, leaks along the staple site, blood clot formation, and wound infections. After surgery, gastric bypass patients can develop micronutrient deficiencies and some bone loss. However, patients can reduce their risk of nutrient deficiencies by taking vitamin and mineral supplements.

The adjustable gastric banding procedure creates a small stomach pouch with an adjustable band instead of fixed surgical staples

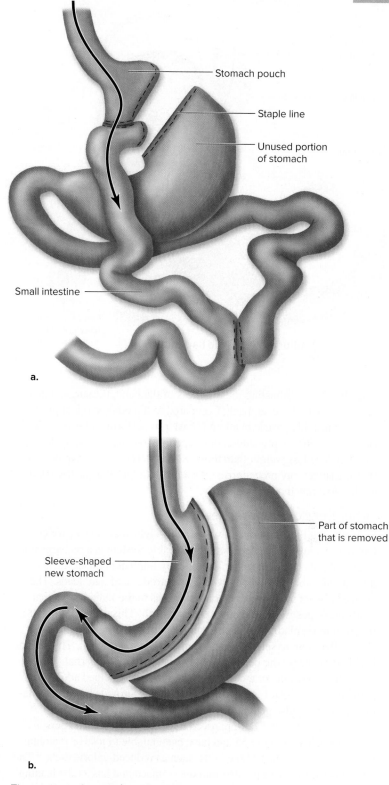

a.
Stomach pouch
Staple line
Unused portion of stomach
Small intestine

b.
Part of stomach that is removed
Sleeve-shaped new stomach

Figure 10.11 Gastric bypass surgeries.

▪ *How do gastric bypass surgeries aid in weight loss?*

bariatric medicine medical specialty that focuses on the treatment of obesity

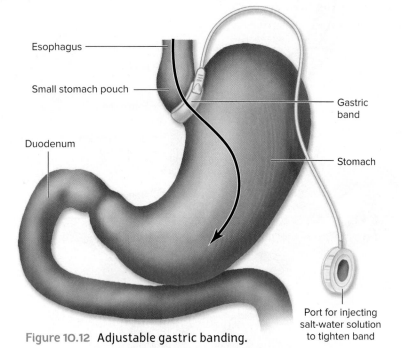

Esophagus

Small stomach pouch

Duodenum

Gastric band

Stomach

Port for injecting salt-water solution to tighten band

Figure 10.12 **Adjustable gastric banding.**

(**Fig. 10.12**). By adjusting the tightness of the band, the surgeon determines the size of the stomach. Compared to the other surgical procedures, adjustable gastric banding is easier to perform and reversible. However, with this procedure, obese people lose weight more slowly and they lose less weight than those who undergo gastric bypass or sleeve gastrectomy procedures.[32] As a result, adjustable gastric banding has lost much of its popularity.

Other Surgical Approaches

Recently, the FDA approved two unique weight-loss devices for certain obese adults. The Maestro Rechargeable System is a rechargeable electrical pulse generator that is surgically implanted under the skin in the patient's abdomen, along with its electrodes and wire leads. The device delivers intermittent electrical pulses to the major nerve that sends messages from the brain to the stomach. This particular nerve is involved in regulating stomach emptying after meals. The nerve also signals the brain to sense that the stomach is empty or full. The patient is able to recharge the pulse generator with a special external charger. According to results of a clinical study, the device helped adult obese patients lose weight, but ongoing research will provide more information about the pulse generator's long-term safety and effectivenss.[33]

AspireAssist is an FDA-approved device for use in obese persons who have BMIs of 35 to 55 and have been unable to lose or maintain weight using nonsurgical methods, such as reduced-calorie diets.[34] The device is surgically implanted into the stomach and has a tube leading from the stomach to an opening "port" that is on the patient's abdominal skin. After a meal, the person is able to open the port and drain a portion of his or her stomach's contents into the toilet. As a result, about 30% of the calories that were consumed do not enter the small intestine and some weight loss occurs.[34]

10.3d Unreliable Weight-Loss Methods

Each year, Americans spend billions of dollars on products and services promoted to help them lose weight. Some people who have excess body fat join commercial weight-loss programs that can be useful for encouraging safe weight loss and maintenance. However, many overweight

fad trendy practice that has widespread appeal for a period, then becomes no longer fashionable

© FoodCollection/StockFood RF

and obese people seek "quick fixes" to lose weight, such as fad diets and dietary supplements promoted to "burn" or "melt" fat fast.

Fad Diets

A **fad** is a trendy practice that has widespread appeal. After a period, however, people lose interest in the practice, and it becomes no longer fashionable. Fad diets often rely on *gimmicks*. A gimmick is an unusual feature or food, such as "raspberry ketones" and "green tea extract," that makes the diet seem to be unique and more likely to work than other diets. Some fad diets use the gimmick of emphasizing one food or food group while excluding almost all others. The grapefruit diet, for example, promotes eating this single food.

Dieters may lose some weight while following eating plans that restrict food variety, but the weight loss occurs because the diet is low in calories, not because grapefruit, açai berries, or other "diet food" contain compounds that cause rapid weight loss. Eventually, dieters abandon such restrictive menu plans because they crave a slice of bread and cannot face another bowl of grapefruit. If they return to their prior eating and other lifestyle habits, fad dieters usually regain much of the weight that they lost while on the diet.

If you examine any diet plan carefully, you can determine whether it's probably a fad. A typical fad diet

- promotes rapid weight loss without calorie restriction and increased physical activity;
- limits food selections from a few food groups and requires specific rituals, such as eating only fruit for breakfast or eating only certain food combinations;
- requires buying a book or various gimmicks, such as expensive dietary supplements, weight-loss patches, or beverages that contain "secret" weight-loss ingredients; or
- relies on testimonials from famous people or connects the diet to trendy places such as Hollywood, California, and South Beach, Florida.

Low-Carbohydrate Approaches

Fad weight-loss diets that limit carbohydrate intakes and are high in protein and saturated fat include the Dr. Atkins' New Diet Revolution, the Scarsdale Diet, and the early phases of the South Beach Diet. A weight-reduction diet is low carbohydrate if it eliminates or severely restricts the intake of carbohydrate-rich foods such as breads, cereals, fruits, vegetables, and sweets.

Low-carbohydrate diets usually produce rapid weight loss initially, primarily because the body loses water. Why? The body produces less glycogen when carbohydrate intake is low and uses much of its stored glycogen to supply glucose for energy. Tissues maintain about 3 grams of water with each gram of glycogen, so a reduction in body glycogen content results in the need for less water to store with it. The kidneys eliminate the excess water in urine.

Carbohydrate-restricted diets often improve high-density lipoprotein ("good cholesterol") and serum triglyceride levels. Such diets can be helpful for losing weight, controlling blood glucose levels, and reducing the risk of CVD.[35] More studies, however, are needed to determine whether low-carbohydrate diets are safe and reduce the risk of CVD when followed for long periods.

Very-Low-Fat Approaches

Very-low-fat diets, such as the Pritikin Diet and the "Eat More, Weigh Less" diet plan, supply approximately 5 to 10% of calories from fat. Such diets generally result in rapid weight loss. Although very-low-fat diets aren't harmful for healthy adults, they are difficult to follow for the long term. Fat contributes to the flavor and texture of foods. Therefore, very-low-fat diets aren't tasty, and they eliminate many foods that are usually high on peoples' favorite foods lists, such as ice cream and meat.

What About Dietary Supplements for Weight Loss?

Many overweight and obese people are attracted to dietary supplements for weight loss because they believe promoters' claims that their products are "magic bullets" for shedding unwanted weight quickly and effortlessly. In general, there's a lack of scientific evidence that supports claims of their effectiveness or long-term safety. At this point, medical experts don't recommend any dietary supplement for weight loss, including products containing green tea extracts, chitosan, or other substances presented in **Table 10.5.**

TABLE 10.5

SELECTED WEIGHT-LOSS SUPPLEMENTS: EFFECTIVE OR NOT EFFECTIVE?

Supplement	Usefulness	Side Effects/Safety Concerns (Usual Doses)
Bitter orange	May increase metabolic rate and suppress appetite. Mixed results concerning weight loss	Some negative effects reported, including chest pain and increased blood pressure and heart rate
Chitosan	Little effect on weight loss	May cause gastrointestinal discomfort including nausea, constipation, and intestinal gas
Chromium	May enhance weight loss to a small extent	Headache, diarrhea, dizziness
Conjugated linoleic acid	Has minimal effect on reducing body weight	Appears to be safe, but can cause gastrointestinal upset
Ephedrine (ma huang, ephedra, ephedra sinica, sida cordifolia, pinellia, and ephedrine with caffeine)	Ephedrine-containing products promote short-term weight loss but also increase risk of serious side effects. Ephedra-containing dietary supplements are banned in the United States.	May cause rapid heart rate, elevated blood pressure, dizziness, sweating, headache, and sleep disturbances. Linked to heart attacks, strokes, and deaths
Garcinia cambogia (hydroxycitric acid, HCA)	Overall evidence does not suggest usefulness	May cause headache, nausea, and gastrointestinal discomfort
Glucomannan	Little or no effect on body weight	Tablet forms can block the esophagus. Diarrhea, intestinal gas, and abdominal discomfort
Green tea and green tea extracts	May enhance weight loss to a small extent	Contains caffeine. Concentrated extracts linked to severe liver damage
Guar gum	Not effective	May cause diarrhea and intestinal gas
Hoodia	Few studies involving humans have been conducted; not effective	Increases blood pressure and heart rate
Pyruvate	Possible minimal effect of weight loss	None reported but may reduce "good" cholesterol levels
Raspberry ketone	More research is needed.	Unknown
Yohimbe	Not effective	Serious negative effects, including hypertension and rapid heart rate

Source: National Institutes of Health, Office of Dietary Supplements: *Dietary supplements for weight loss.* Updated 2015. https://ods.od.nih.gov/factsheets/WeightLoss-HealthProfessional/ Accessed: May 26, 2016.

What *IS* That? - - - - - - - - - - - - →

Promoters of products that contain açai, such as açai juice, claim the tropical fruit has numerous healthful benefits, including stimulating weight loss. Although açai is a source of antioxidants that may reduce inflammation, there is little scientific evidence to support any claims for weight loss.[36]

© Wendy Schiff

Analyzing Advertising Hype

Be wary of weight-loss claims that the product or service

- *Causes rapid and extreme weight loss.* Ads commonly use outrageous claims such as "Lose up to 18 pounds in one week!" to attract consumers. The use of the modifier "up to" means that the person using the product could lose considerably less than 18 pounds a week.

- *Requires no need to change dietary patterns or physical activity.* Principles of energy balance don't support claims such as "Lose weight without dieting or strenuous exercise" and "Eat as much as you want—the more you eat, the more you'll lose."

- *Results in permanent weight loss.* Claims such as "Discover the secret to permanent weight loss" and "Lose weight and keep it off" often appear in ads. These claims target consumers who have lost weight but gained it back and are wary of weight-loss products. Long-term weight loss is difficult to achieve without calorie reduction and regular exercise, and claims that permanent weight loss can result simply from using a product are questionable.

- *Is scientifically proven or doctor endorsed.* Some ads claim their product or service has been "clinically tested," "scientifically proven," or "physician recommended." Scientific testing of the product or service supposedly occurred at "leading" medical centers or universities. However, most ads don't provide information about testing sites or journals where the results were published. Endorsements by medical professionals can be misleading.

- *Displays before-and-after photos.* If you read carefully, you may find disclaimers in small print, such as "results not typical," at the bottom of the "after" photo.

- *Includes a money-back guarantee.* Consumers should recognize that a product doesn't necessarily work just because it's guaranteed. The FTC frequently sues companies that fail to return money to dissatisfied consumers as their ads guarantee.

- *Is safe or natural.* Ads may include safety-related claims, such as "proven 100% safe" or "safe, immediate weight loss." Despite such assurances, weight-loss supplement manufacturers usually have little scientific evidence to support safety claims, particularly concerning long-term use of their products. Furthermore, "natural" doesn't indicate safety. Mushrooms are natural, but many kinds of mushrooms are highly toxic and even deadly.

- *Is supported by satisfied customers.* Testimonials generally provide little reliable information about what consumers can expect from using the product.

10.3e Gaining Weight

In 2011–2012, 2.5% of Americans who were 20 to 39 years of age were underweight.[37] An underweight individual has a BMI that's less than 18.5. Many underweight individuals want to gain weight, especially muscle mass.

For an underweight person, gaining weight can be just as challenging as losing weight is for an overfat person. To gain weight, underweight adults can gradually increase their consumption of calorie-dense foods, especially those high in healthy fats. Fatty fish (such as salmon), olives, avocados, seeds, low-fat cheeses, nuts and nut butters, bananas, and granola made with dried fruit, seeds, and nuts are high-calorie nutritious food choices with low saturated-fat content. Additionally, underweight people can replace beverages such as soft drinks with more nutritious calorie sources, such as 100% fruit juices, smoothies, and milk shakes made with peanut butter and fat-reduced ice cream. Encouraging a regular meal and snack schedule also aids in weight gain and maintenance.

© fStop/Getty Images RF

Module 10.4

Disordered Eating and Eating Disorders

© McGraw-Hill Education. Lars A. Niki, photographer

10.4 - Learning Outcomes

After reading Module 10.4, you should be able to

1. Define all of the key terms in this module.

2. Explain why disordered eating practices and eating disorders are common among young Americans.

3. Identify major kinds of eating disorders, and discuss signs and symptoms, risk factors, and treatments for these conditions.

With the prevalence of obesity rising rapidly in the United States, it isn't surprising that many American adolescents and young adults are concerned about their body shape and weight. Furthermore, the media constantly bombard us with images of the "ideal" body. Television shows and movies often portray thin women or muscular men as happy and successful. Excessive concern about body size and social pressure to avoid weight gain can lead to abnormal food-related practices such as skipping meals, limiting food choices, following fad diets, and bingeing on food. Such disordered eating behaviors are temporary and often occur when a person is under a lot of stress or wants to lose weight to improve his or her appearance. When a person adopts disordered eating behaviors as a lifestyle, the practices can become harmful and difficult-to-treat eating disorders.

Eating disorders are psychological disturbances that lead to serious health problems. In the United States, physicians can diagnose three major types of eating disorders: anorexia nervosa, bulimia nervosa, and binge-eating (overeating) disorder.[38] The causes of eating disorders are unknown, but genetic, social, and psychological factors contribute to their development.

Anorexia nervosa and bulimia nervosa are more likely to develop during adolescence. Binge-eating disorder tends to occur during the adult years. However, these conditions can begin at any age.

Known risk factors for eating disorders include

- sex (females are more likely to develop eating disorders),

- having a history of frequent dieting to control weight,

- being overly concerned or dissatisfied with body shape and weight,

- having low self-esteem and a poor self-image,

- being in a sport or occupation that emphasizes a lean body,

- having a history of being a victim of sexual abuse,[39] and

- being from a dysfunctional family.

Hollywood often portrays thin women or muscular men as happy and successful. This can create unrealistic attitudes toward body image, especially in young people.

© Ingram Publishing/SuperStock RF

eating disorders psychological disturbances that lead to certain physiological changes and serious health complications

297

© Alex Cao/Getty Images RF

10.4a Binge-Eating Disorder

People with binge-eating disorder (BED) often eat an unusually large amount of food at one time (bingeing). People with binge-eating disorder also may eat

- more quickly than usual during binge episodes,
- until they feel uncomfortably full,
- excessive amounts of food even when they're not hungry, and
- alone, because they're embarrassed about their overeating behavior.

After overeating, persons with BED feel disgusted, depressed, or guilty. Individuals with the disorder often feel they cannot control their eating behavior. Unlike someone with bulimia nervosa, a person who has BED doesn't purge (try to eliminate the excess calories) following an episode of binge eating.

In the United States, BED is the most common eating disorder.[40] An estimated 3.5% of American women and 2% of American men have binge-eating disorder. Although anyone can have BED, the disorder is more common in people who are extremely obese.

10.4b Bulimia Nervosa

Bulimia nervosa (**BN**) is characterized by reoccurring episodes of bingeing. Food binges often consist of high-calorie foods and are followed by attempts to purge the calories consumed during binges by self-induced vomiting, as well as abusing laxatives, diuretics, or enemas. Repeated vomiting can cause

- blood chemistry abnormalities; blood potassium can drop dramatically, altering heartbeat and increasing risk of sudden death;
- swelling of the throat;
- tears and bleeding of the esophagus;
- sores or scars on the knuckles (from self-induced vomiting); and
- tooth decay (from self-induced vomiting).

The person with BN feels a lack of control over the purging behaviors. In the United States, about 1.5% of women and 0.5% of men develop BN during their lifetimes.[39]

People with BN are often disgusted with their binge-purge practices. As a result, they often try to hide these behaviors from others. Individuals who have bulimia may be difficult to identify by their appearance because they tend to have BMIs in the healthy range.[41] However, they may view themselves as being overweight and rely excessively on body shape and weight to judge themselves. It is important to recognize that people with bulimia may have a history of anorexia nervosa.

10.4c Anorexia Nervosa

Anorexia nervosa (**AN**) is a severe psychological disturbance characterized by self-imposed starvation that results in malnutrition and extreme underweight. A person with AN maintains a body weight that's 15% or more below the normal weight for his or her height.[42] In the United States, 0.3% of men and 0.9% of women develop AN during their lifetimes.[39]

People with AN

- limit calorie intake, which leads to very low body weight;
- are emotionally disturbed about their body weight and shape;
- have an intense fear of gaining weight or becoming fat, despite their very low weight; and
- deny that they have a serious illness.

In 2010, French model Isabelle Caro died as a result of complications from severe anorexia nervosa. She was 28 years of age.

© Mercier Serge/ZUMAPRESS/Newscom

bulimia nervosa (BN) eating disorder characterized by cyclic episodes of bingeing and calorie-restrictive dieting

anorexia nervosa (AN) severe psychological disturbance characterized by self-imposed starvation

In addition to extreme thinness, signs and symptoms of AN generally include

- confusion or slowed thinking;
- widespread delicate, dense, white hairs on the skin;
- shrunken breasts and buttocks;
- emotional depression;
- low blood potassium levels; and
- tooth decay (from self-induced vomiting).

To lose weight or prevent weight gain, people with AN often avoid eating, especially in front of others, and they may engage in one or more of the following practices:

- self-induced vomiting,
- abuse of laxatives or diuretics,
- excessive exercise regimens, and
- use of appetite suppressants.

With treatment, patients may recover and achieve a healthy weight, but it's not unusual for them to return to their unhealthy eating and physical activity practices. At least 5 to 6% of people with AN eventually die as a result of the disorder.[43]

Other Related Conditions: The Female Athlete Triad

Females participating in appearance-based competitive sports that require low body mass, such as gymnastics, swimming, and figure skating, are at risk of developing the **female athlete triad**.[44] This condition is characterized by low energy intakes, abnormal menstrual cycles, and bone mineral irregularities. Severe food restriction can result in lower blood estrogen levels that, in turn, can cause the absence of menstrual cycles. Young women with low estrogen levels have bones that are less dense and weaker than normal. As a result, these women have an increased risk of bone fractures such as "stress" fractures. For more information about this condition, visit the Female Athlete Triad Coalition at http://www.femaleathletetriad.org/.

10.4d Treating Eating Disorders

A team of health professionals, including registered dietitians, physicians, nurses, and mental health counselors, are usually involved in the treatment of eating disorders. A key goal of therapy is for patients to achieve and maintain healthy BMIs without using unhealthy practices.

Treatment for eating disorders generally includes *cognitive behavioral therapy,* which teaches people ways to monitor their eating behavior and change their unhealthy eating habits. Such therapy also helps patients develop move positive feelings about their body shape and weight. Medication, particularly antidepressants, may also be included as part of treatment.

If you or someone you know has an eating disorder, it's important to seek help for the condition as early as possible—before the affected person's life is at risk. Professional help is often available at student health centers and student guidance/counseling facilities on college campuses.

female athlete triad condition characterized by low energy intakes, abnormal menstrual cycles, and bone mineral irregularities

Psychological counseling can help patients with eating disorders learn to change unhealthy beliefs about themselves.

© David Buffington/Getty Images RF

Module 10.5

Get Moving; Get Healthy!

© Pixtal/AGE Fotostock RF

10.5 - Learning Outcomes

After reading Module 10.5, you should be able to

1. Define all of the key terms in this module.

2. List five health benefits of a physically active lifestyle.

3. Distinguish moderate-intensity activities from vigorous-intensity activities.

4. Plan nutritionally adequate, high-carbohydrate menus.

5. Estimate an athlete's energy and protein needs.

6. List at least five ergogenic aids that athletes often use, and describe their effects on health and physical performance.

The human body is designed for **physical activity**—movement that results from skeletal muscle contraction. Most of the physical activities you perform each day are unstructured, for example, shopping for groceries or doing household tasks. **Exercise** refers to physical activities that are usually planned and structured for a particular purpose, such as having fun, losing weight, or increasing muscle mass. Both forms of physical activity can benefit your health.

10.5a Health Benefits of Regular Exercise

Millions of Americans suffer from chronic illnesses that can be prevented or improved by exercising more often. Exercising regularly can help

- control your weight,

- reduce your risk of CVD,

- reduce your risk for type 2 diabetes,

- reduce your risk of colon and breast cancer,

- strengthen your bones and muscles,

- improve your psychological well-being, and

- increase your chances of enjoying a longer, healthy life.[45]

Performing household chores often involves low-intensity physical activity.

10.5b What's Physical Fitness?

Physical fitness is the ability to perform moderate- to vigorous-intensity activities without becoming excessively tired. If you're physically fit, you have the strength, endurance, flexibility, and balance to meet the physical demands of daily living, exercise, and sports. Proper nutrition is essential for optimal physical fitness and sports performance.

Determining the Intensity of Physical Activity

Intensity refers to the level of exertion (physical effort) used to perform an activity. Duration and type of physical activity, as well as body weight, influence the intensity of skeletal muscle movement. Thus, activities such as walking and swimming can be classified as either moderate- or vigorous-intensity physical activity, depending on the rate at which the activities are performed as well as the weight of the person performing them.

Low-intensity, unstructured physical activities include your usual daily living activities, such as routine household chores. Moderate-intensity activities make your muscles work harder than usual and cause your breathing and heart rates to increase above their usual rates. When doing a moderate-intensity activity, you can talk but you can't sing.[46] When performing a vigorous-intensity activity, you're breathing much faster than usual, and you can't say more than a few words without trying to catch your breath. For examples of physical activities that are generally classified as moderate or vigorous intensity, visit http://www.cdc.gov /physicalactivity/basics/measuring/index.html .

The Physical Activity Pyramid

The physical activity pyramid shown in **Figure 10.13** serves as a visual model to help people add more physical activity into their daily routines. This pyramid presents various activities that need to be performed regularly and discourages physical inactivity.

Performing *aerobic exercise* at least three times a week raises your heart rate, giving your heart a more effective workout. **Aerobic exercise** involves sustained, rhythmic contractions of large muscle groups in the legs and arms. Running, jogging, rapid walking, and swimming are aerobic activities. Performing resistance exercises, such as weight lifting, increases muscle mass and strength, and can also increase bone mass. Stretching activities improve flexibility. You may achieve even greater health benefits by increasing the duration, frequency, and intensity of your exercise routine. For example, you'll exert more physical effort and expend more energy if you "jog" instead of "walk" the dog.

Recommendations for Physical Activity

According to recommendations issued by the American College of Sports Medicine,

healthy adults under 65 years of age should perform at least

- moderate-intensity physical activity for 150 minutes a week,

or

- vigorous-intensity physical activity for 75 minutes a week,

and

- muscle-strengthening exercises (moderate to vigorous) focusing on all major muscle groups on at least 2 days a week.[47] Strengthening activities should give your major muscle groups a workout.

Performing a minute of vigorous-intensity physical activity equals two minutes of moderate-intensity physical activity.[47] Each session of moderate- or vigorous-intensity activities should last at least 10 minutes. It's also a good idea to spread the activities out over a week.

physical activity movement resulting from contraction of skeletal muscles

exercise physical activities that are usually planned and structured for a purpose

physical fitness ability to perform moderate- to vigorous-intensity activities without becoming excessively fatigued

intensity degree of effort used to perform a physical activity

aerobic exercise physical activities that involve sustained, rhythmic contractions of large muscle groups

Sedentary Activity (occasionally)
Sitting, driving, watching TV, using a computer, texting or talking on a phone

Light Recreational Activity (2–3 days/week)
Bowling, walking (fast pace), line dancing, and doing yoga

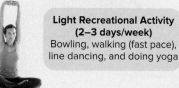

Moderate-Intensity Aerobic Exercise (3–5 days/week, for a total of 150 minutes)
Running, cycling, in-line skating, stair stepping

Flexibility Exercise (2–3 days/week)
Static stretching of major muscle groups. Holding each stretch for 10–30 seconds.

Strength Exercise (2–3 days/week, 8–10 exercises 1 set of 8–12 reps)
Bicep curls, tricep presses, squats, lunges, push-ups

Activities of Daily Living (Most days of the week, accumulate 30+ minutes)
Gardening, raking leaves, mowing the lawn, walking the dog, cleaning the house, playing with your children

Figure 10.13 A physical activity pyramid.

Man exercising with weights: © Ingram Publishing RF; Man at desk, Woman holding basket of flowers: © Stockdisc/PunchStock RF; Woman doing yoga: © Fancy Collection/SuperStock RF; Man on mountain bike: © Photodisc/Getty Images RF; Woman doing forward lunge, Man using weight machine: © Ingram Publishing/Alamy RF; Mother with stroller: © Ingram Publishing/Fotosearch RF

10.5c Fueling Exercise

As mentioned in Unit 4, cells obtain energy by means of a series of chemical reactions ("metabolic pathways") that break down macronutrients to release the energy that's stored within them. Cells capture some of the energy in special compounds such as adenosine triphosphate (ATP). ATP is the primary source of direct energy for all cells.

Aerobic Versus Anaerobic Conditions

In **aerobic** conditions, muscle cells have plenty of oxygen. As a result, the cells can metabolize glucose completely to CO_2 and H_2O. Aerobic conditions enable cells to produce far more ATP-energy than the amount cells can produce when oxygen isn't available. The ability to obtain this amount of energy is useful for endurance athletes because it allows their muscle cells to contract repeatedly for hours.

Gram for gram, fat supplies more ATP-energy than carbohydrate. Fatty acids, however, aren't a very useful fuel for intense, brief exercise, such as a 100-meter sprint. Why? A fatty acid molecule has fewer oxygen atoms in relation to carbon atoms than there are in a glucose molecule. Thus, cells need more oxygen to metabolize a fatty acid molecule than to burn a glucose molecule. During a brief bout of intense exercise, the heart and lungs don't have enough time to deliver much oxygen to muscles. When cells don't have much oxygen (**anaerobic conditions**), glucose is a major source of energy. Under these conditions, muscle cells, however, lack enough oxygen to metabolize glucose completely. **Essential Concept 10.1** illustrates what happens under anaerobic conditions and how your body forms glucose from another substance.

Essential Concept

10.1 Glucose Recycling

1 Cells convert glucose to **pyruvate** and then convert pyruvate to **lactic acid**.

Glucose

Pyruvate

Pyruvate

Lactic acid

ATP

Inside cell

Glucose

Lactic acid

2 The breakdown of glucose to lactic acid produces a small amount of ATP—only enough to sustain maximum physical exertion for 10 seconds to 3 minutes.[48] Lactic acid accumulates in muscles and converts to a related substance, lactate.

H^+

H^+

Lactate

4 The liver can convert lactate into glucose. The liver can then release the glucose into the bloodstream to help meet muscles' demand for fuel or use the simple sugar to make glycogen.

3 Although certain muscle cells can use lactate as a fuel, some of the compound enters the bloodstream.

Lactate

Glucose

Liver

Glycogen

Blood vessel

Lactate

Lactate

aerobic conditions that include oxygen

anaerobic conditions that lack oxygen

pyruvate compound that results from anaerobic breakdown of glucose

lactic acid compound formed from pyruvate during anaerobic metabolism

*Protein supplies a minor percentage of energy.
**Fat use generally is higher because much of the time spent weight lifting is for rest periods.
†The values shown are for a runner consuming carbohydrate during the run; more fat and less carbohydrate would be used if carbohydrates were not consumed.

Figure 10.14 **Carbohydrate or fat?**

Fat or Carbohydrate for Fuel?

The intensity and duration of a physical activity largely influence the relative amounts of fatty acids and glucose that muscles metabolize for energy. Fat is the primary fuel that muscles use while resting or engaged in low- to moderate-intensity physical activities. During prolonged high-intensity exercise, muscles use more glucose than fat for energy. To supply glucose, muscles and the liver break down glycogen. The chart in **Figure 10.14** illustrates rough estimates of carbohydrate and fat metabolism during six forms of exercise.

10.5d General Dietary Advice for Athletes

Compared to nonathletes, athletes generally need more energy to support their physically active lifestyles. Athletes who don't consume enough food energy can lose muscle mass and bone density, experience fatigue and menstrual problems (females), and be at risk of injury.[48]

Male athletes who train or compete aerobically for more than 90 minutes daily need at least 50 kcal/kg/day; their female counterparts need 45 to 50 kcal/kg/day.[49] Thus, athletes may require 3000 kcal/day or more to support their energy needs and maintain their weight. **Table 10.6** presents three sample daily menus that are nutritionally adequate, high in carbohydrates, and supply approximately 3000, 4000, and 5000 kcal/day. Unit 3 provides general information to help you plan nutritious menus using MyPlate.

TASTY Tidbits

A pedometer is a small device that records the number of steps a person takes while engaging in physical activities. A reasonable goal is to take at least 10,000 steps per day. You can purchase an inexpensive pedometer online or at a sporting goods store.

© Wendy Schiff

TABLE 10.6

SAMPLE DAILY 3000, 4000, AND 5000 KCAL MENUS

3000 kcal 62% carbohydrate 20% fat 18% protein	4000 kcal 66% carbohydrate 19% fat 15% protein	5000 kcal 62% carbohydrate 21% fat 17% protein
Breakfast Fat-free milk, 1 cup Cheerios, 2 cups Bagel, 1 Cherry preserves, ½ Tbsp Oat bran muffin, 1 Low-fat cream cheese, 1 Tbsp	**Breakfast** Fat-free milk, 1 cup Cheerios, 2 cups Bran muffins, 2 Orange, 1	**Breakfast** Fat-free milk, 1 cup Cheerios, 2 cups Bran muffins, 2 Orange, 1
Snack Oatmeal-raisin cookie, 1	**Snack** Chopped dates, 1 cup	**Snack** Low-fat plain yogurt, 1 cup Chopped dates, 1 cup
Lunch Chicken breast, skinless roasted, 2 oz Whole-wheat bread, 2 slices Provolone cheese, 1 oz Mayonnaise, 1 tsp Raisins, ½ cup Cranberry juice, 1½ cups Low-fat vanilla yogurt, 1 cup	**Lunch** Macaroni and cheese, 2 cups Leaf lettuce, 2 cups Garbanzo beans, 1 cup Grated carrots, ½ cup French dressing, 2 Tbsp Apple juice, 1 cup	**Lunch** Chicken enchilada, with beans and cheese, 2 Leaf lettuce, 2 cups Garbanzo beans, 1 cup Shredded carrots, ¾ cup Chopped celery, ½ cup Seasoned croutons, ½ cup French dressing, 2 Tbsp Whole-wheat bread, 2 slices Butter or soft margarine, 1 Tbsp
Snack Banana, 1 Oatmeal-raisin cookie, 1	**Snack** Whole-wheat bread, 2 slices Peanut butter, 1 Tbsp Grape jelly, 2 Tbsp Fat-free milk, 1 cup	**Snack** Banana, 1 Bagel, 1 Cream cheese, 1 Tbsp Fat-free milk, 1 cup
Dinner Lean broiled beef, 3 oz Leaf lettuce, 2 cups Garbanzo beans, ½ cup Italian dressing, 2 Tbsp Spinach egg noodles, cooked, 1 cup Butter or soft margarine, 1 tsp Green beans, 1 cup Fat-free milk, ½ cup	**Dinner** Skinless, roasted turkey breast, 2 oz Mashed potatoes, 1 cup Peas 1 cup Butter or soft margarine, 2 tsp Fat-free milk, 1 cup	**Dinner** Lean broiled beef or pot roast, 6 oz Mashed potatoes, 2 cups Butter or soft margarine, 2 tsp Spinach egg noodles, cooked, 1½ cups Grated parmesan cheese, ¼ cup Green beans, 1 cup Oatmeal-raisin cookies, large, 3 Fat-free milk, 1 cup
	Snack Pasta, 1 cup cooked Parmesan cheese, 2 Tbsp Cranberry juice, 1 cup	**Snack** Whole-wheat bagel, 1 Peanut butter, 1 Tbsp Raisins, ½ cup Cranberry juice, 1½ cups

© Wendy Schiff

Focusing on Carbohydrate Intake

Recall from Unit 5 that carbohydrate "spares" protein from being used for energy. If your diet doesn't supply enough carbohydrate to burn for energy, your cells may break down protein into amino acids to use for fuel. Thus, having an adequate carbohydrate intake enables you to conserve the protein in your muscles.

Recommended diets for athletes should supply adequate amounts of energy from carbohydrates. To maintain adequate muscle glycogen, endurance athletes should consume 3 to 10 grams of carbohydrate per kilogram of body weight daily.[48] Athletes who obtain more than 4 hours of moderate- to high-intensity exercise daily may need as much as 12 grams of carbohydrate per kilogram of body weight. **Table 10.7** lists energy and macronutrient information for several carbohydrate-rich foods. By consuming several servings of grains, starchy vegetables, and fruits daily, an athlete can obtain enough carbohydrate to maintain adequate liver and muscle glycogen stores.

What's Carbohydrate (Glycogen) Loading?

Endurance athletes who have more glycogen in their muscles at the start of an event may be able to exercise longer than those who don't have as much muscle glycogen. Carbohydrate, or glycogen, loading involves altering dietary and physical activity patterns a few days before an event to increase muscle glycogen stores well above the normal range. The practice may help delay fatigue in athletes participating in events lasting more than 90 minutes.[48]

© Keith Ovregaard/Cole Group/Getty Images RF

TABLE 10.7

CARBOHYDRATE-RICH FOODS

Food and Amount	kcal	Carbohydrate (g)	Protein (g)	Fat (g)
Macaroni, plain, cooked, 1 cup	221	43.20	8.12	1.30
Spaghetti, cooked, 1 cup	220	42.83	8.12	1.30
Rice, instant, white, cooked, 1 cup	194	41.16	4.60	0.58
Egg noodles, cooked, 1 cup	221	40.26	7.26	3.31
Baked potato, ½ large	139	31.62	3.74	0.19
Corn, canned, drained, 1 cup	133	30.49	4.30	1.64
Bagel, ½, 4" diam.	144	28.04	5.51	0.84
Grapes, 1 cup	104	27.33	1.09	0.24
Banana, 1 med. (approx. 7" long)	105	26.95	1.29	0.39
Baked beans, ½ cup	119	26.85	6.03	0.47
Crackers, 6 rectangular saltines	154	25.53	3.32	4.09
Orange juice, unsweetened, 1 cup	110	25.05	1.99	0.69
Cornflakes, 1 cup	101	24.28	1.88	0.03
Pretzels, 1 oz	108	22.61	2.93	0.75
Cooked oatmeal, plain, 1 cup	129	22.44	5.43	2.13
Yogurt, low-fat, plain, 1 cup	154	17.25	12.86	3.80
English muffin, ½	67	13.11	2.53	0.51
Bread, white, 1 slice	66	12.65	2.19	0.82
Fat-free milk, 1 cup	83	12.15	8.26	0.20
Tortilla, corn, ready-to-cook, 6" diam. (1)	58	12.12	1.48	0.65
Soy milk, 1 cup	127	12.08	10.98	4.70

© Wendy Schiff

Placemat: © McGraw-Hill Education. Mark A. Dierker, photographer

Consuming Carbohydrate During Events

While performing prolonged physical activity (active for 1 to 2.5 hours), athletes can delay fatigue by consuming 30 to 60 g of carbohydrate per hour of activity.[48] Athletes who engage in ultra-endurance exercise (active for more than 2.5 hours) should aim to consume as much as 90 grams of carbohydrates per hour of activity. Commercially available sports drinks are often used as a source of carbohydrates during physical activity. These beverages are usually sweetened with nutritive sweeteners such as sucrose, glucose, fructose, or maltodextrin. Sports drinks typically provide 15 to 27 g of carbohydrate per 12-ounce serving. Sports gels are also good sources of simple carbohydrate, but they generally supply very little fluid. Therefore, it's important for athletes who consume these products to drink enough water to maintain proper hydration during endurance events.

Carbohydrates for Exercise Recovery

After completing exhaustive physical activity, trained athletes can replenish their glycogen stores by consuming approximately 1.0 to 1.2 grams of carbohydrate per kilogram of body weight per hour during the first 4 to 6 hours after the activity.[48] To restore their supply of muscle glycogen quickly after an event, athletes can consume sports drinks, fruit, or fruit juices. During a post-event meal, starchy foods such as whole-grain bread, mashed potatoes, rice, and pasta can be served to boost athletes' carbohydrate consumption.

What About Energy Bars?

Energy, or sports, bars are essentially cookies made from soy and milk proteins that are fortified with vitamins, minerals, and fiber. Sugary

syrups hold these ingredients together. Proteins aren't "quick energy" sources because the liver must process amino acids before they can be used for energy. Granola bars, oatmeal cookies, and fresh or dried fruits are less expensive and more natural sources of energy and nutrients than are energy or sports bars.

Protein Intake

Under normal conditions, carbohydrate and fat are the primary fuels for cellular activity. Protein provides no more than 15% of the body's energy needs. During prolonged physical activity, muscles lose some protein because they metabolize certain amino acids for energy. Therefore, the RDA for protein may not apply to athletes involved in training or competition. Athletes should consume more protein than the RDA of 0.8 grams per kilogram of body weight. According to a recent review, an additional 0.3 grams of protein per kilogram of body weight should be consumed after exercising.[48] Ideal sources of protein include foods such as milk, lean meats, and dietary supplements that contain whey, casein, soy, and egg proteins.

Replenishing Fluids

Athletes should avoid losing more than 2% of their body weight during exercise.[48] Athletes can weigh themselves prior to exercising and then calculate 2% of their body weight. After working out, athletes should weigh themselves again. If the difference between preexercise and postexercise body weights is more than 2%, fluid replacement is needed during such activities. In general, you can replace each pound of water lost during exercise by drinking about 2.5 to 3 cups of a suitable replacement fluid.[48]

Sports drinks provide some nutritional benefits beyond those of plain water. These beverages usually contain simple carbohydrates and electrolytes, such as sodium, that can enhance performance during endurance activities. Recommended products contain about 21 g of carbohydrate per 12-ounce serving, or about 6% carbohydrate by weight. Drinks with a sugar content above 10%, such as soft drinks or fruit juices, aren't recommended because they may cause intestinal discomfort. Sodium and other electrolytes in sports beverages help maintain blood volume, enhance the absorption of water and carbohydrate from the intestinal tract, and stimulate thirst.

TASTY Tidbits

Compared to commercially available sports drinks, diluted fruit juices with added sugar and salt are less expensive sources of water, sodium, and simple sugars. You can prepare your own "sports" drink by adding ¼ cup of orange juice, ¼ cup of sugar, and ⅛ tsp of table salt to 30 oz of water or club soda. Pour the beverage into a quart pitcher, cover, and refrigerate until needed.

Should you drink water or a sports drink during competition? According to experts with the American College of Sports Medicine, sports drinks can improve physical performance when vigorous-intensity activities last more than an hour.[50] Although electrolytes are lost in sweat, the quantities lost in shorter periods can be easily replaced by consuming foods and beverages, such as water or fruit juice, after the event.

Water Intoxication

Water intoxication can occur when people drink too much water, which dilutes the level of sodium in their blood. Although sports drinks generally contain sodium, these beverages are mostly water; therefore, consuming excessive amounts of sports drinks can contribute to overload. Signs and symptoms of water intoxication include confusion, nausea or vomiting, weight gain, and muscle cramps. If not treated promptly, death can result. To avoid water intoxication, athletes should drink water according to their thirst. Don't consume more than a quart of fluid during each hour of exercise.[50]

Heat-Related Illness

Even a small degree of dehydration can lead to declines in an athlete's endurance, strength, and overall performance. Moreover, body temperature rises when dehydration occurs, increasing the risk of heat-related illness, including heat exhaustion and heat stroke. **Table 10.8** presents warning signs and symptoms of heat-related illnesses.

Heatstroke is a medical emergency that needs to be treated by trained medical staff. If you suspect that a person has heatstroke, summon emergency medical assistance immediately (call 911) and move the victim to a cool environment. Cool the person by any means possible. You can spray or sponge him or her with cool water.[51] To reduce the risk of heat illnesses, you should avoid exercising under extremely hot, humid conditions. Furthermore, you should replace fluid losses that occur during prolonged exertion.

heatstroke most dangerous form of heat-related illness

ergogenic aids foods, devices, dietary supplements, or drugs used to improve physical performance

© Rubberball/Getty Images RF

Heat exhaustion can occur after heavy exercise in warm conditions, especially when fluid and salt intakes have been inadequate.

TABLE 10.8 HEAT-RELATED ILLNESSES: WARNING SIGNS AND SYMPTOMS

Heat cramps	Heat exhaustion	Heatstroke
Painful muscle spasms ("heat cramps")	Dark urine	High fever (over 104°F)
Very heavy sweating	Cool, moist skin	Red, hot, dry skin
Tiredness	Weakness	Rapid, shallow breathing
Thirst	Nausea, dizziness, vomiting	Confusion
	Headache	Seizures
		Loss of consciousness

Source: National Library of Medicine, MedlinePlus: *Heat emergencies.* Updated November 2015. https://medlineplus.gov/ency/article/000056.htm Accessed: July 31, 2016

10.5e Ergogenic Aids: Separating Fact from Fiction

Athletes often use **ergogenic aids**—foods, devices, dietary supplements, and even drugs ("doping")—to improve their physical performance. Bee pollen, dried adrenal glands from cattle, seaweed, freeze-dried liver food, and ginseng are among the dietary supplements that athletes consume as they hope to gain the competitive edge over their rivals. However, no reliable scientific evidence supports the effectiveness of most dietary supplements purported to have ergogenic effects. Nevertheless, many athletes firmly believe in the value of

caffeine naturally occurring stimulant drug

the performance-enhancing aids that they use. **Table 10.9** summarizes science-based findings regarding some dietary supplements and ergogenic aids that are popular among athletes.

A few dietary practices can enhance physical performance. These ergogenic aids include consuming sufficient water, electrolytes, and carbohydrates, and eating a balanced, varied diet consistent with MyPlate recommendations. For athletes, meeting carbohydrate and fluid needs—along with overall nutrient needs—is the most important ergogenic aid.

"Energy" Drinks

Sugar-sweetened energy drinks provide calories, but their quick "energy" boost is a result of **caffeine** or other stimulants that are in the products. Caffeine is naturally in coffee and tea. When consumed in moderate amounts, caffeine can increase alertness and decrease fatigue. Some energy drinks also contain the amino acid *taurine* and herbal substances such as ginseng. Although your body uses taurine, humans don't require the compound. Ginseng may enhance the stimulating effects of caffeine.

Caffeine Toxicity

Excess caffeine is toxic. Toxicity signs and symptoms include heartbeat irregularities, increased blood pressure, dehydration, and sleep disturbances. As the popularity of energy drinks increased in the United States, so has the number of people seeking emergency room treatment after consuming the beverages. In 2011, 1 in 10 Americans 12 years of age or older who visited emergency rooms for energy drink–related health problems required hospitalization.[52] In 2011, a 14-year-old girl with a heart condition died after consuming two 24-ounce energy drinks.

The practice of combining energy drinks with alcohol is very dangerous. The caffeine in the energy drink masks the central nervous system depressant effects of the alcohol. As a result, the drinker doesn't realize his or her level of intoxication and consumes too much alcohol.

Football player: © Purestock/SuperStock RF; Energy drinks: © Wendy Schiff; Guarana, (*Paullinia cupana*): © flowerphotos/Alamy

TASTY **Tidbits**

The seeds of the Brazilian shrub *guarana* (*Paullinia cupana*) are a concentrated source of caffeine. At present, the FDA doesn't require manufacturers to include information on food or beverage labels concerning amounts of caffeine provided by guarana or other herbal ingredients.

TABLE 10.9

EVALUATION OF SOME POPULAR ERGOGENIC SUPPLEMENTS/AIDS

Substance	Claim	Current Science-Based Findings Concerning Claims	Side Effects
Caffeine	Enhances fat metabolism Increases alertness	Increases alertness and decreases fatigue, but doesn't increase fat metabolism during exercise	High doses can cause increased heart rate, nervousness, shakiness. May contribute to death when consumed in high amounts.
Creatine	Enhances muscular endurance and strength Increases lean muscle mass	Increases lean and total body mass, improves performance for intense activities that aren't endurance activities, increases strength Such positive effects are not consistent among athletes.	May cause weight gain and gastrointestinal upset
Beta-alanine	May enhance training capacity and improve performance during brief bouts of intense exercise	Seems to be effective	May cause tingling sensation in skin of the face, neck, and hands
Sodium bicarbonate (baking soda)	Reduces lactic acid accumulation	May enhance performance	May cause nausea and vomiting
Beta-hydroxy-beta-methylbutyrate (HMB)	Decreases protein metabolism, increasing muscle mass	May increase muscle mass, but evidence is weak	None reported, but results of long-term use are unknown
Branched chain amino acids (BCAA)	Provide energy for muscles	May enhance muscle recovery after intense physical activity	None reported
Calcium pyruvate	Increases endurance and promotes weight loss	Not effective	Gastrointestinal upset May be harmful
Chromium	Increases lean mass	No benefit	Toxic level: intakes above 400 mcg daily
Coenzyme Q_{10}	Enhances cardiac function, delays fatigue	No benefit	Long-term safety is unknown.
Nitrate	Improves exercise tolerance and performance	Benefits aren't as evident in highly trained athletes.	Concentrates, such as beetroot juice, may cause intestinal upset and red urine.
Ginseng	Combats fatigue and improves stamina	Doesn't improve performance but may decrease muscle damage during exercise	May cause gastrointestinal upset, itching, sleeplessness, and, in rare cases, allergic reactions and liver damage

Sources: Position of the Academy of Nutrition and Dietetics, Dietitians of Canada, and the American College of Sports Medicine: Nutrition and athletic performance. *Journal of the Academy of Nutrition and Dietetics* 116(3):501, 2016; Trexler E T and others: International society of sports nutrition position stand: Beta-alanine. *Journal of the International Society of Sports Nutrition* 12 (1), 2015. doi:10.1186/s12970-015-0090-y; Kreider RB and others: ISSN exercise and sport nutrition review: research and recommendations. *Journal of the International Society of Sports Nutrition* 7 (7):1, 2010; NIH, *Medline Plus: American ginseng* 2015. https://www.nlm.nih.medlineplus/druginfo/natural/967.html Accessed: May 27, 2016.

TABLE 10.10

CAFFEINE CONTENT OF SELECTED BEVERAGES

Beverage (8 fl oz)	Kcal	Caffeine (mg)
Coffee, brewed from grounds, unsweetened***	2	95
AMP Energy Strawberry Limeade**	110	78
Caffé Latte, Starbucks*	100	75
Red Bull***	106	71
Coffee, instant plain, prepared***	5	62
Tea, black, brewed, unsweetened***	2	47
Mountain Dew**	110	36
Cola, sweetened with caffeine***	103	22
Tea, Arizona, ready-to-drink***	95	12
Chocolate drink, milk-based, 8 oz***	120	2

*Nutrition information. http://www.starbucks.com/.

**Nutrition information: http://www.pepsicobeveragefacts.com/.

***U.S. Department of Agriculture, Agricultural Research Service, *USDA National nutrient database for standard reference, release 28.* Nutrient Data Laboratory Home Page. Accessed: May 26, 2016.

Table 10.10 compares the caffeine and calorie contents of popular beverages, including some energy drinks.

10.5f Physically Active for a Lifetime

When developing your personal physical fitness plan, first consider your fitness goals. For example, if you want to lose weight, how much do you want to lose and how many weeks will it take to lose that amount? Do you want to focus more on strengthening your muscles or on improving your aerobic capacity? Then determine when you can work out and whether you'll need to join a fitness facility such as a gym or purchase special equipment, such as handheld weights. For a comprehensive fitness program, make sure to include aerobic, resistance, and stretching activities in your weekly exercise regimen. Consider the following tips:

1. *Choose* physical activities that you enjoy and can do without the need for expensive equipment.

2. *Increase* the time you spend walking each day. Keep walking shoes where you can see them.

3. *Reduce* the amount of time you spend sitting. For example, do more household chores yourself.

4. *Take* stairs instead of elevators or escalators whenever possible.

5. *Park* your car farther from your destination and walk, if you feel it's safe to do so.

6. *Lift* handheld weights while watching television.

7. *Adopt* moderate-intensity activities for your leisure time. For example, join a co-ed volleyball club or take a ballroom dancing class.

In a **Nutshell**

© McGraw-Hill Education. Mark A. Dierker, photographer

Module 10.1 Overweight or Obese?

- A person who's overweight has extra body weight that's contributed by bone, muscle, body fat, and/or body water. Obesity is a condition characterized by excessive and unhealthy amounts of body fat. Obese people have a greater risk of developing type 2 diabetes, hypertension, and cardiovascular disease than people who aren't obese.

- Obesity is the most prevalent nutritional disorder in the United States. In 2013–2014, almost 38% of American adults 20 years of age and older were obese. The prevalence of obesity among American children is a public health concern. Obese children have higher risk of maturing into obese adults than children who aren't obese. Rates of overweight and obesity are also increasing rapidly throughout the world ("globesity").

- Your body has fat-free mass and total body fat, which includes "essential fat" and fat (adipose) tissue. In addition to storing and releasing energy as fat, adipose cells secrete numerous proteins, some of which have roles in regulating food intake, glucose metabolism, and immune responses.

- Subcutaneous fat helps insulate your body against cold temperatures and protects muscles and bones from bumps and bruises. Visceral fat protects abdominal organs.

- Excess body fat distribution influences the risk of obesity-related diseases. People with "apple" body fat distribution have higher risks of CVD and type 2 diabetes than people with "pear" body shapes. Fat cells, particularly visceral fat, make substances that cause inflammation in the body.

- The BMI is a numerical value based on the relationship between body weight and risk of chronic health problems associated with excess body fat. Healthy BMIs range from 18.5 to 24.9. As BMI increases, the risks of serious chronic health problems increase. BMIs shouldn't be applied to highly muscular individuals, people who are elderly, or chronically ill persons.

- Bioelectrical impedance and skinfold thickness measurements are practical ways to estimate your percentage of body fat. A man is overweight when his body is 22 to 25% fat; a woman is overweight when her body is 32 to 37% fat. A man is obese when fat comprises 26% or more of his body; a woman is obese when fat makes up 38% or more of her body. Adults tend to gain fat tissue as they age, but for older adults, some additional fat doesn't necessarily contribute to serious health problems.

Module 10.2 Factors That Influence Your Body Weight

- Your cells generally metabolize primarily glucose and fatty acids, but small amounts of amino acids are also used for energy. Metabolism refers to all chemical changes, or reactions, that constantly occur in living cells. Anabolic reactions require energy to occur; catabolic reactions release energy. Basal metabolism generally accounts for most of the body's total energy use. Numerous factors can influence your metabolic rate, including thyroid hormone production, body composition, sex, age, and calorie intake.

© Rachel Weill/UpperCut Images /Getty Images RF

- The amount of energy expended for a particular physical activity depends largely on the weight of the person, type of activity, and its duration and intensity.

- Total daily energy expenditure equals the sum of kilocalories burned for basal metabolism, physical activity, and TEF in a day. Energy balance occurs when calorie intake from food and beverages equals calorie output for basal metabolism, physical activity, and TEF. A negative energy state occurs when calorie intake is lower than calorie output. A state of positive energy state occurs when calorie intake is greater than calorie output.

- One pound of body fat represents about 3500 kcal. Losing weight requires a negative energy state.

- Hunger and satiety regulate eating behavior. Ghrelin stimulates eating behavior; leptin reduces hunger and inhibits body fat storage. Having a thrifty metabolism enables the body to store more excess energy as fat. According to the set-point theory, the body's fat content is genetically predetermined. Oversized portions of many restaurant foods may contribute to the widespread obesity problem in the United States.

© Purestock/SuperStock RF

Module 10.3 Managing Your Weight Safely

- By losing 5 to 10% of excess body fat, an overfat person can increase beneficial high-density lipoprotein levels, reduce elevated blood pressure, and lower blood glucose and triglyceride levels. There are no quick cures for overweight and obesity.

- A reliable weight-loss plan has several features, including being safe and effective; meeting the dieter's nutritional, psychological, and social needs; including nutritious foods from all food groups; and encouraging regular physical activity. Successful weight loss and long-term weight maintenance involve motivation, calorie reduction, regular physical activity, and changing food-related behaviors.

- Actions that can help you lose excess weight and maintain a lower, healthier body weight include planning menus, monitoring food intake, shopping carefully, preparing and serving your food, and keeping nutrient-dense, low-calorie snacks on hand.

- At present, the FDA has approved few medications for long-term weight loss. Medications don't replace the need to reduce calorie intake and increase physical activity. The most common surgical procedures for weight loss drastically reduce the size of an obese person's stomach, markedly limiting food intake.

Bananas: © Burke/Triolo Productions/Getty Images RF; Apple and slices: © Photodisc/ Getty Images RF; Raisins: © McGraw-Hill Education. Jacques Cornell, photographer

- Many overfat people use fad diets to lose weight. A typical fad diet promotes rapid, dramatic weight loss without calorie restriction and increased physical activity. Low-carbohydrate diets usually produce rapid weight loss initially, primarily because the body loses water. At this point, medical experts don't recommend any dietary supplement for weight loss.

- An underweight individual has a BMI that's less than 18.5. Many underweight individuals want to gain weight, especially muscle mass. To gain weight, underweight adults can gradually increase their consumption of calorie-dense foods, especially those high in healthy fats.

Module 10.4 Disordered Eating and Eating Disorders

- Disordered eating involves temporary chaotic and abnormal food-related practices. The practices can become harmful and difficult-to-treat eating disorders.

- Eating disorders are psychological disturbances that often lead to serious health complications. Anorexia nervosa, bulimia nervosa, and binge-eating disorder are major types of eating disorders. The causes of eating disorders are unknown, but genetic, social, and psychological factors contribute to their development.

- Treatment of eating disorders is complex, involving more than just dietary counseling. It's important to seek professional help for an eating disorder as early as possible—before the behavior becomes highly ingrained or the affected person's life is at risk.

© Wendy Schiff

Module 10.5 Get Moving; Get Healthy!

- You can manage your weight more effectively and reduce your risk of developing the major causes of death and disability by becoming physically active. Healthy adults under 65 years of age should perform moderate-intensity aerobic activity for 150 minutes a week or vigorous-intensity activities for 75 minutes a week. In addition to aerobic activities, adults should perform strength training and flexibility exercises. Most people can achieve even greater health benefits by increasing the duration, frequency, and intensity of their physical activities.

- Regular exercise provides many benefits, such as reducing the risk of heart disease, diabetes, and certain cancers; aiding weight-control efforts; and promoting psychological well-being.

- ATP is the major form of direct energy used by cells. To generate ATP, muscle cells can metabolize carbohydrate, fat, and protein. In muscle cells, glucose molecules are broken down through a series of steps to yield lactic acid (in anaerobic conditions) or CO_2 and H_2O (in aerobic conditions).

- Fat is a key aerobic fuel for muscle cells, especially at rest and during low-intensity exercise. Little protein generally is used to fuel muscles. Under anaerobic conditions, muscle cells metabolize glucose rather than fat for energy, but their ability to sustain the release of energy for intense activity is limited. Muscle cells can obtain far more energy when in aerobic conditions.

- High-carbohydrate diets can be beneficial for athletes, and carbohydrate-rich foods should form the foundation of pre-event meals. Many athletes need more protein than the RDA.

- Physically active people need to be concerned about their fluid intakes. Fluid replacement should be based on thirst and loss of body weight while exercising. Consuming a source of electrolytes, such as a sports drink, can be helpful, especially when the duration of intense exercise exceeds 60 minutes. It's important to avoid overconsumption of water because of the risk of water intoxication.

- Athletes often ingest certain substances, including herbal products, because they believe these substances have ergogenic effects. Scientific evidence, however, doesn't suggest that most of these substances are effective. Furthermore, long-term safety of many ergogenic aids has not been determined.

© Stockbyte/Getty Images RF

Consider This...

1. Why is it usually difficult to pinpoint a cause of obesity?

2. Why are most people who lose weight unable to maintain the lower body weight over time?

3. If your BMI is within the overweight or obese range, discuss your reasons for being interested or not interested in losing weight. If you want to lose weight, what lifestyle changes can you make to meet your weight-loss goal?

4. If your BMI is within the underweight range, discuss your reasons for being interested or not

interested in gaining weight. If you want to gain weight, what lifestyle changes will you make?

5. If your BMI is in the healthy range, discuss steps you can take to maintain a healthy body weight as you grow older.

6. Analyze your weekly physical activity habits. Does your participation in various physical activities meet the minimum recommendations? If not, which physical activities are you willing to include in your weekly routine to improve your fitness level?

© Realistic Reflections RF

Test Yourself

Select the best answer.

1. _____ fat is in a layer under the skin.
   a. Subcutaneous
   b. Visceral
   c. Cellulite
   d. Metabolic

2. Basal metabolism includes energy needs for
   a. breathing and circulating blood.
   b. performing physical activity.
   c. digesting food.
   d. absorbing nutrients.

3. Which of the following statements is true?
   a. Women generally have higher metabolic rates than men.
   b. Thyroid hormone levels influence the metabolic rate.
   c. A person who has more muscle mass will have a lower metabolic rate than someone with less muscle tissue.
   d. When your thyroid gland produces too much thyroid hormone, your metabolic rate drops below normal.

4. A negative energy state occurs when
   a. your body needs more calories than the diet supplies.
   b. fat storage in your body increases.
   c. your energy intake is higher than your energy output.
   d. the thermic effect of your food equals NEAT.

© FoodCollection /Stockfood RF

5. _____ is a hormone that reduces hunger and inhibits fat storage in your body.
   a. Glucosamine
   b. Leptin
   c. Ghrelin
   d. Creatine

6. Members of the National Weight Control Registry tend to
   a. weigh themselves once a month.
   b. follow low-carbohydrate/ high-protein diets.
   c. exercise 2 to 3 times per week.
   d. eat breakfast.

© Wendy Schiff

7. Joseph's BMI is 23. When he's under a lot of stress, he eats a large amount of cookies and ice cream. Soon after eating these foods, he goes to a bathroom and makes himself vomit. Based on this information, Joseph probably has

   a. glycogen storage disease.

   b. anorexia nervosa.

   c. cystic fibrosis.

   d. bulimia nervosa.

8. Miranda is physically fit. Based on this information, she has

   a. an increased risk of osteoporosis.

   b. the strength, endurance, and flexibility to meet the demands of daily living.

   c. a greater need for vitamins and minerals than other women.

   d. more muscle and less bone tissue than other women who are her age.

9. Aerobic activities

   a. enable muscles to use less oxygen than normal.

   b. don't require voluntary muscular contractions.

   c. force muscle cells to use more vitamins and minerals for energy.

   d. involve sustained, rhythmic contractions of certain large skeletal muscles.

10. Which of the following statements is true?

   a. Resistance exercises don't help build bone mass.

   b. Sedentary activities don't require much energy to perform.

   c. Healthy adults should obtain at least 1 hour of vigorous-intensity activity daily.

   d. Older adults can reduce their metabolic rates by exercising regularly.

11. Amy is studying quietly. Under these conditions, her muscles are using primarily _____ for energy.

   a. fat

   b. glucose

   c. amino acids

   d. ketone bodies

12. Which of the following beverages is a common source of caffeine?

   a. Mineral water

   b. Iced tea

   c. Lite beer

   d. Orange drink

13. Under aerobic conditions, cells break down glucose to form

   a. carbon dioxide and water.

   b. nitrogen and DNA.

   c. beta-carotene and vitamin B-6.

   d. sodium and ATP.

14. _____ is an immediate and direct source of energy for cells.

   a. DNA

   b. Glycogen

   c. ATP

   d. Phospholipid

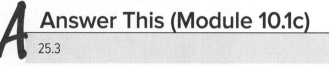

Answer This (Module 10.1c)

25.3

© Brand X Pictures/PunchStock RF

References ➡ See Appendix F.

STUDY TIP: Quickly create a customized practice quiz for this chapter by going to your Connect SmartBook "My Reports" section.

Don't have SmartBook and want to learn more? Go to **whysmartbook.com**.

Nutrition for Your Life, Environment, and World

What's on the Menu?

Module 11.1
Nutrition for a Lifetime

Module 11.2
How Safe Is My Food?

Module 11.3
Dietary Adequacy: A Global Concern

"I can't seem to exercise and eat the way I did before Elijah was born. I find myself snacking with him regularly, plus I don't have the time to work out. When I structure my time and my diet, I feel energetic, but it doesn't last. Within a few weeks, I'm feeling heavy again. I can't keep off the extra pounds I've gained. . . . it's driving me crazy!

We try to 'eat smart,' but planning meals and snacks is very much a challenge. Eating healthy foods has to become a habit with me, so my son will know what's good for him as he grows."

Theresa Washington

© Wendy Schiff

© Blend Images/Getty Images RF

Theresa Washington is a 42-year-old, nontraditional college student, majoring in Business Administration at St. Louis Community College. Her busy lifestyle makes it difficult for her to "eat right," but she's determined to make the effort because she wants to lose weight and set a good example for her 3-year-old son. Is snacking such a bad practice? What can parents and other caregivers do to improve their children's eating habits?

This unit covers three major topics that are important for you and your future. The first part of this unit focuses on nutrition during specific periods of the life cycle, including infancy and the older adult years. Then we'll discuss food-borne illness and the safety of our food supply—concerns of all Americans, regardless of their ages. Finally, we'll provide some basic information about global nutrition, including ways to produce enough nutritious food for the world's population without destroying the Earth's valuable natural resources.

Module 11.1

Nutrition for a Lifetime

11.1- Learning Outcomes

After reading Module 11.1, you should be able to

1. Define all of the key terms in this module.

2. Discuss why proper nutrition is important for having a healthy pregnancy and baby.

3. Classify weight gained during pregnancy according to recommendations that are based on a woman's weight before pregnancy.

4. List nutrients that may need to be supplemented during pregnancy.

5. Describe major physical processes involved in lactation and breastfeeding.

6. Compare the nutritional composition of infant formula with breast milk, and identify at least three advantages of breastfeeding.

7. Explain the rationale for delaying the introduction of solid foods to infants until they're 4 to 6 months of age.

8. Summarize practical suggestions for encouraging healthy eating habits among children.

9. Identify some major nutrition-related health concerns facing American children and teenagers.

10. Identify at least three physical changes that occur during the normal aging process.

11. Explain how growing older affects your nutrient needs.

© Purestock/SuperStock RF

If you are a woman, are you pregnant or considering pregnancy? Do you already have children? If you have children, were they breastfed or fed a synthetic beverage that simulates human milk (**infant formula**)? Do you live with and help to care for an elderly parent or grandparent? These may seem to be very personal questions, but many undergraduate college students don't fit the stereotype of being 18 to 22 years of age, having no children, and residing away from home. Most of the nutrition recommendations presented in this textbook apply to people who are "adults"—loosely defined as the period when a person is 19 to 70 years of age.[1] A person's nutrient needs, however, vary according to life stage. This module focuses on the differing nutrition needs and health concerns of people who are in specific life stages—the **prenatal period** (from conception to birth), pregnancy, **lactation** (milk production for breastfeeding), infancy, childhood, and older adulthood.

Why is it important to learn some basic information about nutrition-related concerns during the life cycle? If you don't have children, you may become a parent in the future. If your parents and grandparents are relatively young and vigorous now, you can expect them to experience declining physical functioning as they grow older. Finally, you need to recognize that most of these changes are normal and will occur in you as well.

11.1a The Prenatal Period

The prenatal period begins with conception and ends with birth. This stage of life lasts about 40 weeks and is often divided into three, 13-week trimesters. During the first 8 weeks, the fertilized egg divides rapidly to form a mass of cells that increases in size and begins to form organs. At this stage, the developing human being is an **embryo.** From 8 weeks after conception until birth, the developing human being is referred to as a **fetus.** During the second and third trimesters, the fetus continues to develop and grow to the point that it's physically mature enough to be born. Birth ends the prenatal period.

The first trimester is a critical stage because nutrient deficiencies or excesses and exposure to toxic compounds, such as alcohol, are most likely to have devastating effects on the embryo/fetus. However, many women who are in their first trimester don't realize they're pregnant.

Throughout the prenatal period, the embryo/fetus develops in the uterus and depends entirely on its mother for survival. During most of the pregnancy, the expectant mother nourishes her embryo/fetus through the **placenta,** the organ of pregnancy that connects the mother's uterus to the embryo/fetus via the umbilical

infant formula synthetic beverage that simulates human milk

prenatal period time between conception and birth

lactation milk production

embryo human organism during the first 8 weeks after conception

fetus human organism from 8 weeks after conception until birth

placenta organ of pregnancy that connects the uterus to the embryo/fetus via the umbilical cord

premature describes infant born before 37 weeks of pregnancy

low-birth-weight (LBW) infant generally weighing less than 5½ pounds at birth

Figure 11.1 Getting ready for birth. (a) The placenta transfers nutrients and oxygen from the mother's bloodstream to the fetus. This organ of pregnancy also conveys waste products from the fetus to the mother's bloodstream for elimination. **(b)** This illustration shows the position of a full-term fetus and its mother's abdominal organs.

■ *Why is having a healthy placenta critical for having a healthy baby?*

cord (**Fig. 11.1**). The role of the placenta is to transfer nutrients and oxygen from the mother's bloodstream to the embryo/fetus. Additionally, the placenta transfers wastes from the embryo/fetus to the mother's bloodstream, so her body can eliminate them. The placenta, however, doesn't allow the mother's blood to mix with the blood of her fetus.

Unfortunately, the placenta doesn't filter many infectious agents and toxic substances, such as alcohol and nicotine, from the mother's blood. Thus, the embryo/fetus can become harmed or killed by infectious diseases and poisonous chemicals that are in her bloodstream.

What's Prematurity?

A developing human being generally needs to spend at least 37 weeks within the uterus to survive after birth without the need for special care. A fetus that's born before the 37th week of prenatal period is **premature**. In 2015, about 10% of American infants were born prematurely.[2] When compared to "full-term" infants (babies born between 39 and 41 weeks of pregnancy), premature infants are more likely to die before their first birthday.

The Importance of Birth Weight

Birth weight is another major factor that determines whether a baby is healthy and survives his or her first year of life. At birth, a healthy, mature fetus usually weighs about 6 to 8 pounds and is 19 to 21 inches long. **Low-birth-weight (LBW)** infants generally weigh less than 5½ pounds. In 2015, 8% of infants born in the United States were low birth weight.[2] A fetus's weight depends on the supply of nutrients that it receives through the placenta. If the placenta fails to grow properly, the developing fetus may be premature and be lighter than average at birth. Low birth weight and prematurity are among the leading causes of death among American infants who are less than 1 year of age.[3]

11.1b Nutrition in Pregnancy

During pregnancy, a woman's body undergoes major physical changes, such as increased blood volume and breast size, increased absorption of many nutrients and higher levels of several hormones. These adaptations enable her body to nourish and maintain the developing embryo/fetus, as well as produce milk for her infant after its birth. However, some of the changes are troublesome and even dangerous for the pregnant woman.

Premature baby being cared for in a special hospital nursery

© Royalty-Free/Corbis RF

TABLE 11.1	COMPARING SELECTED DRIs: 25-YEAR-OLD NONPREGNANT AND PREGNANT WOMEN		
	Energy/Nutrient*	Nonpregnant	Pregnant
	Kilocalories	Estimated Energy Requirement (EER)	First trimester = EER + 0 Second trimester = EER + 340 Third trimester = EER + 452
	Protein	46 g/day	71 g/day
	Vitamin C	75 mg/day	85 mg/day
	Thiamin	1.1 mg/day	1.4 mg/day
	Niacin	14 mg/day	18 mg/day
	Folate	400 mcg/day	600 mcg/day
	Vitamin D	15 mcg/day	15 mcg/day
	Calcium	1000 mg/day	1000 mg/day
	Iron	18 mg/day	27 mg/day
	Iodine	150 mcg/day	220 mcg/day

*RDA

Source of data: Institute of Medicine: *Dietary Reference Intakes.* Available from *Nutrient recommendations: Dietary Reference Intakes (DRIs).* http://ods.od.nih.gov/Health_Information/Dietary_Reference_Intakes.aspx.

Eating for Two?

The mother-to-be should follow a diet that meets her own nutritional needs as well as those of her developing offspring. Otherwise, she's likely to become deficient in certain nutrients, especially iron and calcium, as her fetus removes them from her bloodstream to meet its needs. Depending on the trimester, an expectant woman's requirements for energy (calories), protein, and many other nutrients are greater than her needs were prior to pregnancy. Nevertheless, a pregnant woman doesn't need to double her usual food intake just because she is "eating for two." **Table 11.1** compares Recommended Dietary Allowances (RDA) for energy and selected nutrients that apply to healthy 25-year-old nonpregnant and pregnant women.

Folate and Iron Needs

As Table 11.1 indicates, a pregnant woman's requirements for folate and iron are 50% higher than those of a nonpregnant woman. It's important for women to enter pregnancy with adequate folate status because embryos need the vitamin to support rapid cell division. Pregnant women who are folate deficient have high risk of giving birth to infants with neural tube defects, such as spina bifida (see Unit 8).

During pregnancy, a woman's blood volume expands. Thus, her need for iron increases because her body must use the iron to make more hemoglobin for the extra red blood cells. Additionally, the woman's body transfers iron to the fetus to build its stores of the mineral. If women fail to meet their iron needs during pregnancy, they can develop iron deficiency anemia. Pregnant women who are iron deficient have high risk of giving birth prematurely and having low-birth-weight infants.[4] According to the Dietary Guidelines for Americans, iron is a nutrient of public health concern for pregnant women.

To obtain adequate folate and iron, pregnant women should include food sources of the micronutrients in their diets. Units 8 and 9 provide information about foods that supply these micronutrients. Most physicians also recommend prenatal multiple vitamin/mineral supplements that contain folate and iron for their pregnant patients.

What's Morning Sickness?

During the first trimester, most women experience physical signs that they're pregnant, such as "morning sickness." The name **morning sickness** is misleading because the queasy stomach and vomiting can occur at any time of the day. Some women find that eating crackers and drinking some water helps to reduce the likelihood of feeling nauseated, especially before they get out of bed in the morning. Furthermore, eating

morning sickness nausea and vomiting associated with pregnancy

Placemat: © McGraw-Hill Education. Mark A. Dierker, photographer; Orange juice, Prenatal vitamins: © Wendy Schiff smaller but more frequent meals and nutritious snacks can be helpful. If the vomiting is severe, the pregnant woman should check with her physician. In most instances, morning sickness ends by the beginning of the second trimester.

What About Cravings?

The stereotype of a pregnant woman who craves pickles and ice cream isn't simply a myth. Food cravings are common during this stage of life and aren't limited to any particular food. Ask pregnant women to identify the foods they crave and you're likely to get a variety of responses. The causes of cravings are unknown, but they may be responses to the hormonal changes associated with pregnancy or to the emotional state of the mother-to-be. Unless food cravings supply too many empty calorie foods or contribute to excess weight gain, they're generally harmless.

Some women develop **pica**, the craving of nonfood items such as laundry starch, chalk, cigarette ashes, and soil. Pica may be linked with iron and zinc deficiency, but it's not clear if pica is the result or the cause of such deficiencies. Pregnant women should avoid practicing pica, especially eating clay or soil. Soil may contain substances that interfere with the absorption of minerals in the intestinal tract. Furthermore, eating soil can be harmful because the dirt may be contaminated with toxic substances, such as lead and pesticides, and disease-causing microbes.

11.1c Weight Gain During Pregnancy

pica craving nonfood items

high-birth-weight (HBW) newborn generally weighing more than 8.8 pounds at birth

Nearly all pregnant women experience weight gain. In fact, gaining an appropriate amount of weight is crucial during pregnancy. Women who don't gain enough weight during pregnancy have a high risk of giving birth to a LBW baby. On the other hand, women who gain too much weight during pregnancy can develop serious health problems and may have difficulty losing the excess weight after delivery. **Table 11.2** indicates the typical distribution of weight that's gained during this life stage.

How much weight a woman should gain depends on her prepregnancy weight and the number of fetuses she is carrying. **Table 11.3** presents recommended ranges of weight that women should gain during pregnancy (single fetus). Weight gain recommendations are higher for women who are pregnant with more than one fetus. For example, a healthy woman who is carrying twins may gain as much as 54 pounds during pregnancy.[5]

Women who are obese when they become pregnant are more likely to give birth to **high-birth-weight** (HBW) babies.[6] HBW newborns generally weigh more than 8.8 pounds. Pregnant women with poorly controlled diabetes have a higher risk of giving birth to a HBW infant than mothers who don't have this disorder.

When compared to newborns with healthy weights, HBW infants have higher risk of being injured during the birth process and of having birth defects.[6] Furthermore, HBW infants are more likely to develop childhood obesity.[7]

Soft serve ice cream cone: © Brand X Pictures/PunchStock RF; Jar of pickles: © Photodisc/Alamy RF; Mother holding twin baby socks: © JGI/Blend Images LLC RF

TABLE 11.2	DISTRIBUTION OF WEIGHT GAIN DURING PREGNANCY	
	Tissue	**Approximate Pounds**
	Maternal	
	Blood	3
	Breasts	2
	Uterus	2
	Fat, protein, and retained fluid	11
	Fetus	6–8
	Placenta	1.5
	Amniotic fluid*	2.0

*Fluid that surrounds fetus.

Adapted from http://www.marchofdimes.com/pregnancy/yourbody_weightgain.html.

TABLE 11.3	RECOMMENDED RANGES OF WEIGHT GAIN DURING PREGNANCY	
	Prepregnancy BMI Category	**Recommended Range of Weight Gain (lb)**
	Underweight	28–40
	Healthy weight	25–35
	Overweight	15–25
	Obese	11–20

Source: The American College of Obstetricians and Gynecologists: *Committee opinion: weight gain during pregnancy.* 2013. http://www.acog.org/Resources-And-Publications/Committee-Opinions/Committee-on-Obstetric-Practice/Weight-Gain-During-Pregnancy Accessed: May 27, 2016

Twins!

Figure 11.2 **Rate of weight gain in a healthy pregnancy.**

◼ *Why is it important to monitor a woman's weight gain during pregnancy?*

Rate of Weight Gain

For an expectant mother, the rate of the weight gain is important, as well as the amount of weight gained. Pregnant women usually gain up to 4 pounds of weight during the first trimester. Throughout the rest of their pregnancies, women typically gain at a faster rate—about 1 pound per week. **Figure 11.2** charts the course of weight gain in a healthy pregnancy.

What Is Gestational Hypertension?

High levels of certain hormones can cause various tissues to retain fluid during pregnancy. Although the extra fluid causes some minor swelling (mild edema), especially in the hands and feet, the condition is normal. Rapid weight gain, especially after the fifth month of pregnancy, could be a sign of a serious type of hypertension called **gestational hypertension**. Gestational hypertension is commonly referred to as **preeclampsia** (*pre-e-klamp'-see-a*). Preeclampsia is characterized by sudden, dramatic increase in weight that is due to edema, particularly of the hands or face; hypertension; and protein in urine (**Fig. 11.3**).[8] Treatment often includes bedrest and medications to control high blood pressure. If a woman suffering from preeclampsia develops convulsions, her condition is called **eclampsia** (*e-klamp'-see-a*). In the United States, eclampsia is the second-leading cause of death among pregnant women.[9]

The only effective, emergency treatment for eclampsia is delivering the fetus, but infants born before the 24th week of pregnancy are unlikely to survive. If the fetus is older than 24 weeks, its mother may be hospitalized for treatment. This practice helps physicians monitor the mother's condition and enables the fetus to mature until it has a better chance of surviving after birth.

Figure 11.3 **Signs and symptoms of preeclampsia.**

◼ *What is the only effective treatment for eclampsia?*

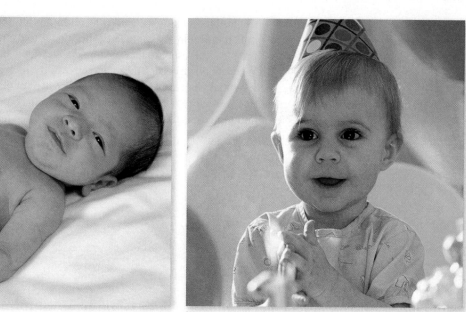

Figure 11.4 Babies' rapid growth rate. (a) Healthy newborn; (b) 1-year-old child.

■ *If this healthy baby weighs 6 pounds, 8 ounces at birth, how much would you expect her to weigh on her first birthday?*

11.1d Infant Nutrition

Rapid physical growth characterizes infancy, the life stage that extends from birth to about 1 year of age. During the first 4 to 6 months of life, a healthy baby doubles its birth weight, and by 1 year of age, an infant's birth weight has tripled. Additionally, an infant's length increases by 50% during its first year of life. Thus, if a baby girl weighs 7 pounds and is 20 inches long at birth, you would expect her to weigh 21 pounds and be 30 inches long by her first birthday (**Fig. 11.4**).

Compared to older children, an infant needs more energy and nutrients per pound of body weight to support its rapid growth. If an infant's diet lacks adequate energy and nutrients, the baby's growth may slow or even stop. Furthermore, the child's brain development might be negatively affected. The following sections take a closer look at infant nutrition, including breastfeeding and other infant feeding practices.

Understanding Lactation

Lactation is a complex process that occurs after a woman gives birth. During the first couple of days after her baby is born, the new mother's breasts produce **colostrum** (*co-loss'-trum*), a yellowish fluid that doesn't look like milk.

Colostrum is a very important first food for babies because the fluid contains antibodies and immune system cells that can be absorbed by the infant's immature digestive tract. Colostrum also contains a substance that encourages the growth of a type of bacteria, *Lactobacillus bifidus*, in the infant's GI tract. Such biologically active substances help an infant's body fight infections and hasten the maturation of the baby's immune system. Thus, breastfed infants, especially those who are exclusively breastfed, have lower risks of allergies and gastrointestinal, respiratory, and ear infections than do formula-fed infants.[10]

By the end of the first week of lactation, colostrum has become mature milk. Breast milk is more watery than cow's milk and may have a slightly bluish color.

Human milk is a rich source of lipids, including cholesterol, and fatty acids such as linoleic acid, arachidonic acid (AA), and docosahexaenoic acid (DHA). An infant's nervous system, especially the brain and eyes, depends on AA and DHA for proper development. Furthermore, the fat in breast milk helps supply the energy needed to maintain the infant's overall growth.

Q Answer This

A healthy newborn's length is 18 inches. What should be the baby's approximate length when he or she is 12 months of age? You can find the answer on the last page of this unit.

Breastfeeding may enhance a new mother's emotional bonding to her baby.

The Lactation Process

When an infant suckles, nerves in the mother's nipple signal her brain to release **prolactin** and **oxytocin** (*ox-e-toe'-sin*) into her bloodstream. Prolactin stimulates specialized cells in breasts to form milk. These cells carry out the lactation process by making some nutrients and removing others from the mother's bloodstream and adding them to her milk. Oxytocin plays a different role in establishing successful lactation. This hormone signals breast tissue to "let down" milk. The **let-down reflex** enables milk to travel in several tubes, called ducts, to the nipple area. A reflex is a physical response that's automatic and not under conscious control. When let-down occurs, the infant removes the milk by continued sucking. **Essential Concept 11.1** shows the major steps of the the lactation process. Shortly before the flow of milk begins, the lactating woman often feels a tingling sensation in her nipples, a signal that let-down is occurring.

Essential Concept

11.1   The Lactation Process

1 A baby's sucking stimulates nerves in the nipple that signal the pituitary gland in the mother's brain.

2 The pituitary gland releases prolactin and oxytocin into her bloodstream.

4 Oxytocin triggers breast tissue to "let down" milk, a process that enables milk to travel via ducts to the nipple area.

3 Prolactin stimulates milk-producing cells in breasts to form milk.

Mother's brain

Nerve signals

Pituitary gland

Oxytocin

Prolactin

Adipose tissue

Nipple

Milk duct

© Royalty-Free/ Corbis RF

Embarrassment, emotional stress and tension, pain, and fatigue can easily block the let-down reflex. For example, if a lactating mother is tense or upset, let-down doesn't occur, and her infant will not be able to obtain milk when it suckles. When this happens, the hungry infant becomes frustrated and angry, and the mother may respond by becoming even more tense and upset, setting up a vicious cycle. At this point, new mothers often give up breastfeeding, reporting that they tried to suckle their babies but were unable to "produce" milk. It helps if new mothers are in a comfortable, relaxed environment when they breastfeed their babies.

It may take a few weeks for the new mother to feel confident as a member of a successful breastfeeding team with her baby. Milk production relies on "supply and demand." The more the infant suckles (demand), the more milk its mother's breasts produce (supply). However, if milk isn't fully removed from the breasts, milk production soon ceases. This is likely to occur when infants aren't hungry because they have been given baby food and formula to supplement breast milk feedings.

Diet for a Lactating Woman

No special foods are necessary to sustain milk production. However, a lactating woman should drink fluids to keep her body properly hydrated. For as long as she breastfeeds her baby, the lactating mother should limit her intake of alcohol-containing beverages because her body secretes the drug into her milk. A woman who breastfeeds her baby should also check with her physician before using any medications, even over-the-counter and herbal products, because such substances may also end up in her breast milk.

Breast Milk Is Best Milk

Breastfeeding offers several advantages for mother and child.[11]

For infants, human milk

- is free of bacteria as it leaves the breast;
- supplies antibodies and immune cells;
- is easily digested;
- reduces risk of food allergies, especially to proteins in infant formulas and cow's milk;
- changes in composition over time to meet the changing needs of a growing infant;
- contains zinc, iron, and other minerals in highly absorbable forms;
- decreases risks of ear, intestinal, and respiratory infections; and
- may reduce the risk of asthma, obesity, and type 1 diabetes in childhood.

For new mothers, breastfeeding

- reduces uterine bleeding after delivery,
- promotes shrinkage of the uterus to its prepregnancy size,
- decreases the risk of breast cancer (before menopause) and ovarian cancer,
- may promote maternal weight loss,
- may enhance emotional bonding with the infant, and
- is less expensive and more convenient than feeding infant formula.

For more information about breastfeeding, visit http://www.cdc.gov/breastfeeding/.

prolactin hormone that stimulates milk production after delivery

oxytocin hormone that causes the "let-down" response and the uterus to contract

let-down reflex automatic physical response to a breastfeeding infant that enables milk to reach the nipple area

A father can help meet his baby's nutritional needs by giving the infant breast milk that's been placed in a bottle. © Getty Images RF

Is Breast Milk a Complete Food?

Registered dietitians and pediatricians generally recommend that new mothers breastfeed their infants exclusively during their babies' first 6 months of life.[11] It's not necessary to supplement young infants' diets with other fluids, such as water, infant formula, and juices, or with solid foods, such as baby food. However, it is important to obtain prompt professional medical care to prevent a baby from becoming dehydrated, particularly if the infant is suffering from diarrhea, vomiting, or fever.

Although breast milk is highly nutritious, it's not a complete food for all infants. Human milk may contain inadequate amounts of vitamin D and the minerals iron and fluoride. The American Academy of Pediatrics (AAP) recommends all breastfed infants be given a supplement that supplies 400 IU of vitamin D per day.[11] Healthy breastfed newborns generally don't need an iron supplement until they're 4 months of age.[12] A fluoride supplement may be necessary for breastfed babies if the mother's water supply isn't fluoridated. Before giving any dietary supplements to their baby, parents or caregivers should discuss their infant's nutritional needs with the child's physician.

After an infant reaches 6 months of age, breastfeeding should continue, but the infant can also be offered some appropriate solid foods, especially foods that are sources of iron. Breastfeeding may be combined with infant foods until the child's first birthday. However, there's no reason why children cannot be breastfed for longer periods. Throughout the world, many mothers continue to nurse their babies well past the babies' first birthdays, but in the United States, this practice is uncommon.

Quitting Too Soon

Nearly all healthy women are physically capable of breastfeeding their infants. In 2013, 81% of American women started breastfeeding their babies soon after birth.[13] By their first birthday, only about 31% of the babies were still being nourished with their mother's milk.

Women who breastfeed their newborns often stop the practice within 6 months. There are many reasons why women discontinue nursing their infants too soon. New mothers often quit because they lack information about and support for breastfeeding their babies. Hospitals may employ lactation consultants who are trained to provide information and advice about breastfeeding to new mothers. An additional resource is La Leche League, an international organization dedicated to providing education and support for breastfeeding women (www.llli.org/).

Some women discontinue breastfeeding because of uncertainty over how much milk their babies are consuming. Baby bottles are marked to indicate ounces, so a mother who bottle-feeds her infant can easily measure the amount of formula consumed. A lactating mother, however, has to observe her baby for cues indicating the child's stomach is full. When a breastfeeding baby is no longer interested in nursing and stops, its mother has to assume the infant has had enough milk.

A well-nourished breastfed infant will gain weight normally and generally have six or more wet diapers as well as one or two bowel movements that consist of soft stools per day. Parents or caregivers who are concerned about their infants' food intake or nutritional status should consult their physician immediately.

Many new mothers discontinue breastfeeding too soon because they need to return to work and have caregivers feed their babies. Lactating women can learn to express milk from their breasts and chill it for later feedings (**Fig. 11.5**). However, many workplaces don't have comfortable, private facilities for women to express milk and then store it safely.

11.1e Infant Nutrition: Formula Feeding

Not every woman wants to breastfeed her baby and, in some instances, people other than the new mother must feed the infant when breast milk is not available. Infant formulas are nutritionally adequate and safe alternatives to mother's milk. Their nutrient compositions, however, aren't identical to human milk (**Table 11.4**). Furthermore, infant formulas do not supply human antibodies and other unique immune system factors that are in breast milk.

Figure 11.5 Expressing milk. This new mother is expressing milk in a special room that was set up for this purpose at her workplace. She'll refrigerate the milk and take it home for later bottle feeding.

Baby: © Kwame Zikomo/Purestock/SuperStock RF; Expressing milk with pump: © Wendy Schiff

The fat content of human milk changes during each feeding, which usually lasts about 20 minutes. In the beginning of the session, the mother's milk is low in fat, but as her infant continues to suckle, the fat content of her milk gradually increases.[14] The higher fat content of the "hind milk" may make the baby feel satisfied and, as a result, discontinue feeding. Infant formulas, however, have uniform composition; that is, they don't change their fat content during a feeding session. Thus, the mother or infant caregiver is more likely to control the amount of formula the baby consumes, possibly leading to overfeeding.

Caregivers should provide an iron-fortified infant formula for babies who aren't breastfed. Not all infant formulas contain iron, so it's important to read the product's label before purchasing it. Formula-fed babies may also need a source of fluoride, but using municipal tap water that has been fluoridated to prepare concentrated infant formulas can ensure adequate fluoride intake.

Why Not Use Cow's Milk as a Formula?

Whole cow's milk shouldn't be fed to infants until they're 1 year of age.[12] Cow's milk is too high in minerals and protein, and it doesn't contain enough carbohydrate and essential fatty acids to meet an infant's needs. Essential fatty acids are critical for the development of an infant's nervous system, which includes the brain.

Infants have more difficulty digesting **casein** (*kay'-seen*), the major protein in cow's milk, than the major proteins in human milk. Cow's milk can also contribute to intestinal bleeding and iron deficiency.[16] Fat-reduced and fat-free cow's milk are too low in energy to be given to most children until they're 2 years of age. By then, the child should be eating a wide variety of foods in addition to milk, including sources of healthy fats and complex carbohydrates.

What About Formula Allergies?

Compared to breastfed infants, formula-fed babies have a greater risk of developing allergies to the formula.[17] Signs and symptoms of such allergies typically include the following:

- vomiting, intestinal pain, diarrhea or constipation;
- itchy, swollen, or reddened skin; and
- runny nose and breathing difficulties, such as asthma.

For babies who are allergic to infant formulas made from cow's milk proteins, similar products made with soy or other proteins are available.

Microwave: © Steve Wisbauer/Getty Images RF; Placemat: © McGraw-Hill Education. Mark A. Dierker, photographer; Pasteurized milk carton, Skim milk carton, Similac, Isomil: © Wendy Schiff

TASTY **Tidbits**

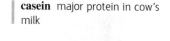

It's generally not recommended to heat bottles containing infant formula or human milk in a microwave oven. The heat can destroy immune factors in human milk and may create hot spots that can scald an infant's tongue. Instead, gently warm a bottle of breast milk or formula by running warm tap water over it or placing the bottle in a pan of warm water for a few minutes.[15] After heating, swirl the fluid in the bottle. To make sure the beverage is not too warm, test its temperature by shaking a drop or two onto your wrist or hand.

casein major protein in cow's milk

TABLE 11.4	COMPARING APPROXIMATE COMPOSITIONS OF HUMAN MILK AND IRON-FORTIFIED INFANT FORMULAS (PER OUNCE)						
Milk or Iron-Fortified Formula	**Energy (kcal/oz)**	**Protein (g/oz)**	**Carbohydrate (g/oz)**	**Fat (g/oz)**	**Cholesterol (mg/oz)**	**Iron (mg/oz)**	**Calcium (mg/oz)**
Human milk	22.5	0.32	2.12	1.35	4.00	0.01	10.0
Cow's milk protein-based formulas							
Similac	20.0	0.41	2.10	1.08	1.00	0.36	16.0
Enfamil	20.0	0.42	2.25	1.06	0.00	0.36	16.0
Soy protein-based formulas							
ProSobee	19.0	0.50	1.86	1.07	0.00	0.36	21.0
Isomil	20.0	0.49	2.04	1.09	0.00	0.36	21.0

extrusion reflex involuntary response in which a young infant thrusts its tongue forward when a solid or semisolid object is placed in its mouth

weaning gradual process of shifting from breastfeeding or bottle-feeding to drinking from a cup and eating solid foods

11.1f Infant Nutrition: Solid Foods

Many new parents are anxious to start feeding their young infants solid food. Solid foods shouldn't be introduced to infants until they're 4 to 6 months of age.[17] Why? An infant's digestive tract cannot readily digest starch before the child is 3 months old. Furthermore, infants are born with the **extrusion reflex**, an involuntary response that occurs when a solid or semisolid object is placed in an infant's mouth. As a result of this reflex, a young baby thrusts its tongue forward, pushing the object out of its mouth. Thus, trying to feed the young infant solid foods is a messy, frustrating process, because the child's tongue automatically pushes the food out of its mouth. Liquid foods, such as breast milk or infant formula, don't elicit the extrusion reflex, so the baby swallows fluids.

As the infant reaches 4 to 6 months of age, the extrusion reflex disappears. Moreover, a 6-month-old infant can usually sit up with back support and coordinate muscular control over his or her mouth and neck movements. These signs indicate the baby is ready physically to eat solid foods, is less likely to choke on such foods, and can turn his or her head away from food when full.

Weaning is the gradual process of shifting an infant from breastfeeding or bottle-feeding to drinking from a cup and eating solid foods. According to current recommendations, caregivers should begin introducing single-ingredient foods, along with breastmilk or formula, when the baby is between 4 to 6 months of age.[17] Typical first foods include rice cereal ("baby cereal"), ground meat or chicken mixed with breastmilk or formula, pureed green beans or squash ("baby vegetables"), and mashed bananas. If, after the child consumes the food for about 3 to 5 days, the new food appears to be tolerated by the baby, the caregiver should introduce another new food and watch the infant for any negative reactions, such as diarrhea, vomiting, skin rash, or runny nose.

In the past, highly allergenic foods, such as peanut butter, fish, and eggs, weren't introduced into a baby's diet until the child was at least 1 year of age. However, results of current studies indicate that *delaying* such foods may *increase* the child's risk of food allergies.[17] For example, feeding peanut butter to a baby who is 6 months of age may prevent the infant from developing peanut allergy later in childhood. Foods that are often thought to be allergenic can be introduced to a baby in very small amounts after the typical first foods have been consumed without causing health problems.[17] If the infant doesn't show signs of an allergic reaction to the food, the child can be fed higher amounts of the item. Caregivers should always check with the infant's physician for advice on when to start feeding a new food to the child.

At about 6 to 8 months of age, the baby's first set of teeth, the "primary teeth," begin to appear. These teeth are important for proper nutrition because they help the child bite and chew food. By 8 to 12 months of age, most infants can use their fingers to pick up and chew "finger foods" such as crackers, toast, and cooked string beans. Babies can also hold a bottle and practice drinking from a special cup ("sippy cup") that has a lid with a spout (**Fig. 11.6**). By about 10 months of age, many infants are mastering self-feeding and making the transition from baby foods to menu items the rest of the family enjoys. Babies need to practice self-feeding skills, even if it means playing with food and creating messes.

Figure 11.6 **Drinking from a "sippy cup."** Such cups as well as baby bottles can also provide food for molds and other microbes, so clean them thoroughly after each use.

Nutrition Fact or Fiction?

Adding solid foods to infants' diets helps babies sleep through the night.

This common belief isn't true. The developmental milestone of "sleeping through the night" generally occurs around 3 to 4 months of age, regardless of what infants are eating.

What Not to Feed Infants

Certain foods and beverages are not appropriate for infants. Avoid feeding

- *Honey*. This product may contain spores of *Clostridium botulinum*, which can produce a potentially fatal toxin in children who are under 1 year old (see Unit 5).

- *Semisolid baby cereal in a baby bottle that has the nipple opening enlarged*. This practice contributes to overfeeding and doesn't help the child learn self-feeding skills.

- *Candy, flavored gelatin water, or soft drinks*. These items provide few micronutrients and displace more nutritious fluids and foods from the infant's diet.

- *Small pieces of hard or coarse foods*. Foods such as hot dogs cut into "coin" shapes, whole nuts, grapes, chunks of cooked meat, raw carrots, popcorn, and peanut butter can cause choking. Caregivers should supervise meals to keep young children from stuffing too much food in their mouths.

- *Excessive amounts of apple or pear juice*. The fructose and sorbitol, a sugar alcohol, contained in these juices can lead to diarrhea. Also, if the infant drinks fruit juice or fruit drinks rather than breast milk or infant formula, the child may not be receiving adequate amounts of calcium and other essential minerals.

- *Unpasteurized (raw) milk or juices*. Unpasteurized milk and juice may be contaminated with bacteria or viruses.

- *Goat's milk*. Goat's milk is low in iron, folate, and vitamins C and D.

pasteurization process that kills the disease-causing microbes in foods and beverages as well as many microbes responsible for spoilage

Very young children can choke on grapes.

TASTY Tidbits

Pasteurization is a special heating process that's used by many commercial food producers to kill disease-causing microbes. In the United States, for example, most raw milk has been pasteurized before it's marketed. The heat treatment doesn't reduce levels of most vitamins that are in the raw milk.[18]

MILK
Ultra-Pasteurized
Vitamin D

11.1g Nutrition for a Healthy Childhood

Childhood can be divided into the preschool period (2 to 5 years of age), the school-age period (6 to 11 years of age), and adolescence (12 to 19 years of age). The rapid growth rate that characterizes the first 12 months of life tapers off quickly during the preschool years and proceeds at a slow but steady rate until the end of the school-age period.

When a child's growth rate slows, the youngster's appetite decreases because he or she doesn't need as much food. Caregivers must recognize that children don't have the stomach capacity to eat adult-size portions of foods. When planning meals for children, caregivers should emphasize nutrient-dense foods, such as lean meats, low-fat dairy products, whole-grain cereals, fruits, nuts, and vegetables. Although many ready-to-eat cereals are sweetened with sugar, it's not necessary to eliminate such foods. Caregivers, however, should read product labels and choose varieties with less added sugar. Additionally, it's important to monitor children's intake of sweets because sugary items can crowd out more nutritious foods from their diets.

During adolescence, the child experiences **puberty,** the stage of life in which a person reaches physical maturity and is capable of reproduction. Adolescence also features a period of dramatic increases in height and weight that's referred to as the **adolescent growth spurt.** To provide the energy and nutrients needed to support such rapid growth rates, a youngster's food intake increases accordingly. If maturing boys and girls choose to eat nutritious foods and maintain a high level of physical activity, they can take advantage of their increased hunger and gain lean body mass without gaining excess body fat. The MyPlate food guide can provide the basis for healthy adolescents to plan nutritionally adequate meals and snacks.

Theresa, the mother featured in the unit opener, is concerned about the influence she has over her young child's snacking habits. She's his role model for food choices and physical activity habits. If she eats a variety of nutrient-dense foods and is more physically active, he's more likely to eat such foods and be active as well.

TASTY Tidbits

Many teenagers (and adults) have acne—pimples, blackheads, and reddening of the skin—that often occurs on the face, upper back, and chest. The cause of acne is unknown, but hormonal, emotional, and genetic factors may contribute to the condition's development.[19] In the past, dermatologists (physicians who treat skin disorders) didn't think diet played much of a role in acne. According to a recent report of the American Academy of Dermatology, however, diets that have a low glycemic index may reduce acne breakouts.[19] See Unit 5 for information about the glycemic index.

What About Snacks?

Snacking isn't necessarily a bad habit, especially if snacks are nutrient dense and fit into the child's overall diet and energy needs. Young children have relatively small stomachs, so nutritious snacks can be offered at midmorning or midafternoon, when the child is likely to become hungry between meals. Some nutritious snacks that preschool age and older children tend to like include

- peanut butter spread on graham crackers;
- fruit smoothies made with no added sugars;
- fruit salad, dried fruit, or cut-up fruit;
- mini-pizzas (half an English muffin, topped with tomato sauce and Mozzarella cheese, and heated in toaster oven or microwave oven);
- plain, low-fat yogurt topped with granola or fresh fruit;
- pasta salad;
- peanuts, cashews, or sunflower seeds;
- fruit juice "Popsicle";
- quick breads, such as banana bread;

puberty stage of life in which a person matures physically and is capable of reproduction

adolescent growth spurt period associated with puberty when a child's height and weight rapidly increases

Boy drinking orange juice: © Fancy Collection/SuperStock RF; Acne: © McGraw-Hill Education; Smiling girl eating cereal and fruit: © McGraw-Hill Education. Eclipse Studios, photographer

- cheese melted on whole-wheat crackers;
- trail mix;
- ready-to-eat cereal; and
- vegetable sticks dipped in hummus.

Fostering Positive Eating Behaviors

Parents often refer to their young children as "picky eaters" because the youngsters don't eat everything offered to them. Furthermore, it's not unusual for preschool children to have "food jags," periods in which they refuse to eat a food that they liked in the past or want to eat only a particular food, such as peanut butter and jelly sandwiches or cereal and milk.

Picky eating and food jags may be expressions of a child's growing need for independence. It's important to recognize that everyone, including a child, is entitled to dislike certain foods. Caregivers should avoid nagging, forcing, and bribing children to eat. Instead, caregivers can offer the children a variety of healthy foods each day and allow the youngsters to choose which items and how much to eat.

Healthy children aren't in danger of starving if they skip a meal. A child who isn't hungry at mealtimes may have eaten a snack before the meal at a friend's home. If a child's lack of appetite persists, caretakers should consult the child's physician to rule out illness.

The following tips can help you improve your child's diet:

- Use the recommendations of MyPlate (see Unit 3) to guide your family's food choices and avoid dictating what they eat.

- Eat meals together as a family as often as possible.

- Reduce amounts of saturated and trans fats in your family's diet.

- Don't place your child on a restrictive diet unless the diet is recommended by the child's physician.

- Avoid using food as a reward or punishment.

- Encourage your child to drink water instead of sugar-sweetened beverages.

- Keep healthy snacks on hand.

- Serve at least five servings of fruits and vegetables each day.

- Discourage eating meals or snacks while watching TV.

- Encourage your child to eat a nutrient-dense breakfast daily.

Common Nutrition-Related Concerns

Nutrition-related problems that often affect children are iron deficiency, poor calcium intake, and obesity.

Iron Deficiency

Iron deficiency can lead to decreased physical stamina, learning ability, and resistance to infection. The best way to prevent iron deficiency in children is to provide foods that are good sources of iron, such as lean meat and enriched breads and cereals. Unit 9 provides more information about iron deficiency.

Poor Calcium Intakes

Over the last 20 years, many adolescents have switched from drinking milk to drinking soft drinks, including energy drinks. Dietitians and other nutrition experts are concerned that many adolescents have inadequate calcium intakes because of this practice. Inadequate calcium intake during adolescence is associated with decreased bone mass and increased likelihood of bone fractures later in life. Adolescents should consume 3 cups/day of fat-free or low-fat milk or equivalent dairy products daily. Furthermore, teenagers need to be aware that physical activity can strengthen bones, whereas smoking cigarettes is a risk factor for osteoporosis (see Unit 9).

TASTY **Tidbits**

The MyPlate website has a special series of web pages for children over 5 years of age. Children can visit the website and play the interactive "Blast Off Game." To test this game and others, visit http://www.choosemyplate.gov/games.

Source: USDA, ChooseMyPlate.gov website, http://www.fns.usda.gov/multimedia/Games/Blastoff/BlastOff_Game.html Accessed: May 28, 2016.

Adolescents should consume 3 cups/day of fat-free or low-fat milk or equivalent dairy products daily.

Obesity

The prevalence of obesity has increased for all American children over the past few decades. One in six children and adolescents is obese.[20] Obese children often have higher-than-normal blood pressure, cholesterol, and glucose levels.[21] Obese youngsters are also more likely to have low self-esteem, sleep apnea, heartburn, and musculoskeletal problems. Such children are at risk to develop hypertension, heart disease, and type 2 diabetes later in life. Furthermore, obese children are more likely to mature into obese adults than children who have healthy body weights.[21]

There's no single cause of excess body fat in children, but researchers have identified factors that are associated with the development of the condition. These factors include having a family history of excess body fat, high birth weight, and obese family members. Furthermore, youngsters who consume too many energy-dense, empty-calorie foods and beverages are also at risk of gaining excess fat in childhood.[21]

A major challenge is preventing childhood obesity without negatively affecting normal growth and development. Caregivers may need to limit the obese child's intakes of empty-calorie foods. These items often replace more nutrient-dense or lower-calorie foods in children's diets.

Aside from making poor dietary choices, physical inactivity also contributes to excessive weight gain in childhood. For many children, media use, such as viewing television programs and playing computer games, replaces physical activities that burn more energy. Children who spend more than 2 hours a day watching TV or using a computer are more likely to be overweight or obese than children who spend less than 2 hours a day using such entertainment media.[22]

Public health efforts to prevent childhood obesity often focus on ways for children to be more physically active. Children need at least 60 minutes of aerobic physical activity daily.[23] If children are not obtaining enough physical activity while at school, their caregivers can enroll them in after-school sports or community-based exercise programs. Being physically active will help children not only to attain healthy body weights but also to maintain healthy body weights later in life.

When helping a child lose weight, caregivers should avoid scolding or nagging the youngster because doing so can make the child rebel against adults, feel unloved and depressed, and dislike his or her body shape. As a result of harboring such negative feelings, an obese child may become vulnerable to developing disordered eating practices or eating disorders.

11.1h Nutrition for Older Adults

In 2014, 14.5% of the U.S. population was 65 years of age or older.[24] By 2060, government experts estimate that 25% of Americans will be in this age group. Americans who are 90 years of age and older comprise fastest-growing segments of the U.S. population.[25]

Although many Americans are living longer than their ancestors, they aren't necessarily living well. Chronic diseases are among the leading causes of death in the United States (see Fig. 1.2). These diseases are associated with lifestyles that include smoking, eating a poor diet, and being physically inactive. The following sections take a closer look at the physical changes associated with the normal aging process and how growing older may affect your nutritional status.

The Aging Process

The aging process begins at conception and is characterized by numerous predictable physical changes. Your body ages, regardless of the dietary and other health-related practices you are following. By the time you're 70 years of age, you'll have reached the final life stage—older adulthood. Growing old is a normal and natural process. **Table 11.5** presents some of the physical changes you can expect to occur as your body ages.

As the human body ages, its need for energy decreases; muscle mass declines as some muscle cells shrink or die. The age-related loss of muscle mass (*sarcopenia*) leads to a decrease in muscular strength and basal metabolism. The aging body typically loses lean tissue and gains fat tissue. Increased body fat results from overeating and lack of physical activity, but even athletic men and lean women usually gain some central body fat after they're 50 years of age. Being overweight or obese may increase the bone density of older adults and result in stronger bones, but having too much body fat increases the risk of type 2 diabetes, hypertension, cardiovascular disease, and osteoarthritis.

TABLE 11.5 AGING: NORMAL PHYSICAL CHANGES

Body System	Changes
Digestive	Reduced saliva and stomach acid secretion; increased heartburn and constipation
Skin, hair, and nails (integument)	Graying hair; drier skin and hair; skin loses elasticity and forms wrinkles; skin bruises easily
Musculoskeletal	Bone-forming cells become less active, resulting in bone loss that can lead to tooth loss and bones that fracture easily; fractures heal more slowly; joints become stiff and painful; muscle mass declines, resulting in loss of strength and stamina
Nervous	Decreased brain weight, reduced production of chemicals that transmit information between nerves, delayed transmission of nervous impulses, loss of short-term memory, and reduced sensory abilities (e.g., vision, hearing, smell, and taste)
Lymphatic (immune)	Reduced functioning resulting in increased vulnerability to cancer and infections
Circulatory	Hardening of the arteries, reduced heart output, increased risk of blood clots
Endocrine	Decreased production of reproductive, growth, and thyroid hormones
Respiratory	Reduced lung capacity, increased vulnerability to respiratory infections
Urinary	Increased loss of functional kidney cells, resulting in decreased blood filtration rate; loss of bladder control

Physical Inactivity

Many of the undesirable physical changes we associate with growing old are the result of a lifetime of physical inactivity. A physically active lifestyle increases muscle strength and mobility, improves balance, slows bone loss, and boosts emotional well-being. Before embarking on a program to increase physical fitness, however, sedentary older adults should consult their physicians concerning appropriate activities.

Older Adults: Common Nutrition-Related Concerns

Compared to younger persons, older adults have greater risk of nutritional deficiencies because their food intake tends to decrease as their metabolic rates and physical activity levels decline. Despite having lower energy needs, however, older adults need the same or even higher amounts of vitamins and minerals. Meeting micronutrient needs while eating less food can be difficult for older persons to accomplish. Older adults tend to consume more than recommended

TASTY Tidbits

A few foods interfere with prescribed drugs. Grapefruit juice, for example, can alter the potency of certain medications that are used to lower blood pressure or cholesterol. Therefore, people who take such medications should avoid consuming grapefruits and grapefruit juice.

© Wendy Schiff

amounts of sodium, saturated fat, and added sugars. Their diets, however, generally don't provide enough fiber, calcium, magnesium, potassium, zinc, and vitamins A, B-6, C, D, E, and folate.[26]

MyPlate can provide the basis for planning nutritionally adequate meals and snacks for healthy older adults. However, amounts of foods recommended in these diet plans may not provide enough vitamin D and calcium for elderly persons. In many instances, older adults can also benefit from taking a daily multiple vitamin/mineral supplement. Older adults who live at home may need professional help planning nutritionally adequate diets.

Numerous factors can negatively influence an older person's nutritional status, including medications, lack of social support, and low income. Many older adults take one or more prescription drugs and/or herbal dietary supplements daily. Such medications and products may interfere with the body's absorption and/or use of certain nutrients. Older people who live alone and on fixed incomes are at risk of undernutrition. Social isolation and low incomes are associated with emotional depression and inability to afford adequate amounts of nutritious food.

Physical factors associated with the aging process also affect food intake. Older adults may eat less because they have lost the ability to taste, smell, and/or chew food. People who lack normal cognitive functioning (thought processes) may be unable to make decisions regarding planning nutritious meals, as well as to shop for and prepare food. Chronic health problems such as arthritis and osteoporosis can interfere with mobility and flexibility, and can also interfere with food shopping and preparation activities.

In many instances, very old people refuse to eat and, as a result, lose considerable amounts of weight—a situation that hastens their death. Monitoring the elderly individual's weight can indicate whether long-term food intake has been adequate. If weight loss becomes significant, a physician should be consulted to determine the cause.

Nutrition Services for Older Adults

You can obtain information regarding locally available nutrition services for older people from medical clinics, private practitioners, hospitals, and health maintenance organizations in your area. To learn more about nutrition-related programs for older adults, visit the following websites: National Institute on Aging, www.nia.nih.gov/; American Geriatrics Society, www.americangeriatrics.org/; and Administration on Aging, www.aoa.gov/.

Module 11.2

How Safe Is My Food?

11.2 - Learning Outcomes

After reading Module 11.2, you should be able to

1. Define all of the key terms in this module.
2. Discuss the government's role in protecting the food supply.
3. List some common types and sources of pathogens that can cause food-borne illness.
4. Describe signs and symptoms of common food-borne illnesses.
5. Identify sources of contaminants in food.
6. Describe ways you can reduce the risk of food-borne illness.

Food-borne illness occurs when microscopic agents (microbes) or their toxic by-products enter food and they're consumed. Each year, one in six Americans becomes sick from various food-borne illnesses.[27] Of those persons who contract such ailments, 128,000 require hospitalization and over 3000 die. In the United States, water-borne disease-causing agents aren't major health threats because municipal water supplies follow government guidelines for sanitation.

Which foods are most likely to be responsible for food-borne illness? How can you reduce the risk of contracting one of these illnesses? Which government agencies monitor the safety of the U.S. food supply? After reading Module 11.2, you'll know answers to these questions.

TASTY **Tidbits**

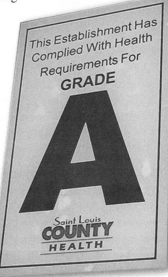

You cannot always rely on your senses to judge the wholesomeness of a food. A food can taste, smell, and appear safe to eat, but it may contain pathogens and/or their toxic by-products.

11.2a The Role of Government Agencies in Food Safety

The United States has one of the safest food supplies in the world, primarily the result of efforts conducted by cooperating governmental agencies that regulate and monitor the production and distribution of food. The Food and Drug Administration (FDA) of the U.S. Department of Health and Human Services and the U.S. Department of Agriculture (USDA) are the key federal agencies that protect consumers by regulating the country's food industry. Your local health department is responsible for inspecting grocery stores, dairy farms, food processing companies, and restaurants. In many communities, restaurants are required to post their sanitation rating where customers can easily see it.

After you obtain foods and bring them into your home, it becomes your responsibility to reduce the risk of food-borne illness by handling the items properly. However, if you suspect that something you consumed made you or a family member very sick, you should contact your physician for treatment. The physician may decide to report the case of food-borne illness to local public health officials so they can investigate and determine the source of your infection.

food-borne illness infection caused by microscopic disease-causing agents in food

This Establishment Has Complied With Health Requirements For
GRADE
A
Saint Louis
COUNTY
HEALTH

In many communities, local health departments inspect restaurants for food-related safety problems. The restaurants must display their rating for sanitation where customers can see it.

Sushi: © Royalty-Free/Corbis RF; Nose: © Ingram Publishing RF;
FDA logo: Source: FDA; Sanitation rating notice: © Wendy Schiff

What *IS* That? ------------------→

Genetic modification involves scientific methods that alter an animal or plant's hereditary material (genes or DNA). For example, genes that produce a desirable trait are transferred from one organism into the DNA of a second organism, altering its genes. **Genetically modified organisms (GMOs)** are often used for feeding livestock, and some foods that people consume contain ingredients from GMOs. According to a report published by the National Academy of Sciences in 2016, there's no scientific evidence that indicates genetically engineered foods are unsafe for humans to consume or harmful to the environment.[28]

11.2b Potential Dangers in Your Food

For thousands of years, people have used certain microbes to produce a variety of foods, including hard cheeses, raised breads, pickled foods, and alcoholic beverages. Other kinds of microbes grow and multiply in food, but their metabolic by-products spoil the food, making it unfit for human consumption. In some instances, disease-causing agents (**pathogens**) contaminate the food. When pathogens enter your food, they can cause vomiting, diarrhea, intestinal cramps, and other signs and symptoms of food-borne illness.

Food-borne pathogens include the following disease-causing agents.

- **Bacteria**—single-cell microorganisms, such as forms of *Clostridium* (*kloss-trid'-ee-um*), *Escherichia* (*esh'-er-ee'-she-ah*), and *Salmonella* (*sall'-mo-nell'-ah*).

- **Viruses**—microscopic agents that can cause infections, such as norovirus and the virus that causes hepatitis A.

- **Molds (fungi)**—simple microbes that live on dead or decaying organic matter. Some fungi are beneficial and edible, such as button mushrooms and the mold in blue cheese. Other fungi contain toxins that can cause organ failure or liver cancer.

- **Protists**—generally single-cell organisms that can have the characteristics of animals, plants, or fungi. *Giardia* (*jee-ar'-dee-ah*) is a single-celled protist that often contaminates natural water sources such as ponds and lakes (**Fig. 11.7**).

- **Parasitic worms**—worms that may be harmful to health because they live in the body. *Trichinella* (*trick'-in-el'-lah*) and *Anisakis* (*ah'-nah-say'-kis*) (**Fig. 11.8**) are parasitic worms that are food-borne pathogens.

Many kinds of food-borne pathogens can infect your digestive tract, inflaming the tissues and causing an "upset stomach" within a few hours after being ingested. A few types of food-borne pathogens multiply in your intestinal tract, enter your bloodstream, and cause general illness when they invade other tissues. Other pathogens don't sicken you directly, but these microbes contaminate food and secrete poisons (toxins). When you eat the contaminated food, the toxins irritate your intestinal tract and cause a type of food-borne illness called **food intoxication** ("food poisoning"). Many of the foods you eat regularly, such as meats, eggs, milk, and products made from milk, are high-risk foods because they support the growth of food-borne pathogens.

Figure 11.7 *Giardia.*

Figure 11.8 *Anisakis.*

genetically modified organisms (GMOs) living things that had alterations made to their hereditary material as a result of biotechnological activity

pathogens disease-causing microbes

bacteria simple single-celled microorganisms

viruses microscopic agents that can cause infections

fungi simple organisms that live on dead or decaying organic matter

protists tiny organisms that can have the characteristics of animals, plants, or fungi

food intoxication illness that results when poisons produced by certain microbes contaminate food and irritate the intestinal tract

parasitic worms worms that are pathogens because they live in the body

incubation period a length of time in which pathogens need to multiply in food or the digestive tract before they can cause illness

11.2c Signs and Symptoms of Common Food-Borne Illnesses

In most cases, otherwise healthy individuals who suffer from common types of food-borne illness recover completely and without professional medical care within a few days. However, vomiting, diarrhea, and other signs of illness can be so severe that the patient requires hospitalization. You should consult a physician when an intestinal disorder is accompanied by one or more of the following signs:

- fever (oral temperature above 101.5°F),
- bloody bowel movements,
- prolonged vomiting that reduces fluid intake,
- diarrhea that lasts more than 3 days, and
- dehydration.[27]

Some food-borne illnesses develop within 1 to 12 hours after eating the contaminated food.

© C. Zachariasen/PhotoAlto RF

Most pathogens have an **incubation period**, a length of time in which they grow and multiply in food or the digestive tract before they can cause illness. Thus, if you develop signs and symptoms of a food-borne illness, you might have difficulty identifying the source of the infection or intoxication. Was the vomiting and diarrhea that you experienced at 7 A.M. the result of eating soft-cooked eggs 24 hours earlier or the sliced deli chicken you ate for lunch two days ago?

Many people mistakenly report that they have the "stomach flu," when they're actually suffering from a food- or water-borne illness. "Flu," or influenza, is an infectious disease caused by specific viruses that invade the respiratory tract. Influenza is characterized by coughing, fever, weakness, and body aches. On the other hand, food-borne illness primarily affects the digestive system and not the respiratory system. Intestinal cramps, diarrhea, and vomiting aren't typical signs and symptoms of influenza, and coughing isn't a usual sign of a food-borne illness. Thus, it's inaccurate to call a bout of diarrhea and intestinal cramps the "stomach flu."

Table 11.6 provides a summary of some common pathogens and signs and symptoms of the food-borne illnesses they cause.

Staphylococcus aureus

© Eye of Science/Science Source

TABLE 11.6

COMMON SOURCES OF FOOD-BORNE ILLNESS

Pathogen	High-Risk Foods	Approx. Time of Onset	Typical Signs and Symptoms
Bacteria			
Campylobacter jejuni	Raw, undercooked poultry; raw milk; contaminated water	2–5 days	Diarrhea (often bloody), abdominal cramping, vomiting, fever
Clostridium botulinum (toxin)	Vacuum-packed foods, improperly canned foods, garlic-in-oil mixtures. Honey may contain spores.	18–36 hours	Vomiting, diarrhea, blurry or double vision, difficulty swallowing, muscular weakness. Can be fatal
Clostridium perfringens (toxin)	Cooked meat, poultry, casseroles, gravies	8–22 hours	Watery diarrhea, severe abdominal cramps
Escherichia coli O157:H7 (toxin)	Raw ground beef, raw seed sprouts, raw leafy greens, fresh fruit, raw milk, unpasteurized juices, foods contaminated with feces	2 hours to 6 days	Intestinal cramps, diarrhea, bloody diarrhea, kidney failure. Can be fatal
Listeria monocytogenes	Raw meat and poultry, raw milk, fresh soft cheese made from raw milk, liver paté, smoked seafood, deli meats and salads, hot dogs, produce	Unknown but probably more than 12 hours for GI tract signs and symptoms; probably a few days to 3 weeks for invasive disease	Fever, muscular aches, vomiting, diarrhea. In pregnant women, the infection can lead to stillbirth (birth of a dead fetus) or premature birth.

TABLE 11.6

COMMON SOURCES OF FOOD-BORNE ILLNESS *(Continued)*

Pathogen	High-Risk Foods	Approx. Time of Onset	Typical Signs and Symptoms
Bacteria (continued)			
Salmonella species	Raw or undercooked meat, poultry, seafood, and eggs; raw seed sprouts; raw vegetables; unpasteurized juice	6 hours–2 days	Nausea, vomiting, fever, chills, headache, abdominal cramps, diarrhea Infection can be fatal in infants, older adults, and people with serious chronic illness.
Staphylococcus aureus (toxin)	Meats, poultry, and eggs; foods made with eggs, such as potato, egg, macaroni, and egg salads; certain homemade ice creams, custards, and cream-filled pastries Cooked foods are often contaminated as a result of improper food handling practices.	1–6 hours	Diarrhea, nausea, vomiting, abdominal cramps, weakness
Viruses			
Hepatitis A *(HAV)*	Food or water that has been contaminated with HAV from feces	2–6 weeks	Fever, loss of appetite, nausea, vomiting, diarrhea, muscle aches, general weakness; may have yellow discoloration of skin and whites of eyes, liver enlargement, and dark-colored urine
Norovirus	Food or water that has been contaminated with infected feces, enabling the virus to be spread person-to-person	1–2 days	Vomiting; watery, nonbloody diarrhea; abdominal cramps; nausea; low-grade fever (occasionally)
Protists			
Cryptosporidium	Foods prepared with contaminated water or by people whose hands were contaminated with infected feces	2–10 days	Profuse, watery diarrhea; abdominal pain; fever; nausea; vomiting; weight loss
Giardia	Consumption of contaminated water, including water from lakes, streams, swimming pools High-risk groups include travelers to certain countries, hikers, and people who swim in or camp by lakes and streams.	1–2 weeks	Diarrhea, abdominal pain, loss of appetite
Toxoplasma	Raw or partially cooked infected meat, especially pork, lamb, or deer meat Accidentally ingesting infected cat feces	Difficult to determine because of uncertain timing of exposure	Fever, headache, muscle aches, rash Pregnant women should avoid contact with cat feces because the pathogen can infect their unborn offspring, causing eye or brain damage.
Parasitic worms			
Anisakis	Raw or undercooked infected seafood	1 hour to 2 weeks	Tickling sensation in throat during or after eating raw/undercooked seafood Severe abdominal pain that may be mistaken for appendicitis Vomiting or coughing up the worm may prevent infection.
Trichinella	Raw or undercooked infected meat, especially pork, bear, seal, and walrus meat	1–2 days	Initially: nausea, vomiting, diarrhea, fatigue, fever, abdominal discomfort Later: headaches, chills, cough, eye swelling, muscle and joint pain In severe cases, death can occur.

© Tetra Images/Alamy RF

Figure 11.9 Dangerous food preparation practice.

■ *From a food safety standpoint, what's wrong with this photo?*

11.2d How Do Pathogens Get into Your Food?

Pathogens are found throughout your environment. Therefore, you need to be aware of how they can enter foods to prevent becoming sick as a result.

- Animals (*vermin*) that live around sewage or garbage, such as flies, cockroaches, mice, and rats, often carry pathogens on their bodies or in their urine and feces. When the vermin come in contact with food, they can transfer the pathogens to humans.

- Poor personal hygiene practices, especially failing to wash your hands frequently, can transmit pathogens to yourself and others.

- Improper food handling frequently results in food-borne illness. A common practice is failing to wash cutting boards and food preparation utensils after they come in contact with raw meat or poultry. The contaminated boards and utensils are then used to prepare other foods. As a result of this practice, **cross-contamination** is likely to occur because the pathogens in one food are transferred to another food, contaminating it. If that food is eaten raw, such as carrots in a salad, it carries a high risk of food-borne illness (**Fig. 11.9**).

- Failing to cook and store foods properly can also increase the likelihood of food-borne illness.

11.2e Preventing Food-Borne Illness

Pathogens usually grow well when the temperature of a high-risk food is between 40°F and 140°F—the "danger zone" (**Fig. 11.10**).[29] Cooking foods to the proper temperature destroys food-borne viruses and bacteria. To be safe, a product must be cooked to an internal temperature that's high enough to destroy harmful pathogens and certain bacterial toxins. Using a meat thermometer is a reliable way to ensure that meat, poultry, and thick pieces of cooking foods have

Figure 11.10 Temperature guide for food safety.

TABLE 11.7

USDA Recommended Safe Minimum Internal Temperatures

Food	Safe Minimum Internal Temperature (°F)
Beef steaks and roasts	145
Fish	145
Pork	145
Ground beef, pork, lamb, and veal	160
Egg dishes	160
Poultry products	165

© FoodCollection/StockFood RF

reached the proper internal temperature without overcooking. **Table 11.7** indicates recommended minimum internal temperatures for cooking these foods.

Chilling food slows the growth of microbes in the items, but some bacteria can grow even at proper refrigeration temperatures. Freezing doesn't kill bacteria or inactivate viruses in food; the process just halts the microbes' ability to multiply.[30] As frozen food thaws, the bacteria and viruses resume their activities and can cause illness.

To reduce your risk of food-borne illness when purchasing food, take the following steps.

- Select frozen foods and highly perishable foods, such as meat, poultry, or fish, last.
- Check "best by" dates on packaged perishable foods. Choose meats and other animal products with the latest dates.
- Don't buy food in damaged containers; for example, avoid containers that leak, bulge, or are severely dented, or jars that are cracked or have loose or bulging lids.
- Open egg cartons and examine eggs; don't buy cartons that have cracked eggs.
- Purchase only pasteurized milk, cheese, and fruit and vegetable juices (check the label).
- Purchase only the amount of produce needed for a week's menus. The longer you keep fresh fruits and vegetables, the more likely they're to spoil.
- Pack meat, fish, and poultry in separate plastic bags, so their drippings don't contaminate each other and your other groceries.
- Take groceries home immediately. Refrigerate or freeze meat, fish, egg, and dairy products promptly.
- Store whole eggs in their cartons, even if your refrigerator has a place for storing eggs. Egg cartons are designed to keep eggs fresh longer than a refrigerator's egg compartment.

Contaminated hands and food preparation surfaces spread pathogens.

The following tips can help reduce your risk of food-borne illness.

- Wash your hands before preparing food, especially after using the toilet, changing a baby's soiled diaper, or playing with pets.
  - Wash your hands in very warm, soapy water for at least 20 seconds before and after touching food. If clean water for hand washing isn't available, use sanitizing hand gels or wipes.
  - Use a fresh paper towel or clean hand towel to dry hands. Reserve dish towels for drying pots, pans, and cooking utensils that aren't washed and dried in a dishwasher.

TASTY Tidbits

When using a meat thermometer, place the thermometer in the thickest part of the muscle tissue, away from bone, fat, or gristle. If the thermometer is inserted incorrectly or placed in the wrong area, the reading may not accurately reflect the internal temperature of the product.

© Wendy Schiff

- Before preparing food, clean food preparation surfaces, including kitchen counters, cutting boards, dishes, knives, and other food preparation equipment, with hot, soapy water.

  - The FDA recommends cutting boards with unmarred surfaces made of easy-to-clean, nonporous materials, such as plastic, marble, or glass. If you prefer to use wooden cutting boards, make sure they're made of a nonabsorbent hardwood, such as oak or maple, and have no obvious seams or cracks.

  - You can kill most pathogens when you clean and sanitize food preparation surfaces and utensils with a solution made by adding a tablespoon of bleach to 1 gallon of water. You can also sanitize kitchen sponges with the dilute bleach solution.

  - Replace cutting boards when they become streaked with cuts because these grooves can be difficult to clean thoroughly and may harbor bacteria.

- Use a solution of 1 tablespoon of bleach mixed in 1 gallon of water to sanitize food preparation surfaces and equipment that have come in contact with raw meat, fish, poultry, and eggs. You can sanitize moist kitchen sponges by heating them in a microwave oven for 1 minute or by washing them in a dishwasher that has a heated dry cycle.[31] In addition, wash kitchen towels frequently.

- Before preparing fresh produce, carefully wash the foods under running water to remove dirt and bacteria clinging to the surface. Bacteria can be sticky, so scrub the peel with a vegetable brush. Even if you plan to remove the skin or peel, wash the produce before you cut it.

To reduce your risk of food-borne illness when preparing and serving food, take the following steps.

- Don't use foods from damaged containers and safety seals or expired "use by" dates.

- Don't taste or use food that spurts liquid or has a bad odor when the can is opened.

- Read product labels to determine whether foods need to be refrigerated after their packages are opened.

- Always thaw high-risk foods in the refrigerator, under cold running water, or in a microwave oven.

- Cook foods immediately after thawing.

- Marinate food in the refrigerator, and if marinating meat, fish, or poultry, discard the marinade.

- Chilled foods should be kept covered and served from a shallow container filled with ice. Hot foods should be kept covered and be served from shallow, heated pans. The best simple advice to follow: "*Keep hot foods hot and cold foods cold.*"

- Avoid eating moldy foods.

- Don't allow hot foods to cool on the counter—place in refrigerator directly.

- When in doubt, throw the food out.

To reduce your risk of food-borne illness when cooking foods, take the following steps.

- Cook beef, poultry, pork, thick pieces of fish, and egg-containing dishes thoroughly, using a meat thermometer to check for doneness.

- Bake stuffing separately from poultry or wash the poultry cavity thoroughly and stuff the bird immediately before cooking. Make sure the temperature of the stuffing reaches 165°F. After cooking, transfer the stuffing to a clean bowl for serving or storage.

Washing hands: © McGraw-Hill Education. Rick Brady, photographer; Clorox bleach: © Wendy Schiff; Cutting board: © Pixtal/Punchstock RF; Ground beef: © John A. Rizzo/Getty Images RF

TASTY Tidbits

Ground meat and poultry are highly perishable and must be thoroughly cooked to avoid being a source of food-borne illness. The interior portion of an intact piece of raw animal flesh is free of bacteria because the tissues aren't exposed to air. However, ground meat and poultry products are often contaminated with microbes in the air and on the grinding equipment.

Nutrition Fact or Fiction?

Food that drops on the floor will not pick up microbes if it's picked up within 5 seconds.

Studies have determined that this is a food-related myth. As soon as food touches a contaminated surface such as a floor, some microbes adhere to it.[32]

TASTY **Tidbits**

Microwave cooking often heats food unevenly, so microbes can survive in the cool spots. While cooking food in a microwave oven, stop the oven occasionally and stir the food to reduce uneven heating. Microwave cooking isn't recommended for stuffed foods because during cooking, the temperature of the stuffing may not be high enough to kill pathogens.[33]

- Serve meat, poultry, and fish on a clean plate. Never use the same plate that held the raw product. When grilling hamburgers, for example, don't put cooked items on the same plate that was used to carry the raw meat to the grill.

- Give picnic foods special attention because outdoor temperatures may favor rapid bacterial growth. Keep cold salads and desserts on ice. Meats should be cooked completely at a picnic site. Don't partially cook foods in advance and plan to finish cooking them at the picnic.

To reduce your risk of food-borne illness when storing and reheating food, take the following steps.

- Cover leftovers and refrigerate or freeze them as soon as you have finished eating, or within 2 hours. If environmental temperatures are above 90°F, refrigerate the leftovers within 1 hour.[34] It's dangerous to let hot foods cool before chilling or freezing them.

- Keep all foods, including leftovers, covered while they're in the refrigerator. Store raw meats, fish, poultry, and shellfish on lower shelves of the refrigerator, so they're separated from foods that are to be eaten raw.

- Check your refrigerator's temperature regularly to make sure it stays below 41°F. Keep the refrigerator as cold as possible without freezing milk and lettuce.

- Cook ground meats and poultry soon after purchasing. If this isn't possible, freeze the ground items.

- Note that raw fish, shellfish, and poultry are highly perishable. It's best to cook these foods or freeze them the day they're purchased.

- Use refrigerated ground meat and patties within 1 to 2 days, and use frozen meat and patties within 3 to 4 months after purchasing them. **Table 11.8** presents recommended time limits for refrigeration and freezer storage of foods. Foods that are stored in the freezer for longer than recommended periods often develop unappealing flavors.

- Use refrigerated leftovers within 4 days.

- Reheat leftovers to 165°F; reheat gravy to a rolling boil to kill pathogenic bacteria that may be present.

TABLE 11.8

COLD STORAGE TIME LIMITS FOR PERISHABLE FOODS

Product	Storage Period in Refrigerator (40°F)	Storage Period in Freezer (0°F)
Fresh meat		
Ground meat	1–2 days	3–4 months
Steaks and roasts	3–5 days	4–12 months
Fresh pork		
Chops	3–5 days	4–6 months
Ground	1–2 days	3–4 months
Roasts	3–5 days	4–6 months
Cured meats		
Luncheon meat (deli sliced or open package)	3–5 days	1–2 months
Luncheon meat (unopened package)	2 weeks	1–2 months
Sausage, raw	1–2 days	1–2 months
Gravy	3–4 days	2–3 months
Fresh fish		
Lean (such as cod, flounder, haddock)	1–2 days	—
Fatty (such as perch, salmon)	1–2 days	—
Fresh chicken or turkey		
Whole	1–2 days	12 months
Parts	1–2 days	9 months
Prestuffed, uncooked chicken breasts	1 day	Not recommended
Leftovers		
Cooked meat	3–4 days	2–3 months
Casseroles that contain meat	3–4 days	2–3 months
Eggs		
Fresh, in shell	3–5 weeks	—
Hard-cooked	1 week	—

Source: USDA, Food Safety and Inspection Service: *Basics of handling foods safely: Cold storage chart.* Updated 2015. http://www.fsis.usda.gov/wps/portal/fsis/topics/food-safety-education/get-answers/food-safety-fact-sheets/safe-food-handling/basics-for-handling-food-safely/ct_index/ Accessed: August 1, 2016

Food safety educators with the federal government have condensed food safety rules into four simple actions:

1. **CLEAN.** Wash hands and surfaces often.
2. **SEPARATE.** Do not cross-contaminate.
3. **COOK.** Cook to proper temperatures.
4. **CHILL.** Refrigerate promptly

For general food safety questions, you can call FDA's food safety hotline at 1-888-723-3366.

What About Restaurant Foods?

In many instances, you cannot control the safety of foods that are prepared in restaurants or other places outside your home. However, you can greatly reduce your risk of food-borne illness by following some important rules, most of which require changing risky food selection, preparation, and storage practices. Be alert for signs of unsafe food handling practices when you eat out. The following tips also apply to foods prepared for dormitory residents:

- Make sure tabletops, dishes, and eating utensils are clean.

- Make sure servers who handle food directly are wearing gloves.

- Check custard, pudding, pies, and salad bar foods to make sure they're chilled and kept on ice.

- Make sure hot foods are served hot or served from a heated food bar.

- If your serving of meat, poultry, or fish doesn't appear to be thoroughly cooked, ask the waiter to return the item to the kitchen to be heated again.

- Be wary of perishable foods in vending machines, especially those that sell sandwiches.

If you or someone you know develops signs and symptoms of food-borne illness that probably resulted from products eaten at a restaurant or sold in a vending machine, call your physician or 911 for emergency care. For nonemergency cases involving food-borne illnesses, contact the staff of your local health department or FDA office (http://www.fda.gov/Safety/ReportaProblem/ucm059044) to report your experience.

TASTY Tidbits

The process of food irradiation preserves food by using a high amount of energy to kill pathogens. The energy passes through the food, as in microwave cooking, and no radioactive material is left behind. It's important to recognize that even when foods, especially meats, have been irradiated, once their packaging has been opened, the foods can still become contaminated.

Radura symbol

11.2f Emergency Food Supply

Hurricanes, tornadoes, earthquakes, "superstorms"—enduring a natural disaster can easily disrupt your access to safe food. Therefore, you should store at least a three-day supply of food for emergency use. Choose foods that have a long storage life, require no refrigeration, and can be eaten without cooking, such as canned meats, fruits, and vegetables. If you have infants, you should also keep a supply of baby foods. **Table 11.9** lists foods that can be included in your emergency food supply. Also store a manual can opener, paper plates, and eating utensils. For more information about emergency preparedness, visit the Centers for Disease Control and Prevention's website: https://emergency.cdc.gov/disasters/.

Aftermath of Super Storm Sandy (2012)

© McGraw-Hill Education.
Mark A. Dierker, photographer

TABLE 11.9	FOODS TO STORE FOR EMERGENCY SITUATIONS
	Bottled water
	Canned meats, fish, fruits, and vegetables
	Canned fruit juices
	Unopened boxes of cereal, low-salt crackers, and trail mix
	Prewrapped fruit-filled granola bars
	Peanut or other nut butters
	Raisins and other dried fruit
	Dry milk powder

Source: Liz Roll/FEMA

This farmworker is wearing protective gear as he handles a pesticide.

Source: Tim McCabe, courtesy of the USDA Natural Resources Conservation Service

11.2g What About Pesticides in Food?

Pesticides can contaminate foods, especially produce. A **pesticide** is any substance that people use to control or kill unwanted insects, weeds, rodents, fungi, or other organisms. The use of pesticides in modern farming practices has helped increase crop yields, reduce food costs, and protect the quality of many agricultural products. However, many pesticides leave small amounts (pesticide residues) in or on treated crops, including fruits, vegetables, and grains, even when they're applied correctly. Concentrations of pesticide residues often decrease as food crops are washed, stored, processed, and prepared. Nevertheless, some of these substances may remain in fresh produce, such as apples or peaches, as well as in processed foods, such as canned applesauce or peaches.

The Environmental Protection Agency (EPA) regulates the proper use of pesticides. The agency can limit the amount of a pesticide that's applied on crops, restrict the frequency or location of the pesticide's application, or require the substance be used only by specially trained, certified persons. The EPA also sets **pesticide tolerances**, maximum amounts of pesticide residues that can be in or on each treated food crop.

How Safe Are Pesticides?

The potential harmful effects of a pesticide in food depend on

- the particular chemical's toxicity,
- how much of it is eaten and how often, and
- a person's life stage and age. Pregnant women, children, those who are sick, and older adults may be more vulnerable to pesticide residues than others.[35]

Tolerable legal amounts of pesticide residues on or in foods are extremely small. However, it's possible that regular exposure to small amounts of these chemicals may enable the substances to accumulate in the body and produce toxicity or initiate cancer. Environmental health experts will continue to monitor the effects of pesticides on humans.

TASTY Tidbits

The Environmental Working Group (EWG) is a nonprofit organization that includes scientists who use data from government sources to protect consumers. The EWG uses the results of government testing to make a list that ranks produce according to amounts of pesticide residues. In 2016, strawberries were at the top of the list of produce because they had the highest pesticide residue levels. Onions were among the produce that contained the lowest pesticide residues. To access the produce list, visit https://www.ewg.org/foodnews /dirty_dozen_list.php.

pesticide substance that people use to kill or control unwanted insects, weeds, or other organisms

pesticide tolerances maximum amounts of pesticide residues that can be in or on each treated food crop

Module 11.3

Dietary Adequacy: A Global Concern

© Digitial Vision/PunchStock RF

11.3 - Learning Outcomes

After reading Module 11.3, you should be able to

1. Define all of the key terms in this module.

2. List factors that contribute to undernutrition in developing countries.

3. Describe how undernutrition during pregnancy and childhood can affect children.

4. Describe efforts to increase the supply of nutritious food in countries where undernutrition is widespread.

5. Identify major federally subsidized food programs in the United States.

6. Discuss how sustainable agriculture can improve the environment.

Undernutrition occurs when long-term energy and nutrient intakes are insufficient to meet an individual's needs. Throughout the world, approximately 800 million people were chronically undernourished in 2016.[36] Regional food shortages contribute to undernutrition. Such shortages can result from traditional dietary practices, crop failures, local warfare, and political instability and corruption. Poverty and undernutrition are commonplace in many developing countries. Impoverished people must also cope with infectious diseases, overcrowded and unsafe housing conditions, and polluted water supplies (**Fig. 11.11**). The following section provides some general information about undernutrition; Unit 10 discussed overnutrition. Unit 7 includes information about protein malnutrition.

Figure 11.11 Factors that contribute to undernutrition. Many factors, including war, disease, and overpopulation, contribute to undernutrition.

11.3a Undernutrition

In chronically undernourished children, nutrient deficiencies are responsible for poor physical growth, delayed physical development, blindness, impaired intellectual development, and premature death. Chronic undernutrition also depresses the body's immune functioning, increasing the risk of death from infectious diseases, such as measles, especially in childhood. Each year, undernutrition contributes to 3.1 million deaths of children who are under 5 years of age.[37] The vast majority of childhood deaths associated with undernutrition occurs among poor populations in developing countries, particularly in Sub-Saharan Africa and parts of Asia.[37]

Undernutrition During Pregnancy

Undernutrition can be very harmful when it occurs during periods of rapid growth, such as pregnancy, infancy, and childhood. Women who are undernourished during pregnancy are more likely to die while giving birth than pregnant women who are adequately nourished. Furthermore, malnourished pregnant women have a high risk of giving birth to infants that are born prematurely. These babies often suffer from breathing problems and have low birth weights—conditions that increase their risk of dying during their first year of life.

undernutrition state of health that occurs when long-term energy and nutrient intakes are insufficient to meet an individual's needs

345

What *IS* That? - - - - - - - - - - - - - →

In parts of Africa, Cambodia, and the Philippines, many people eat locusts, especially when the insects are plentiful. Popular ways to cook locusts include frying with seasonings or placing locusts on skewers and roasting them over hot embers. The legs and wings are removed from the grilled insects before they are cooked or eaten. Over 60% of the dry weight of a locust is protein, so the insect is an excellent source of the macronutrient.[38]

© IT Stock/Alamy RF

kwashiorkor form of protein-energy malnutrition that occurs when a child is abruptly weaned from breast milk and consumes inadequate amounts of high-quality protein

marasmic kwashiorkor form of protein-energy malnutrition that's characterized by edema and wasting

marasmus severe form of protein-energy malnutrition that causes extreme weight loss; starvation

Undernutrition During Infancy

As explained in Module 11.1, breast milk is the best food for young infants because it's sanitary, is nutritionally adequate, and provides babies with immunity to some infectious diseases. Throughout the world, only about 36% of babies consume only breast milk during their first 6 months of life.[39] Infant formulas are nutritious substitutes for breast milk, but they are generally more expensive. To extend infant formulas, poor parents in developing countries often add excessive amounts of water. This practice dilutes the nutritional value of the formula and increases the likelihood of contaminating it with disease-causing microbes. In infants, the diarrhea that results from drinking formula mixed with unsanitary water can rapidly cause loss of body water (dehydration) and death.

Dietitians and physicians recommend that infants be breastfed exclusively for the first 6 months of life. Ideally, babies should continue to receive breast milk in addition to solid foods well into their second year, especially in places where clean water is unavailable. Protein malnutrition typically occurs soon after impoverished children are weaned abruptly from breast milk and introduced to far-less-nourishing solid foods.

Undernutrition During the Preschool Years

The brain grows rapidly during the first 5 years of life. When undernutrition occurs during this period, the effects can be devastating to the child's brain and result in permanent learning disabilities. Additionally, chronically undernourished children don't grow normally and tend to be shorter—if they survive to adulthood.

In the United States and other developed countries, children are usually well nourished and vaccinated against common childhood diseases, including measles. In poorer nations, however, many children are malnourished and not protected from the virus that causes measles. Measles is a life-threatening illness for malnourished children because their immune systems don't function normally.

What's Protein-Energy Malnutrition?

Protein-energy malnutrition (PEM) affects people whose diets lack adequate amounts of protein as well as energy. Kwashiorkor, marasmic kwashiorkor, and marasmus are forms of PEM. **Kwashiorkor** (*qwash'-ee-or'-kor*) primarily occurs in developing countries where mothers commonly breastfeed their infants until they give birth to another child. The older youngster, who's usually a toddler, is fairly healthy until abruptly weaned from its mother's milk to make way for the younger sibling. Although the toddler may obtain adequate energy by consuming a traditional diet of cereal grains, the diet lacks enough complete protein to meet the youngster's high needs. The signs and symptoms of kwashiorkor occur as a result of the child's poor diet.

Children with kwashiorkor have stunted growth; unnaturally blond, sparse, and brittle hair; and patches of skin that have lost their normal coloration. The children also have swollen cheeks, arms, legs, and bellies that make them look well fed, but their appearance is misleading. During starvation, levels of proteins in blood that maintain proper fluid balance decline, resulting in edema (see Unit 7). The edema makes the protein-deficient child look plump and overfed instead of thin and undernourished.

In many cases, the child suffering from kwashiorkor doesn't obtain enough energy and eventually develops **marasmic kwashiorkor**, a condition characterized by edema and wasting (**Fig. 11.12**). Wasting is the loss of organ and muscle proteins as the body tears down these tissues to obtain amino acids for energy.

Severe PEM causes extreme weight loss and a condition called **marasmus** (*mah-raz'-mus*), which is commonly referred to as starvation. Obvious signs of marasmus are weakness and wasting. People suffering from marasmus avoid physical activity to conserve energy, and they're often irritable. The following section describes efforts that can reduce the occurrence of PEM in the world.

Figure 11.12 This photo of undernourished children was taken during a civil war in Nigeria (late 1960s).

Source: Centers for Disease Control/ Dr. Lyle Conrad RF

11.3b World Food Crisis: Finding Solutions

Reducing protein-energy malnutrition through food aid programs is a major goal of the United Nations. The World Food Program and United Nations Children's Fund (UNICEF) are agencies within the United Nations that provide high-quality food for undernourished populations. UNICEF also supports the development and distribution of ready-to-use, therapeutic food (RUTF) to treat severe undernutrition among young children in developing countries. Plumpy'nut, for example, is an energy- and nutrient-dense paste made from a mixture of peanuts, powdered milk, oil, sugar, vitamins, and minerals. During processing, the paste is placed in foil packets to keep the food clean and make it easy to transport to remote places without refrigeration. In 2010, UNICEF supplied nearly 21,000 metric tons of RUTFs to feed starving children in developing nations.[40]

11.3c Does Undernutrition Occur in the United States?

You may be surprised to learn that some people are undernourished in wealthy, developed nations such as the United States. Poverty is often responsible for undernutrition in any country. In 2015, 13.5% of the U.S. population was living at or below the U.S. Department of Health and Human Services poverty guideline.[41] In 2016, the poverty guideline was $24,300 for a family of four.[42]

Most American households are **food secure**, which means the people in those households have access to and can purchase sufficient food to lead healthy, active lives. In 2015, food insecurity was reported in about 13% of all households in the United States.[43] **Food insecurity** describes individuals or families who are concerned about running out of food or not having enough money to buy more food. People who are unemployed, work in low-paying jobs, or have excessive medical and housing expenses often experience food insecurity. Food insecurity may also affect older adults who live on fixed incomes, especially if they're forced to choose between purchasing nutritious food and buying life-extending medications.

Table 11.10 lists major federally supported food programs in the United States. Such programs provide food for people in need. However, not every eligible food-insecure person has access to or takes advantage

food secure describes households in which the residents have access to and can purchase sufficient food to lead healthy, active lives

food insecurity describes individuals or families who are concerned about running out of food or not having enough money to buy more food

TABLE 11.10

MAJOR FEDERALLY SUBSIDIZED FOOD PROGRAMS IN THE UNITED STATES

Program	General Eligibility Requirements	Description
Supplemental Nutrition Assistance Program (formerly called the Food Stamp Program)	Low-income individuals and families	Participants use an Electronic Benefit Transfer (debit) card to purchase allowable food items.
Commodity Supplemental Food Program	Certain low-income groups, including pregnant women, preschool-age children, and the elderly	In some states, state agencies distribute USDA surplus foods to eligible people.
Special Supplemental Nutrition Program for Women, Infants, and Children (WIC)	Low-income pregnant or breastfeeding women, infants, and children under 5 years of age who are at nutritional risk	Participants receive checks or vouchers to purchase milk, cheese, fruit juice, certain cereals, infant formula, and other specific food items at grocery stores. Nutrition education is also provided.
National School Lunch Program	Low-income children of school age	Certain schools receive subsidies from the government to provide free or reduced-price nutritionally balanced lunches.
School Breakfast Program	Low-income children of school age	Certain schools receive subsidies from the government to provide free or reduced-price nutritionally balanced breakfasts.
Child and Adult Care Food Program	Children enrolled in organized childcare programs and seniors in adult care programs	Sites receive reimbursement for nutritious meals supplied to participants.
The Nutrition Program Congregate Meals for the Elderly	Age 60 or older (no income guidelines)	Sites provide free, nutritious noon meals. Participant can contribute money for cost of the meal.
Home-Delivered Meals (Meals on Wheels)	Age 60 or older but unable to leave home	At least 5 days a week, volunteers deliver a noon meal to the participant's home. Meal is free, or participant can contribute money for the cost of the meal.
Food Distribution Program on Indian Reservations	Low-income American Indian or non-Indian households on reservations; members of federally recognized Native-American tribes	Distribution of monthly food packages. This program is an alternative to the Supplemental Nutrition Assistance Program and includes nutrition education component.

of the aid. For more information about the federal government's nutrition assistance programs, visit http://www.nutrition.gov/food-assistance-programs.

There are actions you can take to help relieve the problem of hunger in your community. You can stimulate student interest by researching the extent of food insecurity in the area and then writing an article about the situation for the campus newspaper. You can help food-insecure people directly by volunteering to prepare or serve food at a soup kitchen or homeless shelter in your community. You can also initiate and coordinate a canned food drive on your campus to benefit a local food pantry.

11.3d Feeding the World, Protecting Natural Resources

The world's population is estimated to be over 6.5 billion people. If the present rate of population growth doesn't slow, an estimated 9.7 billion people will be living on Earth in 2050.[44] By 2050, agricultural efforts will need to double their current level of production to meet the population's demand for more food.[45]

Replacing forests with new farmlands often harms the environment.

© McGraw-Hill Education. Barry Barker, photographer

Our current system of food production relies primarily on conventional agricultural methods. In general, conventional farming requires considerable amounts of water and pesticides that can harm our environment. Irrigation systems often remove fresh water from rivers and other natural sources at a faster rate than it's restored. This activity reduces water flow to many communities. The water that runs off conventional farms can carry precious topsoil with it and pesticides that pollute waterways. Such farming methods also release greenhouse gases, especially carbon dioxide and methane, which contribute to global warming. Furthermore, the need for new farmland often requires cutting down trees so that forests can be converted to croplands. The loss of forests eliminates wild animal and plant habitats. About 40% of the Earth's land (excluding Greenland and Antarctica) is used for food production; very little suitable land remains to be farmed.[45] What can be done to feed the world's population without destroying the Earth's natural resources?

What's Sustainable Agriculture?

Sustainable agriculture involves farming methods that meet the demand for more food without depleting natural resources and harming the environment. The challenge is finding ways to have farmers and ranchers make the conversion from primarily conventional farming techniques to sustainable agriculture. Farming needs to be profitable for farmers and ranchers, so any switch from conventional to sustainable agricultural methods must not reduce their profit margins.

To solve the problems created by conventional agricultural methods, an international team[45] developed the following five points for establishing a universal policy:

- *Stop expanding agricultural activity, especially into tropical forests and grasslands.*

- *Find ways to improve crop yields on existing farms.*

  - Biotechnology in agriculture has led to the development of crops that supply higher yields, resist pests, or are tolerant of drought conditions. **Biotechnology** involves the use of living things—plants, animals, microbes—to manufacture new products.

  - By increasing food production or modifying the nutritional content of foods, biotechnology offers a way of reducing the world food crisis.

sustainable agriculture farming methods that don't deplete natural resources while meeting the demand for food

biotechnology the use of living things to manufacture new products

© Steven Schleuning RF

- *Find ways to use natural resources and pesticides more efficiently.*
  - Use irrigation systems that apply water directly to a plant's base instead of spraying it into the air, where much of the water evaporates.
  - Rely more on nonchemical methods of pest management or **integrated pest management (IPM)**. IPM involves using a variety of methods for controlling pests while limiting damage to the environment. IPM methods include growing pest-resistant crops, using certain helpful insects to control crop-destroying bugs, and trapping adult insect pests before they can reproduce (**Fig. 11.13**).

- *Eat less meat.* Sixty percent of the world's crops (primarily grains) are grown for human consumption.[45] Most of the remaining crops are used to feed cattle and other farm animals. It takes about 30 pounds of grains to produce each pound of hamburger.[45] By eating less meat, especially beef, more grains could be produced to feed people. Grass-fed beef also spares grains for human consumption, because grass isn't eaten by people.

- *Reduce food waste.* About 30% of food is wasted.[45] In many instances the food spoils before you can eat it or it's thrown out as garbage. Reducing portion sizes and better menu planning can reduce the amount of food that you waste each day.

Taking Action

Poverty and hunger have always plagued humankind; the causes of poverty and hunger are complex and, therefore, are difficult to eliminate. Nevertheless, certain social, political, economic, and agricultural changes can reduce the number of people who are chronically hungry. In the short run, wealthy countries can provide food aid to keep impoverished people from starving to death. Families and small farmers in underdeveloped nations need to learn new and more efficient methods of growing, processing, preserving, and distributing nutritious regional food products. Additionally, governments can support programs that encourage breast-feeding and fortify locally grown or commonly consumed foods with vitamins and minerals that are often deficient in local diets.

In the long run, population control is critical for preserving the Earth's resources for future generations. Impoverished parents in poor countries often have many children because they expect only a few to survive and reach adulthood. When people are financially secure, adequately nourished, and well educated, they tend to have fewer, healthier children. Thus, long-term ways to slow population growth include providing well-paying jobs, improving public education, and increasing access to health care services.

Source: ARS/USDA

Figure 11.13 **Helpful insect.** The spined soldier bug (left) makes a meal of a Mexican bean beetle larva. Bean beetle larvae are pests of snap beans and soybeans.

integrated pest management (IPM) nonchemical methods of agricultural pest management

What steps can you take to reduce the amount of food that you waste?

© Wendy Schiff

In a **Nutshell**

© McGraw-Hill Education.
Mark A. Dierker, photographer

Module 11.1 Nutrition for a Lifetime

- The first trimester of pregnancy is a critical stage of prenatal development. The placenta transfers nutrients and oxygen from the mother's bloodstream to the embryo/fetus. The placenta also transfers wastes from the embryo/fetus to the mother's bloodstream, so her body can eliminate them.

- During pregnancy, a woman's body undergoes major physical changes that enable her body to nourish and maintain the developing embryo/fetus, as well as produce milk for her infant after its birth. Depending on the trimester, an expectant woman's requirements for energy, protein, and many other nutrients are greater than her needs prior to pregnancy.

- The amount of weight a woman should gain during pregnancy depends on her prepregnancy weight and the number of fetuses she's carrying. Women who gain excess weight during pregnancy are likely to retain the extra pounds after giving birth.

- Rapid weight gain, especially after the fifth month of pregnancy, could be a sign of gestational hypertension. If a woman with gestational hypertension develops convulsions, her condition is called eclampsia. In the United States, eclampsia is the second-leading cause of death among pregnant women.

- During the first 4 to 6 months of life, a healthy baby doubles its birth weight, and by 1 year of age, an infant's birth weight has tripled. Additionally, an infant's length increases by 50% during its first year of life. If an infant's diet lacks adequate energy and nutrients, the baby's growth may slow or even stop.

- Prolactin stimulates specialized cells in breasts to form milk. Oxytocin signals breast tissue to "let down" milk. The let-down reflex enables milk to travel in ducts to the nipple area.

- Breastfeeding offers several advantages for the infant and its mother. Colostrum contains antibodies, immune system cells, and a substance that encourages the growth of *Lactobacillus bifidus* in the infant's GI tract. Breastfed infants, especially those who are exclusively breastfed, have lower risks of allergies and gastrointestinal, respiratory, and ear infections than do formula-fed infants.

© BananaStock/PictureQuest RF

- Although iron-fortified infant formulas are nutritionally adequate and safe, their nutrient compositions aren't identical to human milk. Infant formulas don't supply immune system factors that are in breast milk. Human milk may contain inadequate amounts of vitamin D and the minerals iron and fluoride.

- Healthy babies are physically mature enough to consume solid baby foods by 4 to 6 months of age. After an infant reaches 6 months of age, breastfeeding should continue, but the infant can also be offered some appropriate solid foods. Breastfeeding can be combined with providing a variety of tolerated foods until the child's first birthday.

- Whole cow's milk shouldn't be fed to infants until they're 1 year of age. Fat-reduced cow's milk and fat-free cow's milk are too low in energy to be given to most children until they're 2 years of age.

- The rapid growth rate that occurs during a child's first 12 months of life tapers off quickly during the preschool years. When a child's growth rate slows, the youngster's appetite decreases because he or she doesn't need as much food. When planning meals for children, caregivers should emphasize nutrient-dense foods, such as lean meats, low-fat dairy products, whole-grain cereals, fruits, nuts, and vegetables.

- During adolescence, the child experiences puberty and the adolescent growth spurt. To provide the energy and nutrients needed to support such rapid growth rate, an adolescent's food intake increases accordingly. Nutrition-related problems that often affect young children and adolescents are iron deficiency, poor calcium intakes, and obesity.

- The aging process begins at conception and is characterized by numerous predictable physical changes, including the need for fewer calories later in life. Many of the undesirable physical changes associated with growing old are the result of a lifetime of physical inactivity.

- Compared to younger persons, older adults have greater risk of nutritional deficiencies. Diets of older adults often provide inadequate amounts of vitamins and minerals.

- Factors that can influence an older person's nutritional status include medications, lack of social support, low income, lack of mobility, and tooth loss. People who have impaired cognitive and physical functioning may be unable to make decisions regarding planning nutritious meals, as well as to shop for and prepare food.

Module 11.2 How Safe Is My Food?

- Food-borne illness occurs when pathogens or their toxic by-products enter food and they're consumed. The United States has one of the safest food supplies in the world. The FDA and the USDA are the key federal agencies that protect consumers by regulating the country's food industry.

- Food-borne pathogens include bacteria, viruses, molds, protists, and parasitic worms. Food-borne pathogens may infect your digestive tract, inflaming the tissues. Some food-borne pathogens multiply in your intestinal tract, enter your bloodstream, and cause general illness when they invade other tissues. Other pathogens contaminate food and secrete poisons that irritate your intestinal tract and cause food intoxication. Protein-rich foods are more likely to support the growth of food-borne pathogens than other foods.

- Signs and symptoms of food-borne illness typically include vomiting, diarrhea, and intestinal cramps. Influenza is a respiratory tract infection, so it's inaccurate to call a bout of diarrhea and intestinal cramps the "stomach flu."

- Pathogens are found throughout your environment. Poor personal hygiene practices and improper food handling frequently result in food-borne illness. Failing to cook and store foods properly can also increase the likelihood of food-borne illness. The "danger zone" for high-risk foods is between 40°F and 140°F. Cooking foods to the proper temperature destroys food-borne viruses and bacteria. Chilling food slows the growth of microbes.

- Pesticides can contaminate foods, especially produce. Concentrations of pesticide residues often decrease as food crops are washed, stored, processed, and prepared. The EPA regulates the proper use of pesticides and sets pesticide tolerances.

© Susan Thompson Photography/Flickr/ Getty Images RF

Module 11.3 Dietary Adequacy: A Global Concern

- Undernutrition occurs when long-term energy and nutrient intakes are insufficient to meet an individual's needs. Poverty and undernutrition are common in countries where people must cope with infectious diseases, overcrowded and unsafe housing conditions, and polluted water supplies.

- In chronically undernourished children, nutrient deficiencies are responsible for stunted physical growth, delayed physical development, reduced immune system function, blindness, impaired intellectual development, and premature death. The vast majority of childhood deaths associated with undernutrition occur among poor populations in developing countries, particularly in parts of Africa and Asia.

- Undernourished pregnant women are more likely to die while giving birth than are adequately nourished pregnant women. Furthermore, malnourished pregnant women have a high risk of giving birth prematurely.

- In developing countries, poor parents often add excessive amounts of water to infant formula, which dilutes the nutritional value of the formula and increases the likelihood of contaminating it with disease-causing microbes. Babies should continue to receive breast milk in addition to solid foods well into their second year, especially in places where clean water is unavailable. Protein malnutrition typically occurs soon after impoverished children are weaned abruptly from breast milk and introduced to far less-nourishing solid foods.

- In 2015, 13.5% of the U.S. population lived at or below the poverty guidelines. Food insecurity affected almost 13% of all households in the United States in 2015. In the United States, several federally supported food programs provide food for people in need.

- An estimated 9.7 billion people will be living on Earth in 2050. Agricultural efforts will need to double their current level of production to meet the population's demand for more food. Our current system of food production relies primarily on conventional agricultural methods that use considerable amounts of water and pesticides and create greenhouse gases.

- Sustainable agriculture involves farming methods that meet the demand for more food without depleting natural resources and harming the environment. Steps to solve the problems created by conventional agricultural methods should include: stopping the expansion of agricultural activity into tropical forests and grasslands; improving crop yields, for example by using biotechnology in agriculture; being more efficient with the use of natural resources and pesticides; eating less meat; and reducing food waste.

- Certain social, political, economic, and agricultural changes can reduce the number of people who are chronically hungry. Population control is critical for preserving the Earth's resources for future generations. Long-term ways to slow population growth include providing well-paying jobs, improving public education, and increasing access to health care services.

Consider This...

1. One of your friends just found out that she is pregnant. Although her BMI is within the healthy range, she's concerned about gaining too much weight during pregnancy. What advice would you provide your friend concerning the need to gain some weight during this life stage? If your friend's prepregnancy weight was 125 pounds, how much weight would be appropriate for her to gain during pregnancy?

2. Your pregnant friend wants your advice concerning whether she should breastfeed or formula-feed her baby. After reading Unit 11, what information would you provide to help your friend decide to breastfeed?

3. Olivia is a healthy 2-month-old baby. Olivia's mother, Kara, wants to replace Olivia's iron-fortified infant formula with the same fresh fluid

2% milk that she drinks. What advice would you give to Kara concerning the appropriateness of making such a decision?

4. Are your parents, grandparents, and/or great-grandparents still alive? If any of your ancestors died before they were 60 years of age, can you identify their causes of death and factors that contributed to their deaths? What lifestyle changes can you make now that can help you achieve a longer, healthier lifetime?

5. Consider your usual food preparation and storage practices. From what you learned after reading Unit 11, list any practices you have that are unsafe.

6. What steps can you take to reduce the amount of food that you waste?

Test Yourself

Select the best answer.

1. The embryo/fetus develops most of its organs during the
   a. preconception period.
   b. first trimester.
   c. second trimester.
   d. third trimester.

2. Preeclampsia is a form of _____ that can develop during pregnancy.
   a. hypertension
   b. diabetes
   c. hypertriglyceridemia
   d. anemia

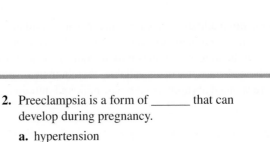

3. A healthy infant who weighs 6.5 pounds at birth can be expected to weigh _____ pounds by her first birthday.
   a. 13.0   c. 19.5
   b. 16.5   d. 23.5

4. Breastfed infants are _____ than babies who are fed infant formula.
   a. more likely to have diarrhea
   b. less likely to have sickle cell disease
   c. more likely to have respiratory infections
   d. less likely to have ear infections

5. Which of the following factors can influence an older adult's nutritional status?
   a. Illnesses
   b. Medications
   c. Income level
   d. All of the above are correct.

6. Food-borne illnesses are usually characterized by
   a. flu-like signs and symptoms.
   b. coughing, sneezing, and respiratory inflammation.
   c. megaloblastic anemia and nervous system defects.
   d. abdominal cramps, diarrhea, and vomiting.

7. Which of the following practices doesn't help reduce the growth of food-borne pathogens?
   a. Washing hands before preparing food
   b. Keeping cold foods cold and hot foods hot
   c. Cooking foods to proper internal temperatures
   d. Storing cooked meat at room temperature

8. Which of the following temperatures is recommended for storing chilled foods in a refrigerator?
   a. 40°F
   b. 50°F
   c. 60°F
   d. 70°F

9. The _____ Program enables eligible low-income participants to use a special debit card to purchase food at authorized stores.
   a. Nutritious Food Purchase
   b. Supplemental Nutrition Assistance
   c. Healthy Diets for All
   d. Eat Better for Less

10. Which of the following actions is not a solution to the problems created by conventional agricultural methods?
    a. Cut down tropical forests to make way for more farmland.
    b. Improve crop yields through biotechnological advancements.
    c. Use integrated pest management methods.
    d. Eat less red meat.

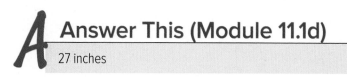

Answer This (Module 11.1d)

27 inches

References ➡ See Appendix F.

STUDY TIP: Quickly create a customized practice quiz for this chapter by going to your Connect SmartBook "My Reports" section.

Don't have SmartBook and want to learn more? Go to **whysmartbook.com**.

Appendixes

Appendix A	English-Metric Conversion and Metric-to-Household Units	A-3
Appendix B	Canada's Food Guide	A-4
Appendix C	Daily Values (DVs) Table	A-11
Appendix D	The Basics of Energy Metabolism	A-12
Appendix E	Answers to *Test Yourself* Questions	A-14
Appendix F	References	A-15
Appendix G	Dietary Reference Intake (DRI) Tables	A-29
Appendix H	Stretching Your Food Dollars	A-35
Appendix I	Modifying Recipes for Healthy Living	A-39

© C. Squared Studios/Getty Images RF

Appendix A

English-Metric Conversion and Metric-to-Household Units

LENGTH

ENGLISH (USA)		METRIC
inch	=	2.54 cm (centimeter)
foot	=	0.30 m (meter)
0.039 inches	=	millimeter (mm)
0.390 inches	=	centimeter (cm)
39.4 inches	=	meter (m)

WEIGHT

ENGLISH (USA)		METRIC
ounce	=	28.35 g
pound	=	0.45 kg
2.2 lb	=	kilogram

VOLUME

ENGLISH (USA)		METRIC
teaspoon	=	5 milliliters (ml)
tablespoon	=	15 ml
fluid ounce	=	30 ml
quart	=	0.95 liter (L)
cup	=	237 ml

VOLUME

ENGLISH (USA)		METRIC
1.06 quart	=	liter

HOUSEHOLD UNITS

3 teaspoons (tsp)	=	1 tablespoon (tbsp)
4 tbsp	=	¼ cup (c)
5 tbsp + 1 tsp	=	⅓ c
8 tbsp	=	½ c
16 tbsp	=	1 c

HOUSEHOLD UNITS

1 c	=	8 fluid ounces
1 c	=	½ pint
2 c	=	1 pint
4 c	=	1 quart
2 pints	=	1 quart
4 quarts	=	1 gallon

Appendix B

Canada's Food Guide

This appendix includes recommendations developed by the Canadian government regarding Canadian dietary patterns, as well as some regulations that apply to food labeling in that country. For more information about this guide, visit http://hc-sc.gc.ca/fn-an/food-guide-aliment/order-commander /eating_well_bien_manger-eng.php. The Dietary Reference Intakes (DRIs) that apply to Canadian and U.S. citizens are provided in Appendix G.

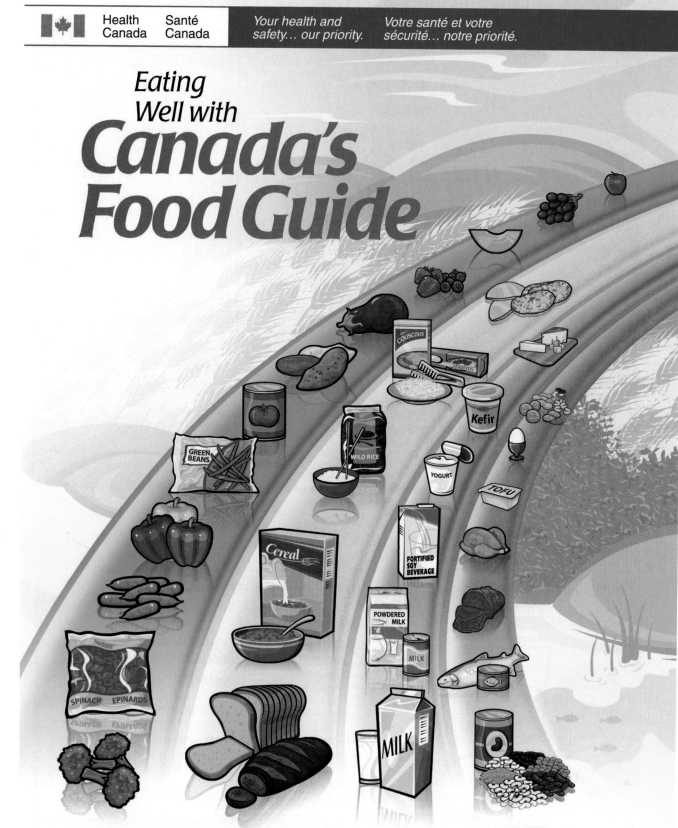

Advice for different ages and stages...

Children

Following *Canada's Food Guide* helps children grow and thrive.

Young children have small appetites and need calories for growth and development.

- Serve small nutritious meals and snacks each day.

- Do not restrict nutritious foods because of their fat content. Offer a variety of foods from the four food groups.

- Most of all... be a good role model.

Women of childbearing age

All women who could become pregnant and those who are pregnant or breastfeeding need a multivitamin containing **folic acid** every day. Pregnant women need to ensure that their multivitamin also contains **iron**. A health care professional can help you find the multivitamin that's right for you.

Pregnant and breastfeeding women need more calories. Include an extra 2 to 3 Food Guide Servings each day.

Here are two examples:
- Have fruit and yogurt for a snack, or
- Have an extra slice of toast at breakfast and an extra glass of milk at supper.

Men and women over 50

The need for **vitamin D** increases after the age of 50.

In addition to following *Canada's Food Guide*, everyone over the age of 50 should take a daily vitamin D supplement of 10 µg (400 IU).

How do I count Food Guide Servings in a meal?

Here is an example:

Vegetable and beef stir-fry with rice, a glass of milk and an apple for dessert		
250 mL (1 cup) mixed broccoli, carrot and sweet red pepper	=	2 **Vegetables and Fruit** Food Guide Servings
75 g (2 ½ oz.) lean beef	=	1 **Meat and Alternatives** Food Guide Serving
250 mL (1 cup) brown rice	=	2 **Grain Products** Food Guide Servings
5 mL (1 tsp) canola oil	=	part of your **Oils and Fats** intake for the day
250 mL (1 cup) 1% milk	=	1 **Milk and Alternatives** Food Guide Serving
1 apple	=	1 **Vegetables and Fruit** Food Guide Serving

Recommended Number of *Food Guide Servings* per Day

	Children			Teens		Adults			
Age in Years	2-3	4-8	9-13	14-18		19-50		51+	
Sex	Girls and Boys			Females	Males	Females	Males	Females	Males
Vegetables and Fruit	4	5	6	7	8	7-8	8-10	7	7
Grain Products	3	4	6	6	7	6-7	8	6	7
Milk and Alternatives	2	2	3-4	3-4	3-4	2	2	3	3
Meat and Alternatives	1	1	1-2	2	3	2	3	2	3

The chart above shows how many Food Guide Servings you need from each of the four food groups every day.

Having the amount and type of food recommended and following the tips in *Canada's Food Guide* will help:

• Meet your needs for vitamins, minerals and other nutrients.

• Reduce your risk of obesity, type 2 diabetes, heart disease, certain types of cancer and osteoporosis.

• Contribute to your overall health and vitality.

What is One Food Guide Serving?
Look at the examples below.

Fresh, frozen or canned vegetables
125 mL (½ cup)

Leafy vegetables
Cooked: 125 mL (½ cup)
Raw: 250 mL (1 cup)

Fresh, frozen or canned fruits
1 fruit or 125 mL (½ cup)

100% Juice
125 mL (½ cup)

Bread
1 slice (35 g)

Bagel
½ bagel (45 g)

Flat breads
½ pita or ½ tortilla (35 g)

Cooked rice, bulgur or quinoa
125 mL (½ cup)

Cereal
Cold: 30 g
Hot: 175 mL (¾ cup)

Cooked pasta or couscous
125 mL (½ cup)

Milk or powdered milk (reconstituted)
250 mL (1 cup)

Canned milk (evaporated)
125 mL (½ cup)

Fortified soy beverage
250 mL (1 cup)

Yogurt
175 g
(¾ cup)

Kefir
175 g
(¾ cup)

Cheese
50 g (1 ½ oz.)

Cooked fish, shellfish, poultry, lean meat
75 g (2 ½ oz.)/125 mL (½ cup)

Cooked legumes
175 mL (¾ cup)

Tofu
150 g or
175 mL (¾ cup)

Eggs
2 eggs

Peanut or nut butters
30 mL (2 Tbsp)

Shelled nuts and seeds
60 mL (¼ cup)

Oils and Fats

- Include a small amount – 30 to 45 mL (2 to 3 Tbsp) – of unsaturated fat each day. This includes oil used for cooking, salad dressings, margarine and mayonnaise.
- Use vegetable oils such as canola, olive and soybean.
- Choose soft margarines that are low in saturated and trans fats.
- Limit butter, hard margarine, lard and shortening.

Make each Food Guide Serving count...
wherever you are – at home, at school, at work or when eating out!

▸ **Eat at least one dark green and one orange vegetable each day.**
- Go for dark green vegetables such as broccoli, romaine lettuce and spinach.
- Go for orange vegetables such as carrots, sweet potatoes and winter squash.

▸ **Choose vegetables and fruit prepared with little or no added fat, sugar or salt.**
- Enjoy vegetables steamed, baked or stir-fried instead of deep-fried.

▸ **Have vegetables and fruit more often than juice.**

▸ **Make at least half of your grain products whole grain each day.**
- Eat a variety of whole grains such as barley, brown rice, oats, quinoa and wild rice.
- Enjoy whole grain breads, oatmeal or whole wheat pasta.

▸ **Choose grain products that are lower in fat, sugar or salt.**
- Compare the Nutrition Facts table on labels to make wise choices.
- Enjoy the true taste of grain products. When adding sauces or spreads, use small amounts.

▸ **Drink skim, 1%, or 2% milk each day.**
- Have 500 mL (2 cups) of milk every day for adequate vitamin D.
- Drink fortified soy beverages if you do not drink milk.

▸ **Select lower fat milk alternatives.**
- Compare the Nutrition Facts table on yogurts or cheeses to make wise choices.

▸ **Have meat alternatives such as beans, lentils and tofu often.**

▸ **Eat at least two Food Guide Servings of fish each week.***
- Choose fish such as char, herring, mackerel, salmon, sardines and trout.

▸ **Select lean meat and alternatives prepared with little or no added fat or salt.**
- Trim the visible fat from meats. Remove the skin on poultry.
- Use cooking methods such as roasting, baking or poaching that require little or no added fat.
- If you eat luncheon meats, sausages or prepackaged meats, choose those lower in salt (sodium) and fat.

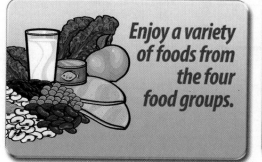

Enjoy a variety of foods from the four food groups.

Satisfy your thirst with water!

Drink water regularly. It's a calorie-free way to quench your thirst. Drink more water in hot weather or when you are very active.

* Health Canada provides advice for limiting exposure to mercury from certain types of fish. Refer to www.healthcanada.gc.ca for the latest information.

Eat well and be active today and every day!

The benefits of eating well and being active include:

- Better overall health.
- Lower risk of disease.
- A healthy body weight.
- Feeling and looking better.
- More energy.
- Stronger muscles and bones.

Be active

To be active every day is a step towards better health and a healthy body weight.

Canada's Physical Activity Guide recommends building 30 to 60 minutes of moderate physical activity into daily life for adults and at least 90 minutes a day for children and youth. You don't have to do it all at once. Add it up in periods of at least 10 minutes at a time for adults and five minutes at a time for children and youth.

Start slowly and build up.

Eat well

Another important step towards better health and a healthy body weight is to follow *Canada's Food Guide* by:

- Eating the recommended amount and type of food each day.
- Limiting foods and beverages high in calories, fat, sugar or salt (sodium) such as cakes and pastries, chocolate and candies, cookies and granola bars, doughnuts and muffins, ice cream and frozen desserts, french fries, potato chips, nachos and other salty snacks, alcohol, fruit flavoured drinks, soft drinks, sports and energy drinks, and sweetened hot or cold drinks.

Read the label

- Compare the Nutrition Facts table on food labels to choose products that contain less fat, saturated fat, trans fat, sugar and sodium.
- Keep in mind that the calories and nutrients listed are for the amount of food found at the top of the Nutrition Facts table.

Nutrition Facts
Per 0 mL (0 g)

Amount	% Daily Value
Calories 0	
Fat 0 g	0 %
Saturates 0 g	0 %
+ Trans 0 g	
Cholesterol 0 mg	
Sodium 0 mg	0 %
Carbohydrate 0 g	0 %
Fibre 0 g	0 %
Sugars 0 g	
Protein 0 g	

Vitamin A	0 %	Vitamin C	0 %
Calcium	0 %	Iron	0 %

Limit trans fat

When a Nutrition Facts table is not available, ask for nutrition information to choose foods lower in trans and saturated fats.

Take a step today...

✓ Have breakfast every day. It may help control your hunger later in the day.

✓ Walk wherever you can – get off the bus early, use the stairs.

✓ Benefit from eating vegetables and fruit at all meals and as snacks.

✓ Spend less time being inactive such as watching TV or playing computer games.

✓ Request nutrition information about menu items when eating out to help you make healthier choices.

✓ Enjoy eating with family and friends!

✓ Take time to eat and savour every bite!

For more information, interactive tools, or additional copies visit Canada's Food Guide on-line at:
www.healthcanada.gc.ca/foodguide

or contact:

Publications
Health Canada
Ottawa, Ontario K1A 0K9
E-Mail: publications@hc-sc.gc.ca
Tel.: 1-866-225-0709
Fax: (613) 941-5366
TTY: 1-800-267-1245

Également disponible en français sous le titre : Bien manger avec le Guide alimentaire canadien

This publication can be made available on request on diskette, large print, audio-cassette and braille.

Appendix C

Daily Values (DVs) Table

Source: Modified from the FDA.

Nutrition Facts
3 1/2 servings per container
Serving size 1/2 cup (126g)

Amount per serving
Calories 40

	% Daily Value*
Total Fat 0g	0%
Saturated Fat 0g	0%
Trans Fat 0g	
Cholesterol 0mg	0%
Sodium 50mg	0%
Total Carbohydrate 6g	2%
Dietary Fiber 2g	2%
Total Sugars 4g	7%
Includes 0g Added Sugars	
Protein 4g	0%
Vitamin D 0mcg	0%
Calcium 26mg	2%
Iron 0mg	0%
Potassium 300mg	6%

* The % Daily Value (DV)... In a serv... nutrient... 2,000... vice.

DIETARY COMPONENT	UNIT OF MEASURE	CURRENT DAILY VALUES FOR PEOPLE OVER 4 YEARS OF AGE
Total fat*	g	78
Saturated fatty acids*	"	20
Protein*	"	50
Cholesterol	mg	300
Total carbohydrate*	g	275
Fiber	"	28
Added sugars	"	50
Vitamin A	mcg (RAEs)	900
Vitamin D	mcg	20
Vitamin E	mg	15
Vitamin K	mcg	120
Vitamin C	mg	90
Folate	mcg	400
Thiamin	mg	1.2
Riboflavin	"	1.3
Niacin	"	16
Vitamin B-6	"	1.7
Vitamin B-12	mcg	2.4
Biotin	mcg	30
Pantothenic acid	mg	5
Calcium	"	1300
Phosphorus	"	1250
Iodine	mcg	150
Iron	mg	18
Magnesium	"	420
Copper	"	0.9
Zinc	"	11
Sodium	"	2300
Potassium	"	4700
Chloride	"	2300
Manganese	"	2.3
Selenium	mcg	55
Chromium	"	35
Molybdenum	"	45

*These Daily Values are based on a 2000 kcal diet.

Appendix D

The Basics of Energy Metabolism

Energy-investment steps

Glucose

1
ATP
ADP

ATP Yield

−2 ATP

Glucose 6-phosphate

Fructose 6-phosphate

2
ATP
ADP

Fructose 1, 6-biphosphate

3

2X Glyceraldehyde 3-phosphate

Energy-harvesting steps

2P
2X NAD⁺
4
2X NADH + H⁺

2X 1, 3-bisphosphoglycerate

+2 ATP

5
2 ADP
2 ATP

2X 3-phosphoglycerate

H₂O
6

2X Phosphoenolpyruvate

+2 ATP

2 ADP
7
2 ATP

2 ATP

8 2X Pyruvate

(Net Gain ATP)

1 Adding phosphate to glucose using ATP produces an activated molecule.

2 Rearrangement, followed by a second addition of phosphate using ATP, produces fructose 1, 6-biphosphate.

3 The 6-carbon molecule is split into two 3-carbon-phosphate molecules.

4 Oxidation, followed by the addition of phosphate produces 2 NADH + 2H⁺ molecules and two 3-carbon-phosphate-phosphate molecules.

5 Removal of 2 phosphate groups by 2 ADP molecules produces 2 ATP molecules and two 3-carbon-phosphate molecules.

6 Removal of water produces two 3-carbon-phosphate molecules.

7 Removal of 2 phosphate groups by 2 ADP molecules produces 2 ATP molecules.

8 Pyruvate is the end product of this metabolic pathway.

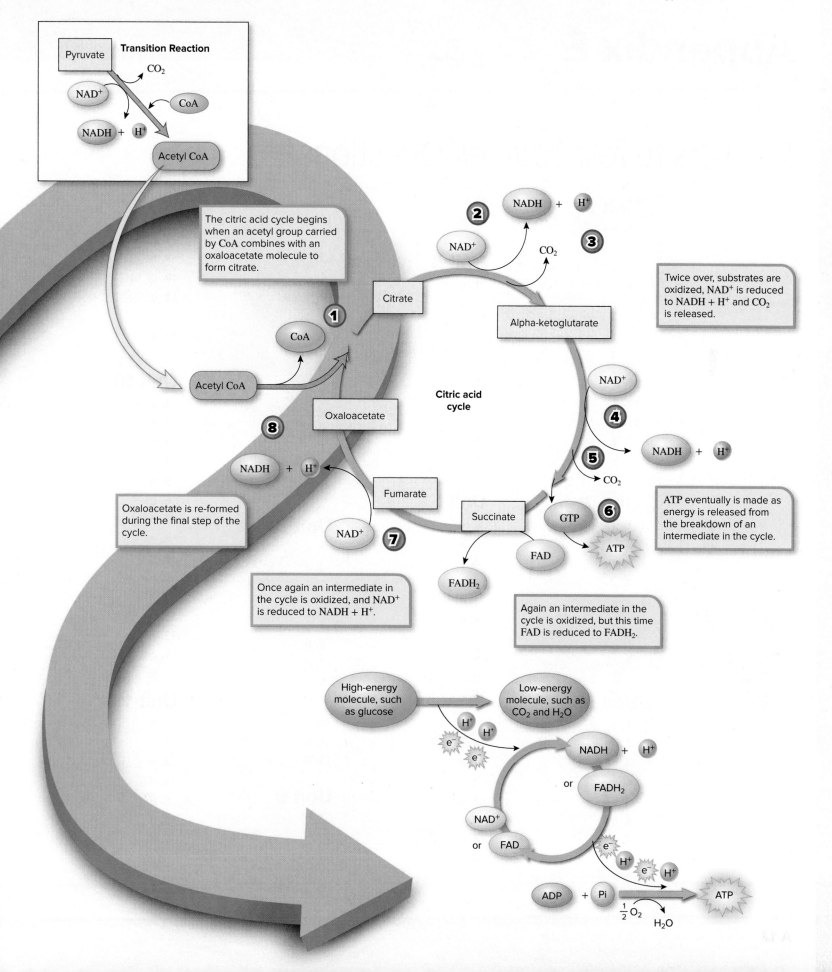

Transition Reaction

Pyruvate

CO$_2$

NAD$^+$

CoA

NADH + H$^+$

Acetyl CoA

The citric acid cycle begins when an acetyl group carried by CoA combines with an oxaloacetate molecule to form citrate.

Citric acid cycle

CoA

Acetyl CoA

Oxaloacetate

Fumarate

Citrate

Alpha-ketoglutarate

Succinate

GTP

FAD

FADH$_2$

ATP

NADH + H$^+$

NAD$^+$

CO$_2$

NADH + H$^+$

NAD$^+$

CO$_2$

NADH + H$^+$

NAD$^+$

1
2
3
4
5
6
7
8

Twice over, substrates are oxidized, NAD$^+$ is reduced to NADH + H$^+$ and CO$_2$ is released.

ATP eventually is made as energy is released from the breakdown of an intermediate in the cycle.

Again an intermediate in the cycle is oxidized, but this time FAD is reduced to FADH$_2$.

Once again an intermediate in the cycle is oxidized, and NAD$^+$ is reduced to NADH + H$^+$.

Oxaloacetate is re-formed during the final step of the cycle.

High-energy molecule, such as glucose

Low-energy molecule, such as CO$_2$ and H$_2$O

H$^+$ H$^+$

e$^-$ e$^-$

NADH + H$^+$

or

FADH$_2$

NAD$^+$

or

FAD

e$^-$

H$^+$ e$^-$ H$^+$

ADP + Pi

$\frac{1}{2}$O$_2$

H$_2$O

ATP

Appendix E

Answers to *Test Yourself* Questions

Unit 1
1. b
2. c
3. a
4. d
5. d
6. b
7. b
8. a
9. a
10. d
11. b
12. d
13. b

Unit 2
1. a
2. c
3. d
4. a
5. b
6. d
7. a
8. c

Unit 3
1. a
2. d
3. c
4. c
5. b
6. d
7. d
8. a
9. c
10. a

11. c
12. b

Unit 4
1. b
2. a
3. b
4. a
5. b
6. d
7. a
8. d
9. a
10. b

Unit 5
1. d
2. a
3. b
4. a
5. c
6. d
7. b
8. d
9. a
10. c

Unit 6
1. c
2. a
3. a
4. b
5. d
6. b
7. c
8. b

9. d
10. d

Unit 7
1. a
2. a
3. d
4. b
5. c
6. b
7. d
8. c
9. c
10. b
11. a
12. d

Unit 8
1. a
2. a
3. c
4. b
5. c
6. b
7. d
8. c
9. b
10. b
11. c
12. d

Unit 9
1. c
2. b
3. d
4. d
5. a

6. b
7. b
8. a
9. b
10. c
11. d
12. a
13. a

Unit 10
1. a
2. a
3. b
4. a
5. b
6. d
7. d
8. b
9. d
10. b
11. a
12. b
13. a
14. c

Unit 11
1. b
2. a
3. c
4. d
5. d
6. d
7. d
8. a
9. b
10. a

Appendix F

References

Unit 1

1. Centers for Disease Control and Prevention: *Tobacco use*. 2015. http://www.cdc.gov/WinnableBattles/Tobacco/index.html Accessed: May 1, 2016
2. U.S. Department of Health and Human Services, U.S. Department of Agriculture: *2015–2020 Dietary Guidelines for Americans*. 2015. http://health.gov/dietaryguidelines/2015/guidelines/ Accessed: May 1, 2016
3. U.S. Department of Health and Human Services, National Institutes of Health, Office of Dietary Supplements: *Dietary Supplement Health and Education Act of 1994. Public Law 103-417, 103rd Congress*. https://ods.od.nih.gov/About/DSHEA_Wording.aspx Accessed: May 1, 2016
4. Vadeboncoeur C and others: A meta-analysis of weight gain in first year university students: Is freshman 15 a myth? *BMC Obesity* 2:22, 2015. Published online May 28, 2015. doi: 10.1186/s40608-015-0051-7 PMCID: PMC4511069
5. U.S. Department of Agriculture, ChooseMyPlate.gov: *Supertracker*. Updated April 13, 2016. http://www.choosemyplate.gov/tools-supertracker Accessed: May 1, 2016
6. Purdue University Horticulture: *Lychee*. http://www.hort.purdue.edu/newcrop/morton/lychee.html Accessed: May 1, 2016
7. Position of the Academy of Nutrition and Dietetics: Functional foods. *Journal of the Academy of Nutrition and Dietetics*. 113(8):1096, 2013. doi: 10.1016/j.jand.2013.06.002

Unit 2

1. Benedetti F and others: How placebos change the patient's brain. *Neuropsychopharmacology* 36(1):339, 2011.
2. National Institutes of Health, National Center for Complementary and Integrative Health: *Pomegranate*. Last modified May 10, 2016. https://nccih.nih.gov/health/pomegranate/at-a-glance Accessed: May 28, 2016
3. National Institutes of Health, National Center for Complementary and Integrative Health: *Ginger*. Modified April 2016. https://nccih.nih.gov/health/ginger Accessed: May 3, 2016
4. Marshall BJ and others: Pyloric *Campylobacter* infection and gastroduodenal disease. *Medical Journal of Australia* 142(8):439, 1985.
5. Federal Trade Commission (November 2011). *Miracle Health Claims*. http://www.consumer.ftc.gov/articles/0167-miracle-health-claims Accessed: May 3, 2016
6. Federal Trade Commission: *Marketers of unproven weight-loss products ordered to pay nearly $2 million*. 2010. https://www.ftc.gov/news-events/press-releases/2010/01/marketers-unproven-weight-loss-products-ordered-pay-nearly-2 Accessed: May 3, 2016

Unit 3

1. Institute of Medicine: *Dietary Reference Intakes for vitamin C, vitamin E, selenium, and carotenoids*. Washington, DC: National Academies Press, 2000.
2. Oregon State University, Linus Pauling Institute, Micronutrient Information Center: *Vitamin C*. Updated 2014. http://lpi.oregonstate.edu/mic/vitamins/vitamin-C Accessed: May 4, 2016

3. Otten JJ and others (eds): *Dietary Reference Intakes: The essential guide to nutrient requirements.* Institute of Medicine of the National Academies. Washington, DC: National Academies Press, 2006.

4. Barr SI and others: Interpreting and using the Dietary Reference Intakes in dietary assessment of individuals and groups. *Journal of the American Dietetic Association* 102(6):780, 2002.

5. FDA provides guidance on "whole grain" for manufacturers. *FDA News*, P06-23 (last update April 2013). http://www.fda.gov/NewsEvents/Newsroom/PressAnnouncements/2006/ucm108598.htm Accessed: May 5, 2016

6. U.S. Department of Agriculture, ChooseMyPlate.gov: *All about the fruit group.* Last updated March 2016. http://www.choosemyplate.gov/fruit Accessed: May 5, 2016

7. U.S. Department of Agriculture, ChooseMyPlate.gov: *Fruits: Tips to help you eat fruits.* http://www.choosemyplate.gov/fruits-tips Accessed: May 5, 2016

8. U.S. Department of Agriculture, ChooseMyPlate.gov: *All about oils: What are oils?* Updated March 2016. http://www.choosemyplate.gov/oils Accessed: May 5, 2016

9. U.S. Department of Agriculture: *Introduction to organic practices.* 2015. https://www.ams.usda.gov/sites/default/files/media/Organic%20Practices%20Factsheet.pdf Accessed: May 5, 2016

10. Johansson E and others: Contribution of organically grown crops to human health. *International Journal of Environmental Research and Public Health* 11:3870, 2014. doi:10.3390/ijerph110403870

11. U.S. Departments of Health and Human Services and Agriculture: *2015–2020 Dietary Guidelines for Americans.* 2015. http://health.gov/dietaryguidelines/2015/guidelines/ Accessed: May 1, 2016

12. U.S. Department of Agriculture, Choosemyplate.gov: *Empty calories: fats and sugars: know your limits.* Updated: March 2016. http://www.choosemyplate.gov/preschoolers-empty-calories Accessed: June 3, 2016

13. U.S. Food and Drug Administration: *How to understand and use the Nutrition Facts label.* Last updated January 2015. http://www.fda.gov/food/ingredientspackaginglabeling/labelingnutrition/ucm274593.htm Accessed: May 5, 2016

14. U.S. Government Publishing Office, Electronic Code of Federal Regulation: *Title 21: Food and drugs, part 101–food labeling, subpart A-general provisions, §101.14 Health claims: General requirements.* May 9, 2016. http://www.ecfr.gov/cgi-bin/text-idx?SID=1aec8849e2bf8bd210e518715257e6ff&mc=true&node=se21.2.101_114&rgn=div8 (4) Accessed: May 11, 2016

15. National Center for Complementary and Integrative Health: *Using dietary supplements wisely.* Last updated June 2014. https://nccih.nih.gov/health/supplements/wiseuse.htm Accessed: May 5, 2016

16. National Center for Complementary and Integrative Health: *Vitamins and minerals.* Modified 2015. https://nccih.nih.gov/health/vitamins Accessed: May 5, 2016

17. National Center for Complementary and Integrative Health: *Use of complementary health approaches in the U.S., What complementary and integrative approaches do Americans use? Key findings from the 2012 National Health Interview Survey.* Last updated 2015. https://nccih.nih.gov/research/statistics/NHIS/2012/natural-products Accessed: May 5, 2016

18. National Center for Complementary and Integrative Health: *Herbs at a Glance: Echinacea.* 2012. https://nccih.nih.gov/health/echinacea/ataglance.htm Accessed: May 4, 2016

19. Bradley J: *NBJ: 'The US supplement industry is $37 billion, not $12 billion.'* June 1, 2015. http://www.nutraingredients-usa.com/Markets/NBJ-The-US-supplement-industry-is-37-billion-not-12-billion Accessed: May 8, 2016

20. Huang H-Y and others: The efficacy and safety of multivitamin and multimineral supplement use to prevent cancer and chronic disease in adults: A systematic review for a National Institutes of Health State-of-the-Science Conference. *Annals of Internal Medicine* 145(5):372, 2006.

Unit 4

1. National Institutes of Health, National Institute of Diabetes and Digestive and Kidney Diseases: *Ulcerative colitis*. 2014. https://www.niddk.nih.gov/health-information/health-topics/digestive-diseases/ulcerative-colitis/Pages/facts.aspx Accessed: November 3, 2016
2. Besnard P: Taste of fat: a sixth taste modality? *Physiological Reviews*. 96(1):151, 2016. doi: 10.1152/physrev.00002.2015
3. Saladin KS: *Anatomy & physiology*. 7th ed. Boston: McGraw-Hill Publishing Company, 2015.
4. National Institutes of Health, U.S. National Library of Medicine: Choking—adult or child over 1 year. *Medline Plus*. Last updated 2015. http://www.nlm.nih.gov/medlineplus/ency/article/000049.htm Accessed: May 7, 2016
5. Machado MV and Cortez-Pinto H: Diet, microbiota, obesity, and NAFLD: A dangerous quartet. *International Journal of Molecular Sciences* 1:17(4): pii: E481, 2016. doi: 10.3390/ijms17040481
6. Hooman A and Hazen SL: Contribution of gut bacteria to lipid levels: Another metabolic role for microbes? *Circulation Research* 117:750, 2015. doi:10.1161/CIRCRESAHA.115.307409
7. The basics of probiotics. *NIH Medline Plus* 10(4): 22, 2016. https://www.nlm.nih.gov/medlineplus/magazine/issues/winter16/articles/winter16pg22.html Accessed: May 7, 2016
8. American Gastroenterological Association: *Understanding constipation*. January 2013. http://www.gastro.org/info_for_patients/2013/6/6/understanding-constipation Accessed: May 7, 2016
9. Mayo Clinic: Diseases and conditions: *Diverticulitis*. 2014. http://www.mayoclinic.org/diseases-conditions/diverticulitis/basics/definition/CON-20033495?p=1 Accessed: May 7, 2016
10. National Institutes of Health, U.S. National Library of Medicine: Nausea and vomiting—adults. *Medline Plus*. Updated 2015. http://www.nlm.nih.gov/medlineplus/ency/article/003117.htm Accessed: May 7, 2016
11. National Institutes of Health, National Institute of Diabetes and Digestive and Kidney Diseases: *Gastroesophageal reflux (GER) and gastroesophageal reflux disease (GERD) in adults*. 2014. http://www.niddk.nih.gov/health-information/health-topics/digestive-diseases/ger-and-gerd-in-adults/Pages/overview.aspx Accessed: May 7, 2016
12. National Institutes of Health, National Institute of Diabetes and Digestive and Kidney Diseases: *Peptic ulcer disease*. 2014. http://www.niddk.nih.gov/health-information/health-topics/digestive-diseases/peptic-ulcer/Pages/overview.aspx Accessed: May 7, 2016
13. National Institutes of Health, National Institute of Diabetes and Digestive and Kidney Diseases: *Irritable bowel syndrome (IBS)*. 2015. https://www.niddk.nih.gov/health-information/health-topics/digestive-diseases/irritable-bowel-syndrome/Pages/overview.aspx Accessed: October 2, 2016
14. National Institutes of Health, National Institute of Diabetes and Digestive and Kidney Diseases: *Irritable bowel syndrome*. 2015. https://www.nlm.nih.gov/medlineplus/ency/article/000246.htm Accessed: May 7, 2016
15. National Institutes of Health, National Institute of Diabetes and Digestive and Kidney Diseases: *Ulcerative colitis and colon cancer*. 2014. http://www.niddk.nih.gov/health-information/health-topics/digestive-diseases/ulcerative-colitis/Pages/facts.aspx#10 Accessed: May 7, 2016
16. American Cancer Society: *What is colorectal cancer?* Revised January 2016. http://www.cancer.org/cancer/colonandrectumcancer/detailedguide/colorectal-cancer-what-is-colorectal-cancer Accessed: May 7, 2016

Unit 5

1. U.S. Department of Agriculture, Economic Research Service: *Sugar and sweeteners yearbook tables, U.S. sugar supply and use*. Tables 51, 52, and 53. Last updated May 4, 2016. http://www.ers.usda.gov/data-products/sugar-and-sweeteners-yearbook-tables.aspx#25456 Accessed: May 8, 2016
2. Causes of ADHD. *MedlinePlus* Spring 2014. https://www.nlm.nih.gov/medlineplus/magazine/issues/spring14/articles/spring14pg15-16.html Accessed: May 8, 2016

3. Horton J: The truth about agave. 2014. *WebMD.* http://www.webmd.com/diet/the-truth-about-agave Accessed: May 8, 2016

4. Position of the Academy of Nutrition and Dietetics: Use of nutritive and nonnutritive sweeteners. *Journal of the Academy of Nutrition and Dietetics* 112(5):739, 2012; Erratum vol. 112(8):1279.

5. Swithers SE: Artificial sweeteners produce the counterintuitive effect of inducing metabolic derangements. *Trends in Endocrinology & Metabolism* 24(9):431, 2013. doi: 10.1016/j.tem.2013.05.005\

6. Centers for Disease Control and Prevention: *Botulism.* Last updated May 2016. http://www.cdc.gov/botulism/index.html Accessed: June 20, 2016

7. U.S. Food and Drug Administration: Code of Federal Regulations: *21 CFR172.804 Title 21, volume 3* (Revised 2015). http://www.accessdata.fda.gov/scripts/cdrh/cfdocs/cfcfr/CFRSearch.cfm?fr=172.804 Accessed: May 9, 2016

8. Otten JJ and others, eds: *Dietary Reference Intakes: The essential guide to nutrient requirements.* Washington, DC: National Academies Press, 2006.

9. U.S. Department of Agriculture, Agricultural Research Service: *What We Eat in America, NHANES 2013–2014: Nutrient Intakes from food and beverages: Mean amounts consumed by individuals: By gender and age.* 2016. https://www.ars.usda.gov/ARSUserFiles/80400530/pdf/1314/Table_1_NIN_GEN_13.pdf Accessed: November 14, 2016

10. U.S. Departments of Agriculture and Health and Human Services: *2015–2020 Dietary Guidelines for Americans.* 2015. http://health.gov/dietaryguidelines/2015/guidelines/ Accessed: May 9, 2016

11. U.S. Department of Agriculture, Agricultural Research Service: *What's in the food you eat search tool, 5.0.* http://www.ars.usda.gov/Services/docs.htm?docid=17032 Accessed: May 9, 2016

12. Joslin Diabetes Center: *Goals for blood glucose control.* 2016. http://www.joslin.org/info/Goals-for-Blood-Glucose-Control.html Accessed: May 10, 2016

13. Bray GA: Energy and fructose from beverages sweetened with sugar or high-fructose corn syrup pose a health risk for some people. *Advances in Nutrition* 4(2):220, 2013. doi: 10.3945/an.112.002816

14. Funtikova AN and others: Soft drink consumption is positively associated with increased waist circumference and 10-year incidence of abdominal obesity in Spanish adults. *The Journal of Nutrition* 145(2):328, 2015.

15. Centers for Disease Control and Prevention: Estimates of diabetes and its burden in the United States, 2014. Last updated May 2015. *National Diabetes Statistics Report* http://www.cdc.gov/diabetes/data/statistics/2014StatisticsReport.html Accessed: May 10, 2016

16. Centers for Disease Control and Prevention, National Diabetes Prevention Program: *About diabetes.* Page last updated January 2016. http://www.cdc.gov/diabetes/prevention/prediabetes-type2/index.html Accessed: May 10, 2016

17. National Institutes of Health, National Institute of Diabetes and Kidney and Digestive Diseases: *Causes of diabetes.* 2014. http://www.niddk.nih.gov/health-information/health-topics/Diabetes/causes-diabetes/Pages/index.aspx Accessed: May 10, 2016

18. Centers for Disease Control and Prevention: *Diabetes and pregnancy.* 2015. http://www.cdc.gov/pregnancy/diabetes.html Accessed: May 10, 2016

19. National Institutes of Health, National Institute of Diabetes and Kidney and Digestive Diseases: *The A1c test and diabetes.* 2014. http://www.niddk.nih.gov/health-information/health-topics/diagnostic-tests/a1c-test-diabetes/Pages/index.aspx Accessed: May 10, 2016

20. Carter P and others: Dietary recommendations for the prevention of type 2 diabetes: What are they based on? *Journal of Nutrition and Metabolism* 2012 Article ID: 847202 doi:10.1155/2012/847202

21. Maki KC and Phillips AK: Dietary substitutions for refined carbohydrate that show promise for reducing risk of type 2 diabetes in men and women. *The Journal of Nutrition* 145:159S, 2015.

22. American Diabetes Association: *Hypoglycemia (low blood glucose).* Updated 2015. http://www.diabetes.org/living-with-diabetes/treatment-and-care/blood-glucose-control/hypoglycemia-low-blood.html Accessed: May 10, 2016

23. U.S. Department of Health and Human Services, National Heart Lung and Blood Institute: *What is metabolic syndrome?* 2015. http://www.nhlbi.nih.gov/health/health-topics/topics/ms/ Accessed: May 10, 2016

24. National Institutes of Health, Institute of Diabetes and Digestive and Kidney Diseases: *Nonalcoholic steatohepatitis.* 2014. http://www.niddk.nih.gov/health-information/health-topics/liver-disease/nonalcoholic-steatohepatitis/Pages/facts.aspx Accessed: June 22, 2016

25. National Institutes of Health, National Institute of Diabetes and Kidney and Digestive Diseases: *What is lactose intolerance?* 2014. http://www.niddk.nih.gov/health-information/health-topics/digestive-diseases/lactose-intolerance/Pages/facts.aspx Accessed: May 10, 2016

26. Maagaard L and others: Follow-up of patients with functional bowel symptoms treated with a low FODMAP diet. *World Journal of Gastroenterology* 22(15): 4009, 2016. http://dx.doi.org/10.3748/wjg.v22.i15.4009

27. Position of the Academy of Nutrition and Dietetics: Health implications of dietary fiber. *Journal of the Academy of Nutrition and Dietetics* 115(11):1861, 2015.

Unit 6

1. U.S. Departments of Health and Human Services and Agriculture: *2015–2020 Dietary Guidelines for Americans.* 2015. http:// health.gov/dietaryguidelines/2015/guidelines/ Accessed: April 30, 2016

2. Federal Trade Commission: *FTC settlement prohibits marketers of children's vitamins from making deceptive health claims about brain and eye development.* 2011. https://www.ftc.gov/news-events/press-releases/2010/12/ftc-settlement-prohibits-marketers-childrens-vitamins-making Accessed: May 2, 2016

3. U.S. Food and Drug Administration: *Talking about trans fat: What you need to know.* http://www.fda.gov/Food/ResourcesForYou/Consumers/ucm079609.htm Updated May 2016 Accessed: November 4, 2016

4. U.S. Food and Drug Administration, FDA News Release: The *FDA takes step to remove artificial trans fat in processed foods.* 2015. http://fda.gov/NewsEvents/Newsroom/PressAnnouncements/ucm451237.htm Accessed: June 25, 2016

5. Zeisel, SH: Nutrition in pregnancy: The argument for including a source of choline. *International Journal of Women's Health* 5:193, 2013.

6. National Center for Health Statistics: *Health, United States, 2015: With special feature on racial and ethnic disparities.* Table 19. Hyattsville, MD, 2016.

7. Saladin KS: *Anatomy & physiology.* 7th ed. Boston: McGraw-Hill Publishing Company, 2015.

8. Klop B and others: Dyslipidemia in obesity: Mechanisms and potential targets. *Nutrients* 5:1218, 2013. doi:10.3390/nu5041218

9. Lubrano V and Balzan S: Consolidated and emerging inflammatory markers in coronary artery disease. *World Journal of Experimental Medicine* 5(1):21, 2015. doi: 10.5493/wjem.v5.i1.21

10. National Institutes of Health, National Heart, Lung, and Blood Institute: *Who is at risk for atherosclerosis?* Updated 2015. http://www.nhlbi.nih.gov/health/health-topics/topics/atherosclerosis/atrisk Accessed: May 12, 2016

11. Position of the Academy of Nutrition and Dietetics: Dietary fatty acids for healthy adults. *Journal of the Academy of Nutrition and Dietetics* 114(1): 136, 2014.

12. Widmer RJ and others: The Mediterranean diet, its components, and cardiovascular disease. *The American Journal of Medicine* 128(3):229, 2015.

13. National Institutes of Health, National Center for Alternative and Complementary Medicine: *Herbs at a glance: Garlic.* 2012. http://nccam.nih.gov/health/garlic/ataglance.htm Accesssed: May 13, 2016

14. U.S. Department of Agriculture, Agricultural Research Service: *What We Eat in America, NHANES 2013–2014: Nutrient Intakes from food and beverages: Mean amounts consumed by individuals: By gender and age.* 2016. https://www.ars.usda.gov/ARSUserFiles/80400530/pdf/1314/Table_1_NIN_GEN_13.pdf Accessed: November 14, 2016

15. National Institutes of Health, National Center for Complementary and Integrative Health: *Omega-3 supplements: In depth.* Updated 2015. https://nccih.nih.gov/health/omega3/introduction.htm Accessed: May 14, 2016

16. American Heart Association: *Drug therapy for cholesterol.* 2014. http://www.heart.org /HEARTORG/Conditions/Cholesterol/PreventionTreatmentofHighCholesterol/Drug-Therapy -for-Cholesterol_UCM_305632_Article.jsp#.VzecA-T8S88 Accessed: May 14, 2016

17. Rong Y and others: Egg consumption and risk of coronary heart disease and stroke: Dose-response meta-analysis of prospective cohort studies. *British Medical Journal* 346:e8539, Published online 2013, January 7. doi:10.1136/bmj.e8539

Unit 7

1. U.S. Department of Agriculture, Agricultural Research Service: *What We Eat in America, NHANES 2013–2014: Nutrient Intakes from food and beverages: Mean amounts consumed by individuals: By gender and age.* 2016. https://www.ars.usda.gov/ARSUserFiles/80400530/ pdf/1314/Table_1_NIN_GEN_13.pdf Accessed: November 14, 2016

2. U.S. Department of Agriculture, Center for Nutrition Policy: *Protein contributed from major foods groups.* 2014. http://www.cnpp.usda.gov/reports-publications Accessed: May 16, 2016

3. U.S. Departments of Agriculture and Health and Human Services: *2015–2020 Dietary Guidelines for Americans.* 2015. http://health.gov/dietaryguidelines/2015/guidelines/ Accessed: May 9, 2016

4. Oelke EA and others: *Quinoa. Alternative field crops manual.* University of Wisconsin-Extension, University of Minnesota: Center for Alternative Plant & Animal Productions, and the Minnesota Extension Service. (ND) http://www.hort.purdue.edu /newcrop/afcm/quinoa.html Accessed: May 16, 2016

5. Gallup.com: *In U.S., 5% of Americans consider themselves vegetarians.* July 26, 2012. http://www.gallup.com/poll/156215/consider-themselves-vegetarians.aspx Accessed: May 16, 2016

6. Le L T and Sabaté J: Beyond meatless, the health effects of vegan diets: Findings from the Adventist cohorts. *Nutrients* 6:2131, 2014. doi:10.3390/nu6062131

7. Rizzo NS and others: Nutrient profiles of vegetarian and nonvegetarian dietary patterns. *Journal of the Academy of Nutrition and Dietetics* 113(12):1610, 2013. doi: 10.1016/j .jand.2013.06.349. Epub 2013, August 27

8. Kocaoglu C and others: Cerebral atrophy in a vitamin B12-deficient infant of a vegetarian mother. *Journal of Health, Population and Nutrition* 32(2):367, 2014.

9. Position of the American Dietetic Association: Vegetarian diets. *Journal of the American Dietetic Association* 109(7):1266, 2009.

10. Cuenca-Sánchez M and others: Controversies surrounding high-protein diet intake: Satiating effect and kidney and bone health. *Advances in Nutrition* 6(3):260, 2015. doi: 10.3945/an.114.007716

11. Delimaris I: Adverse effects associated with protein intake above the recommended dietary allowance for adults. *ISRN Nutrition* 2013, Article ID 126929, 6 pages. http://dx.doi .org/10.5402/2013/126929

12. Position of the Academy of Nutrition and Dietetics, Dietitians of Canada, and the American College of Sports Medicine: Nutrition and athletic performance. *Journal of the Academy of Nutrition and Dietetics* 116(3):501, 2016.

13. Witard WC and others: Protein considerations for optimizing skeletal muscle mass in healthy young and older adults. *Nutrients* 8:181, 2016. doi:10.3390/nu8040181

14. Naclerio F and Larumbe-Zabala E: Effects of whey protein along or as part of a multi-ingredient formulation on strength, fat-free mass, or lean body mass in resistance-trained individuals: A meta-analysis. *Sports Medicine* 46(1):125, 2016. doi:10.1007/s40279-015-0403-y

15. World Health Organization: *Global health observatory (GHO): Underweight in children.* 2016. http://www.who.int/gho/mdg/poverty_hunger/underweight_text/en/ Accessed: May 17, 2016

16. National Institute of Allergy and Infectious Disease: *Food allergy.* Updated May 9, 2016. http://www.niaid.nih.gov/topics/foodallergy/Pages/default.aspx Accessed: May 17, 2016

17. McHenry M and Watson W: Impact of primary food allergies on the introduction of other foods amongst Canadian children and their siblings. *Allergy, Asthma & Clinical Immunology* 10:26, 2014. doi:10.1186/1710-1492-10-26

18. National Institutes of Health, National Institute of Diabetes and Digestive and Kidney Diseases: *Definition and facts for celiac disease.* Updated June 2016. https://www.niddk.nih.gov/health-information/health-topics/digestive-diseases/celiac-disease/Pages/definition-facts.aspx Accessed: November 4, 2016

19. Gaesser GA, Angadi SS: Gluten-free diet: Imprudent dietary advice for the general population? *Journal of the Academy of Nutrition and Dietetics* 112 (9): 1330, 2012.

Unit 8

1. U.S. Department of Agriculture, Agricultural Research Service: *What We Eat in America, NHANES 2013–2014: Nutrient Intakes from food and beverages: Mean amounts consumed by individuals: By gender and age.* 2016. https://www.ars.usda.gov/ARSUserFiles/80400530/pdf/1314/Table_1_NIN_GEN_13.pdf Accessed: November 14, 2016

2. World Health Organization: *Micronutrient deficiencies: Vitamin A deficiency.* (ND) http://www.who.int/nutrition/topics/vad/en/index.html Accessed: May 18, 2016

3. National Institutes of Health, Office of Dietary Supplements: *Vitamin A: Factsheet for professionals.* Updated February 2016. https://ods.od.nih.gov/factsheets/VitaminA-HealthProfessional/ Accessed: May 18, 2016

4. Nowak JZ: AMD—the retinal disease with an unprecised etiopathogenesis: In search of effective therapeutics. *Acta Poloniae Pharmaceutica—Drug Research* 71(6): 900, 2014.

5. National Institutes of Health, Office of Dietary Supplements: *Vitamin D: Factsheet for professionals.* Updated February 2016. https://ods.od.nih.gov/factsheets/VitaminD-HealthProfessional/ Accessed: May 18, 2016

6. Wacker M, Holick MF: Sunlight and vitamin D: Global perspective for health. *Dermato-Endocrinology* 5(1):51, 2013.

7. National Institutes of Health, Office of Dietary Supplements: *Vitamin E.* Updated May 9, 2016. https://ods.od.nih.gov/factsheets/VitaminE-HealthProfessional/ Accessed: May 18, 2016

8. National Institutes of Health, Office of Dietary Supplements: *Vitamin K.* Updated February, 2016. https://ods.od.nih.gov/factsheets/VitaminK-HealthProfessional/ Accessed: May 18, 2016

9. National Institutes of Health, Medline Plus: *Niacin and niacinamide (vitamin B3).* 2015. https://www.nlm.nih.gov/medlineplus/druginfo/natural/924.html Accessed: May 19, 2016

10. National Institutes of Health, Office of Dietary Supplements: *Vitamin B6.* Updated February 2016. https://ods.od.nih.gov/factsheets/VitaminB6-HealthProfessional/ Accessed: May 19, 2016

11. National Institutes of Health, Office of Dietary Supplements: *Vitamin B12.* February 2016. https://ods.od.nih.gov/factsheets/VitaminB12-HealthProfessional/ Accessed: May 19, 2016

12. Dali-Youcef N, Andrès R: An update on cobalamin deficiency in adults. *Quarterly Journal of Medicine* 102(1):17, 2009.

13. Centers for Disease Control and Prevention: *Spina bifida: Data and statistics.* Updated December 2015. http://www.cdc.gov/ncbddd/spinabifida/data.html Accessed: May 19, 2016

14. National Institutes of Health, Office of Dietary Supplements: *Vitamin C.* Updated February 2016. https://ods.od.nih.gov/factsheets/VitaminC-HealthProfessional/ Accessed: May 19, 2016

15. Oregon State University, Linus Pauling Institute, Micronutrient Information Center: *Vitamin C.* Updated 2014. http://lpi.oregonstate.edu/mic/vitamins/vitamin-C Accessed: May 19, 2016

16. National Institutes of Health, National Cancer Institute: *Risk factors for cancer.* Updated December 2015. http://www.cancer.gov/about-cancer/causes-prevention/risk Accessed: May 20, 2016

17. Colditz GA and Sutcliffe S: The preventability of cancer. *JAMA Oncology.* Published online May 19, 2016. doi:10.1001/jamaoncol.2016.0889

18. National Institutes of Health, National Cancer Institute: *Alcohol and cancer risk*. 2013. http://www.cancer.gov/about-cancer/causes-prevention/risk/alcohol/alcohol-fact-sheet Accessed: May 20, 2016

19. National Institutes of Health, National Cancer Institute: *Diet*. 2015. http://www.cancer.gov /about-cancer/causes-prevention/risk/diet Accessed: May 20, 2016

20. American Cancer Society: *Common questions about diet and cancer*. Revised February 2016. http://www.cancer.org/healthy/eathealthygetactive /acsguidelinesonnutritionphysicalactivityforcancerprevention/acs-guidelines-on-nutrition -and-physical-activity-for-cancer-prevention-common-questions Accessed: May 20, 2016

Unit 9

1. U.S. Department of Health and Human Services: *Bone health and osteoporosis: A report of the Surgeon General*. Rockville, MD: U.S. Department of Health and Human Services, Office of the Surgeon General, 2004. http://www.surgeongeneral.gov/library/reports /bonehealth/ Accessed: May 21, 2016

2. U.S. Department of Agriculture, Agricultural Research Service: *What We Eat in America, NHANES 2013–2014: Nutrient Intakes from food and beverages: Mean amounts consumed by individuals: By gender and age*. 2016. https://www.ars.usda.gov/ARSUserFiles/80400530/ pdf/1314/Table_1_NIN_GEN_13.pdf Accessed: November 14, 2016

3. Office of Dietary Supplements, National Institutes of Health: *Dietary supplement fact sheet: Calcium*. Updated February 2016. http://ods.od.nih.gov/factsheets/Calcium -HealthProfessional/ Accessed: May 21, 2016

4. National Institutes of Health, Medline Plus: *Osteoporosis*. Last updated May 13, 2016. https://www.nlm.nih.gov/medlineplus/osteoporosis.html Accessed: May 21, 2016

5. International Osteoporosis Foundation: *Facts & statistics*. 2015. http://www.iofbonehealth .org/facts-statistics Accessed: May 21, 2016

6. National Institutes of Health, Osteoporosis and Related Bone Diseases National Resource Center: *Osteoporosis: Peak bone mass in women*. 2015. http://www.niams.nih.gov/Health_ Info/Bone/Osteoporosis/bone_mass.asp Accessed: May 21, 2016

7. National Institutes of Health, Osteoporosis and Related Bone Diseases National Resource Center: *Osteoporosis overview*. 2015. http://www.niams.nih.gov/Health_Info/Bone /Osteoporosis/overview.asp#c Accessed: May 21, 2016

8. National Institutes of Health, Medline Plus: *Calcium carbonate with magnesium overdose*. 2015. https://www.nlm.nih.gov/medlineplus/ency/article/002539.htm Accessed: May 21, 2016

9. Centers for Disease Control and Prevention, Community Water Fluoridation: *2014 Water fluoridation statistics*. http://www.cdc.gov/fluoridation/statistics/2014stats.htm Accessed: May 22, 2016

10. National Institutes of Health, Medline Plus: *Potassium*. Updated March 2016. https://www .nlm.nih.gov/medlineplus/potassium.html Accessed: May 22, 2016

11. Cleveland Clinic: *Salt substitutes*. ND. http://my.clevelandclinic.org/services/heart /prevention/nutrition/food-choices/salt-substitutes Accessed: May 22, 2016

12. Centers for Disease Control and Prevention: *Hypertension*. Last reviewed May 5, 2016. http://www.cdc.gov/bloodpressure/ Accessed: May 22, 2016

13. Centers for Disease Control and Prevention, High Blood Pressure: *High blood pressure risk factors*. 2014. http://www.cdc.gov/bloodpressure/risk_factors.htm Accessed: May 22, 2016

14. American Heart Association: *Frequently asked questions (FAQs) about sodium*. Last reviewed 2014. http://www.heart.org/HEARTORG/HealthyLiving/HealthyEating /HealthyDietGoals/Frequently-Asked-Questions-About-Sodium_UCM_306840_Article. jsp#.V0IFTeT8T-U Accessed: May 22, 2015

15. U.S. Departments of Agriculture and Health and Human Services: *2015–2020 Dietary Guidelines for Americans*. 2015. http://health.gov/dietaryguidelines/2015/guidelines/ Accessed: May 9, 2016

16. U.S. Department of Agriculture, Agricultural Research Service: *USDA national nutrient database for standard reference, release 28.* Updated May 20, 2016. http://www.ars.usda.gov/Services/docs.htm?docid=8964 Accessed: May 22, 2016

17. Oregon State University, Linus Pauling Institute, Micronutrient Information Center: *Iron.* 2009. http://lpi.oregonstate.edu/infocenter/minerals/iron/ Accessed: May 22, 2016

18. National Institutes of Health, Office of Dietary Supplements: *Iron.* Updated February 2016. https://ods.od.nih.gov/factsheets/Iron-HealthProfessional/#h5 Accessed: May 22, 2016

19. National Institutes of Health, Medline Plus: *Iron deficiency anemia.* Updated 2015. https://www.nlm.nih.gov/medlineplus/ency/article/000584.htm Accessed: May 22, 2016

20. American Red Cross: *Eligibility requirements.* ND. http://www.redcrossblood.org/donating-blood/eligibility-requirements Accessed: May 22, 2016

21. Office of Dietary Supplements, National Institutes of Health: *Magnesium.* Updated February 2016. https://ods.od.nih.gov/factsheets/Magnesium-HealthProfessional/ Accessed: May 22, 2016

22. National Institutes of Health, Office of Dietary Supplements: *Selenium.* Updated February 2016. https://ods.od.nih.gov/factsheets/Selenium-HealthProfessional/ Accessed: May 22, 2016

23. National Institutes of Health, Office of Dietary Supplements: *Iodine.* Updated 2011. https://ods.od.nih.gov/factsheets/Iodine-HealthProfessional/ Accessed: May 22, 2016

24. Mayo Clinic: What's the difference between sea salt and table salt? *Nutrition and healthy eating.* May 2016. http://www.mayoclinic.org/healthy-lifestyle/nutrition-and-healthy-eating/expert-answers/sea-salt/faq-20058512 Accessed: May 22, 2016

25. National Institutes of Health, Office of Dietary Supplements: *Zinc.* Updated February 2016. https://ods.od.nih.gov/factsheets/Zinc-HealthProfessional Accessed: May 22, 2016

26. Office of Dietary Supplements, National Institutes of Health: *Chromium.* 2013. https://ods.od.nih.gov/factsheets/Chromium-HealthProfessional/#h5 Accessed: May 23, 2016

27. Saladin KS: *Anatomy & physiology.* 7th ed. Boston: McGraw-Hill Publishing Company, 2015.

28. Valtrin H: "Drink at least eight glasses of water a day." Really? Is there evidence for "8×8"? *American Journal of Physiological Regulation and Integrative Comparative Physiology* 283:R993, 2002.

29. Food and Nutrition Board, Institute of Medicine: *Dietary Reference Intakes for water, potassium, sodium, chloride, and sulfate.* Washington, DC: National Academies Press, 2004.

30. Shah MK and others: Hypernatremia in the geriatric population. *Clinical Interventions in Aging* 9:1987, 2014. doi: 10.2147/CIA.S65214. eCollection 2014

31. Mayo Clinic Staff: *Hangovers: Definition.* 2014. http://www.mayoclinic.org/diseases-conditions/hangovers/basics/definition/con-20025464 Accessed: May 23, 2016

32. Mayo Clinic: *Hyponatremia.* 2014. http://www.mayoclinic.org/diseases-conditions/hyponatremia/basics/symptoms/con-20031445 Accessed: May 23, 2016

33. Centers for Disease Control and Prevention: *Binge drinking.* Updated 2015. http://www.cdc.gov/alcohol/fact-sheets/binge-drinking.htm Accessed: May 23, 2016

34. Centers for Disease Control and Prevention: *Excessive alcohol use.* Last update December 2015. http://www.cdc.gov/chronicdisease/resources/publications/aag/alcohol.htm Accessed: May 23, 2016

35. American Cancer Society: *Alcohol use and cancer.* Last revised 2014. http://www.cancer.org/cancer/cancercauses/dietandphysicalactivity/alcohol-use-and-cancer Accessed: May 24, 2016

36. American Heart Association: *Alcohol and heart health.* ND. http://www.heart.org/HEARTORG/HealthyLiving/HealthyEating/Nutrition/Alcohol-and-Heart-Health_UCM_305173_Article.jsp#.V0R7-fkrLIU Accessed: May 24, 2016

Unit 10

1. National Institutes of Health, National Heart, Lung, and Blood Institute: *Why is a healthy weight important?* ND. http://www.nhlbi.nih.gov/health/educational/lose_wt/index.htm Accessed: May 24, 2016

2. Fryar CD and others: *Prevalence of overweight, obesity, and extreme obesity among adults aged 20 and over: United States, 1960–1962 through 2013–2014.* July 18, 2016. http://www.cdc.gov/nchs/data/hestat/obesity_adult_13_14/obesity_adult_13_14.htm Accessed: November 28, 2016

3. Centers for Disease Control and Prevention: *Childhood obesity facts: Prevalence of childhood obesity in the United States, 2011–2014.* November 17, 2016. http://www.cdc.gov/obesity/data/childhood.html Accessed: November 28, 2016

4. World Health Organization, Media Centre: *Obesity and overweight.* Updated 2015. http://www.who.int/mediacentre/factsheets/fs311/en/ Accessed: May 24, 2016

5. Naaz A and others: Loss of cyclin-dependent kinase inhibitors produces adipocyte hyperplasia and obesity. *The FASEB Journal* 18:1925, 2004.

6. Saladin KS: *Anatomy & Physiology* 7th ed. Boston: McGraw-Hill Publishing Company, 2015.

7. Bray GA, Champagne CM: Dietary patterns may modify central adiposity. *Journal of the American Dietetic Association* 109:1354, 2009.

8. Avram, MM: Cellulite: A review of its physiology and treatment. *Journal of Cosmetic and Laser Therapy* 6:181, 2004.

9. Centers for Disease Control and Prevention: *Overweight & obesity: Adult obesity causes & consequences.* Updated 2015. http://www.cdc.gov/obesity/adult/causes.html Accessed: May 24, 2016

10. Puhl RM, Heuer CA: Obesity stigma: Important considerations for public health. *American Journal of Public Health* 100(6): 1019, 2010. doi: 10.2105/AJPH.2009.159491

11. Han TS, Lean MEJ: A clinical perspective of obesity, metabolic syndrome and cardiovascular disease. *Journal of the Royal Society of Medicine Cardiovascular Disease* 5:1, 2016. doi: 10.1177/204800401663337

12. National Institutes of Health, National Heart, Lung, and Blood Institute: *Guidelines on overweight and obesity: Electronic textbook.* ND. http://www.nhlbi.nih.gov/health-pro/guidelines/current/obesity-guidelines/e_textbook/txgd/4142.htm Accessed: May 24, 2016

13. National Institutes of Health, National Heart, Lung, and Blood Institute: *Assessing your weight and health risk.* ND. http://www.nhlbi.nih.gov/health/educational/lose_wt/risk.htm Accessed: May 24, 2016

14. Garcia AL and others: Improved prediction of body fat by measuring skinfold thickness, circumferences, and bone breadths. *Obesity Research* 13:626, 2005.

15. Food and Nutrition Board, National Institute of Health: *Dietary Reference Intakes for energy, carbohydrate, fiber, fat, fatty acids, cholesterol, protein, and amino acids (macronutrients).* Washington, DC: National Academies Press, 2005.

16. Williams MH and others: *Nutrition for health, fitness & sport.* 11th ed. New York: McGraw-Hill, 2017.

17. Knudsen N and others: Small differences in thyroid function may be important for body mass index and the occurrence of obesity in the population. *Journal of Clinical Endocrinology & Metabolism* 90:4019, 2006.

18. Haugen HA and others: Variability of measured resting metabolic rate. *American Journal of Clinical Nutrition* 78:1141, 2005.

19. Hall KD and others: Energy balance and its components: Implications for body weight regulation. *American Journal of Clinical Nutrition* 95(4):989, 2012. doi: 10.3945/ajcn.112.036350 PMCID: PMC3302369

20. Tremblay MA and others: Systematic review of sedentary behaviour and health indicators in school-aged children and youth. *International Journal of Behavioral Nutrition and Physical Activity* 8:98, 2011. doi: 10.1186/1479-5868-8-98

21. Inoue S and others: Television viewing time is associated with overweight/obesity among older adults, independent of meeting physical activity and health guidelines. *Journal of Epidemiology* 22(1):50, 2012. doi:10.2188/jea.JE20110054

22. National Institutes of Health, National Heart Lung and Blood Institute: *How can overweight and obesity be prevented?* 2012. http://www.nhlbi.nih.gov/health/health-topics/topics/obe/prevention Accessed: May 25, 2016

23. Jequier E: Leptin signaling, adiposity, and energy balance. *Annals of the New York Academy of Sciences* 967:379, 2002.

24. Rolls BJ: What is the role of portion control in weight management? *International Journal of Obesity (London)* 38(Suppl 1): S1, 2014. doi: 10.1038/ijo.2014.82

25. National Institutes of Health, National Heart Lung and Blood Institute: *How are overweight and obesity treated?* 2012. http://www.nhlbi.nih.gov/health/health-topics /topics/obe/treatment.html Accessed: May 25, 2016

26. National Institutes of Health, National Institute of Diabetes and Digestive and Kidney Diseases: *Very low-calorie diets.* 2012. http://www.niddk.nih.gov/health-information /health-topics/weight-control/very-low-calorie-diets/Pages/very-low-calorie-diets.aspx Accessed: May 25, 2016

27. Kraschnewski JL and others: Long-term weight loss maintenance in the United States. *International Journal of Obesity (London)* 34 (11):1634, 2010. doi:10.1038/ijo.2010.94

28. National Weight Control Registry: *NWCR facts.* ND. http://www.nwcr.ws/Research/default .htm Accessed: June May 25, 2016

29. Mayo Clinic, Weight loss: *Common weight loss drugs.* 2015. http://www.mayoclinic.org /healthy-lifestyle/weight-loss/in-depth/weight-loss-drugs/art-20044832?pg=2 Accessed: May 25, 2016

30. National Institutes of Health, National Institute of Diabetes and Digestive and Kidney Diseases, Weight-Control Information Network: *Bariatric surgery for severe obesity.* 2011. http://win.niddk.nih.gov/publications/gastric.htm Accessed: May 25, 2016

31. Lee WJ, Almulaifi A: Recent advances in bariatric/metabolic surgery: Appraisal of clinical evidence. *Journal of Biomedical Research* 29(2):98, 2015. doi: 10.7555/JBR.28.20140120

32. Sundbom M: Laparoscopic revolution in bariatric surgery. *World Journal of Gastroenterology* 20(41): 15135, 2014.

33. U.S. Food and Drug Administration, FDA News Release: *FDA approves first-of-kind device to treat obesity.* January 14, 2015. http://www.fda.gov/NewsEvents/Newsroom /PressAnnouncements/ucm430223.htm Accessed: May 25, 2016

34. U.S. Food and Drug Administration, FDA News Release: *FDA approves AspireAssist obesity device.* June 14, 2016. http://www.fda.gov/newsevents/newsroom /pressannouncements/ucm506625.htm Accessed: June 17, 2016

35. Dyson P: Low carbohydrate diets and type 2 diabetes: What is the latest evidence? *Diabetes Therapy* 6:411, 2015. doi: 10.1007/s13300-015-0136-9

36. Devalaraja S and others: Exotic fruits as therapeutic complements for diabetes, obesity and metabolic syndrome. *Food Research International* 44(7): 1856, 2011. doi: 10.1016 /j.foodres.2011.04.008 PMCID: PMC3156450

37. Centers for Disease Control and Prevention, National Center for Health Statistics: *Prevalence of underweight among adults aged 20 and over: United States, 1960–1962 through 2011–2012.* 2015. http://www.cdc.gov/nchs/data/hestat/underweight_adult_11_12 /underweight_adult_11_12.htm Accessed: May 25, 2016

38. American Psychiatric Association: *Diagnostic and statistical manual of mental disorders,* 5th ed. Arlington, VA: American Psychiatric Publishing, 2013.

39. American Dietetic Association: Position of the American Dietetic Association: Nutrition intervention in the treatment of eating disorders. *Journal of the American Dietetic Association* 111(8):1236, 2011.

40. National Institutes of Health, National Institute of Diabetes and Digestive and Kidney Diseases: *Binge eating disorder.* 2012. http://www.niddk.nih.gov/health-information/health-topics/weight-control/binge_eating/Pages/binge-eating-disorder.aspx Accessed: May 26, 2016

41. National Institutes of Health, National Library of Medicine: Bulimia. *MedlinePlus.* Updated May 3, 2016. http://www.nlm.nih.gov/medlineplus/ency/article/000341.htm Accessed: May 26, 2016

42. National Institutes of Health, National Library of Medicine: Anorexia nervosa. *MedlinePlus.* Updated March 2014. https://www.nlm.nih.gov/medlineplus/ency /article/000362.htm Accessed: May 26, 2016

43. Campbell K, Peebles R: Eating disorders in children and adolescents: State of the art review. *Pediatrics* 134(3): 582, 2014. doi: 10.1542/peds.2014-0194

44. American College of Sports Medicine: *Female athlete triad.* 2011. https://www.acsm.org /docs/brochures/the-female-athlete-triad.pdf Accessed: May 26, 2016

45. Centers for Disease Control and Prevention: *Physical activity and health: The benefits of physical activity*. Updated 2015. http://www.cdc.gov/physicalactivity/basics/pa-health /index.htm Accessed: May 26, 2016

46. National Heart Lung and Blood Institute: *Types of physical activity*. 2015. http://www.nhlbi.nih .gov/health/health-topics/topics/phys/types Accessed: May 26, 2016

47. National Heart Lung and Blood Institute: *Recommendations for physical activity*. 2015. http://www.nhlbi.nih.gov/health/health-topics/topics/phys/recommend.html Accessed: May 26, 2016

48. Position of the Academy of Nutrition and Dietetics, Dietitians of Canada, and the American College of Sports Medicine: Nutrition and athletic performance. *Journal of the Academy of Nutrition and Dietetics* 116(3):501, 2016.

49. Economos CD and others: Nutritional practices of elite athletes: Practical recommendations. *Sports Medicine* 16:381, 1993.

50. American College of Sports Medicine: *Selectively and effectively using hydration for fitness*. 2011. https://www.acsm.org/docs/brochures/selecting-and-effectively-using -hydration-for-fitness.pdf Accessed: May 26, 2016

51. Centers for Disease Control and Prevention: *Heat stress*. Last updated May 23, 2016. http:// www.cdc.gov/niosh/topics/heatstress/ Accessed: May 26, 2016

52. Substance Abuse and Mental Health Services Administration: *The Dawn Report: 1 in 10 energy drink-related emergency department visits results in hospitalization*. March 13, 2014. http://www.samhsa.gov/data/sites/default/files/spot124-energy-drinks-2014.pdf Accessed: May 26, 2016

Unit 11

1. Otten JJ and others (eds.): Institute of Medicine: *Dietary Reference Intakes: The essential guide to nutrient requirements*. Washington, DC: National Academies Press, 2006.

2. Hamilton BE and others: Births: Preliminary data for 2015. *National Vital Statistics Reports* 65(3): 1, 2016.

3. Centers for Disease Control and Prevention, Reproductive Health: *Infant mortality*. Last updated January 2016. http://www.cdc.gov/reproductivehealth/MaternalInfantHealth /InfantMortality.htm Accessed: May 27, 2016

4. National Institutes of Health, National Heart, Lung, and Blood Institute: *Your guide to anemia*. 2011. http://www.nhlbi.nih.gov/files/docs/public/blood/anemia-yg.pdf Accessed: May 27, 2016

5. March of Dimes: *Weight gain during pregnancy*. 2009. http://www.marchofdimes.org /pregnancy/weight-gain-during-pregnancy.aspx Accessed: May 27, 2016

6. Position of the Academy of Nutrition and Dietetics: Obesity, reproduction, and pregnancy outcomes. *Journal of the Academy of Nutrition and Dietetics* 116(4): 667, 2016.

7. Yi Z and others: Pre-pregnancy body mass index in relation to infant birth weight and offspring overweight/obesity: A systematic review and meta-analysis. *PLoS One* 16;8(4), 2013: e61627. doi: 10.1371/journal.pone.0061627

8. National Institutes of Health, National Heart Lung and Blood Institute, MedlinePlus: *Preeclampsia*. Updated 2014. https://www.nlm.nih.gov/medlineplus/ency/article/000898 .htm Accessed: May 27, 2016

9. National Institutes of Health, National Heart Lung and Blood Institute: *High blood pressure in pregnancy*. ND. http://www.nhlbi.nih.gov/health/resources/heart/hbp -pregnancy Accessed: May 27, 2016

10. Lessen R, Kavanagh K: Position of the Academy of Nutrition and Dietetics: Promoting and supporting breastfeeding. *Journal of the Academy of Nutrition and Dietetics* 115(3):444, 2015. doi: 10.1016/j.jand.2014.12.014

11. American Academy of Pediatrics: Policy statement: Breastfeeding and the use of human milk. *Pediatrics* 129(3): e827, 2012. doi:10.1542/peds.2011-3552

12. Baker RD, Greer, FR: Diagnosis and prevention of iron deficiency and iron-deficiency anemia in infants and young children (0–3 years of age). *Pediatrics* 126(5): 1040, 2010.

13. Centers for Disease Control and Prevention: *Breastfeeding, CDC National Immunization Survey.* Last updated August 2016. http://www.cdc.gov/breastfeeding/data/NIS_data/index.htm Accessed: November 9, 2016

14. Saarela T and others: Macronutrient and energy contents of human milk fractions during the first six months of lactation. *Acta Paediatricia* 94(9):1176, 2005.

15. U.S. Food and Drug Administration: *Food safety for moms to be: Once baby arrives.* Last updated April 2016. http://www.fda.gov/Food/ResourcesForYou/HealthEducators/ucm089629.htm Accessed: May 27, 2016

16. Fomon SJ: Infant feeding in the 20th century: Formula and beikost. *Journal of Nutrition* 131:409S, 2001.

17. Fleischer DM and others: Adverse reactions to foods committee report: primary prevention of allergic disease through nutritional interventions: Guidelines for healthcare professionals. *Journal of Allergy and Clinical Immunology: In Practice* 1:29, 2013. https://www.aaaai.org/Aaaai/media/MediaLibrary/PDF%20Documents/Libraries/Preventing-Allergies-Healthcare-15.pdf Accessed: May 28, 2016

18. Macdonald LE and others: A systematic review and meta-analysis of the effects of pasteurization on milk vitamins, and evidence for raw milk consumption and other health-related outcomes. *Journal of Food Protection* 74(11):1814, 2011.

19. American Academy of Dermatology: *Growing evidence suggests possible link between diet and acne.* 2013. https://www.aad.org/media/news-releases/growing-evidence-suggests-possible-link-between-diet-and-acne Accessed: May 28, 2016

20. Centers for Disease Control and Prevention: *Childhood overweight and obesity.* Updated 2015. http://www.cdc.gov/obesity/childhood/index.html Accessed: May 28, 2016

21. Centers for Disease Control and Prevention: *Childhood obesity causes & consequences.* Updated June 2015. http://www.cdc.gov/obesity/childhood/causes.html Accessed: May 28, 2016

22. Centers for Disease Control and Prevention, National Center for Health Statistics: *TV watching and computer use in U.S. youth aged 12–15, 2012. NCHS Data Brief No. 157,* July 2014. http://www.cdc.gov/nchs/data/databriefs/db157.htm Accessed: May 28, 2016

23. Centers for Disease Control and Prevention: *Tips for parents—ideas to help children maintain a healthy weight.* Updated 2015. http://www.cdc.gov/healthyweight/children/index.html Accessed: May 28, 2016

24. U.S. Census Bureau: *FFF: Older Americans Month: May 2016.* 2016. http://www.census.gov/newsroom/facts-for-features/2016/cb16-ff08.html Accessed: May 28, 2016

25. U.S. Census Bureau: *90+ in the United States: 2006–2008.* 2011. http://www.census.gov/prod/2011pubs/acs-17.pdf Accessed: May 28, 2016

26. Deierlein AL and others: Diet quality of urban older adults aged 60–99: The cardiovascular health of seniors and built environment study. *Journal of the Academy of Nutrition and Dietetics* 114(2):279, 2014. doi:10.1016/j.jand.2013.09.002

27. Centers for Disease Control and Prevention, Healthy Living: *Be food safe: Protect yourself from food poisoning.* Updated April 2016. http://www.cdc.gov/Features/BeFoodSafe/ Accessed: May 29, 2016

28. The National Academy of Sciences, Board on Agriculture and Natural Resource, Report in Brief: *Genetically engineered crops: Experiences and prospects.* 2016. http://nas-sites.org/ge-crops/2016/05/16/report-in-brief/ Accessed: May 29, 2016

29. U.S. Department of Agriculture, Food Safety and Inspection Service: *"Danger Zone" (40 °F – 140 °F).* 2013. http://www.fsis.usda.gov/wps/portal/fsis/topics/food-safety-education/get-answers/food-safety-fact-sheets/safe-food-handling/danger-zone-40-f-140-f/ct_index Accessed: July 31, 2016

30. U.S. Department of Agriculture, Food Safety and Inspection Service: 2013. *Freezing and food safety.* http://www.fsis.usda.gov/wps/portal/fsis/topics/food-safety-education/get-answers/food-safety-fact-sheets/safe-food-handling/freezing-and-food-safety/CT_Index Accessed: July 31, 2016

31. U.S. Department of Agriculture, Agricultural Research Service: *Best ways to clean kitchen sponges.* 2007. http://www.ars.usda.gov/is/pr/2007/070423.htm Accessed: May 29, 2016

32. Miranda RC, Schaffner DW: Longer contact times increase cross-contamination of *Enterobacter aerogenes* from surfaces to food. *Applied and Environmental Microbiology* 82(21):6490, 2016.

33. U.S. Department of Agriculture, Food Safety and Inspection Service: *Cooking safely in the microwave oven.* Last modified 2013. http://www.fsis.usda.gov/wps/portal/fsis/topics /food-safety-education/get-answers/food-safety-fact-sheets/appliances-and-thermometers /cooking-safely-in-the-microwave/cooking-safely-in-the-microwave-oven Accessed: May 29, 2016

34. U.S. Department of Agriculture, Food Safety and Inspection Service: *Basics for handling food safely.* Last modified 2015. http://www.fsis.usda.gov/wps/portal/fsis/topics/food -safety-education/get-answers/food-safety-fact-sheets/safe-food-handling/basics-for -handling-food-safely/ct_index Accessed: May 29, 2016

35. National Pesticide Information Center: *Pesticides and human health.* Updated 2015. http:// npic.orst.edu/health/humhealth.html Accessed: May 30, 2016

36. World Health Organization, Nutrition: *Malnutrition in the crosshairs.* December 1, 2016. http://www.who.int/nutrition/pressrelease-FAOWHO-symposium-malnutrition/en/ Accessed: December 3, 2016

37. World Food Program: *Hunger statistics.* ND. http://www.wfp.org/hunger/stats Accessed: May 30, 2016

38. Food and Agricultural Organization of the United Nations, Locust Watch: *Frequently asked questions (FAQs) about locusts.* 2009. http://www.fao.org/ag/locusts/en/info/info/faq/ Accessed: May 30, 2016

39. World Health Organization: *Infant and young child feeding.* Updated January 2016. http:// www.who.int/mediacentre/factsheets/fs342/en/ Accessed: May 30, 2016

40. United Nations Children's Fund: *Nutrition and micronutrients.* Updated 2011. http:// www.unicef.org/supply/index_39993.html Accessed: May 30, 2016

41. Proctor BD and others: Income and poverty in the United States: 2015. *Current Population Reports.* P60–256(RV), U.S. Government Printing Office, Washington, DC, 2016.

42. U.S. Department of Health and Human Services: *HHS poverty guidelines for 2016.* January 2016. https://aspe.hhs.gov/poverty-guidelines Accessed: December 2, 2016

43. Coleman-Jensen A and others: Household food security in the United States in 2015. *Economic Research Report No.* (ERR-215), September 2016.

44. United Nations: *World population projected to reach 9.7 billion by 2050.* July 2015. http:// www.un.org/en/development/desa/news/population/2015-report.html Accessed: May 30, 2016

45. Foley JA: Can we feed the world & sustain the planet? *Scientific American* 305(5):60, 2011.

Appendix G
Dietary Reference Intake (DRI) Tables

Dietary Reference Intakes (DRIs): Recommended Intakes for Individuals, Vitamins
Food and Nutrition Board, Institute of Medicine, National Academies

Life Stage Group	Vitamin A (µg/d)[a]	Vitamin C (mg/d)	Vitamin D (µg/d)[b,c]	Vitamin E (mg/d)[d]	Vitamin K (µg/d)	Thiamin (mg/d)	Riboflavin (mg/d)	Niacin (mg/d)[e]	Vitamin B-6 (mg/d)	Folate (µg/d)[f]	Vitamin B-12 (µg/d)	Pantothenic Acid (mg/d)	Biotin (µg/d)	Choline (mg/d)[g]
Infants														
0–6 mo	400*	40*	10	4*	2.0*	0.2*	0.3*	2*	0.1*	65*	0.4*	1.7*	5*	125*
7–12 mo	500*	50*	10	5*	2.5*	0.3*	0.4*	4*	0.3*	80*	0.5*	1.8*	6*	150*
Children														
1–3 y	**300**	**15**	**15**	**6**	30*	**0.5**	**0.5**	**6**	**0.5**	**150**	**0.9**	2*	8*	200*
4–8 y	**400**	**25**	**15**	**7**	55*	**0.6**	**0.6**	**8**	**0.6**	**200**	**1.2**	3*	12*	250*
Males														
9–13 y	**600**	**45**	**15**	**11**	60*	**0.9**	**0.9**	**12**	**1.0**	**300**	**1.8**	4*	20*	375*
14–18 y	**900**	**75**	**15**	**15**	75*	**1.2**	**1.3**	**16**	**1.3**	**400**	**2.4**	5*	25*	550*
19–30 y	**900**	**90**	**15**	**15**	120*	**1.2**	**1.3**	**16**	**1.3**	**400**	**2.4**	5*	30*	550*
31–50 y	**900**	**90**	**15**	**15**	120*	**1.2**	**1.3**	**16**	**1.3**	**400**	**2.4**	5*	30*	550*
51–70 y	**900**	**90**	**15**	**15**	120*	**1.2**	**1.3**	**16**	**1.7**	**400**	**2.4**[h]	5*	30*	550*
>70 y	**900**	**90**	**20**	**15**	120*	**1.2**	**1.3**	**16**	**1.7**	**400**	**2.4**[h]	5*	30*	550*
Females														
9–13 y	**600**	**45**	**15**	**11**	60*	**0.9**	**0.9**	**12**	**1.0**	**300**	**1.8**	4*	20*	375*
14–18 y	**700**	**65**	**15**	**15**	75*	**1.0**	**1.0**	**14**	**1.2**	**400**[i]	**2.4**	5*	25*	400*
19–30 y	**700**	**75**	**15**	**15**	90*	**1.1**	**1.1**	**14**	**1.3**	**400**[i]	**2.4**	5*	30*	425*
31–50 y	**700**	**75**	**15**	**15**	90*	**1.1**	**1.1**	**14**	**1.3**	**400**[i]	**2.4**	5*	30*	425*
51–70 y	**700**	**75**	**15**	**15**	90*	**1.1**	**1.1**	**14**	**1.5**	**400**	**2.4**[h]	5*	30*	425*
>70 y	**700**	**75**	**20**	**15**	90*	**1.1**	**1.1**	**14**	**1.5**	**400**	**2.4**[h]	5*	30*	425*
Pregnancy														
≤18 y	**750**	**80**	**15**	**15**	75*	**1.4**	**1.4**	**18**	**1.9**	**600**[j]	**2.6**	6*	30*	450*
19–30 y	**770**	**85**	**15**	**15**	90*	**1.4**	**1.4**	**18**	**1.9**	**600**[j]	**2.6**	6*	30*	450*
31–50 y	**770**	**85**	**15**	**15**	90*	**1.4**	**1.4**	**18**	**1.9**	**600**[j]	**2.6**	6*	30*	450*
Lactation														
≤18 y	**1200**	**115**	**15**	**19**	75*	**1.4**	**1.6**	**17**	**2.0**	**500**	**2.8**	7*	35*	550*
19–30 y	**1300**	**120**	**15**	**19**	90*	**1.4**	**1.6**	**17**	**2.0**	**500**	**2.8**	7*	35*	550*
31–50 y	**1300**	**120**	**15**	**19**	90*	**1.4**	**1.6**	**17**	**2.0**	**500**	**2.8**	7*	35*	550*

mg = milligram, µg = microgram

NOTE: This table (taken from the DRI reports; see **www.nap.edu**) presents Recommended Dietary Allowances (RDAs) in **bold type** and Adequate Intakes (AIs) in ordinary type followed by an asterisk (*). RDAs and AIs may both be used as goals for individual intake. RDAs are set to meet the needs of almost all (97 to 98%) individuals in a group. For healthy breastfed infants, the AI is the mean intake. The AI for other life stage and gender groups is believed to cover needs of all individuals in the group, but lack of data or uncertainty in the data prevents being able to specify with confidence the percentage of individuals covered by this intake.

[a] As retinol activity equivalents (RAEs). 1 RAE = 1 µg retinol, 12 µg β-carotene, 24 µg α-carotene, or 24 µg β-cryptoxanthin. To calculate RAEs from REs of provitamin A carotenoids in foods, divide the REs by 2. For preformed vitamin A in foods or supplements and for provitamin A carotenoids in supplements, 1 RE = 1 RAE.

[b] cholecalciferol. 1 µg cholecalciferol = 40 IU vitamin D.

[c] In the absence of adequate exposure to sunlight.

[d] As α-tocopherol. α-Tocopherol includes RRR-α-tocopherol, the only form of α-tocopherol that occurs naturally in foods, and the 2R-stereoisomeric forms of α-tocopherol (RRR-, RSR-, RRS-, and RSS-α-tocopherol) that occur in fortified foods and supplements. It does not include the 2S-stereoisomeric forms of α-tocopherol (SRR-, SSR-, SRS-, and SSS-α-tocopherol), also found in fortified foods and supplements.

[e] As niacin equivalents (NE). 1 mg of niacin = 60 mg of tryptophan; 0–6 months = preformed niacin (not NE).

[f] As dietary folate equivalents (DFE). 1 DFE = 1 µg food folate = 0.6 µg of folic acid from fortified food or as a supplement consumed with food = 0.5 µg of a supplement taken on an empty stomach.

[g] Although AIs have been set for choline, there are few data to assess whether a dietary supply of choline is needed at all stages of the life cycle, and it may be that the choline requirement can be met by endogenous synthesis at some of these stages.

[h] Because 10 to 30% of older people may malabsorb food-bound B-12, it is advisable for those older than 50 years to meet their RDA mainly by consuming foods fortified with B-12 or a supplement containing B-12.

[i] In view of evidence linking folate intake with neural tube defects in the fetus, it is recommended that all women capable of becoming pregnant consume 400 µg from supplements or fortified foods in addition to intake of food folate from a varied diet.

[j] It is assumed that women will continue consuming 400 µg from supplements or fortified food until their pregnancy is confirmed and they enter prenatal care, which ordinarily occurs after the end of the periconceptional period—the critical time for formation of the neural tube.

Adapted from the *Dietary Reference Intakes* series, National Academies Press. Copyright 1997, 1998, 2000, 2001, 2011, by the National Academy of Sciences. The full reports are available from the National Academies Press at **www.nap.edu.**

Dietary Reference Intakes (DRIs): Recommended Intakes for Individuals, Elements
Food and Nutrition Board, Institute of Medicine, National Academies

Life Stage Group	Calcium (mg/d)	Chromium (µg/d)	Copper (µg/d)	Fluoride (mg/d)	Iodine (µg/d)	Iron (mg/d)	Magnesium (mg/d)	Manganese (mg/d)	Molybdenum (µg/d)	Phosphorus (mg/d)	Selenium (µg/d)	Zinc (mg/d)
Infants												
0–6 mo	200*	0.2*	200*	0.01*	110*	0.27*	30*	0.003*	2*	100*	15*	2*
7–12 mo	260*	5.5*	220*	0.5*	130*	11	75*	0.6*	3*	275*	20*	3
Children												
1–3 y	700	11*	340	0.7*	90	7	80	1.2*	17	460	20	3
4–8 y	1000	15*	440	1*	90	10	130	1.5*	22	500	30	5
Males												
9–13 y	1300	25*	700	2*	120	8	240	1.9*	34	1250	40	8
14–18 y	1300	35*	890	3*	150	11	410	2.2*	43	1250	55	11
19–30 y	1000	35*	900	4*	150	8	400	2.3*	45	700	55	11
31–50 y	1000	35*	900	4*	150	8	420	2.3*	45	700	55	11
51–70 y	1000	30*	900	4*	150	8	420	2.3*	45	700	55	11
>70 y	1200	30*	900	4*	150	8	420	2.3*	45	700	55	11
Females												
9–13 y	1300	21*	700	2*	120	8	240	1.6*	34	1250	40	8
14–18 y	1300	24*	890	3*	150	15	360	1.6*	43	1250	55	9
19–30 y	1000	25*	900	3*	150	18	310	1.8*	45	700	55	8
31–50 y	1000	25*	900	3*	150	18	320	1.8*	45	700	55	8
51–70 y	1200	20*	900	3*	150	8	320	1.8*	45	700	55	8
>70 y	1200	20*	900	3*	150	8	320	1.8*	45	700	55	8
Pregnancy												
≤18 y	1300	29*	1000	3*	220	27	400	2.0*	50	1250	60	12
19–30 y	1000	30*	1000	3*	220	27	350	2.0*	50	700	60	11
31–50 y	1000	30*	1000	3*	220	27	360	2.0*	50	700	60	11
Lactation												
≤18 y	1300	44*	1300	3*	290	10	360	2.6*	50	1250	70	13
19–30 y	1000	45*	1300	3*	290	9	310	2.6*	50	700	70	12
31–50 y	1000	45*	1300	3*	290	9	320	2.6*	50	700	70	12

NOTE: This table presents Recommended Dietary Allowances (RDAs) in **bold type** and Adequate Intakes (AIs) in ordinary type followed by an asterisk (*). RDAs and AIs may both be used as goals for individual intake. RDAs are set to meet the needs of almost all (97 to 98%) individuals in a group. For healthy breastfed infants, the AI is the mean intake. The AI for other life stage and gender groups is believed to cover needs of all individuals in the group, but lack of data or uncertainty in the data prevents being able to specify with confidence the percentage of individuals covered by this intake.

Sources: Dietary Reference Intakes for Calcium, Phosphorus, Magnesium, Vitamin D, and Fluoride (1997); *Dietary Reference Intakes for Thiamin, Riboflavin, Niacin, Vitamin B-6, Folate, Vitamin B-12, Pantothenic Acid, Biotin, and Choline* (1998); *Dietary Reference Intakes for Vitamin C, Vitamin E, Selenium, and Carotenoids* (2000); *Dietary Reference Intakes for Vitamin A, Vitamin K, Arsenic, Boron, Chromium, Copper, Iodine, Iron, Manganese, Molybdenum, Nickel, Silicon, Vanadium, and Zinc* (2001); and *Dietary Reference Intakes for Calcium and Vitamin D* (2011). These reports may be accessed via **www.nap.edu.**

Adapted from the *Dietary Reference Intake series*, National Academies Press. Copyright 1997, 1998, 2000, 2001, and 2011 by the National Academy of Sciences. The full reports are available from the National Academies Press at **www.nap.edu.**

Dietary Reference Intakes (DRIs): Recommended Intakes for Individuals, Macronutrients
Food and Nutrition Board, Institute of Medicine, National Academies

Life Stage Group	Carbohydrate (g/d)	Total Fiber (g/d)	Fat (g/d)	Linoleic Acid (g/d)	α-Linolenic Acid (g/d)	Protein[a] (g/d)
Infants						
0–6 mo	60*	ND	31*	4.4*	0.5*	9.1*
7–12 mo	95*	ND	30*	4.6*	0.5*	11.0
Children						
1–3 y	130	19*	ND[b]	7*	0.7*	13
4–8 y	130	25*	ND	10*	0.9*	19
Males						
9–13 y	130	31*	ND	12*	1.2*	34
14–18 y	130	38*	ND	16*	1.6*	52
19–30 y	130	38*	ND	17*	1.6*	56
31–50 y	130	38*	ND	17*	1.6*	56
51–70 y	130	30*	ND	14*	1.6*	56
>70 y	130	30*	ND	14*	1.6*	56
Females						
9–13 y	130	26*	ND	10*	1.0*	34
14–18 y	130	26*	ND	11*	1.1*	46
19–30 y	130	25*	ND	12*	1.1*	46
31–50 y	130	25*	ND	12*	1.1*	46
51–70 y	130	21*	ND	11*	1.1*	46
>70 y	130	21*	ND	11*	1.1*	46
Pregnancy						
14–18 y	175	28*	ND	13*	1.4*	71
19–30 y	175	28*	ND	13*	1.4*	71
31–50 y	175	28*	ND	13*	1.4*	71
Lactation						
14–18 y	210	29*	ND	13*	1.3*	71
19–30 y	210	29*	ND	13*	1.3*	71
31–50 y	210	29*	ND	13*	1.3*	71

NOTE: This table presents Recommended Dietary Allowances (RDAs) in **bold type** and Adequate Intakes (AIs) in ordinary type followed by an asterisk (*). RDAs and AIs may both be used as goals for individual intake. RDAs are set to meet the needs of almost all (97 to 98%) individuals in a group. For healthy breastfed infants, the AI is the mean intake. The AI for other life stage and gender groups is believed to cover needs of all individuals in the group, but lack of data or uncertainty in the data prevents being able to specify with confidence the percentage of individuals covered by this intake.

[a]Based on 0.8g protein/kg body weight for reference body weight.

[b]ND = not determinable at this time.

Sources: Dietary Reference Intakes for Energy, Carbohydrate, Fiber, Fat, Fatty Acids, Cholesterol, Protein, and Amino Acids (2002). This report may be accessed via **www.nap.edu.** Adapted from the *Dietary Reference Intake* series, National Academies Press. Copyright 1997, 1998, 2000, 2001, by the National Academy of Sciences. The full reports are available from the National Academies Press at **www.nap.edu.**

Dietary Reference Intakes (DRIs): Recommended Intakes for Individuals, Electrolytes and Water
Food and Nutrition Board, Institute of Medicine, National Academies

Life Stage Group	Sodium (mg/d)	Potassium (mg/d)	Chloride (mg/d)	Water (L/d)
Infants				
0–6 mo	120*	400*	180*	0.7*
7–12 mo	370*	700*	570*	0.8*
Children				
1–3 y	1000*	3000*	1500*	1.3*
4–8 y	1200*	3800*	1900*	1.7*
Males				
9–13 y	1500*	4500*	2300*	2.4*
14–18 y	1500*	4700*	2300*	3.3*
19–30 y	1500*	4700*	2300*	3.7*
31–50 y	1500*	4700*	2300*	3.7*
51–70 y	1300*	4700*	2000*	3.7*
> 70 y	1200*	4700*	1800*	3.7*
Females				
9–13 y	1500*	4500*	2300*	2.1*
14–18 y	1500*	4700*	2300*	2.3*
19–30 y	1500*	4700*	2300*	2.7*
31–50 y	1500*	4700*	2300*	2.7*
51–70 y	1300*	4700*	2000*	2.7*
> 70 y	1200*	4700*	1800*	2.7*
Pregnancy				
14–18 y	1500*	4700*	2300*	3.0*
19–50 y	1500*	4700*	2300*	3.0*
Lactation				
14–18 y	1500*	5100*	2300*	3.8*
19–50 y	1500*	5100*	2300*	3.8*

NOTE: The table is adapted from the DRI reports. See **www.nap.edu**. Adequate Intakes (AIs) are followed by an asterisk (*). These may be used as a goal for individual intake. For healthy breastfed infants, the AI is the average intake. The AI for other life stage and gender groups is believed to cover the needs of all individuals in the group, but lack of data prevent being able to specify with confidence the percentage of individuals covered by this intake; therefore, no Recommended Dietary Allowance (RDA) was set.

Source: Dietary Reference Intakes for Water, Potassium, Sodium, Chloride, and Sulfate (2005). This report may be accessed via **www.nap.edu**.

Acceptable Macronutrient Distribution Ranges

Macronutrient	Range (percent of energy)		
	Children, 1–3 y	Children, 4–18 y	Adults
Fat	30–40	25–35	20–35
omega-6 polyunsaturated fats (linoleic acid)	5–10	5–10	5–10
omega-3 polyunsaturated fats[a] (α-linolenic acid)	0.6–1.2	0.6–1.2	0.6–1.2
Carbohydrate	45–65	45–65	45–65
Protein	5–20	10–30	10–35

[a]Approximately 10% of the total can come from longer-chain n-3 fatty acids.

Source: Dietary Reference Intakes for Energy, Carbohydrate, Fiber, Fat, Fatty Acids, Cholesterol, Protein, and Amino Acids (2002). The report may be accessed via **www.nap.edu**.

Adapted from the *Dietary Reference Intakes series*, National Academies Press. Copyright 1997, 1998, 2000, 2001, 2011, by the National Academy of Sciences. The full reports are available from the National Academies Press at **www.nap.edu**.

Dietary Reference Intakes (DRIs): Tolerable Upper Intake Levels (UL[a]), Vitamins
Food and Nutrition Board, Institute of Medicine, National Academies

Life Stage Group	Vitamin A (µg/d)[b]	Vitamin C (mg/d)	Vitamin D (µg/d)	Vitamin E (mg/d)[c,d]	Vitamin K	Thiamin	Riboflavin	Niacin (mg/d)[d]	Vitamin B-6 (mg/d)	Folate (µg/d)[d]	Vitamin B-12	Pantothenic Acid	Biotin	Choline (g/d)	Carotenoids[e]
Infants															
0–6 mo	600	ND[f]	25	ND	ND	ND	ND	ND	ND	ND	ND	ND	ND	ND	ND
7–12 mo	600	ND	38	ND	ND	ND	ND	ND	ND	ND	ND	ND	ND	ND	ND
Children															
1–3 y	600	400	63	200	ND	ND	ND	10	30	300	ND	ND	ND	1.0	ND
4–8 y	900	650	75	300	ND	ND	ND	15	40	400	ND	ND	ND	1.0	ND
Males, Females															
9–13 y	1700	1200	100	600	ND	ND	ND	20	60	600	ND	ND	ND	2.0	ND
14–18 y	2800	1800	100	800	ND	ND	ND	30	80	800	ND	ND	ND	3.0	ND
19–70 y	3000	2000	100	1000	ND	ND	ND	35	100	1000	ND	ND	ND	3.5	ND
>70 y	3000	2000	100	1000	ND	ND	ND	35	100	1000	ND	ND	ND	3.5	ND
Pregnancy															
≤18 y	2800	1800	100	800	ND	ND	ND	30	80	800	ND	ND	ND	3.0	ND
19–50 y	3000	2000	100	1000	ND	ND	ND	35	100	1000	ND	ND	ND	3.5	ND
Lactation															
≤18 y	2800	1800	100	800	ND	ND	ND	30	80	800	ND	ND	ND	3.0	ND
19–50 y	3000	2000	100	1000	ND	ND	ND	35	100	1000	ND	ND	ND	3.5	ND

[a]UL = The maximum level of daily nutrient intake likely to pose no risk of adverse effects. Unless otherwise specified, the UL represents total intake from food, water, and supplements. Due to lack of suitable data, ULs could not be established for vitamin K, thiamin, riboflavin, vitamin B-12, pantothenic acid, biotin, or carotenoids. In the absence of ULs, extra caution may be warranted in consuming levels above recommended intakes.

[b]As preformed vitamin A only.

[c]As α-tocopherol; applies to any form of supplemental α-tocopherol.

[d]The ULs for vitamin E, niacin, and folate apply to synthetic forms obtained from supplements, fortified foods, or a combination of the two.

[e]Beta-Carotene supplements are advised only to serve as a provitamin A source for individuals at risk of vitamin A deficiency.

[f]ND = Not determinable due to lack of data of adverse effects in this age group and concern with regard to lack of ability to handle excess amounts. Source of intake should be from food only to prevent high levels of intake.

Sources: Dietary Reference Intakes for Calcium and Vitamin D (2011); Dietary Reference Intakes for Calcium, Phosphorus, Magnesium, Vitamin D, and Fluoride (1997); Dietary Reference Intakes for Thiamin, Riboflavin, Niacin, Vitamin B-6, Folate, Vitamin B-12, Pantothenic Acid, Biotin, and Choline (1998); Dietary Reference Intakes for Vitamin C, Vitamin E, Selenium, and Carotenoids (2000); and Dietary Reference Intakes for Vitamin A, Vitamin K, Arsenic, Boron, Chromium, Copper, Iodine, Iron, Manganese, Molybdenum, Nickel, Silicon, Vanadium, and Zinc (2001). These reports may be accessed via www.nap.edu.

Dietary Reference Intakes (DRIs): Tolerable Upper Intake Levels (UL[a]), Elements and Electrolytes[b,c]
Food and Nutrition Board, Institute of Medicine, National Academies

Life Stage Group	Arsenic[b]	Boron (mg/d)	Calcium (g/d)	Copper (μg/d)	Fluoride (mg/d)	Iodine (μg/d)	Iron (mg/d)	Magnesium (mg/d)[d]	Manganese (mg/d)	Molybdenum (μg/d)	Nickel (mg/d)	Phosphorus (g/d)	Selenium (μg/d)	Vanadium (mg/d)[e]	Zinc (mg/d)	Sodium (mg/d)	Chloride (mg/d)
Infants																	
0–6 mo	ND[f]	ND	1	ND	0.7	ND	40	ND	ND	ND	ND	ND	45	ND	4	ND	ND
7–12 mo	ND	ND	1.5	ND	0.9	ND	40	ND	ND	ND	ND	ND	60	ND	5	ND	ND
Children																	
1–3 y	ND	3	2.5	1000	1.3	200	40	65	2	300	0.2	3	90	ND	7	1500	2300
4–8 y	ND	6	2.5	3000	2.2	300	40	110	3	600	0.3	3	150	ND	12	1900	2900
Males, Females																	
9–13 y	ND	11	3	5000	10	600	40	350	6	1100	0.6	4	280	ND	23	2200	3400
14–18 y	ND	17	3	8000	10	900	45	350	9	1700	1.0	4	400	ND	34	2300	3600
19–70 y	ND	20	2.5[g]	10000	10	1100	45	350	11	2000	1.0	4	400	1.8	40	2300	3600
>70 y	ND	20	2	10000	10	1100	45	350	11	2000	1.0	3	400	1.8	40	2300	3600
Pregnancy																	
≤18 y	ND	17	3	8000	10	900	45	350	9	1700	1.0	3.5	400	ND	34	2300	3600
19–50 y	ND	20	2.5	10000	10	1100	45	350	11	2000	1.0	3.5	400	ND	40	2300	3600
Lactation																	
≤18 y	ND	17	3	8000	10	900	45	350	9	1700	1.0	4	400	ND	34	2300	3600
19–50 y	ND	20	2.5	10000	10	1100	45	350	11	2000	1.0	4	400	ND	40	2300	3600

[a] UL = The maximum level of daily nutrient intake that is likely to pose no risk of adverse effects. Unless otherwise specified, the UL represents total intake from food, water, and supplements. Due to lack of suitable data, ULs could not be established for arsenic, chromium, and silicon. In the absence of ULs, extra caution may be warranted in consuming levels above recommended intakes.

[b] Although a UL was not determined for arsenic, there is no justification for adding arsenic to food or supplements.

[c] Although silicon has not been shown to cause adverse effects in humans, there is no justification for adding silicon to supplements.

[d] The ULs for magnesium represent intake from a pharmacological agent only and do not include intake from food and water.

[e] Although vanadium in food has not been shown to cause adverse effects in humans, there is no justification for adding vanadium to food and vanadium supplements should be used with caution. The UL is based on adverse effects in laboratory animals and this data could be used to set a UL for adults but not children and adolescents.

[f] ND = Not determinable due to lack of data of adverse effects in this age group and concern with regard to lack of ability to handle excess amounts. Source of intake should be from food only to prevent high levels of intake.

[g] Upper Limit declines to 2 after age 50.

Sources: Dietary Reference Intakes for Calcium and Vitamin D (2011); Dietary Reference Intakes for Calcium, Phosphorus, Magnesium, Vitamin D, and Fluoride (1997); Dietary Reference Intakes for Thiamin, Riboflavin, Niacin, Vitamin B-6, Folate, Vitamin B-12, Pantothenic Acid, Biotin, and Choline (1998); Dietary Reference Intakes for Vitamin C, Vitamin E, Selenium, and Carotenoids (2000); Dietary Reference Intakes for Vitamin A, Vitamin K, Arsenic, Boron, Chromium, Copper, Iodine, Iron, Manganese, Molybdenum, Nickel, Silicon, Vanadium, and Zinc (2001); and Dietary Reference Intakes for Water, Potassium, Sodium, Chloride, and Sulfate (2004). These reports may be accessed via www.nap.edu.

Adapted from the Dietary Reference Intakes series, National Academies Press. Copyright 1997, 1998, 2000, 2001, 2011, by the National Academy of Sciences. The full reports are available from the National Academies Press at www.nap.edu.

Appendix H

Stretching Your Food Dollars

Are you concerned about the high cost of food? If you are, how can you lower your food costs without sacrificing proper nutrition? You can trim food costs, and preserve and even improve the nutritional quality of your diet, by analyzing your food buying practices and making a few changes. This appendix focuses on ways you can eat well for less. Please note that the pricing of products reflects retail food prices during the summer of 2016 in a major Midwestern city, but you should find them useful for comparing current prices where you live.

Where and What You Buy

Where you buy foods and beverages and what you decide to purchase are major factors in determining your overall food expenditures. If you frequently purchase meals and snacks from vending machines, convenience stores, fast-food outlets, and other restaurants, you may be spending too much on such "convenience" foods. In general, the less time you spend preparing food, the more money you'll spend by having someone at a commercial outlet prepare the food for you. Even if a fast-food restaurant hamburger seems like a bargain because it's "only $1.00," you're likely paying a premium for the French fries and soft drink that you purchase to accompany the sandwich. From a nutrition standpoint, fast foods are often energy dense—high in saturated fat and added sugars—and low in micronutrients (except sodium), fiber, and phytochemicals.

You probably already know that supermarkets have the same snack foods and staple items (bread and milk) as convenience stores and usually offer these foods at lower prices. Furthermore, supermarkets have a much larger selection of foods, particularly more nutrient-dense raw or less processed foods, than convenience stores. It may be easier to stop at a convenience store and load up on foods while you load up on gas than to shop in a supermarket. However, you pay extra for the convenience and your diet may suffer as a result of poor food choices.

A good way to save money is to buy foods in large quantities at "bulk" food stores or at smaller, "no frills," cash-only grocery stores. Although shopping at these places can reduce your food costs, food choices are usually more limited than the selection in supermarkets. It's important to recognize that buying food in bulk is a bargain only if you can use the item before it spoils.

© Comstock/PunchStock RF

How to Shop Wisely in Supermarkets

To lower your food costs, plan your meals and snacks before you shop for food. Prepare a shopping list to help avoid needless or impulse purchases and having to return to the store to buy forgotten items. Keep the grocery list in a convenient place, such as on the refrigerator, and jot down items as they become depleted.

When shopping for groceries, you'll need to compare *unit costs* of similar food products. A "unit" of a packaged food item is usually indicated in ounces, pounds, cups, or other serving sizes. Food packages and containers are available in different sizes and hold different amounts of food, which can make comparing costs of similar foods difficult. Using a calculator to compare prices can be helpful. For example, a box of one brand of shredded wheat cereal contains 15.0 ounces of cereal and costs $3.89; a box contains a different brand of shredded wheat that contains 11.5 ounces of cereal costs $3.69. Which box contains cereal that's lower in cost? To answer this question, determine the unit price of the cereal in each box by dividing the cost of the entire package by the number of units of food it contains.

Box #1

$3.89 entire box ÷ 15.0 ounces = approximately $.26/ounce

Box #2

$3.69 entire box ÷ 11.5 ounces = approximately $.32/ounce

In this situation, the larger box of cereal is a better buy, even though it costs more than the smaller box. Some supermarkets indicate unit prices on shelf tags, but the tags may be difficult to read or confusing.

Supermarkets offer a wide variety of prepared foods, including deli items, frozen entrées, fresh cut-up fruit packaged in single-serving plastic bags or bins, and rotisserie chicken. Although these "fast foods" are convenient, food processing and packaging add to the cost of food. Such foods may contain unhealthy amounts of salt, solid fat, or added sugar. To save money and improve your diet, rely less on prepared foods and more on "slow foods"—foods that require some of your time and effort to prepare. Figure H.1 uses various forms of chicken to illustrate this point. A 2.5–lb rotisserie-cooked chicken costs $3.50/lb, but you can save money by purchasing a whole chicken ($2.69/lb) and cooking it yourself. Instead of buying raw, skinless, boneless chicken breasts ($6.19/lb), buy raw split chicken breasts that have the bones and skin ($1.99/lb). Remove the skin and bones after the chicken breasts are cooked. You can use the cooked chicken immediately, freeze the meat in containers for a future meal, or chill the meat before chopping it to make chicken salad.

Eating more fruits and vegetables is the natural way to add micronutrients, fiber, and phytochemicals to your diet. Many supermarkets offer fresh fruit and vegetables that have been trimmed, cut up, and packed into containers. Before you reach for one of these items, compare its price with that of its raw counterpart. For example, a 2.2–oz, single-serving package of sliced apples sells for $1.25, and a pound of raw apples is priced at $1.99. In this case, buying the raw apples and slicing them yourself is a money-saving practice. To make this

(a)

(b)

Comparing apples to apples. The cost of a 2.2–oz package of apple slices (a) is almost five times the cost of the same amount of fresh, bulk, sliced raw apples (b).

determination, you'll need to calculate the unit price of each product. An ounce of the packaged apples costs about 57 cents ($1.25 divided by 2.2 oz/package). A pound of apples equals 16 ounces, so an ounce of these apples costs about 12 cents ($1.99 divided by 16). Thus, the prepackaged sliced apples cost almost five times more than the bulk raw apples.

Produce that's grown in the United States is usually less expensive when it's in season and more plentiful. For example, berries are plentiful in the spring and early summer, tomatoes and melons in late summer, and apples in the fall. "Fresh" produce that's shipped long distances to supermarket suppliers is often picked before its peak ripeness. As a result, the fruits and vegetables may not taste as good or be as nutritious as locally grown produce. Produce, for example, loses some of its vitamin C content when it's bruised or becomes wilted. Therefore, consider buying fresh produce directly from local farmers, if possible. Although you still need to compare prices of farmers' market items with those of fresh produce sold in supermarkets, you may be able to find reasonably priced produce that's grown within 100 miles of your home at farmers' markets. Buying produce from local farmers helps support your community's economy, too.

An alternative to buying produce directly from growers is to purchase frozen or canned fruits and vegetables. These products are often less expensive than their fresh counterparts. Furthermore, produce that's destined to be frozen is generally harvested when ripe and frozen immediately, maximizing much of its vitamin content and fresh flavor.

The following practices can help you save money when shopping for food.

- Use unit pricing to compare costs of similar packaged products.
- Be wary of appealing offers that aren't bargains. For example, items marked "3 for $1.00" or "10 for $10.00" can be confusing to consumers. It's important to understand that you don't need to buy the entire quantity. For example, if a store

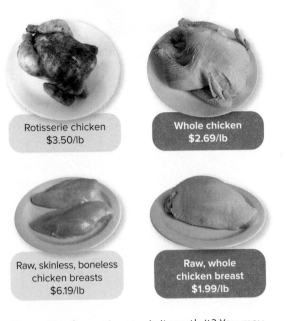

Rotisserie chicken
$3.50/lb

Whole chicken
$2.69/lb

Raw, skinless, boneless
chicken breasts
$6.19/lb

Raw, whole
chicken breast
$1.99/lb

Figure H.1 Convenience—Is it worth it? You may save money by purchasing a raw whole chicken and cutting it into parts or a whole chicken breast and removing the skin and bones.

All: © Wendy Schiff

offers 3 kiwifruits for a dollar, and you cannot use 3 of them, buy one for 34 cents. That price is still a bargain compared to buying kiwifruits that are "2 for $1.00." Also, beware of offers such as "10 oranges for $10." Paying $1 for an orange isn't a bargain! The same store may be selling a bag of 10 oranges for $5. At that price, each orange costs only 50 cents.

- Package sizes can be misleading, so ignore the size of a package and compare net weights of package contents to determine the best value.

- Compare the unit price of organic foods and similar conventionally produced items. If an organic food item is more expensive, consider purchasing the conventional product instead.

- Compare unit prices of preportioned snack foods such as chips or cookies in 100-Calorie packages with prices of the typical, larger package-size products. Such preportioned snacks may be convenient and helpful if you're trying to control your calorie intake, but they're usually more costly per ounce than the same foods purchased in larger packages. Furthermore, people may eat more of the preportioned snack foods, because they think they're lower in calories than the same items packed in larger containers. Make your own preproportioned snacks. For example, buy a large package of oatmeal cookies and place two-cookie portions into reusable storage bags. When you want a snack, eat the two cookies.

- Use coupons when purchasing brand-name items. However, be aware that many stores offer similar products, often referred to as "store brands," that are less expensive than the brand-name items. Although store brand items don't have name recognition, these products are usually just as nutritious as their corresponding brand-name items.

- Limit your carbonated soft drink, commercially prepared coffee, energy drink, and bottled water purchases. When you're thirsty, locate the nearest water fountain and have a drink for free!

- Check "sell by," "best if used by," or "use by" dates on packages of perishable foods such as eggs and dairy products. Compared to canned and frozen foods, perishable foods lose their appealing sensory qualities, such as fresh taste and appearance, more rapidly during storage. The "sell by" date informs store employees about the length of time the product should be displayed for sale. Obviously, it's best to buy foods before the sell-by date. The "best if used by" or "use by" dates indicate the last day to use the product before it loses its best flavor and other sensory qualities. The date doesn't indicate the last day to purchase the food because of safety concerns. Also, read food product labels for storage information. Many products must be refrigerated after opening to delay spoilage. Unit 11 provides more information about proper food storage practices.

- Have at least one vegetarian meal a week.

- Red meats are among the most expensive protein sources, so have more meals in which chicken, turkey, or fish is the main source of animal protein.

- Canned fish can be a less expensive choice than fresh fish, because there's less waste (skin and large bones).

- Remember that any food product isn't a good buy if the item spoils before you can use it.

- Foods that contain a lot of empty calories often look more appealing when your stomach is empty. To reduce the likelihood of buying such foods on impulse, avoid shopping for groceries when you're hungry.

- Be wary of buying food items that are displayed near or along checkout aisles. They're usually energy-dense foods that are sources of empty calories such as candy bars, energy drinks, and baked goods.

- Many perishable foods, such as shredded cheese and fluid fat-free milk, can be frozen.

© Wendy Schiff

Canned fish, such as tuna, salmon, and sardines, can be a less expensive choice than meat or fresh fish.

Prepare a shopping list to help avoid needless or impluse purchases.

© Rob Melyncuk/Getty Images RF

- If you drink coffee, buy a small coffeemaker, a can of ground coffee, and coffee filters to make the beverage. Consider carrying a small thermos of coffee in your backpack. It's much less expensive to make a cup of your own coffee than to buy one from a coffeehouse.

- Canned beans are often sold in large cans that may be cheaper per ounce than beans in smaller cans. If the larger-sized product is less expensive, buy it. After opening the large can of beans, remove the amount needed for the meal, and freeze the remainder in an air-tight container for a future meal.

- For fresh seasonings, grow your own herbs. Basil, oregano, parsley, cilantro, and thyme grow well in flower pots placed in a sunny area. Snip as many leaves as needed for recipes, while keeping the rest of the plants intact.

- Share potluck dinners with friends. Plan the menu and ask your friends to bring certain items, such as vegetable or fruit salads and whole-grain rolls or breads. Inexpensive entrees (the main food items on the menu) include spaghetti and meat sauce, chicken burritos, vegetarian chili, tuna and noodle casserole, and tacos made with canned tuna fish.

For fresh seasonings, grow your own herbs such as basil, oregano, parsley, and thyme.

© Wendy Schiff

Appendix I

Modifying Recipes for Healthy Living

By making minor changes to a recipe, you can improve the product's nutritional quality and make it healthier. Table I-1 provides suggestions for common ingredient substitutions and indicates how the changes improve the nutritional quality of the products. Modifying the type of milk in a waffle recipe, for example, can decrease the product's fat content. As you modify recipes, keep the following tips in mind.

- Don't change every ingredient. Make one or two minor changes each time you try the recipe. For example, if you're making a cake for the first time, don't eliminate all the sugar and fat. These are ingredients that add flavor, color, texture, and moisture to the cake. A cake with no sugar or fat would be dry and almost tasteless.

- Recipes can often be made healthier simply by making minor changes, such as replacing solid fat with canola oil, eliminating some or all of the salt, or reducing the amount of sugar by 25%. You probably will not notice a significant difference in taste or quality if you use ¾ cup of sugar instead of 1 cup or ½ teaspoon of salt instead of 1 teaspoon. Appendix A provides information about household measures, such as cups and teaspoons.

© Onoky/Getty Images

TABLE I-1

RECIPE SUBSTITUTIONS FOR BETTER NUTRITION

RECIPE CALLS FOR	MODIFICATION OR SUBSTITUTION	NUTRITIONAL EFFECTS OF THE CHANGE
All-purpose (white) flour or bread flour	Use ½ whole-wheat flour and ½ all-purpose flour for each cup of all-purpose or bread flour.	Adds fiber
Butter or margarine (in baking)	Replace each quantity of butter or margarine with an equivalent amount of applesauce. Use ½ cup mashed cooked carrots, sweet potato, pumpkin, or squash for each 1 cup butter or margarine in baked goods.	Reduces calories and solid fat ("unhealthy fat"); adds some fiber and vitamins Reduces calories and solid fat; adds some fiber, vitamins, and phytochemicals
Cream	Use whole milk or half-and-half.	Reduces calories and solid fat
Cream cheese, regular	Use fat-free or reduced-fat ("Neufchatel") cream cheese.	Reduces calories and solid fat
Cheese, regular	Use low-fat or nonfat cheese. NOTE: Don't use nonfat cheese in cooked foods, because it won't melt properly.	Reduces calories and solid fat
Enriched pasta or rice	Whole-grain pasta or brown rice. Mix ½ whole-grain pasta with ½ regular pasta.	Adds fiber
Eggs	Use 2 egg whites or ¼ cup egg substitute for each whole egg.	Reduces calories and solid fat
Evaporated milk	Use fat-free evaporated milk.	Reduces calories and solid fat
Condensed milk	Use fat-free evaporated milk. NOTE: Products won't be as sweet.	Reduces calories from solid fat and added sugar

Recipe Calls for	Modification or Substitution	Nutritional Effects of the Change
Fruit canned in heavy sugar syrup	Use fresh or frozen fruit. Use fruit canned in "own juice" or light syrup, or rinse sugar syrup from fruit before using.	Reduces calories and added sugar
Herbs with added salt (i.e., "garlic salt")	Use salt-free ground herbs and spices or fresh herbs and spices such as basil, cilantro, dill, oregano, or paprika.	Reduces sodium
Salt	Don't add to water before cooking vegetables or pasta. Don't add salt to foods before serving them.	Reduces sodium
Sour cream, regular	Use fat-free or low-fat sour cream. Use plain fat-free yogurt.	Reduces calories and solid fat
Sugar, white or brown	Reduce the amount of sugar by 25 to 50%. Use sugar-substitute that's appropriate for preparing baked products.	Reduces calories and sugar
Vegetable oil	Reduce amount by 25%. Use $\frac{3}{4}$ cup mashed cooked carrots, sweet potato, pumpkin, or squash for 1 cup oil in baked goods.	Reduces calories and adds "healthy" fat Reduces calories and fat and adds fiber, vitamins, and phytochemicals
Whole milk, 2% milk	Use fat-free or low-fat milk.	Reduces calories and solid fat

Glossary

A

absorption process by which substances are taken up from the digestive tract and enter the bloodstream or the lymph

absorptive cells digestive tract cells that absorb nutrients

Acceptable Macronutrient Distribution Ranges (AMDRs) macronutrient intake ranges that are nutritionally adequate and may reduce the risk of diet-related chronic diseases

accessory organs organs of the digestive system that assist digestive tract function

acid-base balance maintaining the proper hydrogen concentration of body fluids

added sugars sugars added to foods during processing or preparation

adenosine triphosphate (ATP) "energy currency" of cells

Adequate Intakes (AIs) dietary recommendations that assume a population's average daily nutrient intakes are adequate because no deficiency diseases are present

adipose cells fat cells; specialized cells that store fat

adolescent growth spurt period associated with puberty when a child's height and weight rapidly increases

aerobic conditions that include oxygen

aerobic exercise physical activities that involve sustained, rhythmic contractions of large muscle groups

aerobic metabolism metabolic pathways that require oxygen

alcohol (ethanol) a mind-altering depressant drug that's often classified as a food

alcohol abuser person who experiences problems at home, work, and school that are associated with his or her drinking habits

alcoholic person who is dependent on alcohol and experiences withdrawal signs and symptoms when he or she hasn't consumed the drug

alpha-linolenic acid an essential omega-3 fatty acid

alpha-tocopherol vitamin E

alternative sweeteners substances that are added to sweeten foods while providing few or no kilocalories

amino acids nitrogen-containing chemical units that comprise proteins

anabolic reactions chemical changes in cells that require energy to occur

anabolism metabolic processes that build larger substances from smaller ones

anaerobic conditions that lack oxygen

anaerobic metabolism metabolic pathway that functions without oxygen

anecdotes reports of personal experiences

angina chest pain that results from lack of oxygen to heart muscle tissue

anorexia nervosa (AN) severe psychological disturbance characterized by self-imposed starvation

antibodies proteins that help prevent and fight infection

antioxidant substance that protects cells and their components from being damaged or destroyed by harmful environmental and internal factors

appetite desire to eat appealing food

arachidonic acid (AA) omega-6 fat derived from linoleic acid

ariboflavinosis riboflavin deficiency disease

arterial plaque lipid-filled patch that builds up within the wall of an artery, causing hardening of the artery

arteriosclerosis ("hardening of the arteries") condition that results from atherosclerosis

ascorbic acid vitamin C

atherosclerosis long-term disease process in which plaque builds up inside arterial walls

B

bacteria simple single-celled microorganisms

balance matching calorie intake with calorie expenditure to maintain a healthy weight

bariatric medicine medical specialty that focuses on the treatment of obesity

basal metabolism the minimal number of calories the body uses for vital activities after fasting and resting for 12 hours

beriberi thiamin deficiency disease

beta-carotene carotenoid that the body can convert to vitamin A

bile substance needed for proper fat digestion

bile salts component of bile

bioavailability body's ability to absorb and use a nutrient

bioelectrical impedance technique of estimating body composition in which a device measures the conduction of a weak electrical current through the body

biotechnology the use of living things to manufacture new products

blood alcohol concentration (BAC) estimated percentage of alcohol in blood

body mass index (BMI) numerical value of relationship between body weight and risk of chronic health problems associated with excess body fat

bulimia nervosa (BN) eating disorder characterized by cyclic episodes of bingeing and calorie-restrictive dieting

C

caffeine naturally occurring stimulant drug

calcitonin hormone secreted by the thyroid gland when blood calcium levels are too high

cancer group of diseases characterized by abnormal cell behavior

carbohydrates class of nutrients that is a major source of energy for the body

carcinogen agent that causes cancer

cardiovascular disease (CVD) group of diseases that affect the heart and blood vessels

carotenemia yellowing of the skin that results from excess beta-carotene in the body

carotenoids yellow-orange pigments in fruits and vegetables

casein major protein in cow's milk

catabolic reactions chemical changes in cells that release energy

catabolism metabolic processes that break down larger substances into smaller ones

celiac disease chronic disease characterized by an autoimmune response in the small intestine to the protein gluten

cell smallest living functional unit in an organism

central-body obesity condition characterized by having a large amount of visceral fat and an "apple" shape

chemical digestion chemical breakdown of foods by substances secreted into the digestive tract

cholesterol sterol in animal foods that's made by your body

choline vitamin-like compound in lecithin

chylomicron particle formed by small intestinal cells that transports lipids in the bloodstream

chyme mixture of gastric juice and partially digested food

cirrhosis hardening of tissues

coenzyme ion or small molecule that interacts with enzymes, enabling the enzymes to function

cofactor ion or small molecule that helps an enzyme function

collagen fibrous protein that gives strength to connective tissue

colon major structure of the large intestine

colorectal cancer cancer that starts in either the colon or the rectum

colostrum initial form of breast milk that contains antibodies and immune system cells

complementary combinations mixing certain plant foods to provide all essential amino acids without adding animal protein

constipation condition that occurs when bowel movements occur less frequently than normal and/or are difficult to eliminate

control group group being studied that does not receive a treatment

cornea clear covering over the front of eyeball

cretinism condition that affects babies born to iodine-deficient women

cross-contamination unintentional transfer of pathogenic microbes from one food to another

D

Daily Values (DVs) set of nutrient intake standards developed for labeling purposes

deficiency disease state of health that occurs when a nutrient is missing from the diet

dehydration condition characterized by inadequate body water

diabetes mellitus (diabetes) group of serious chronic diseases characterized by abnormal glucose, fat, and protein metabolism

diastolic pressure pressure in an artery that occurs when the heart relaxes between contractions

diet usual pattern of food choices

dietary fiber (fiber) indigestible plant material; most types are polysaccharides

Dietary Reference Intakes (DRIs) various energy and nutrient intake standards for Americans

dietary supplement product that contains a vitamin, a mineral, an herb or other plant product, an amino acid, or a dietary substance that supplements the diet

digestion process by which large food components are mechanically and chemically broken down

digestive tract muscular tube that extends from the mouth to the anus

disaccharide simple sugar comprised of two monosaccharides

diuretic substance that increases urine production

diverticula small pouches that can form in the lining of the large intestine

DNA master molecule that has the instructions for making proteins

docosahexaenoic acid (DHA) omega-3 fatty acid derived from alpha-linolenic acid

double-blind study experimental design in which neither the participants nor the researchers are aware of each participant's group assignment

duodenum first segment of the small intestine

E

eating disorders psychological disturbances that lead to certain physiological changes and serious health complications

eclampsia condition that occurs when a woman with preeclampsia develops convulsions

edema accumulation of fluid in tissues

eicosapentaenoic acid (EPA) omega-3 fatty acid derived from alpha-linolenic acid

electrolytes minerals that have electrical charges when dissolved in water; ions

embryo human organism during the first 8 weeks after conception

empty calories calories from unhealthy fats, added sugars, and/or alcohol

emulsifier substance that helps fat-soluble and water-soluble compounds mix with each other

energy capacity to perform work

energy balance calorie intake equals calorie output

energy density energy value of a food in relation to the food's weight

energy intake calories from foods and beverages that contain macronutrients and alcohol

energy output calories cells use to carry out their activities

enrichment addition of iron, thiamin, riboflavin, niacin, and folic acid to cereal grain products

enzymes proteins that help chemical reactions occur

epiglottis flap of tissue that folds down over the trachea (windpipe) to keep food from entering the lungs during swallowing

epithelial cells cells that form protective linings of the body

ergogenic aids foods, devices, dietary supplements, or drugs used to improve physical performance

esophagus tubular organ of the digestive tract that connects the back of the mouth with the stomach

essential amino acids amino acids the body cannot make or can't make enough to meet its needs

essential fatty acids lipids that must be supplied by the diet

essential nutrient nutrient that must be supplied by food

Estimated Average Requirement (EAR) amount of a nutrient that meets the needs of 50% of healthy people in a life stage/sex group

Estimated Energy Requirement (EER) average daily energy intake that meets the needs of a healthy person maintaining his or her weight

exercise physical activities that are usually planned and structured for a purpose

experiment a way of testing a scientific question

extracellular water fluid that surrounds cells or is in blood

extrusion reflex involuntary response in which a young infant thrusts its tongue forward when a solid or semisolid object is placed in its mouth

F

fad trendy practice that has widespread appeal for a period, then becomes no longer fashionable

fat-free mass lean tissues

fat-soluble vitamins vitamins A, D, E, and K

Federal Trade Commission (FTC) federal agency that enforces consumer protection laws and investigates health claims

female athlete triad condition characterized by low energy intakes, abnormal menstrual cycles, and bone mineral irregularities

fetal alcohol spectrum disorder (FASD) condition characterized by abnormal physical and intellectual development that affects newborns of women who consumed alcohol during pregnancy

fetus human organism from 8 weeks after conception until birth

folic acid and **food folate** forms of folate

food-borne illness infection caused by microscopic disease-causing agents in food

food insecurity describes individuals or families who are concerned about running out of food or not having enough money to buy more food

food intolerance negative physical reactions to eating a food that don't involve the immune system

food intoxication illness that results when poisons produced by certain microbes contaminate food and irritate the intestinal tract

food secure describes households in which the residents have access to and can purchase sufficient food to lead healthy, active lives

fortification addition of any nutrient to food

free radicals chemically unstable factors that can damage or destroy cells

fructose monosaccharide in fruits, honey, and certain vegetables; "levulose" or "fruit sugar"

fungi simple organisms that live on dead or decaying organic matter

G

galactose monosaccharide that is a component of lactose

gastroesophageal reflux disease (GERD) chronic condition characterized by frequent heartburn

gastroesophageal sphincter ring of muscle in the lower part of the esophagus; controls the opening between the esophagus and stomach

genetically modified organisms (GMOs) living things that had alterations made to their hereditary material as a result of biotechnological activity

gestational hypertension type of hypertension that can develop during pregnancy

ghrelin protein that stimulates eating behavior

glucagon hormone that helps regulate blood glucose levels

glucose monosaccharide that is a primary fuel for muscles and other cells; "blood sugar"

gluten group of related proteins in wheat, barley, and rye

glycemic index (GI) measure of the body's blood glucose response after eating a food that supplies 50 g of digestible carbohydrates as compared to a standard amount of glucose or white bread

glycemic load (GL) value determined by multiplying the glycemic index of a carbohydrate-containing food by the amount of carbohydrate in a typical serving of the food

glycogen storage form of glucose in humans and other animals

goiter enlargement of thyroid gland

H

health claim statement that describes relationship between a food or food ingredient and reduced risk of a nutrition-related condition

heart attack loss of blood flow to a section of the heart muscle, causing the tissue to die

heartburn backflow of irritating stomach contents into the esophagus

heatstroke most dangerous form of heat-related illness

Heimlich maneuver life-saving technique for people who are choking

heme iron-containing portion of hemoglobin

heme iron form of iron that's well absorbed

hemoglobin iron-containing protein in red blood cells that transports oxygen to tissues

hemorrhoids swollen veins in the anal canal that can cause itching and bleeding

hepatitis inflammation of the liver

high-birth-weight (HBW) newborn generally weighing more than 8.8 pounds at birth

high-density lipoprotein (HDL) lipoprotein that transports cholesterol away from tissues and to the liver, where it can be eliminated

high-quality (complete) protein protein that contains all essential amino acids in amounts that support the deposition of protein in tissues and the growth of a young person

homocysteine a toxic amino acid

hormones chemical messengers

hunger uncomfortable feeling that drives a person to consume food

hydration water status

hypertension abnormally high blood pressure levels that persist

hypoglycemia condition that occurs when the blood glucose level is abnormally low

I

ileum last segment of the small intestine

incubation period a length of time in which pathogens need to multiply in food or the digestive tract before they can cause illness

infant formula synthetic beverage that simulates human milk

insoluble fiber forms of dietary fiber that generally don't dissolve in water

insulin hormone that helps regulate blood glucose levels

integrated pest management (IPM) nonchemical methods of agricultural pest management

intensity degree of effort used to perform a physical activity

intracellular water fluid that's inside cells

intrinsic factor (IF) substance produced in the stomach that helps vitamin B-12 absorption

iron deficiency anemia condition characterized by red blood cells that don't contain enough hemoglobin

irritable bowel syndrome (IBS) chronic condition characterized by frequent bouts of intestinal cramps with diarrhea or constipation

J

jejunum middle segment of the small intestine

K

ketone bodies chemicals that result from the incomplete breakdown of fat for energy

kilocalorie (kcal) or **Calorie** unit of measuring food energy

kwashiorkor form of protein-energy malnutrition that occurs when a child is abruptly weaned from breast milk and consumes inadequate amounts of high-quality protein

L

lactase intestinal enzyme that breaks down lactose into glucose and galactose

lactation milk production

lacteal lymphatic system vessel in villus that absorbs most lipids

lactic acid compound formed from pyruvate during anaerobic metabolism

lactose disaccharide comprised of a glucose and a galactose molecule; "milk sugar"

lactose intolerance inability to digest lactose properly

lactovegetarian vegetarian who consumes milk and milk products for animal protein

lactoovovegetarian vegetarian who consumes milk products and eggs for animal protein

lecithin major phospholipid in food

legumes plants that produce pods with a single row of seeds

leptin hormone that reduces hunger and inhibits fat storage in the body

let-down reflex automatic physical response to a breastfeeding infant that enables milk to reach the nipple area

lifestyle way of living that includes diet, physical activity habits, use of tobacco and alcohol, and other typical patterns of behavior

linoleic acid an essential omega-6 fatty acid

lipases enzymes that break down lipids

lipids class of organic nutrients that generally don't dissolve in water (water-insoluble)

lipoprotein structure that transports lipids through the bloodstream and lymph

low-birth-weight (LBW) infant generally weighing less than 5½ pounds at birth

low-density lipoprotein (LDL) lipoprotein that carries cholesterol to tissues

low-quality (incomplete) protein protein that lacks or has inadequate amounts of one or more of the essential amino acids

lymph fluid in the lymphatic system

M

macronutrients nutrients needed in gram amounts daily and that provide energy; carbohydrates, proteins, and fats

major minerals essential mineral elements required in amounts of 100 mg or more per day

malnutrition state of health that occurs when the body is improperly nourished

maltase enzyme that breaks down maltose into two glucose molecules

maltose disaccharide comprised of two glucose molecules; "malt sugar"

marasmic kwashiorkor form of protein-energy malnutrition that's characterized by edema and wasting

marasmus severe form of protein-energy malnutrition that causes extreme weight loss; starvation

mechanical digestion physical breakdown of foods

megadose generally defined as an amount of a vitamin or mineral that greatly exceeds the recommended amount

megaloblastic anemia condition characterized by fewer and abnormal red blood cells

metabolic rate body's rate of energy use a few hours after resting and eating

metabolic syndrome condition that increases risk of CVD

metabolism the sum of all chemical reactions occurring in living cells

micelle lipid-rich particle that is surrounded by bile salts; transports lipids to absorptive cells

micronutrients vitamins and minerals

minerals elements in the Earth's rocks, soils, and natural water sources

moderation consuming foods in reasonable amounts

monoglyceride single fatty acid attached to a glycerol backbone

monosaccharide simple sugar that is the basic molecule of carbohydrates

monounsaturated fatty acid fatty acid that has one double bond within the carbon chain

morning sickness nausea and vomiting associated with pregnancy

mucus slippery fluid that protects certain cells

myoglobin iron-containing protein in muscle cells that controls oxygen uptake from red blood cells

MyPlate USDA's interactive Internet dietary and menu planning guide

N

negative energy state calorie intake is less than calorie output

neural tube embryonic structure that eventually develops into the brain and spinal cord

nonessential amino acids group of amino acids that the body can make

nonexercise activity thermogenesis (NEAT) involuntary skeletal muscular activities such as fidgeting

nonheme iron form of iron in vegetables, grains, meats, and supplements

nonnutritive ("artificial") sweeteners group of manufactured alternative sweeteners that are intensely sweet-tasting compared to sugar

nutrient content claim statement that describes levels of nutrients in a packaged food

nutrient-dense describes foods or beverages that contain more beneficial nutrients in relation to total calories

nutrients life-sustaining chemicals in food that are necessary for proper body functioning

nutrition study of nutrients and how the body uses these substances

Nutrition Facts panel information on food packaging that indicates nutrition information per serving of the food

O

obesity condition characterized by an excessive and unhealthy amount of body fat

omega-3 fatty acid type of polyunsaturated fatty acid that has its first double bond at the number 3 carbon

omega-6 fatty acid type of polyunsaturated fatty acid that has its first double bond at the number 6 carbon

omnivore organism that can digest and absorb nutrients from plants, animals, fungi, and bacteria

organ collection of tissues that function in a related fashion

organ system group of organs that work together for a similar purpose

organic foods foods produced without the use of antibiotics, hormones, synthetic fertilizers and pesticides, genetic improvements, or ionizing radiation

organic nutrients nutrients that have carbon in their chemical structure

osteomalacia adult rickets; condition characterized by poorly mineralized (soft) bones

osteoporosis chronic disease characterized by bones with low mass and reduced structure

overweight having extra weight from bone, muscle, body fat, and/or body water

ovovegetarian vegetarian who eats eggs for animal protein

oxytocin hormone that causes the "let-down" response and the uterus to contract

P

pancreatic lipase digestive enzyme that removes two fatty acids from each triglyceride molecule

parathyroid hormone (PTH) hormone secreted by parathyroid glands when blood calcium levels are too low

partial hydrogenation food manufacturing process that adds hydrogen atoms to liquid vegetable oil, forming trans fats and saturated fats

pasteurization process that kills the pathogens in foods and beverages as well as many microbes responsible for spoilage

pathogens disease-causing microbes

peer review expert critical analysis of a research article before it's published

pesticide tolerance maximum amount of pesticide residue that can be in or on each treated food crop

placebo fake treatment, such as a sham pill, injection, or medical procedure

pellagra niacin deficiency disease

pepsin stomach enzyme that breaks down proteins into polypeptides

peptic ulcer a sore that occurs in the lining of the upper digestive tract

peptide bond chemical attraction that connects two amino acids together

peptides short chains of a few amino acids

peripheral vascular disease (PVD) atherosclerosis affecting a blood vessel that doesn't carry blood to the heart or brain

peristalsis type of muscular contraction of the digestive tract

pernicious anemia condition caused by the lack of intrinsic factor

pesticide substance that people use to kill or control unwanted insects, weeds, or other organisms

pesticide tolerances maximum amounts of pesticide residues that can be in or on each treated food crop

phospholipid type of lipid needed to make cell membranes and for proper functioning of nerve cells

physical activity movement resulting from contraction of skeletal muscles

physical fitness ability to perform moderate- to vigorous-intensity activities without becoming excessively fatigued

phytochemicals compounds made by plants that are not nutrients but may be healthful

pica craving nonfood items

placebo fake treatment, such as a sham pill, injection, or medical procedure

placebo effect response to a placebo

placenta organ of pregnancy that connects the uterus to the embryo/fetus via the umbilical cord

polypeptides chains of two or more amino acids

polysaccharides compounds comprised of more than 10 monosaccharides bonded together

polyunsaturated fatty acid fatty acid that has two or more double bonds within the carbon chain

positive energy state calorie intake is greater than calorie output

prebiotics forms of dietary fiber that promote the growth of healthful intestinal bacteria

preeclampsia form of gestational hypertension

prehypertension persistent systolic blood pressure readings of 120 mm Hg to 139 mm Hg and diastolic readings of 80 mm Hg to 89 mm Hg

premature describes infant born before 37 weeks of pregnancy

prenatal period time between conception and birth; pregnancy

previtamin D inactive form of vitamin D

probiotics live and active cultures of beneficial microbes

prolactin hormone that stimulates milk production after delivery

protein-energy malnutrition (PEM) condition that affects people whose diets lack adequate amounts of protein and energy

proteins large, complex organic nutrients made up of amino acids

protists tiny organisms that can have the characteristics of animals, plants, or fungi

provitamin A carotenoids that the body converts to vitamin A

puberty stage of life in which a person matures physically and is capable of reproduction

pyloric sphincter ring of muscle at the base of the stomach that controls the rate at which chyme leaves the stomach

pyruvate compound that results from anaerobic breakdown of glucose

Q

quackery practicing medicine without the proper training and licensing

R

Recommended Dietary Allowances (RDAs) standards for recommending daily intakes of several nutrients

rectum lower section of the large intestine

requirement smallest amount of a nutrient that maintains a defined level of nutritional health

retinol (preformed vitamin A) form of vitamin A that's in animal sources of food

rickets vitamin D deficiency disorder in children

risk factor personal characteristic that increases a person's chances of developing a disease

S

saliva watery fluid secreted by the salivary glands that mixes with food in the mouth

salivary amylase enzyme secreted by the salivary glands that begins starch digestion in the mouth

satiety sense that enough food or beverages have been consumed to satisfy hunger

saturated fatty acid fatty acid that only has single bonds holding each carbon in the carbon chain together

scurvy vitamin C deficiency disease

semivegetarian or **flexitarian** person who eats eggs, fish, and dairy foods but generally avoids meat

set-point theory scientific notion that body fat content is genetically predetermined

skinfold thickness measurements technique of estimating body composition in which calipers are used to measure the width of skinfolds at multiple body sites

soluble fiber forms of dietary fiber that dissolve or swell in water

solvent substance in which other substances dissolve

spina bifida type of neural tube defect in which the spine doesn't form properly before birth and it fails to enclose the spinal cord

starch storage form of glucose in plants

stroke loss of blood flow to a region of the brain, causing the death of brain cells in that area

structure/function claim statement that describes the role a nutrient plays in maintaining a structure of the body or promoting a normal body function

subcutaneous fat layer of tissue that's under the skin and has more fat cells than other kinds of cells

sucrase enzyme that breaks down sucrose into a glucose and a fructose molecule

sucrose disaccharide comprised of a glucose and a fructose molecule; "table sugar"

sulfites group of sulfur-containing compounds in foods and often added to wines, potatoes, and shrimp as a preservative

sustainable agriculture farming methods that don't deplete natural resources while meeting the demand for food

systolic pressure maximum blood pressure within an artery that occurs when the heart contracts

T

teratogen agent that causes birth defects

testimonial personal endorsement of a product

thermic effect of food (TEF) energy used to digest foods and beverages as well as absorb and further process the macronutrients

thyroid hormone hormone that regulates the body's metabolic rate

tissues masses of cells that have similar characteristics and functions

Tolerable Upper Intake Level (Upper Level or UL) standard representing the highest average amount of a nutrient that's unlikely to be harmful when consumed daily

tolerance state that occurs when the liver adjusts to the usual amount of alcohol that's been consumed and metabolizes it more quickly

total body fat essential fat and storage fat tissue

total water intake refers to water obtained from metabolic and external sources

trace minerals essential mineral elements required in amounts that are less than 100 mg per day

trans fatty acids unsaturated fatty acids that have an unusual structure

treatment group group being studied that receives a treatment

triglyceride lipid that has three fatty acids attached to a three-carbon compound called glycerol; fats and oils

U

ulcerative colitis form of inflammatory bowel disease

undernutrition state of health that occurs when long-term energy and nutrient intakes are insufficient to meet an individual's needs

urea waste product of amino acid metabolism

U.S. Food and Drug Administration (FDA) federal agency that regulates claims on product labels

V

variety including different foods from each food group

vegans vegetarians who eat only plant foods

very-low-density lipoprotein (VLDL) lipoprotein that transports a high proportion of lipids in the bloodstream

vegetarians people who eat plant-based diets

villi (singular, **villus**) tiny, fingerlike projections of the small intestinal lining that participate in digesting and absorbing food

viruses microscopic agents that can cause infections

visceral fat adipose tissue that's under the abdominal muscles, which forms a protective apron over the stomach and intestines

vitamin complex organic molecule that regulates certain metabolic processes

vitamin precursors (provitamins, previtamins) substances in food or the body that cells can convert into active vitamins

W

water intoxication condition that occurs when too much water is consumed in a short time period or the kidneys have difficulty filtering water from blood

water-soluble vitamins thiamin, riboflavin, niacin, vitamin B-6, pantothenic acid, folate, biotin, vitamin B-12, and vitamin C

weaning gradual process of shifting from breastfeeding or bottle-feeding to drinking from a cup and eating solid foods

whole grains the entire, ground, cracked, or flaked seeds of cereal grains, such as wheat, buckwheat, oats, corn, rice, wild rice, rye, and barley

Index

A

AAP (American Academy of Pediatrics), 326
Abdominal fat, 121
Abdominal thrusts, 79, 79f
Absorption
  calcium, 199, 201t
  defined, 75
  digestive system functions, 86f
  in large intestine, 85
  lipids, 83, 83f, 88
  minerals, 233
  of minerals, 233
  phosphorus, 199, 201t
  protein, 164, 165, 166
  in small intestine, 81
  of vitamin B-12, 213
  vitamin E, 202
  of vitamins, 190
  water-soluble nutrients, 83
Absorptive cells, 81, 81f, 83, 139, 140, 140f, 165f, 166f, 178
Academy of Nutrition and Dietetics, 35, 37
Açai, 294, 296
Acceptable Daily Intakes (ADIs) for sweeteners, 109, 109t
Acceptable Macronutrient Distribution Ranges (AMDRs), 44, 44t
  for carbohydrates, 44t
  for fats, 44, 44t, 150
  for proteins, 44t, 176
Accessory organs of digestive system, 76, 84, 84f
Acesulfame-K, 108, 108t, 109t
Acetylcholine, 137
Acid-base balance, 162, 163
Acid group, 130
Acidophilus, 64t
Acid reflux, 89–90
Acne, 330
Added sugars, 105, 106f, 107t, 112, 117
Adenosine triphosphate (ATP), 96, 302
Adequate Intakes (AI), 44
  for fat intake, 150
  iodine, 252, 253
  for manganese, 255t
  for potassium, 240, 243t
  for sodium, 243t
  for vitamin K, 204t
  for water, 259
ADHD (attention deficit hyperactivity disorder), 105
Adipose cells, 141, 141f, 277–278, 277f
Adipose tissue. See Body fat
Adjustable gastric banding, 293–294, 294f
Administration on Aging, 333
Adolescence, 330
Adolescent growth spurts, 330
Adrenaline, 121
Advertising
  food, 288
  weight-loss claims in, 296
Aerobic conditions, 302
Aerobic exercise, 301
Aerobic metabolism, 96
Aflatoxin, 222t
Agave nectar, 106
Age. See also Older adults
  metabolic rate and, 284
  as risk factor for atherosclerosis, 146
Age-Related Eye Disease Study (AREDS), 197
Age-related macular degeneration (AMD), 197
Agriculture, sustainable, 348–349
AI. See Adequate Intakes (AI)
Air, swallowing, 80, 123
Alanine, 163t
Al-Anon/Alateen, 268
Albumin, 162
Alcohol, 262–268

abuse/abuser, 265, 268, 268f
alcohol use disorders, 265, 265t
blood alcohol concentration (BAC), 263–265, 263t, 264f
body's processing of, 263
cancer and, 221, 266
as a carcinogen, 221, 222t
classification of drinkers, 262, 263t
content, in alcoholic beverages, 262
defined, 262, 263
dietary guidelines for, 53
as a diuretic, 260
effect on the body, 266, 267f
empty calories from, 13, 51
fat production and, 141
health benefits of, 268
health problems related to, 266, 267f, 268
nervous system effects, 263, 263t
as a nonnutrient, 10, 262
nutrition and, 266
providing 7 kcal, 9, 262
as risk factor for atherosclerosis, 147
triglycerides and, 146
Alcoholic beverages, 262
Alcoholics/alcoholism, 253, 265–266
Alcoholics Anonymous, 268
Alcoholism test, 265
Alcohol poisoning, 265
Algae, 150t
Allergies
  food, 178–179, 328
  infant formula, 327
  signs and symptoms of food, 178
  skin patch testing for, 179
Allicin, 149
Almonds, 15, 170
Alpha-carotene, 11t
Alpha-linolenic acid, 10t, 133, 133f, 150
Alpha-tocopherol, 201. See also vitamin E
Alternative sweeteners, 108, 108t
Aluminum, antacids and, 90
Alzheimer's disease, 192, 202
AMD (age-related macular degeneration), 197
AMDRs. See Acceptable Macronutrient Distribution Ranges (AMDRs)
American Academy of Pediatrics (AAP), 326
American Cancer Society, 35
American College of Sports Medicine, 301, 307
American Diabetes Association, 118, 119
American Geriatrics Society, 333
American Heart Association, 242
Amino acid metabolism
  vitamin B-6 and, 209
  vitamins for, 191f
Amino acids
  branched chain amino acids (BCAA), 309t
  building proteins with, 166–167
  classification of, 163, 163t
  components of, 163, 163f
  converted into glucose, 116
  defined, 163
  energy from, 116
  essential, 10t, 163, 163t
  excess, 167–168, 176
  limiting, 170
  nitrogen loss and, 168
  nonessential acids, 163, 163t, 168
  peptide bonds between, 164, 164f
  in polypeptides, 164
  protein digestion and, 164–166
  sulfur in, 232
Ammonia, 167, 176, 176f
Amylase, salivary, 113
Anabolic reactions, 283

Anabolism, 96
Anaerobic conditions, 302
Anaerobic metabolism, 96
Anal canal, 85, 85f
Anaphylactic shock, 179
Anecdotes, 23, 24, 30, 34
Anemia, 211
  folate and vitamin B-12 deficiencies, 211, 214–215
  iron deficiency, 246, 320
  megaloblastic, 211, 214
  pernicious, 215
Angina, 144
Animal foods, unhealthy fat in, 48. See also Meat
Animals, experiments on, 24
Anisakis, 335, 335f, 337t
Anorexia nervosa, 298–299
Antacids, 90, 238
Anthocyanins, 11t
Antibodies, 162, 163
Antioxidants
  copper and, 250
  in cruciferous vegetables, 195
  defined, 10, 192
  free radicals protection and, 192
  garlic and, 149
  minerals and, 232f
  phytochemicals, 10, 11t
  reducing risk of CVD and, 147
  selenium and, 250
  Vitamin C and, 217, 219t
  Vitamin E and, 201, 201f, 203t
  vitamins and, 191f
Appetite, 288
Apple juice, 329
Applesauce, 153
"Apple shape" body, 279, 279f
Arachidonic acid (AA), 133, 133f, 323
AREDS (Age-Related eye Disease Study), 197
Arginine, 163t
Ariboflavinosis, 206, 207, 209t
Arsenic, 222t, 231, 231t
Arterial plaque, 143
Arteries
  carotid, 144, 144f
  hardening of. See Atherosclerosis
Artificial sweeteners, 108, 108t, 109, 109t
Ascorbic acid, 217. See also Vitamin C
Asian Diet Pyramid, 56, 56f
Asparagine, 163t
Aspartame, 108, 108t, 109, 109t
Aspartic acid, 163t
AspireAssist device, 294
Asthma, plant-based supplements and, 62
Atherosclerosis
  assessing your risk of, 149
  defined, 142
  lipoproteins and, 144–145, 144f
  oxidized LDL cholesterol and, 146, 146f
  peripheral vascular disease (PVD), 144
  process of, 142–143
  reducing your risk of, 147–149
  risk factors for, 146–147
Athletes
  carbohydrates for, 305–306 305t
  dietary advice for, 303, 305–307
  ergogenic aids, 307–308, 309t
  female athlete triad, 299
  heat-related illnesses in, 307, 307t
  protein intake and, 176–177, 306
  sample meals for, 304t
Atkins diet, 294
ATP (adenosine triphosphate), 96, 302
Attention deficit hyperactivity disorder (ADHD), 105

Autoimmune disease
　celiac disease, 180
　defined, 180
　pernicious anemia, 215
　type I diabetes, 118
Avidin, 216

B

Baby food, homemade, 328
BAC. *See* Blood alcohol concentration (BAC)
Bacteria, 336t–337t
　diarrhea and, 88
　in food, 335, 336t–337t, 338
　food preparation and, 340
　frozen food and, 339
　intestinal, 85
　omnivore diet and, 75
　probiotics, 85, 88
　ulcers and, 29
"Bad foods," 13
Baked beans, calcium in, 236t
Baking soda, 309t
Balance, in healthy diets, 14
Bariatric medicine, 293–294, 293f, 294f
Basal metabolism, 283, 284
Beano®, 123
Beans
　complementary combinations
　　and, 171
　salt and, 172
Beef fat, 132t
Bee pollen, 307
Beer, 262
Belviq, 293
Benzene, 222t
Beriberi, 206–207, 209t
Beta-alanine, 309t
Beta-carotene, 11, 64t, 192, 194, 195, 196
Beta-hydroxy-beta methylbutyrate (HMB), 309t
BHA (buylated hydroxyanisole), 134
BHT (buylated hydroxytoluene), 134
Bias, research, 28
Bile, 84, 91, 123, 190
Bile salts, 138, 139, 141, 141f
Binge drinking, 262, 263t, 265
Binge-eating disorder (BED), 298
Bioavailability of minerals, 233
Bioelectrical impedance, 281, 281f
Biological factors, weight gain and, 287–288
Biological fuels, 95, 97
Biopsy, 93–94
Biotechnology, 348
Biotin, 10t
　deficiency, 216, 216t
　functions of, 191f, 216t
　Recommended Dietary Allowance (RDA), 216t
　sources of, 216t
　toxicity, 216t
　as water-soluble vitamin, 189, 189t, 205
Birth weight, 319
Bisphenol A, 261
Bitter orange, 295t
Bleach, for sanitizing food preparation surfaces, 340
Blindness
　age-related macular degeneration and, 197
　night, 196
　preventing, 196
　vitamin A deficiency and, 196
Blood alcohol concentration (BAC), 263, 263t, 264, 264f
Blood cells, 72, 72f
Blood cholesterol
　fiber and, 123
　nictotinic acid for, 206
　soluble fiber and, 111
Blood clotting. *See* Clots/clotting
Blood donation, 247
Blood glucose
　chromium and, 255
　device used for testing, 118
　diabetes and, 117, 118, 119–120

fasting levels of, 118
　glycemic index (GI) and, 119–120
　hypoglycemia and, 120–121
　maintaining levels of, 114–115
　metabolic syndrome and, 121
　monitoring levels of, 119
Blood pressure. *See also* Hypertension
　diastolic, 241, 242t
　healthy, for 20-30 year olds, 144
　high, metabolic syndrome and, 121
　hypertension levels, 242t
　normal levels, 242t
　prehypertension levels, 242t
　systolic, 241, 242t
Blood proteins, 162
Blood thinners/thinning
　vitamin E supplements and, 202
　vitamin K, 203
Blue agave, 106
BMI. *See* Body mass index (BMI)
Body
　fluid compartments of, 257–258, 257f
　as a "human machine," 95
　organization of your, 72, 73f
　organ systems of, 74
Body composition
　adipose tissue and, 277–278, 277f
　sex differences, 6, 6f
　influencing metabolic rate, 283
Body fat. *See also* Obesity; Overweight
　adipose cells, 277, 277f
　body composition, 6f
　body mass index (BMI) and, 280–281, 281t
　cellulite, 279
　distribution of, 278, 279–280, 279f
　essential fat, 277
　gaining. *See* Weight gain
　health effects of excess, 279–280
　healthy amount of, 282
　measuring, 281–282, 281f, 282f
　reducing. *See* Weight loss
　spot reducing, 290
　subcutaneous fat, 278, 278f, 279, 282, 282f
　total body fat, 277
　visceral fat, 278, 278f, 279
　waist circumference measurement, 280, 280f
　weight classification by percentage of, 282, 282t
Body image, 297
Body mass index (BMI), 280–281, 281t
Body, organization of, 72–74, 74t
Body weight. *See* Weight
Bok choy, 236, 236t
Bone health
　fluoride and, 239
　minerals for, 232f
　osteoporosis, 237–238, 237f
　vitamin D and, 198, 199
　vitamin K and, 203
　vitamins A, D, K, and C for, 191f
Bone remodeling, 234
Bottled water, 261
Botulism poisoning, 109
BPA (bisphenol A), 261
Branched chain amino acids (BCAA), 309t
Bran, wheat, 15, 15f, 123
Brazil nuts, 250
Breastfeeding
　advantages of, 325
　combined with infant food, 326
　for infant's first 6 months, 326
　mother's diet for, 325
　quitting too soon, 326
　relaxed environment for, 325
　vegan diet and, 175
　vitamin D and, 200
　weaning from, 328
Breast milk, 323, 325–326
Broccoli, 236
Brown rice, 123

Brown sugar, nutritional content, 105t
Bruising, 219
Buffer, 163
Bulimia nervosa (BN), 298
Burping, 80
Butter, 148, 151, 152, 153
Butter fat, 132t
Butylated hydroxyanisole (BHA), 134
Butylated hydroxytoluene (BHT), 134
B vitamins, 10t. *See also* Vitamin B-1 (thiamin); Vitamin B-2 (riboflavin); Vitamin B-3 (niacin); Vitamin B-6 (pyridoxine); Vitamin B-12 (cobalamin)
　megadose of, 62
　niacinamide form of, 206
　in protein foods, 48
　as water-soluble vitamins, 189

C

Caffeine, 10
　content in selected beverages, 310t
　defined, 308
　as a diuretic, 260
　in energy drinks, 308
　as ergogenic supplement, 309t
　possible health benefits of, 11t
　sources of, 11t, 105
　toxicity, 308
Calcitonin, 234
Calcium, 10t, 231t
　absorption, 233
　adult Recommended Dietary Allowance (RDA), 239t
　antacids and, 90, 238
　for children, 331
　content in selected foods, 236t
　in dairy foods, 47
　deficiency signs and symptoms, 239t
　dietary sources, 239t
　as electrolyte, 232
　functions of, 232f, 239t
　kidney stones, 62
　megadose of, 62
　MyPlate food sources of, 237f
　for older adults, 333
　osteoporosis and, 237–238
　regulating level of, 234
　sources of, 234–236, 235t, 236t
　supplements, 237
　in tap water, 231
　tips for getting more, 236
　toxicity, 239t
　vegetarian/vegan diet and, 174, 174t
　vitamin D and, 199
Calcium ascorbate, 217
Calcium carbonate, 237
Calcium citrate, 237
Calcium phosphate, 199
Calcium pyruvate, 309t
Caloric intake
　for athletes, 303
　cutting, for weight loss, 286
　in Dietary Guidelines, 52
　macronutrient intakes and, 112f
　metabolic rate and, 284
　reducing, for weight loss, 290
Calories
　defined, 8
　empty, 13, 14, 51, 55, 104
　energy balance and, 286–287, 286f, 287f
　Estimated Energy Requirement (EER), 43
　intake and output, 283–287
　output, for selected physical activities, 285
Campylobacter jejuni, 336t
Cancer
　alcohol and, 221, 266
　carcinogens and, 220, 221
　as chronic disease, 4
　colorectal, 93–94, 93f, 123
　diet and, 221, 222, 222t
　free radical damage and, 192
　metastasis, 93, 221

obesity and, 221
   progression of, 220–221, 220f, 221f
   risk factors for, 221
   skin, 187
   vitamins and, 220–222
Canned beans, 172
Canned fish, 235
Canned foods, 190
Canned fruit, 112
Canola oil, 132t
Capsaicin, 11t
Carbohydrate-restricted diets, 294–295
Carbohydrates, 6, 101–123
   Acceptable Macronutrient Distribution Ranges
     (AMDRs), 44, 44t
Carcinogens, 220, 221, 222t
Cardiovascular disease (CVD), 142–153
   "apple" body shape and, 279
   atherosclerosis. See Atherosclerosis
   deaths from, 142
   defined, 135
   heart healthy food selection and preparation tips,
     151–153
   prescription drugs for, 153
   prevalence of, 142
   reducing your risk of, 147–149
   risk factors of, 146
   saturated and trans fats and, 135
Cardiovascular system, 74f, 74t
Caro, Isabelle, 298
Carotenemia, 196
Carotenoids, 191f, 194, 195, 196, 197
Casein, 327
Catabolic reactions, 283
Catabolism, 96
Celiac disease, 86, 180
Cell(s), 72, 73f
   absorptive, 81, 81f, 83, 139f, 140, 140f,
     166f, 178
   cancer, 220–221, 220f
   defined, 8
   energy and, 102
   epithelial, 194, 195
   functions of a typical human, 8
   glucose and, 116
   muscle, 73
   proteins' role in making and maintaining, 162
   types of, 72, 72f
Cell membranes, phospholipids and, 136
Cellular metabolism, minerals for, 232f
Cellulite, 279
Cellulose, 110, 111t
Centers for Disease Control and Prevention
     (CDC), 35, 343
Central-body obesity, 279
Chapman, Clare, 23, 26, 37
Cheese
   calcium in, 236t
Chicken fat, 132t
Child and Adult Care Food Program, 347t
Children
   acne in, 330
   adolescent growth spurt, 330
   with anemia, 246
   blindness in, 196
   calcium intake, 331
   food allergies in, 178, 179
   fostering positive eating behaviors in, 331
   iron deficiency in, 331
   iron supplements and, 244
   nutrition for, 330–332
   obesity among, 276, 288, 332
   physical activity for, 332
   protein-energy malnutrition (PEM) in, 178
   puberty, 330
   with rickets, 187, 198
   snacking, 330
   undernutrition among, 346–347
   vegan/vegetarian diet and, 175
   vitamin A deficiency in, 196
Chitosan, 295t
Chives, 149

Chloride, 10t, 231t, 255t
   as electrolyte, 232
   function of, 232f
Choking, 79
Cholesterol, 130. See also Lipoproteins
   absorbing and transporting, 140
   alcohol's effect on, 268
   arrangement of carbon atoms, 135f
   body's production of, 135–136
   in breast milk, 323, 327
   carbon atoms, 135f
   cardiovascular disease and, 123, 142–146
   classification of blood lipid levels, 149, 149t
   content in foods, 135t
   definition, 135
   dietary sources of, 135, 135t
   digesting, 138–139
   eggs/egg yolks and, 153
   fiber and, 111
   functions of, 135
   in gallstones, 91, 91f
   health and unhealthy levels of, 149t
   "healthy food" and, 59
   metabolic syndrome and, 121
   oxidized LDL cholesterol, 146, 146f
   plant sterols/stanols and, 146
   prescription drugs for lowering, 153
   recommendations for intake of, 150
   reducing intake of, 53, 153
Choline, 10t, 137, 216, 216t
   functions of, 191f
   as water soluble, 189
Chondroitin sulfate, 64t
Chromium, 10t, 231t, 254, 255t,
     295t, 309t
Chronic diseases, 4
   defined, 4
   family history of, 5
   lifestyle and, 5
   percentage of leading causes of death, 4f
   risk factors increasing your chances of
     developing, 5
Chylomicron, 83, 83f, 140, 140f, 144, 144f
Chyme, 80, 85, 140
Cigarette smoking. See Smoking
Cirrhosis, 266
Cis fatty acids, 133, 134
Claims on food labels, 59, 59f, 61
Clostridium botulinum, 336t
Clostridium perfringens, 336t
Clots/clotting
   alcohol and, 268
   blood vessel obstruction, 143, 144
   heart attacks and, 144
   minerals for, 232f
   proteins and, 162
   strokes and, 144
   vitamin E supplements and, 202
   vitamin K and, 191f
Cobalamin. See Vitamin B-12 (cobalamin)
Cobalt, 232
Cocoa butter, 132t
Coconut oil, 23, 131, 132t
Cod liver oil, 187, 198
Coenzyme Q-10, 64t, 309t
Coenzymes, 205–206, 211
   folate and, 211
   vitamin B-6 and, 209
Cofactor, 232
Cognitive behavioral therapy, 299
Cognitive impairment, 202
Cold storage for food, 339, 341, 342t
Collagen, 162, 217
Colon, 85, 85f
Colon cleansing, 92
Colorectal cancer, 93–94, 93f, 123
Colostrum, 323
Comfrey, 62
Commodity Supplemental Food Program, 347t
Complementary combinations, 171
Complete protein, 170
Congeners, 260

Conjugated linoleic acid, 295t
Constipation, 87, 123
Contrave, 293
Control groups, in human intervention studies, 26
Cooking. See Food preparation
Coomes, Olivia, 161, 177
Copper, 10t, 231t, 232f, 233, 251t, 251t
Corn, 45, 209
Cornea, 196
Corn oil, 132t
Cottage cheese, calcium in, 236t
Country of origin, on food labels, 58
Cow's milk, for infants, 323, 327
Cravings, food, 321
C-reactive protein, 147
Creatine, 309t
Cretinism, 253
Crohn's disease, 94
Croker, Amanda, 58, 187, 200
Cross-contamination, 338, 339
Cruciferous vegetables, 195
Cryptosporidium, 337t
Culture, food choices and, 3
Cured meats, cold storage time
     limits, 342t
Cutting boards, food safety and, 340
Cysteine, 163t, 232
Cystic fibrosis, 190

D

Daily Values (DVs), 58, 61
Dairy. See also Milk
   for adolescents, 331
   magnesium in, 249f
   minerals in, 230f
   MyPlate guidelines, 55t
   nutrients in, 47
   potassium in, 240f
   serving equivalents, 47
   vitamins in, 193f, 206f
Dairy foods
   calcium in, 235–236, 235f, 236t
DASH diet, 242
Death, leading causes of, 4f
Death, pellagra, 207
Deficiencies
   biotin, 216, 216t
   calcium, 239t
   folate, 211, 214–215, 215t
   iron, 246, 246f, 249t, 331
   magnesium, 248, 249t
   power player vitamins, 206, 209t
   protein, 178
   vitamin, 188
   vitamin A, 195–197, 197t
   vitamin B-1, 206, 207, 209t
   vitamin B-2, 206, 207, 209t
   vitamin B-12, 211, 215
   vitamin D, 200–201, 201t
   vitamin E, 202, 203t
   vitamin K, 204
   zinc, 253, 255t
Deficiency diseases, 10, 16, 206–207, 219
Dehydration, 88, 260
Deli meats, 52
Dementia, 207
Dental decay, carbohydrates and, 122
Dental fluorosis, 239, 239t
Dermatitis, 207
DHA. See Docosahexaenoic acid
     (DHA)
Diabetes mellitus, 117–119
   as chronic disease, 4
   classifying according to A1c values,
     119, 119t
   defined, 117
   gestational, 119
   monitoring, 119
   prevalence of, 118
   preventing, 119–120
   as risk factor for atherosclerosis, 146
   signs and symptoms of, 118

Diabetes mellitus (*continued*)
    type 1, 117–118
    type 2, 117, 118, 332
Diarrhea, 88, 207
Diastolic pressure, 241, 242t
Diet
    cancer risk reduction and, 222
    defined, 4
    diet-related carcinogens, 222t
    features of healthy, 14
    heart healthy, 151–153
    individualizing your, 16
    for lactating women, 325
    malnutrition and, 12
    meal planning, 45–56
        Dietary Guidelines, 52, 53, 54t
        food groups, 45–51
        food guide pyramids, 56, 57f
        MyPlate guide, 55, 55f, 55t
    poor, as risk factor for atherosclerosis, 146
    reducing risk of CVD with, 148–149
    requirements and recommendations, 42–44
        Acceptable Macronutrient Distribution Ranges (AMDRs), 44, 44t
        Adequate Intakes (AI), 44
        Dietary Reference Intakes (DRIs), 42
        Estimated Average Requirement (EAR), 43
        Estimated Energy Requirement (EER), 43
        Recommended Dietary Allowance (RDA), 43–44
        Tolerable Upper Intake Level (UL), 44
    role in cancer development, 221, 222t
    supplements. *See* Supplements
Dietary adequacy, 345–349
Dietary fiber, 110
Dietary Guidelines for Americans, 52
    2015-2020 version, 52, 53
    about, 52
    applying, 54
    for fat intake, 150
    healthy eating pattern, 52, 53t
    on iron, 246
    on iron needs, 320
    key recommendations, 53
    on potassium, 240
    on protein intake, 168
    on added sugar intake, 112
    on trans fat intake, 134
Dietary guides, 56. *See also* MyPlate food guide
Dietary Reference Intakes (DRIs), 42–43, 43f, 44. *See also*
        Recommended Dietary Allowance (RDA)
    Adequate Intakes (AI), 44
    Estimated Average Requirement (EAR), 43
    Estimated Energy Requirement (EER), 43
    explained, 42–43
    during pregnancy, 320t
    Recommended Dietary Allowance (RDA), 43–44
    Tolerable Upper Intake Level (UL), 44
Dietary Supplement and Health Education Act (DSHEA), 60
Dietary supplements. *See* Supplements
Dietetics, 37
Diets
    fad, 294–295
    gluten-free, 180, 180t
    high-protein weight-loss, 177
    very-low-calorie, 284, 290
    very low-fat, 295
Digestion
    of carbohydrates, 113, 113f
    chemical, 75
    defined, 75
    in large intestine, 85
    major steps in process of, 86f
    mechanical, 75
    protein, 164–166, 166f
    in the small intestine, 81
    starting in the mouth, 77
    vitamins, 190
Digestive system, 74t. *See also* Digestive tract
    accessory organs, 84, 84f
    major organs and tissues, 74t
    primary functions of, 74t
Digestive system, disorders of
    acid reflux, 89
    colorectal cancer, 93–94
    constipation, 87
    diarrhea, 88

gallstones, 91
GERD (gastroesophageal reflux disease), 89–90
irritable bowel syndrome (IBS), 92
peptic ulcers, 90–91
ulcerative colitis, 92–93
vomiting, 88
Digestive tract
    accessory organs of, 76, 77f, 84
    defined, 75
    esophagus, 78, 78f, 79, 79f
    fiber and, 123
    large intestine, 85
    major organs of, 76
    mouth, 77
    small intestine, 81, 81f
    stomach, 80, 80f
    summary of functions, 86, 86f
    swallowing, 78–79
Dipeptides, 165f
Disaccharides, 104
Disclaimers, 34, 61, 61f
Diuretics, 260
Diverticula, 87
DNA
    antioxidants and, 192f
    cancer and, 220
    defined, 167
    folate and, 211
    illustration of a segment of, 167f
Docosahexaenoic acid (DHA), 133, 133f, 150, 323
Double-blind study, 26
Double bond, in fatty acids, 131, 131f, 133, 133f
Dr. Atkins' New Diet Revolution, 294
DRIs. *See* Dietary Reference Intakes (DRIs)
Dry eye, 196
Duodenum, 81
DVs (Daily Values), 58

E

EAR (Estimated Average Requirements), 43, 43f
Eating disorders, 297–299
    anorexia nervosa, 298–299
    binge-eating disorder, 298
    bulimia nervosa, 298
    causes of, 297
    defined, 297
    female athlete triad, 299
    risk factors for, 297
    treating, 299
    weight loss for children and, 332
"Eat More, Weigh Less" diet plan, 295
Echinacea, 62, 64t
Eclampsia, 322, 323
E. coli bacteria, 88
Edamame, 137
Edema, 162, 162f, 258, 322
EER (Estimated Energy Requirements), 43, 284
EGA (estimated glucose average), 119
Eggs
    avidin in, 216
    cholesterol content, 135t
    cold storage time limits, 342t
    cooking temperatures for, 339t
    eggshell color, nutrient content and, 137
    as emulsifier, 137
    food safety and, 339, 339t
    grading, nutrition content and, 137
Egg substitutes, 153
Egg yolks, cholesterol in, 135t
Eicosapentaenoic acid (EPA), 133,
    133f, 150
Electrolytes
    defined, 232
    hydration and, 258
    minerals functioning as, 232
    sports drinks and, 306, 307
    water loss and, 259
Embryo, 318, 319
Emergency food supply, 343, 343t
Emotional stress
    as risk factor for atherosclerosis, 147
    stomach ulcers and, 29
Empty calories, 13, 14, 51, 55, 104
Emulsifier, 137
Endocrine system, 74t

Endosperm, 15, 15f
Enemas, 92
Energy
    adipose cells and, 141
    alcohol providing, 9
    carbohydrates and, 102
    defined, 95
    Estimated Energy Requirements (EER), 43, 284
    in food, 8
    foods dense in, 14
    forms of, 95
    glucose and, 116
    macronutrients supplying, 9
    metabolism, 95–97, 97f
    negative energy state, 286–287, 287f
    for physical activity, 284
    positive energy state, 287, 287f
    protein-energy malnutrition (PEM), 178, 346
    protein providing, 163
    sources for the body, 9f
Energy balance, 286–287, 286–289, 286f, 289f
Energy bars, 306
Energy dense foods, 14
Energy density, 14
Energy drinks, 308
Energy intake, 283
Energy metabolism, 95–97, 97f
    vitamins for, 191f
Energy output, 283, 290
Energy output (energy expenditure), 283, 284, 285, 285t, 287, 287f
Energy sources, 9f
Enfamil, 327t
Enrichment, 46, 207, 210
Environmental influences, weight gain and, 288
Environmental Protection Agency (EPA), 261, 344
Environmental Working Group (EWG), 344
Enzymes
    coenzyme, 205
    defined, 77
    digestion and, 81
    in mouth, 77
    pancrease and, 86, 86f
    proteins producing, 162
    in stomach, 80
EPA. *See* Environmental Protection Agency (EPA)
Ephedrine, 295t
Epiglottis, 78, 78f
Epinephrine, 121
Epithelial cells, 194, 195
Epoxy resins, BPA and, 261, 261f
Equal®, 108t
Ergogenic aids, 307–308, 309t
Erythritol, 108, 108t
Esophagus, 78, 78f, 79, 79f, 267f
Essential amino acids, 10t, 163, 163t, 170
Essential fat, 277
Essential fatty acids, 133–134, 133f, 150
Essential nutrients, 10, 10t
Estimated Average Requirement (EAR), 43, 43f
Estimated Energy Requirements (EER), 43, 284
Estimated glucose average (eGA), 119
Estrogen, 238
Ethnic background, food choices and, 3
Evening primrose oil, 64t
Exercise. *See also* Physical activity
    aerobic, 301
    bone health and, 238
    constipation and, 87
    defined, 300
    fueling, 302, 302f
    health benefits of regular, 300
Experiment, 24
Extracellular water, 257, 258
Extreme obesity, 278, 281, 293
Extrusion reflex, 328

F

Fad, defined, 294
Fad diets, 294–295
Family history, 5. *See also* Genetics
Fasting blood glucose levels, 118
Fat absorption, 190
Fat, body. *See* Body fat
"Fat cells," 141
Fat (adipose) cells, 277–278, 277f

Fat-free mass, 277
Fat-free milk, 47
Fats, 6, 51. *See also* Lipids
   absorbing and transporting, 140
   Acceptable Macronutrient Distribution Ranges (AMDRs), 44, 44t, 150
   in animal foods, 48
   body composition of, 6f
   calorie percentage in average American diet, 112f
   in dairy foods, 47
   digesting, 138–139
   excess, 141
   excess glucose and, 116
   fatty acid content of, 132t
   food group, 50
   "healthy," 50, 170
   "hidden," 117
   liquid, 133
   as macronutrient, 9
   in protein foods, 48
   recommendations for intake of, 150
   roles of, 130
   saturated, 134–135, 147–148, 151
   solid fats, 51, 133, 148, 153
   storage of, 141, 141f
   total, on food label, 58
   trans, 134–135, 134f
Fat-soluble vitamins, 189, 189t, 190, 193–204
Fatty acids (FAs)
   in breast milk, 323
   in the carbon chain, 131
   chain of carbon atoms, 130, 131f
   chylomicron formation, 140f
   cis, 133, 134
   comparing sources of saturated and unsaturated, 132f
   content of fats and oils, 132t
   effects on LDL and HDL, 148
   essential, 133–134, 133f
   heart-healthy diet and, 148
   metabolism of, 140, 141
   monoglyceride, 139
   relationship among essential, 133f
   saturated fatty acid, 130–131, 131f
   unsaturated
      monounsaturated fatty acid, 131, 131f
      polyunsaturated fatty acid, 131, 131f
"Fatty liver," 122
FDA. *See* Food and Drug Administration (FDA)
Feces, 85
Federal Trade Commission (FTC), 32, 35, 134
Female athlete triad, 299
Female Athlete Triad Coalition, 299
Fermentation, 85
Fetal alcohol spectrum disorder (FASD), 268, 268f
Fetal alcohol syndrome, 268, 268f
Fetus, 319, 319f
Fiber, 110–111
   classification of, 111t
   colorectal cancer and, 123
   constipation and, 87
   dietary content in common foods, 111t
   digestive tract and, 123
   eating excessive amounts of, 123
   heart health and, 123
   increasing intake of, 123
   weight control and, 123
Fibrin, 162
First Amendment, nutrition information and, 31
Fish
   calcium in canned, 235
   cold storage time limits, 342t
   cooking temperatures for food safety, 339t
   increasing intake of, 150
   methylmercury in, 150
   omega-3 fats through, 150, 150t
Fish oil, 64t, 339t
Fish oil supplements, 150
Flatulence, 85, 123
Flaxseed, 64t, 150
Flaxseed oil, 64t
Flexitarian, 173
Fluid balance
   minerals for, 232f
   potassium and sodium and, 240–241, 243t

proteins and, 162
   reasons for necessity of, 258
   water intake and output and, 258, 259f
   weight increase and, 259
Fluid compartments of the body, 257–258, 257f
Fluids, athletes replenishing, 306–307
Fluoride, 231t, 239, 239f, 239t
   in bottled water, 261
   in tap water, 231
Fluorosis, 239
Flu, the, 336
FODMAPs, 122
Folate, 10t
   deficiency, 214, 215t
   defined, 211
   explained, 211
   food sources of, 212, 212t, 215t
   in fruit, 49
   functions of, 191f, 211, 215t
   for pregnant women, 320
   Recommended Dietary Allowance (RDA), 215t
   as water-soluble vitamin, 189, 189t
Folic acid. *See* Folate
Food(s). *See also* specific foods
   advertising, 288
   bacteria in, 335, 336t–337t
   "bad," 13
   carbohydrate-rich, 305t
   cholesterol in, 135t
   contributing to acid reflux, 89
   energy dense, 14
   functional, 17, 146
   "good," 13
   irradiation of, 343
   junk, 13
   nutrient-dense, 13–14
   organic, 51
   pesticides in, 344
   processing of, 15
   "solid," 326, 328, 329
   stored for emergencies, 343, 343t
   substitution suggestions, 54t
   wasting, 349
   "whole," 15
Food advertising, 288
Food allergies, 178–179, 328
Food and Drug Administration (FDA)
   bottled water and, 261
   BPA regulation and, 261
   dietary supplements and, 61–62
   food label regulation, 59
   food safety and, 334
   MedWatch program, 63
   nutrition information and, 31, 35
   partially hydrogenated oils (PHOs) and, 134
   role in food safety, 334
   on stevia, 106
   trans fat labeling and, 134
Food-borne illnesses, 334, 336t–337t
   common sources of, 336t–337t
   defined, 334
   preventing, 338–343, 339t, 342t
   reporting to public health officials, 334
   from restaurants, 343
   sources of, 336t–337t
Food-borne pathogens, 335
Food budget, protein(s) and, 172
Food choices, factors influencing, 3, 3f
Food cravings, 321
Food energy, 8. *See also* Energy
Food folate, 211. *See also* Folate
Food groups
   combination foods, classification of, 51, 52f
   dairy foods, 47
   fruits, 49
   grains, 45–46
   other foods (oils, solid fats, sweets), 50–51
   protein foods, 48
   vegetables, 50
Food insecurity, 347
Food intolerance, 179
Food intoxication (food poisoning), 335
Food irradiation, 343
"Food jags," 331
Food labels, 57f

added sugars in, 106f
   allergen information on, 179, 179f
   bottled water, 261
   claims on, 59, 59f
   Daily Values (DVs), 58
   food allergies and, 179
   "healthy" foods, 59
   ingredients list, 57f, 58, 60, 106, 106f
   Nutrition Facts panel, 57–58, 57f
   for restaurant and vending machine foods, 58–59
   sodium content on, 242
   supplements, 60–61, 61f
Food poisoning, 335
Food preparation
   bacteria and, 340
   carcinogens and, 222
   food safety and, 338, 339–340
   heart healthy tips, 151–153
   by older adults, 333
   preventing food-borne illnesses and, 338–340
   retaining vitamin content of foods and, 190
   Vitamin C and, 218
   Vitamin E and, 202
   for weight loss, 291
Food processing, mineral loss and, 233
Food production, 348–349
Food Pyramids, 56, 56f
Food safety, 334–344
   cold storage time limits, 341, 342t
   food-borne illnesses, 334, 336t–337t
   food preparation and, 338, 339–340
   foods touching the floor and, 341
   four food safety rules, 342
   GMOs and, 335
   government agencies' role in, 334
   how pathogens get in food, 338
   microwave cooking and, 341, 343
   potential dangers in foods, 335
   restaurant foods, 343
   sanitation ratings, 334
   signs and symptoms of illness, 336
Food security, 347
Food shopping, 291, 339
Food stamp program, 347t
Formula feeding, 326–327, 327t
Fortification, 46
Framingham Heart Study, 27
Free radicals, 10, 146
   antioxidants and, 192, 192f
   Vitamin C and, 217
   Vitamin E and, 201
Freeze-dried liver food, 307
Freezing foods, 339, 341, 342t
Frey, McKenzie, 275
Fructose, 103, 105, 122. *See also* High-fructose corn syrup (HFCS)
Fruit juices, 49, 112
Fruits
   adding to water, 112
   canned, 112
   examples, 49
   iron in, 245f
   lychee, 17
   magnesium in, 249f
   minerals in, 230f
   MyPlate guidelines, 55t
   nutrients in, 49
   pomegranate, 27
   potassium in, 240f
   serving equivalents, 49
   as snacks, 53
   storing, 53
   variation in nutritional content, 49
   vitamins in, 193f, 206f
Fruit sugar, 103
FTC (Federal Trade Commission), 32, 35, 134
Functional foods, 17, 146
Fungi, in food, 335

G
Galactose, 103, 113f, 122
Gallbladder, 76, 84, 84f, 91, 91f
Gallstones, 91, 91f
Garcinia cambogia, 295t
Garlic, 62, 64t, 149
Gastric banding, 293–294, 294f

Gastric bypass surgery, 293–294, 293f
Gastric juice, 80
Gastritis, 29
Gastroesophageal reflux (GER), 89
Gastroesophageal reflux disease (GERD), 89–90
Gastroesophageal sphincter, 80, 80f
Genetically modified organisms (GMOs), 335
Genetics
    cardiovascular disease and, 146, 147
    weight gain and, 288
Gestational diabetes, 119
Gestational hypertension, 322, 322f, 323
Ghrelin, 287–288, 293
GI (glycemic index), 119–120
Giardia, 335, 337t
Gimmicks, 294
Ginger, 29, 64t
Ginkgo biloba, 62, 65t
Ginseng, 65t, 307, 308, 309t
GL (glycemic load), 120
"Globesity," 277
Glucagon, 114
Glucomannan, 295t
Glucosamine hydrochloride, 65t
Glucose, 113f, 122
    amino acids converted into, 116
    defined, 103
    for energy, 116
    as essential nutrient, 10t
    excess, 116
    fiber and, 110
    food sources of, 103
    soluble fiber and, 111
    starch and, 110
Glucose molecules, 110, 110f
Glucose recycling, 302
Glutamic acid, 163t
Glutamine, 163t
Gluten-free diet, 180, 180t
Gluten intolerance, 86
Glycemic index (GI), 119–120
Glycemic load (GL), 120
Glycerol, 130, 140, 141
Glycine, 163t
Glycogen, 110, 110f
    athletes and, 305–306
    storage, 116
GMOs (genetically modified organisms), 335
Goat's milk, 329
Goiter, 252, 252f
"Good foods," 13
Government agencies, food safety and, 334
Grains
    Dietary Guidelines on, 53
    enriched, 46, 233
    examples of, 46
    food processing and, 233
    iron in, 233, 245f
    magnesium in, 249f
    minerals in, 230f
    MyPlate guidelines, 55t
    potassium in, 240f
    serving comparisons, 46
    serving equivalents, 46
    as source of protein, 171
    vitamins in, 193f, 206f
    whole, 15, 45, 123
Grapefruit diet, 294
Grapefruit juice, 333
Grapeseed oil, 132t
Green tea/green tea extract, 65t, 294, 295t
Grocery shopping, 291
Ground meat
    cold storage time limit for, 342t
    cooking temperatures for food safety, 339t
    thoroughly cooking, 340
Growth/development
    adolescent growth spurts, 330
    during childhood, 330
    infancy, 323, 323f
    minerals for, 232f
    vitamins for, 191f

Guarana, 308
Guar gum, 295t
Guava, 218
Guinea pigs, 217
Gums, 110, 111t
Gut microbiome, 85

H

Ham, cholesterol in, 135t
Hand washing, food safety and, 339
Hangovers, 260
"Hardening of the arteries." See Atherosclerosis
Hard liquors, 262
"Hard" water, minerals in, 231
HDL (high-density lipoprotein) cholesterol
    alcohol and, 269
    classification of blood lipid levels, 149, 149t
    composition of, 144f
    effects of dietary fatty acids on, 148
    explained, 145
    healthy and unhealthy levels of, 149t
Health
    carbohydrates and, 117–123
    fiber and, 122–123
    sugar and, 122
Health Canada, dietary guide, 56
Health claims, 59
Health departments, local, 334
Healthy eating patterns, 52, 52t
"Healthy" fats, 50, 170
Heart attack, 144, 192
Heartburn, 89–90
Heart disease
    deaths from, 4, 4t, 142
    Framingham Heart Study, 27
    lifestyle and, 5
    risk factors for, 5, 27, 29
Heart health
    alcohol and, 266, 267f
    calcium supplements and, 237
    diet, 56f, 150
    fiber and, 123
    fish oil supplements, 150
    food selection and preparation tips, 151–152
    Mediterranean Diet, 149
Heat cramps, 307t
Heat exhaustion, 307t
"Heat of metabolism," 95–96
Heatstroke, 307, 307t
Heimlich maneuver, 79, 79f
Helicobacter pylori bacterium, 29
Heme, 209
Heme iron, 244
Hemicellulose, 110, 111t
Hemoglobin, 163
    defined, 244
    iron and, 244
    sickle cell disease and, 167
    transporting oxygen in red blood cells, 162, 167
    vitamin B-6 and, 209
Hemorrhoids, 87
Hepatitis, 266
Hepatitis A (HAV), 335, 337t
Herbal supplements, safety and, 62
Herbal teas, 62
High-birth-weight (HBW) babies, 321
High blood pressure. See Hypertension
High-density lipoproteins (HDL). See HDL (high-density lipoprotein) cholesterol
High-fat meats, 48
High-fructose corn syrup (HFCS), 101, 105, 105t, 106, 112
High-protein diets, 176
High-quality protein, 170
Histidine, 10t, 163t
HMB (beta-hydroxy-beta methylbutyrate), 309t
Holidays, weight loss and, 291
Hollywood, California, 297
Homocysteine, 209
Honey, 101, 104, 105, 105t, 106, 109, 118, 329
Hoodia, 295t
Hormones. See also specific hormones
    anabolic reactions and, 96
    cancer development and, 221

    osteoporosis and, 238
    proteins making, 162
    thyroid, 252, 283
Hot dogs, cholesterol in, 135t
H. pylori, 29
Human intervention studies, 26
Hunger, 287, 348, 349
"Husk-tomatoes" (tomatillos), 50
Hydration, 257, 258, 259
Hydrochloric acid (HCl), 80
Hydrogenation, partial, 134
Hyperactivity, sugar and, 105
Hypertension
    blood pressure levels, 242t
    causes of, 242
    danger of, 144
    defined, 144
    gestational, 322, 322f, 323
    "hardening of the arteries" and, 144
    metabolic syndrome and, 121
    as risk factor for atherosclerosis, 146
    sodium and, 241–242
    treatment, 242
Hypoglycemia, 120–121

I

IBS (irritable bowel syndrome), 92
Ice cream
    calcium in, 236t
Ice cream, cholesterol in, 135t
Ileum, 81
Immune function, vitamins for, 191f
Immune system, 74t
Incomplete proteins, 171
Incubation period, 336
India, foods from, 41
Indian reservations, food distribution programs on, 347t
Infant formula, 318
Infant nutrition, 323–329
    cow's milk, 323, 327
    formula feeding, 326–327, 327t
    homemade baby food, 328
    lactation, 323–326, 326f
    rapid growth rate, 323, 323f
    "sleeping through the night" and, 329
    solid foods, 328–329
    supplements, 326
    weaning, 328
    what not to feed infants, 329
Infants
    with cretinism, 253
    rapid growth rate, 323, 323f
    undernutrition in, 346
    Vitamin K-deficient, 204
Inflammatory bowel disease (IBD), 92, 94
Influenza, 336
Ingredients list, on food labels, 57f, 58, 60, 106, 106f
Insoluble fiber, 110, 111t
Insulin, 114, 115, 118, 120, 162, 166
Insulin pump, 118
Integrated pest management (IPM), 349
Integumentary system, 74t
Intensity (physical activity), 300–301
International Units (IUs), 194
Internet, evaluating nutrition information on, 35
Intestinal bacteria, 85, 88
Intestinal gas, 123
Intracellular water, 257, 258
Intrinsic factor (IF), 213
Iodide, 230f, 252
Iodine, 10t, 231t, 252–253, 255t
Iodized salt, 252
Iron, 10t, 231, 231t
    absorption, 233
    adult RDA, 249t
    blood donation and, 247
    cookware, 246
    copper and, 251
    deficiency, 249t, 331
    deficiency-related disorders, 246, 246f
    function of, 232f, 249t
    heme iron, 244
    increasing intake of, 247

megadose of, 62
nonheme iron, 244
for pregnant women, 320
in protein foods, 48
sources of, 244, 245f, 245t, 249t
supplements, 244
toxicity, 249t
vegetarian/vegan diet and, 174, 174t
Iron deficiency anemia, 246, 320
Irradiation of food, 343
Irrigation systems, 348, 349
Irritable bowel syndrome (IBS), 92
Isoflavonoids, 11t
Isoleucine, 10t, 163t
Isomil, 327t
IUs. *See* International Units (IUs)

J
Jejunum, 81
Juices, fruit, 49, 112
"Junk foods," 13

K
Kale, 195, 236
    calcium in, 236t
Kava, 62, 65t
Kefir, 88
Keratin, 162
Ketoacidosis, 116
Ketone bodies, 116
Kidney disease, potassium and, 241
Kidneys
    excess oxalate in, 219
    excess protein and, 176
    water loss and, 259
Kidney stones, 201, 219, 238, 260
Kilocalories (kcal). *See also* Energy; Food energy
    defined, 8
    estimating number in food servings, 9, 9f
    MyPlate daily guidelines, 55t
Kwashiorkor, 346

L
Labels
    claims on food, 59
    dietary supplement, 60–62, 61f
    food, 57–59, 57f
Laboratory experiments, 25
Lactase, 113, 113f, 122
Lactation, 318, 323–325
    advantages of breastfeeding, 325
    diet for, 325
    expressing breast milk, 326, 326f
    process of, 324–325
    quitting breastfeeding too soon, 326
    supplements for infants and, 326
Lacteal, 81, 81f
Lactic acid, 302, 303
Lactobacillus, 64t
Lactobacillus bifidus, 323
Lactoovovegetarian, 173
Lactose, 103, 104, 105, 113, 113f, 122
Lactose intolerance, 122
Lactovegetarian, 173
La Leche League, 326
Lang, Matthew, 71, 92–93
Lard (pork fat), 132t
Large intestine, 85, 85f, 86, 86f, 113f
Larynx, 78f
Lavender, 65t
LDL (low-density lipoprotein)
    atherosclerosis and, 146
    as "bad" cholesterol, 146
    composition of, 144f
    effects of dietary fatty acids on, 148
    explained, 145
    health and unhealthy levels of, 149t
    metabolic syndrome and, 121
    prescription drugs for lowering, 153
Lead, 231
Lecithin, 136–137
Leftovers

cold storage time limits for, 342t
    food safety and, 341
    from restaurants, 291
Legumes
    defined, 169
    as source of protein, 169, 171
Lemonade, 29
Leptin, 288
Let-down reflex, 324–325
Leucine, 10t, 163t
Levulose, 103
Lifecycle nutrition, 318–333
    childhood, 330–332
    infants, 323–329, 323f, 327t
    older adults, 332–333
    pregnancy, 319–322, 320f, 321f
    prenatal period, 318–319, 319f
Lifestyle
    changes in, for weight loss, 290
    defined, 5
    heart disease and, 5
    reducing risk of atherosclerosis and, 147, 153
Light foods, 59
Lignin, 110
Limiting amino acids, 170
Linoleic acids, 10t, 133, 133f, 323
Lipases, 138
Lipids, 6, 128–155. *See also* Cholesterol; Fats; Oils
    absorbing and transporting fat and cholesterol, 140
    absorption of, 83, 83f
    body composition of, 6f
    in breast milk, 323
    cholesterol. *See* Cholesterol
    classification of blood lipid levels, 149, 149t
    defined, 130
    digesting, 138–139
    fats. *See* Fats
    fatty acids. *See* Fatty acids (FAs)
    major functions of, 7
    oils. *See* Oils
    phospholipids, 136–137, 136f, 140, 144f
    roles in body, 130
    stored in fat cells, 141f
    triglycerides, 130–135
    water insolubility of, 130
    as water-insoluble, 130, 130f
Lipoproteins
    atherosclerosis and, 144–146, 146f, 149
    chylomicron, 144f
    chylomicron formation, 140, 140f
    composition and size, 144f
    defined, 140
    high-density lipoprotein (HDL), 144f, 145, 149, 149t
    low-density lipoprotein (LDL). *See* LDL (low-density lipoprotein)
    very-low-density lipoprotein (VLDL), 140, 144f
Listeria monocytogenes, 336t
Lithium, 231t
Liver, 82f, 84, 86, 86f, 140
    alcohol abuse and, 268
    alcohol use/abuse and, 267f
    bile salts and, 141
    cholesterol in, 135t
    digestion of carbohydrates and, 113f
    lipoproteins and, 145
    protein digestion and, 166, 166f
Lobelia, 62
Locusts, 346
Loperamide, 89
Low-birth-weight (LBW), 319
Low-calorie foods, 59
Low-carbohydrate diets, 294–295
Low-density lipoproteins (LDL). *See* LDL (low-density lipoprotein)
Low-fat foods, 59
Low-fat milk, 47
Low-income people, malnutrition among, 12
Low-quality protein, 170
Lubricants, protein, 162
Lutein, 11t, 194
Lychee fruit, 17
Lycopene, 11t, 194
Lymph, 81

Lymphatic system, 74t, 83
Lysine, 10t, 163t, 171

M
Macronutrients, 9. *See also* Carbohydrates; Fats; Protein(s)
    Acceptable Macronutrient Distribution Ranges (AMDRs), 44, 44t
    average intake of, 112f
    in grains, 45
Macular degeneration, 197
Maestro Rechargeable System, 294
Magnesium, 10t, 231, 231t
    adult RDA, 249t
    antacids and, 90, 238
    deficiency, 248, 249t
    as electrolyte, 232
    function of, 232f, 248, 249t
    source of, 248t
    sources of, 249f, 249t
    toxicity, 249t
Ma huang, 62
Major minerals, 231, 231t
Malignant cancer cells, 93, 220, 220f, 221f
Malignant tumors, 220
Malnutrition
    explained, 12
    protein-energy malnutrition (PEM), 178, 346
Maltase, 113
Malt liquors, 262
Maltose, 104
"Malt sugar," 104
Manganese, 10t, 231t, 232f, 255t
Mannitol, 108
Maple syrup, 105t
Marasmic kwashiorkor, 346
Marasmus, 346
Margarine
    containing plant sterols/stanols, 146
    fat in, 151
Margarine substitutes, 17
Margin of safety, 43
Marshall, Barry, 29
Meal planning, 45–56
    Dietary Guidelines, 52, 53, 54t
    food groups, 45–51
    MyPlate guide, 55, 55f, 55t
Meals on Wheels, 347t
Meat. *See also* specific types of meat
    charring of, carcinogens and, 222
    cold storage time limits, 342t
    deli, 52
    heart healthy food selection and preparation, 151
    high-fat, 48
    lean, 48
    red, 170
    sustainable agriculture and, 349
Meat substitutes, 175
Meat thermometer, 338–339
Mechanical digestion, 75
Medications
    foods interfering with, 333
    weight-loss, 293
Medicinal herbs, 62
Mediterranean Diet
    food pyramid, 56, 56f
    for heart health, 149, 150
MedWatch program, 63
Megadoses, 62
    of niacin, 206
    of vitamin C, 219
Megaloblastic, 211
Megaloblastic anemia, 214
Melanin, 200
Melatonin, 65t
Menopause, 238
Menstrual cycle, abnormal, 299
Menu planning, 291
Mercury, 231
Metabolic rate, 283–284
    basal, 284
    calculating an estimate of, 284
    defined, 283
    factors influencing, 283–284

Metabolic syndrome, 121–122
Metabolic water, 258
Metabolism, 8, 283
    aerobic, 96
    amino acid, 191f, 209
    anabolism, 96
    anaerobic, 96
    basal, 283
    "biological" fuels, 95, 97
    catabolism, 96
    defined, 8, 283
    energy, 95–97, 97f, 283–284
    fatty acids, 140, 141
    glucose and, 116
    thrifty, 288
Metastasized, 93, 221, 221f
Methionine, 10t, 163t, 166, 171, 211, 232
Methylmercury, 150
Metric prefixes, 9, 9t
Micelle, 139
Micronutrients, 9. See also Minerals; Vitamin(s)
    in fruits, 49
    in protein foods, 48
    range of safe intake, 16, 16f
Microwaves
    food safety and, 341, 343
    heating infant formula in, 327
Mild cognitive impairment, 202
Milk
    for adolescents, 331
    breast, 323, 325–326
    calcium in, 47, 236, 236t
    for infants, 323, 327
    lactose intolerance and, 122
    low-fat, 47
    pasteurization of, 329
    soy, 47
    unpasteurized, 329
    whole, 47, 135t
Milk allergy, 122
Milk sugar, 104
Minerals, 6, 229–268. See also specific minerals
    absorption, 233
    from animal foods, 48
    body composition of, 6f
    defined, 229
    as essential nutrients, 10, 10t
    functioning as electrolyte, 232
    function of, 7, 232
    major, 231t
    as micronutrient, 9
    MyPlate food sources, 230f
    sources of, 229, 230f, 233
    supplements, 62, 233
    trace, 231, 231t
    water as a source of, 231
Misinformation. See Nutrition information and
        misinformation
Moderation, in healthy diets, 14
Molasses, 105t
Molds, in food, 335
Molecules, 75
Molybdenum, 10t, 231t
"Money back" guarantees, 34
Monk fruit extract, 108
Monoglycerides, 139, 140f
Monosaccharides, 103, 110
Monounsaturated fats, 148
Monounsaturated fatty acid (monounsaturated FA), 131, 132,
        132t, 148
Moreno, Marisa, 3, 15
Morning sickness, 29, 320–321, 321–322
Motion sickness, 29
Mouth, 77, 86, 86f, 113f
Mucilages, 110, 111t
Mucin, 162
Mucus, 80
Multivitamin/multimineral (MV/MM) products, 60, 63
Muscle cells, 72, 72f
Muscle contraction/relaxation, minerals for, 232f
Muscles, fuel for, 302–303
Muscular system, 74t
Mutation, 167
Myoglobin, 244
MyPlate food guide, 15f, 55, 55f, 55t

calcium, 236, 237f
    for children, 331
    fat-soluble vitamins, 193f
    iron, 245f
    magnesium, 249f
    minerals, 230f
    for older adults, 333
    potassium, 240f
    on protein food sources, 168
    recommended amount of fruit, 112
    recommended amounts of food, 55t
    Super Tracker, 287
    using, 55
    vegetarian diet and, 175
    water-soluble vitamins, 206f
    zinc, 253, 254f
MyPyramid Plan, 56

N

Nasal cavity, 78f
National Academy of Sciences, 335
National Heart Lung and Blood Institute, 276
National Institute on Aging, 333
National Osteoporosis Foundation, 35
National School Lunch Program, 347t
National Weight Control Registry, 292
"Natural food," 59
Natural resources, food production and, 348–349
Natural sugars, 105
NatureSmart LLC, 134
NBTY, Inc., 134
Necta Sweet®, 108t
Nectresse™, 108, 108t
Negative energy state, 286–287, 287f
Negative thought patterns, weight loss and, 292
Neotame, 108, 108t
Neotame®, 108t
Nerve cells, 72, 72f
Nervous system, 74t
    blood alcohol concentration (BAC) and, 263, 263t
    major organs and tissues of, 74t
    primary functions of, 74t
Neural tube, 214
Neural tube defects, 214
Nguyen, Damian, 229
Niacin. See Vitamin B-3 (niacin)
Nickel, 231, 231t
Nicotinic acid, 206
Night blindness, 196
Nitrate, 309t
Non-alchoholic fatty liver disease (NAFLD), 122
Nonessential amino acids, 163, 163t, 168
Nonexercise activity thermogenesis (NEAT), 285
Nonfat milk, 47
Nonheme iron, 244
Nonnutrients, 10
Nonnutritive ("artificial") sweeteners, 108–109, 108t, 109t
Norovirus, 337t
"Nursing bottle syndrome," 122
Nut butters, 153. See also Peanut butter
NutraSweet®, 108t
Nutrient content claims, 59
Nutrient-dense food, 13–14
Nutrients
    added to foods (fortification), 46
    body composition of, 6f
    defined, 4
    essential, 10, 10t
    food energy and, 8
    functions of, 7
    organic, 6
    removed by processing of foods, 15
    six classes of, 6
    storage of, 42
    taking supplements vs. natural source of, 63
Nutrient supplements. See Supplements
Nutrition
    alcohol's effect on, 266
    basics of, 6–12
    defined, 4
    key concepts, 13–17
    lifecycle. See Lifecycle nutrition
    reasons for learning about, 4–5
Nutrition experts, 36–37
Nutrition Facts panel, 57–58, 57f

Nutrition information and misinformation
    anecdotes, 23, 24, 30, 34
    on the Internet, critical evaluation of, 35
    mistrust of medical professionals and, 30–31
    from nutrition experts, 36–37
    reasons for misinformation, 31–32
    "red flags" of misinformation, 33–34
    reliability of sources, 30
    research bias and, 28
    skeptical consumerism and, 32–33
    studies establishing cause and effect, 29
    testimonials, 30, 34
Nutritionists, 37
Nutrition Program, Congregate Meals for the Elderly, 347t
Nutrition-related research
    cause/effect and, 29
    conflicting findings in, 28
    Framingham Heart Study, 27
    human intervention studies, 26
    population studies, 27
    research bias and, 28
    scientific method, 24–25
Nutritive sweeteners, 106
Nuts/seeds
    almonds, 15
    energy density and, 14, 15
    fiber through, 123
    omega-3 fats in, 150, 150t
    as source of "healthy" fats, 170
    as source of protein, 169, 171

O

Oatmeal, 113, 123
Obesity
    BMI and, 281t
    cancer development and, 221
    central-body, 279, 280f
    in children, 276, 288, 332
    defined, 276
    extreme, 278, 281, 293
    general attitude toward, 279
    medical treatments for, 293–294, 293f, 294f
    in older adults, 332
    overnutrition and, 12
    percentage of body fat, 282, 282t
    prevalence of, 276–277, 276t, 277f
    race/ethnicity and, 276
    sound weight-loss plan for, 289
    television viewing and, 288
Observation in scientific method, 24
Office of Dietary Supplements, 63
Oils. See also Lipids
    fatty acid content of, 132t
    food group, 50
    MyPlate guidelines, 55t
    oleic, 134
    with omega-3 fatty acids, 150t
    partially hydrogenated, 134
    saturated FAs in, 131
    vitamins in, 193f
Older adults
    nutrition for, 332–333
    nutrition services for, 333
    osteoporosis in, 237–238, 238f
    physical activity/inactivity among, 333
    physical changes in, 332, 333t
    population statistics, 332
    supplemental vitamins for, 63
    vitamin B-12 deficiency in, 215
Oleic oils, 134
Olive oil, 132t
Omega-3 fatty acids
    alpha-linolenic acid, 133, 133f
    defined, 133
    food sources of, 150, 150t
    through fish oil supplements, 150
    vegetarian/vegan diet and, 174, 174t
Omega-6 fatty acids, 133, 133f, 150
Omega end, 130
Omnivore, 75
Onions, 149
Orange juice, 17
Organ, 73
Organic foods, 51
Organic nutrients, 6
Organism, 73f

Organizations, websites sponsored by, 35
Organ system, 73, 73f, 74, 74t
Orlistat, 293
Osteomalacia, 200–201
Osteoporosis, 201, 203, 237–238, 238f
Overfat, 276. *See also* Overweight
Overnutrition, 12
Overweight, 276. *See also* Obesity
    defined, 276
    in older adults, 332
    percentage of body fat and, 282, 282t
    prevalence of, 276t
    use of term, 276
Ovovegetarian, 174
Oxalate, 219
Oxalic acid, 236
Oxidized LDL cholesterol, 146, 146f
Oxytocin, 324

P

Palm kernal oil, 132
Palm oil, 131, 132t
Pancreas, 84, 84f, 138
Pancreatic lipase, 138
Pantothenic acid (Vitamin B-5), 10t, 189, 189t, 191f, 205, 216, 216t
Parasitic worms, 335, 337t
Parathyroid gland, 234, 235f
Parathyroid hormone (PTH), 234
Partially hydrogenated oils (PHOs), 134
Pasteurization, 329
Pathogens, 335
Peanut butter, 136, 137, 169t, 171, 178
Peanut oil, 132t
Peanuts
    allergy to, 179
    protein in, 170
Pear juice, 329
"Pear shape" body, 279, 279f
Pectin, 110, 111t
Pedometer, 303
Peer review, 24, 25
Pellagra, 206, 207f, 209t
Pennyroyal, 62
Peptic ulcers, 90–91, 90f
Peptide bond, 164, 165
Percent of Daily Values (DVs), 58, 61
Peripheral vascular disease (PVD), 144
Peristalsis, 79, 79f
Pernicious anemia, 215
Personal Dietary Analysis, 123
Perspiration, 258, 259f
Pesticides, 344, 349
Pesticides in foods, 344, 344f
Pesticide tolerances, 344
Pest management, 349
Phenylalanine, 10t, 163t
Phenylketonuria (PKU), 109
Phospholipids, 136–137, 136f
Phosphorus, 10t, 231t
    in dairy foods, 47
    function of, 232f
    nutritional information, 255t
    vitamin D and, 199
Physical activity. *See also* Exercise
    among older adults, 333
    caloric output/minute for selected, 285t
    for children, 332
    defined, 300, 301
    developing a plan for, 310
    energy for, 284
    inactivity, as risk factor for atherosclerosis, 146
    intensity of, 300–301
    nonexercise activity thermogenesis (NEAT), 285
    recommendations for, 300
    reducing risk of CVD with, 147
    unstructured, 300
    weight loss and, 290
Physical activity pyramid, 301, 301f
Physical fitness, 300, 301
Physicians, nutrition information/misinformation and, 30, 36
Phytochemicals
    cancer risk reduction and, 222
    defined, 10

dietary supplements and, 63
    food sources, 11t
    in fruit, 49
    health benefits, 11t
    in margarine substitutes, 17
    supplements and, 63
    toxic, 10
    "whole" foods and, 15
Pica, 321
"Picky eaters," 332
Picnic foods, food safety and, 341
Pizza, 51
PKA (phenylketonuria), 109
PKU (phenylketonuria), 109
Placebo effect, 26
Placebos, 26
Placenta, 319, 319f
Planning meals. *See* Meal planning
Plant proteins, 169, 171
Plant sterols/stanols, 146
Platelets, 269
Polypeptides, 164
Polyps, 94
Polysaccharides, 110
Polyunsaturated fats, effect on LDL and LDL, 148
Polyunsaturated fatty acid, 131, 132, 132t, 133, 134, 147, 148
Pomegranate, 27
Popcorn, 152
Population growth, 348, 349
Population studies, 27
Pork
    cold storage time limits, 342t
    cooking temperatures for, 339t
    USDA recommended safe temperatures, 339t
Positive energy state, 287, 287f
Potassium, 10t, 231t
    Adequate Intake (AI), 240, 243t
    in dairy foods, 47
    deficiency signs and symptoms, 243t
    depletion, symptoms of, 240
    as electrolyte, 232
    food sources, 240, 240f, 240t, 243t
    in fruit, 49
    function of, 232f
    functions, 243t
    MyPlate on sources of, 240f
    toxicity, 243t
Poultry
    bacterial contaminants in, 340
    cholesterol in chicken breast, 135t
    cooking temperatures for food safety, 339t
    thoroughly cooking, 340
    USDA recommended safe temperatures, 339t
Poverty guidelines, 347
Poverty, undernutrition and, 345, 347, 349
Power player vitamins, 206–209
Precursors, 188
Pre-diabetes, 118
Preeclampsia, 322, 322f, 323
Prefixes, metric, 9, 9t
Preformed vitamin A, 194
Pregnancy
    cravings during, 321
    diabetes during, 119
    Dietary Reference Intakes (DRIs) during, 320t
    fish intake during, 150
    folate intake and, 214, 320
    iron intake during, 320
    morning sickness during, 320–321
    nutrition during, 319–320, 319t
    preeclampsia during, 322, 322f
    undernutrition during, 345
    vitamin A and, 196
    weight gain during, 321–322, 321t, 322f
Prehypertension, 241, 242t
Premature baby, 319
Prenatal period, 318–319, 319f
Preschool years, undernutrition during, 346
Prescription drugs
    for cardiovascular disease, 153
    herbal supplements and, 62
    for high blood lipid levels, 153
    interfering with absorption of nutrients, 333
Previtamin D, 198
Previtamins, 188

Pritikin Diet, 295
Probiotics, 17, 85, 88
Processed foods, food safety and, 15
Processing of foods, 233
Prolactin, 324
Proline, 163t
ProSobee, 327t
Protein(s), 6, 161–180
    absorption of, 164, 166
    Acceptable Macronutrient Distribution Ranges (AMDRs), 44t, 168, 176
    amino acids. *See* Amino acids
    for athletes, 306
    athletes and, 176–177
    average intake in American diet, 168
    body composition of, 6f
    building with amino acids, 166–167
    calculating recommended intake for, 168
    calorie percentage in average American diet, 112f
    celiac disease and, 180
    choosing variety of, 53
    combining complementary, 171
    complete, 170
    content in common foods, 169t
    in dairy foods, 47
    deficiency of, 178
    defined, 162, 163
    Dietary Guidelines for Americans on sources of, 168
    digestion of, 164–166, 166f
    as essential nutrients, 10t
    excess intake of, 176
    fate of excess, 167–168
    food allergies and, 178–179
    food intolerances and, 179
    food sources of, 161, 169
    function of, 7t
    gluten, 180, 180t
    in grains, 45
    high-protein weight-loss diets and, 177
    high-quality, 170
    incomplete, 170
    iron in, 245f
    low-quality, 170
    as macronutrient, 19
    magnesium in, 249f
    malnutrition and, 178
    minerals in, 230f
    MyPlate guidelines, 55t, 168
    potassium in, 240f
    quality of, 170–171
    Recommended Dietary Allowance (RDA) for, 168, 176
    roles of, 162–163
    satiety and, 179
    serving equivalents, 48
    stretching your food dollars and, 172
    student profile, 161
    supplements, 177
    vegetarianism and, 173–175, 174t
    vitamins in, 193f, 206f
Protein-energy malnutrition (PEM), 178, 346
Protists, 335, 337t
Provitamin A, 194
Provitamins, 188
Puberty, 330
Pyloric sphincter, 80, 80f
Pyridoxine. *See* Vitamin B-6 (pyridoxine)
Pyruvate, 295t

Q

Qsymia, 293
Quackery, 33
Quercetin, 11t
Question, developing in scientific method, 24
Quinoa, 170, 170f

R

Radiation therapy, 94
Radura symbol, 343
Raghothaman, Abby, 41
Rancidity, 134
Raspberry ketones, 294, 295t
Reactive hypoglycemia, 121
Ready-to-use, therapeutic food (RUTF), 346–347
Rebiana, 106, 108t

Recommended Dietary Allowance (RDA), 43–44
  for biotin, 216t
  for calcium, 239t
  for carbohydrates, 116
  for choline, 216t
  for chromium, 255t
  for copper, 251t
  explained, 44–45
  for fat intake, 150
  for fluoride, 239t
  for folate, 215t
  for iodine, 255t
  for iron, 249t
  for magnesium, 249t
  for niacin (vitamin B-3), 209t
  for pantothenic acid, 216t
  for phosphorus, 255t
  power player vitamins, 209t
  for pregnant and nonpregnant women, 320, 320t
  for protein, 168, 176
  for riboflavin (vitamin B-2), 209t
  for selenium, 251t
  for thiamin (vitamin B-1), 209t
  for vitamin A, 197t
  for vitamin B-6, 210t
  for vitamin B-12, 215t
  for vitamin C, 219t
  for vitamin D, 201
  for vitamin E, 203t
  for zinc, 255t
Rectum, 85, 85f, 86, 86f, 113f, 166f
Red blood cell formation, minerals for, 232f
Red blood cells (RBCs)
  hemoglobin transporting oxygen in, 162, 167, 209
  iron deficiency and, 246f
  iron in, 232
  megaloblastic anemia and, 214
  vitamin B-12 and folate for production of, 211, 211f
  vitamins for formation of, 191f
"Red flags" of misinformation, 33–34
Red meat, 170
Reduced-fat foods, 59
Red yeast rice, 65t
Refined sugars, 104
Refrigerated foods, 341, 342t
Registered dietitian (RD), 37
Registered nutritionist dietitian (RDN), 37
Reinhardt, Jason, 265
Reproductive system, 74t
Requirement(s)
  defined, 42, 44
  Dietary Reference Intakes (DRIs), 42–43, 43f
  Estimated Average Requirement (EAR), 43, 43f
  Estimated Energy Requirement (EER), 43, 284
Research bias, 28, 34
Respiratory system, 74t
Restaurants
  food safety and, 343
  sanitation ratings, 334
  weight loss and, 291
Resveratrol, 11t
Retina, 196
Retinoin (Retin-A), 196
Retinol, 194, 196
Retinol activity equivalent (RAE), 195
Retinol binding protein, 162
Rexall Sundown, Inc., 134
Rhizomes, 29
Rhubarb, 236
Riboflavin. See Vitamin B-2 (riboflavin)
Rickets, 187, 198, 198f, 200
Risk factors, 5
Rodents, 24
Roux-en-Y operation, 293, 293f

S
Saccharin, 108, 108t, 109t
Safe Drinking Water Act, 261
Safety, food. See Food safety
Safety issues. See also Food safety
  herbal supplements, 62
  vitamin and mineral supplements, 62
Safflower oil, 132t
Salad dressing, 59, 148, 152
Saliva, 77

Salivary amylase, 113
Salmon
  calcium in, 235
  cholesterol in, 135t
Salmonella, 337t
Salt. See Sodium chloride (salt)
Salt substitutes, 240
Sanitation ratings, 334
Sanitizing food preparation surfaces, 340
Saponins, 11t
Sarcopenia, 332
Sardines
  calcium in, 235, 236t
  cholesterol in, 135t
Sassafras, 62
Satiety, 179, 287
Saturated fats
  cardiovascular disease and, 134–135, 147, 148
  consuming less of, 53
  heart healthy food selection and, 151
Saturated fatty acids, 130–131
  butter and, 151
  comparing sources of unsaturated FAs and, 132
  content in fats and oils, 132t
  Dietary Guidelines recommendation for, 150
  effect on LDL and HDL, 148
  effects on LDL and HDL, 148
  replacing with polyunsaturated FAs, 147, 148
  as solid fat, 133
  sources of, compared with unsaturated FAs, 132
Saxenda, 293
Scare tactics, 30
Scarsdale Diet, 294
Scientific method, steps of, 24–25
Scientific-sounding terms, nutrition misinformation and, 33
Scott, Nancy, 129
Scurvy, 219, 219f
Seafood, omega-3 fats in, 150, 150t
Seaweed, 307
Sedentary, 288
Seeds. See Nuts/seeds
Selenium, 10t, 231t, 250, 250t, 251t
  food processing and, 233
  function of, 232f
  megadose of, 62
Semivegetarians, 173
Serine, 163t
Serving comparisons (equivalents), 45
  dairy, 47
  fruits, 49
  grains, 46
  protein, 48
  vegetables, 50
Serving sizes
  estimating, 51, 52f, 53f
  on food label, 57f, 58, 61
Set-point theory, 288
Shrimp, cholesterol in, 135t
Sickle cell disease, 167
Silicon, 231t
Similac, 327t
Simple carbohydrates
  disaccharides, 104
  monosaccharides, 103
Sippy cups, 328
Skeletal fluorosis, 239
Skeletal system, 74t
Skim milk, 47
Skin cancer, 187
Skinfold thickness measurement, 282, 282f
Sleep apnea, 147
Sleeve gastrectomy, 293, 294
Small intestine, 81, 81f, 85f, 86, 86f
  bile salts and, 141
  digestion of carbohydrates and, 113f
  digestion of lipids and, 135, 138, 140
  protein digestion and, 166f
Smell, sense of, 77
Smoking, 5
  cancer and, 221
  cardiovascular disease and, 147
  osteoporosis and, 331
  oxidized LDL cholesterol and, 146
  as risk factor for atherosclerosis, 146
  vitamin C intake and, 44, 219

Smoothies, homemade, 236
Smooth muscle cells, 72, 72f
Snacks, 330–331
Social support, for weight loss, 292
Sodium, 10t, 231t
  Adequate Intake (AI), 243t
  deficiency signs and symptoms, 243t
  as electrolyte, 232
  extracellular water and, 258
  fluid balance and, 259
  food sources of, 241, 243t
  function of, 232f, 243t
  hypertension and, 241–242
  reducing in diet, 53, 242
  toxicity, 243t
Sodium ascorbate, 217
Sodium bicarbonate (baking soda), 309t
Sodium chloride (salt)
  beans and, 172
  function of, 232f
  iodine and, 252
  in soft water, 231
Sodium Intake Assessment, 242, 243
Soft drinks, 101, 105, 112, 117
Solid fats, 51, 53, 133, 148, 153
Solid foods, 326, 328, 329
Soluble fiber, 110, 111t, 141
Solvent, 257
Sorbitol, 108
South Beach Diet, 294
Soybean oil, 132t
Soybeans (soy), 136, 137, 150, 170, 172
Soy milk, 47, 122
Soy protein, 170
Special Supplemental Nutrition Program for Women, Infants, and
    Children (WIC), 347t
SPF (sun protection factor), 200
Spina bifida, 214, 214f, 320
Spinach, 244
Spined soldier bug, 349f
Splenda®, 108t
Sports drinks, 306, 307
Sports gels, 306
Standard drink, 262
Stanols, 146
Staphylococcus aureus, 337t
Starch, 110
Statins, 153
Sterols, 146
Stevia leaves, 106, 108, 108t
St. John's wort, 65t
Stomach, 80, 80f, 86, 86f
  digestion of carbohydrates and, 113f
  protein digestion and, 166f
Stomach ulcers, 29
Stools, 85
Strokes
  deaths from, 142
  defined, 144
  free radical damage and, 192
Structure/function claim, 59
Stuffing, cooking, 340
Subcutaneous fat, 278, 278f, 279, 282, 282f
Substance Abuse and Mental Health Service Administration,
    National Helpline, 268
Sucralose, 108, 108t, 109t
Sucrase, 113, 162, 166
Sucrose, 104, 113, 162
Sugar alcohols, 108
Sugars
  added, 105, 106f, 107t, 112
  comparison of sweeteners, 105t
  consuming less of added, 53
  disaccharides, 104
  hyperactivity in children and, 105
  "malt," 104
  "milk," 104
  monosaccharides, 103
  natural, 105
  "table," 104
Sugar-sweetened beverages, 112, 117
Sugar-sweetened drinks, 112
Sugar Twin®, 108t
Sugary foods, 51
Sulfites, 179

Sulfur, 10t, 11t, 231, 231t, 255t
Sunett®, 108t
Sunflower seeds, 170
Sunlight, vitamin D and, 187, 198, 200, 200f, 201
Sun protection factor (SPF), 200
Sunscreen, 200
Supplemental Nutrition Assistance Program, 347t
Supplements
    for athletes, 307–308, 309t
    calcium, 237
    cancer risk reduction and, 222
    chromium, 254
    deciding to take, 63
    disclaimers, 61, 61f
    explained, 12, 60
    FDA regulation, 61–62
    fish oil, 150
    individualized needs and, 16
    for infants, 326
    iron, 244
    labels, 60–61, 61f
    megadose of, 62
    minerals, 233
    most commonly used, 60
    not containing vitamins and minerals, 60
    nutrients from foods vs., 16
    popular, 64–65t
    protein, 177
    risks and benefits of, where to find, 63
    safety of herbal, 62
    safety of vitamin and minerals, 62
    vitamin, 134, 220
    vitamin E and, 202
    weight-loss, 295, 295t
Sustainable agriculture, 348–349
Swallowing, 77, 78–79
Swallowing air, 80, 123
Sweeteners
    acceptable daily intakes for nonnutritive, 109t
    agave nectar, 106
    alternative, 108–109, 108t
    on food label, 106f
    high-fructose corn syrup, 101, 105, 105t, 106, 112
    nonnutritive (artificial), 118–119, 118f, 119f
    nutritional comparison of, 105t
    nutritive, 106
    safety of artificial, 109
    in sports drinks, 306
    stevia, 106, 108, 108t
    sugars, 103–105
Sweet Leaf®, 108t
Sweet'N Low®, 108t
Sweet One®, 108t
Swiss cheese, calcium in, 236t
Syrup, in canned fruit, 112
Systolic pressure, 241, 242t

T
Table sugar, 103, 104, 105, 106, 112
Tap water, minerals in, 231, 239
Tarragon, 242
Taste, 77
Taste buds, 77
Taurine, 308
Teeth, dental fluorosis and, 239, 239f
Television programming, weight gain and, 288, 332
Testimonials, 30, 34
Testing questions, in scientific method, 25
Tetratogen, 106
"Tex-Mex" food, 3
Thermic effect of food (TEF), 285
Thiamin. See Vitamin B-1 (thiamin)
Thirst, 260
Threonine, 10t, 163t, 171
Thrifty metabolism, 288
Thyroid gland, 234, 235f, 252, 253
Thyroid hormone, 252, 253, 283
Tissues, 73f
Tofu, 172, 236, 236t
Tolerable Upper Intake Level (Upper Level), 44
Tomatillos, 50
Tomatoes, 196
Tooth decay, 122
Total body fat, 277
Total carbohydrates, on food label, 58

Total fats, on food labels, 58
Total water intake, 258
Toxicity
    caffeine, 308
    calcium, 239t
    choline, 216t
    chromium, 255t
    fluoride, 239t
    iodine, 255t
    magnesium, 248
    power player vitamins, 209t
    vitamin, 189
    vitamin A, 196
    vitamin D, 201
    vitamin E, 202, 203t
    water, 260
    zinc, 255t
Toxicity disorder, 44
Toxic phytochemicals, 10
Toxins, in food, 335
Toxoplasma, 337t
Trace minerals, 231, 231t
Trachea, 78
Trans fats
    cardiovascular disease and, 135
    consuming less of, 53
    eating fewer foods containing, 148
    effect on LDL and HDL, 148
    explained, 134
    in processed foods, 134
Trans fatty acids, 134–135, 148
Transport proteins, 163
Treatment groups, in human intervention studies, 26
Tretinoin (Retin-A), 196
Trichinella, 335, 337t
Triglycerides, 130–135, 140f. See also Fats; Oils
    alcohol and, 266
    basic parts of, 130f
    cardiovascular disease and, 146
    chylomicron formation, 140f
    composition of, 130, 130f
    defined, 130
    healthy and unhealthy levels of, 149t
    high, as risk factor for atherosclerosis, 147
    metabolic syndrome and, 121
Tripeptides, 164, 165f
Tropical plant oils, 131
Truvia®, 108t
Tryptophan, 10t, 163t, 171
Tubers, 110
Tumors, 220–221, 220f, 221f
Turkey, cholesterol in, 135t
Type 1 diabetes, 117–118
Type 2 diabetes, 117, 118, 332
Tyrosine, 163t

U
UL. See Upper Limit (UL)
Ulcerative colitis, 92–93
Ulcers, 29, 90–91
Umami taste, 77
Undernutrition, 345–349
    defined, 345
    explained, 12
    factors contributing to, 345, 345f
    federally supported programs for, 347–348, 347t
    during infancy, 346
    population growth and, 348
    during pregnancy, 345
    during preschool years, 346
    protein deficiency and, 178
    protein-energy malnutrition, 346
    solutions for, 346–347, 349
    sustainable agriculture and, 348–349
    in the United States, 347–348
Underweight children, 178
Underweight people, 296
UNICEF (United Nations Children's Fund), 346–347
Unpasteurized (raw) milk/juice, 329
Unsaturated fatty acids, 130, 133
    content in fats and oils, 132t
    egg yolks and, 153
    as liquid fat, 133
    monounsaturated FA, 131, 132, 132t, 148
    polyunsaturated FA, 131

sources of, compared with saturated FAs, 132
    trans fatty acids, 134–135, 134f
Upper Limit (UL)
    for calcium, 239t
    for chloride, 255t
    for copper, 251t
    for fluoride, 239t
    for folate, 215t
    for iodine, 255t
    for iron, 249t
    for magnesium, 249t
    for manganese, 255t
    for niacin, 209t
    for phosphorus, 255t
    for selenium, 251t
    for sodium, 243t
    for thiamin, 209t
    for vitamin A, 197t
    for vitamin B-6, 210t
    for vitamin C, 219t
    for vitamin D, 201t
    for vitamin E, 203t
    for vitamin K, 204t
    for water, 260
    for zinc, 255t
Urea, 176
Urinary system, 74t
Urine, 259, 260
U.S. Department of Agriculture (USDA), 14
    2015–2020 Dietary Guidelines for Americans. See Dietary Guidelines for Americans
    food standards, 45
    organic foods and, 51
    role in food safety, 334
    website, 51
U.S. Department of Health and Human Services (USDHHS)
    2015–2020 Dietary Guidelines for Americans. See Dietary Guidelines for Americans
    poverty guidelines, 347
    role in food safety, 334

V
Valerian, 62, 65t
Valine, 10t, 163t
Vanadium, 231t
Variety, food, 14, 52, 55
Vegans, 173, 174, 175, 215
Vegetable oils, 53
Vegetables
    cruciferous, 195
    fiber in, 111t, 123
    iron in, 245f
    magnesium in, 249f
    minerals in, 230f
    MyPlate guidelines, 55t
    potassium in, 240f
    retaining vitamin content in, 190
    serving equivalents, 50
    steaming, 190
    vitamins in, 193f, 206f
Vegetarianism, 173–175
    children and, 175
    commercially prepared foods, 175
    food suggestions for protein intake and, 175
    lactoovovegetarian, 173
    lactovegetarianism, 173
    meat substitutes and, 175
    nutritional benefits of, 174, 174t
    nutritional disadvantages of, 174, 174t
    ovovegetarian, 173
    semivegetarians, 173
    types of diets, 173
    vitamin B-12 and, 215
Very-low-calorie diet, 284, 290
Very-low-density lipoprotein (VLDL), 140, 144f, 145
Very-low-fat diets, 295
Villi/villus, 81, 81f, 82
Viruses, in foods, 335, 337t
Visceral fat, 278, 278f, 279, 280
Vitamin(s), 6, 187–223. See also specific vitamins
    absorption of, 190
    body's requirements of, 188
    cancer and, 220–222
    classifying, 189, 189t
    conserving in your food, 190

Vitamin(s) (continued)
deficiencies in, 188, 266
defined, 188
as essential nutrients, 10, 10t
fat-soluble, 189, 189t, 190, 193–204
functions of, 7, 191f
International Units (IUs), 194
megadose, 62
as a micronutrient, 9, 188
"power player," 206–209, 207t–208t, 209t
roles of, 191–192
supplements, 60, 60f, 62, 63, 134, 220
toxicities, 189
water-soluble, 189, 189t, 205–219
Vitamin A, 10t, 194–197
in dairy foods, 47
deficiencies, 195–197, 197t
as fat-soluble vitamin, 189
food sources of, 194–195, 195t
functions of, 191–192, 191f, 194, 197t
megadose of, 62
preformed, 194
provitamin A, 194
Recommended Dietary Allowance (RDA), 197t
sources of, 194, 195, 195t, 196, 197t
summary, 197
toxicity of, 196, 197t
Vitamin B-1 (thiamin), 10t
deficiency, 206, 207, 209t
food sources of, 207t, 209t
functions of, 191f, 206, 209t
Recommended Dietary Allowance (RDA), 209t
toxicity, 209t
as water-soluble vitamin, 189, 189t
Vitamin B-2 (riboflavin), 10t
in dairy foods, 47
deficiency, 206, 207, 209t
food sources of, 207, 208f, 209t
functions of, 191f, 206, 209t
Recommended Dietary Allowance (RDA), 209t
toxicity, 209t
as water-soluble vitamin, 189, 189t
Vitamin B-3 (niacin), 10t
corn and, 209
deficiency, 206, 207, 209t
food sources of, 207, 208t, 209t
functions of, 191f, 206, 209t
megadose of, 62
Recommended Dietary Allowance (RDA), 209t
toxicity, 209t
as water-soluble vitamin, 189, 189t
Vitamin B-5. See Pantothenic acid (Vitamin B-5)
Vitamin B-6 (pyridoxine)
food sources of, 210, 210t
functions of, 191f, 209, 210t
megadose of, 62
Recommended Dietary Allowance (RDA), 210t
toxicity, 210t
Vitamin B-12 (cobalamin)
absorption of, 213
cobalt in, 232
deficiency, 215, 215t
food sources of, 212, 212t, 215t
functions of, 191f, 211, 215t
Recommended Dietary Allowance (RDA), 215t
storage of excess, 214
vegan diet and, 175
vegetarian diet and, 174, 174t
as water-soluble vitamin, 189, 189t
Vitamin C
as an antioxidant, 192
in apples vs. oranges, 49
cigarette smoking and, 219
collagen and, 217
deficiency of, 219, 219t
food sources of, 218, 218t, 219t
in fruit, 49
functions of, 191f, 217, 219t
iron and, 244
megadose of, 62
prevention of colds and, 217
Recommended Dietary Allowance (RDA), 219t
requirement for, 42
supplements, 62, 62f

toxicity, 219, 219t
as water-soluble vitamin, 189, 189t
Vitamin D, 10, 198–201
bone health and, 238
in dairy foods, 47
deficiencies, 187, 188, 200–201, 201t
as fat-soluble vitamin, 189
function of, 199
functions of, 191f, 201t
how your body makes, 198
megadose of, 62
for older adults, 333
previtamin D, 198
Recommended Dietary Allowance (RDA), 201t
sources of, 199, 199t, 201t
student profile on, 187, 200
sunlight and, 187, 198, 200, 200f, 201
supplement, 237
supplement for infants, 326
toxicity, 201, 201t
two major forms of, 199
vegetarian/vegan diet and, 174, 174t
vitamin D₂, 199
vitamin D₃, 199
Vitamin E, 62
alpha-tocopherol form, 201
as an antioxidant, 192
antioxidant activity, 201f
deficiencies, 202, 203t, 204t
as fat-soluble vitamin, 189
function of, 191f, 201, 203t, 204t
Recommended Dietary Allowance (RDA), 203t
sources of, 202, 202t, 203t, 204t
supplements, 62, 202
toxicity, 202, 203t, 204t
Vitamin C and, 217
Vitamin K
clots/clotting and, 202, 203, 203f
deficiencies, 204
as fat-soluble vitamin, 189
function of, 191f, 203
functions of, 191f
sources of, 204, 204t
vitamin E and, 202
VLDL (very-low-density lipoprotein), 140, 144, 145
Vomiting, 89, 320–321, 327, 336

W

Waist circumference measurement, 280, 280f
Walnut oil, 132t
Walnuts, 150
Warfarin, 203
Warren, Robin, 29
Warrington, Neill, 101
Washington, Theresa, 317
Wasting food, 349
Water, 6, 256–261
adding fruit to, 112
Adequate Intake, 259
Adequate Intake (AI), 259
alcohol and body, 266
body composition of, 6f
body's fluid compartments and, 257–258, 257f
body's loss of, 259–260
bottled, 261
daily water balance, 258, 259f
dehydration and, 20
as essential nutrient, 10, 10t, 256
extracellular, 257
flavored beverages, 261
fluid balance and, 257–258
fluoridation of, 239
in food and beverages, 256, 256t
functions in body, 7, 257
intracellular, 257
necessity of, 256
public water supplies, 239, 261
recommended daily intake of, 259
replenishing fluids, 306–307
Safe Drinking Water Act, 261
softening, 231
tap, 261
total water intake, 258

toxicity, 260
urine and, 260
Water-insoluble nutrients, 83
Water intake, constipation and, 87
Water intoxication, 260, 307
Water-soluble nutrients, 82, 83
Water-soluble vitamins, 189, 189t, 205–219
Weaning, 328
Weight. See also Obesity; Overweight; Weight gain; Weight loss
body mass index (BMI), 280–281, 281t
caloric input and ouput, 283–285, 283–287, 285t, 287f
classification by percentage of body fat, 282, 282t
energy balance and, 276–287, 286–287, 286f
factors influencing, 283–287, 286f
underweight, 178, 296
Weight-bearing activities, 238
Weight control, fiber and, 123
Weight gain
carbohydrates and, 117
in college students, 12
energy balance and, 286–287
factors influencing, 287–289
during pregnancy, 321–322, 321t, 322f
sugar-sweetened soft drinks and, 117
television and, 288
temporary, from salty foods, 259
for underweight people, 296
Weight loss, 269
advertisers claims, 296
energy balance and, 286–287
gluten-free diet and, 180
high-protein diets, 177
lifestyle changes and, 290
medically sound plan for, 289
medications, 293
in older adults, 333
setting goals for, 290
suggested practices for, 291–292
"3500-kcal-rule-of-thumb" for, 286
unreliable methods for, 294–296, 295f
weight gain following, 288, 291
Weight-loss diet, high-protein, 177
Weight-loss supplements, 295, 295t
Well water, 239
Wheat bran, 15, 15f, 123
Wheat germ, 15, 15f, 123, 136, 137
Whey protein, 177
White blood cells, 72
White flour, 15, 15f
White granulated sugar, 105t
"Whole" foods, 15
Whole grains, 15, 45, 52, 53, 123
Whole milk, 47, 135t
Wine, 262
World Food Program, 346
World Health Organization (WHO)
on overweight/obese adults, 277
on underweight children, 178
Worms, parasitic, 335, 337t

X

Xylitol, 108

Y

Yogurt, 17, 85, 88, 152, 236t
Yohimbe, 295t

Z

Zeaxanthin, 194
Zetia®, 153
Zinc, 10t, 231, 231t, 253, 253t, 254f, 255t
absorption, 233
copper and, 251
deficiency, 253, 255t
food processing and, 233
function of, 232f
functions of, 255t
in "hard" water, 231
ingesting more than 150 mg per day, 253
in protein foods, 48
Recommended Dietary Allowance (RDA), 255t
sources of, 253, 253t, 254f, 255t
toxicity, 255t